RECENT ADVANCES IN HIP AND KNEE ARTHROPLASTY

Edited by **Samo K. Fokter**

Recent Advances in Hip and Knee Arthroplasty
Edited by Samo K. Fokter

Published by InTech

Janeza Trdine 9, 51000 Rijeka, Croatia

Publishing Process Manager Adriana Pecar

Technical Editor Teodora Smiljanic

Cover Designer InTech Design Team

Additional hard copies can be obtained from orders@intechopen.com

Recent Advances in Hip and Knee Arthroplasty, Edited by Samo K. Fokter
p. cm.
ISBN 978-953-307-841-0

For EU product safety concerns:
IN TECH d.o.o., Prolaz Marije Krucifikse Kozulić 3, 51000 Rijeka, Croatia,
info@intechopen.com or visit our website at intechopen.com.

Meet the editor

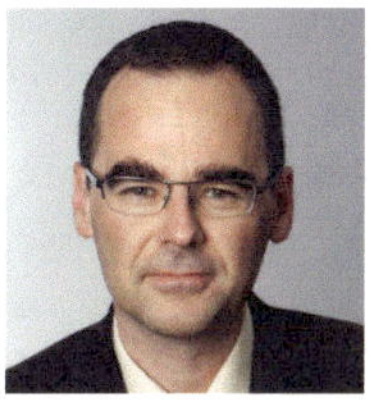

Dr Samo K. Fokter obtained his medicine degree in 1985 at the Medical Faculty of Ljubljana University in Slovenia, where he also completed his residency in orthopaedics. He was a research fellow at the Orthopaedic Clinic of Zagreb, Croatia, visiting fellow in Basel, Switzerland, and Koeln, Germany. He is currently appointed as Assistant Professor of Surgery at the Medical Faculty of Maribor University, and Assistant Professor of Orthopaedic Surgery at the Medical Faculty of Ljubljana University. He works as Head of Department of Orthopaedic Surgery and Sports Trauma at Celje Teaching Hospital, and is the current Immediate Past President of the Slovenian Orthopaedic Society at the Slovenian Medical Association. He is a Board member of the European Association of Research Groups for Spinal Osteosynthesis (ARGOSPINE), and an Assistant Editor in Chief of HYPERLINK "http://www.springerlink.com/content/101157/" \n _blankEuropean Journal of Orthopaedic Surgery and Traumatology (EJOST). He dedicated a large part of his free time to active voluntary work at the Mountain Rescue Service of Slovenia.

Contents

Preface XI

Part 1 Hip Arthroplasty 1

Chapter 1 **Degenerative Hip Joint Pain – The Non-Arthroplasty Surgical Options 3**
Ahmed Alghamdi and Martin Lavigne

Chapter 2 **Hip Arthroplasty 27**
N. A. Sandiford, U. Alao, J. A. Skinner and S. R. Samsani

Chapter 3 **Hip Fracture in the Elderly: Partial or Total Arthroplasty? 43**
Samo K. Fokter and Nina Fokter

Chapter 4 **Why Minimally Invasive Surgery in Hip Arthroplasty? 55**
Antonio Silvestre, Fernando Almeida, Pablo Renovell, Raúl López, Laura Pino and Luis Puertes

Chapter 5 **Minimally Invasive Total Hip Arthroplasty 69**
Mel S. Lee

Chapter 6 **The Effect of Drainage After Hip Arthroplasty 85**
Andrej Strahovnik and Samo K. Fokter

Chapter 7 **Rehabilitation of Patients Following Arthroplasty of the Hip and Knee 99**
Magdalena Wilk-Frańczuk

Chapter 8 **Methods for Optimising Patient Function After Total Hip Arthroplasty 119**
Tosan Okoro, Andrew Lemmey, Peter Maddison and John G. Andrew

Part 2 Special Topics in Hip Arthroplasty 133

Chapter 9 **Planning of Arthroplasty in Dysplastic Hips 135**
Nevzat Selim Gokay, Alper Gokce, Bulent Alp and Fahri Erdogan

Chapter 10 **Hip Arthroplasty in Highly Dislocated Hips 153**
Zoran Bascarevic, Zoran Vukasinovic, Violeta Bascarevic and Vladimir Bascarevic

Chapter 11 **Modular Femoral Neck Fracture After Total Hip Arthroplasty 169**
Igor Vučajnk and Samo K. Fokter

Chapter 12 **Surface Replacement of Hip Joint 181**
Hiran Amarasekera and Damian Griffin

Chapter 13 **Retrograde Stem Removal Techniques in Revision Hip Surgery 191**
Kálmán Tóth

Part 3 Knee Arthroplasty 201

Chapter 14 **History of Condylar Total Knee Arthroplasty 203**
Luca Amendola, Domenico Tigani, Matteo Fosco and Dante Dallari

Chapter 15 **The UniSpacer™: Correcting Varus Malalignment in Medial Gonarthrosis 223**
Joern Bengt Seeger and Michael Clarius

Chapter 16 **Posterior Stabilized Total Knee Arthroplasty 231**
Fabio Orozco and Alvin Ong

Chapter 17 **Mobile Bearing Concept in Knee Arthroplasty 241**
Nahum Rosenberg, Arnan Greental and Michael Soudry

Chapter 18 **Soft Tissue Balance in Total Knee Arthroplasty 249**
Tomoyuki Matsumoto, Hirotsugu Muratsu, Seiji Kubo, Masahiro Kurosaka and Ryosuke Kuroda

Chapter 19 **The Role of Drainage After Total Knee Arthroplasty 267**
Ta-Wei Tai, Chyun-Yu Yang and Chih-Wei Chang

Chapter 20 **Proximal Tibiofibular Joint in Knees with Arthroplasty 275**
Hakan Boya

Part 4 Special Topics in Knee Arthroplasty 281

Chapter 21 **Special Situations in Total Knee Arthroplasty 283**
Orlando M. de Cárdenas Centeno and Felix A. Croas Fernández

Chapter 22 **Patient-Specific Patellofemoral Arthroplasty 301**
Domenick J. Sisto, Ronald P. Grelsamer and Vineet K. Sarin

Chapter 23 **Fixation of Periprosthetic Supracondylar Femur Fractures Above Total Knee Arthroplasty – The Indirect Reduction Technique with the Condylar Blade Plate and the Minimally Invasive Technique with the LISS 315**
K. Kolb, P.A. Grützner, F. Marx and W. Kolb

Chapter 24 **Knee Arthrodesis with the Ilizarov External Fixator as Treatment for Septic Failure of Knee Arthroplasty 343**
M. Spina, G. Gualdrini, M. Fosco and A. Giunti

Part 5 Computer Assisted Total Knee Arthroplasty 355

Chapter 25 **Strategies to Improve the Function, Kinematic and Implants' Positioning of a TKA with Minimally Invasive Computer-Assisted Navigation 357**
Nicola Biasca and Matthias Bungartz

Chapter 26 **Possibilities of Computer Application in Primary Knee Replacement 381**
František Okál, Adel Safi, Martin Komzák and Radek Hart

Chapter 27 **Concepts in Computer Assisted Total Knee Replacement Surgery 397**
M. Fosco, R. Ben Ayad, R. Fantasia, D. Dallari and D. Tigani

Chapter 28 **Computer Assisted Orthopedic Surgery in TKA 421**
Eun Kyoo Song and Jong Keun Seon

Chapter 29 **Computer Assisted Total Knee Arthroplasty – The Learning Curve 443**
Jean-Claude Bové

Preface

The purpose of this book is to offer an exhaustive overview of recent insights into the current state of the art in most performed arthroplasties of large joints in lower extremities.

The tremendous long term success of Sir Charnley's total hip arthroplasty has encouraged many researchers, physicians, surgeons, and technicians to search for new applications, designs, technology, and surgical exposures to treat pain, improve function, and create solutions for a higher quality of life. Indeed, the story of success was repeated very soon with knee arthroplasty. Moreover, the number of knee arthroplasties has shown almost exponential growth worldwide, and has exceeded the number of total hip arthroplasties in many clinics in the Western countries within the past decade.

The treatment options in degenerative joint disease have evolved very quickly. Many surgical procedures are quite different today than they were only five years ago. In this book, we endeavor to provide a comprehensive, up-to-date analysis and description of the treatment of joint disease. Although nonsurgical measures are mentioned, the emphasis is on hip and knee problems that require surgical treatment.

In an effort to be comprehensive, this book addresses hip arthroplasty with special emphasis on evolving minimally invasive surgical techniques. Some challenging topics in hip arthroplasty are additionally covered in a special section. Regarding knee arthroplasty, particular attention is given to different designs of endoprostheses and soft tissue balance. Special situations in knee arthroplasty are covered in a special section. Recent advances in computer technology created the possibility for the routine use of navigation in knee arthroplasty. This remarkable success is covered in depth as well.

Each chapter includes current philosophies, techniques, and an extensive review of the literature. We have been as fortunate as to have an outstanding group of arthroplasty specialists from all over the world contributing to this text. Some current topics have been discussed by several authors, therefore, repetition is inevitable. However, as the problems are illuminated from different points of view, this brings an added value to the book.

We especially wish to acknowledge the contributing authors. Without them, a work of this magnitude would simply not be feasible. We thank them for allocating much of their very valuable time to this project. Not only do we appreciate their participation, but also their adherence as a group to the time parameters set for this publication.

Dr. Samo K. Fokter, MD,
Assist. Professor and Chairman,
Dept. for Orthopaedic Surgery and Sports Trauma,
Celje Teaching Hospital
Slovenia

Part 1

Hip Arthroplasty

1

Degenerative Hip Joint Pain – The Non-Arthroplasty Surgical Options

Ahmed Alghamdi and Martin Lavigne
Université de Montréal
Canada

1. Introduction

Degenerative Hip Joint Pain (DHJP) is a major cause of functional limitation in both young active and old sedentary patients. Total hip arthroplasty (THA) is one of the most successful surgical procedures performed in orthopaedics. Sir John Charnley introduced the concept of low friction arthroplasty for end stage hip arthritis. The rewarding result of this procedure makes THA the gold standard for the treatment of end stage degenerative hip disease. In a recent retrospective study to establish the implant survivorship after THA in young patient at 25 years follow up, up to 89% (80%-98%) survivorship was reported among patients who were diagnosed with developmental dysplasia, 85% (77%-93%) in patients diagnosed with rheumatoid arthritis and 74% (61%-87%) in patients group with idiopathic degenerative arthritis of the hip[1]. Despite improved surgical technique, implant biomaterial and prosthesis design, complications such as recurrent dislocation, osteolysis and loosening still exist. Failure of THA may present with particular problems when revision arthroplasty is needed in young patient, which makes hip joint preservation techniques still actual in this population (hip arthroscopy, surgical dislocation with osteochondroplasty, periacetabular osteotomy, proximal femur osteotomy), and put back on track older surgical procedures such as hip fusion or resection arthroplasty for certain rare indications.

2. Evaluation of painful hip joint

Evaluation of painful hip joint starts with history and physical examination followed by imaging study and laboratory investigation, as needed. Patient with DHJP presents with acute or insidious onset pain, usually with a recurring pattern. It is critical to differentiate sources of hip pain originating from intra-articular pathology from those secondary to extra articular pathology. Intra-articular pathology usually causes deep-seated pain, localized in the anterior groin or inguinal region, although pain of intra-articular origin may be felt at any area around the hip joint. Individuals with symptoms secondary to Femoroacetabular impingements (FAI) might indicate the location of pain by gripping the lateral hip, just above the greater trochanter, between the abducted thumb and index finger. This is known as C-sign[2]. Other symptoms of intra-articular pathology include catching, popping and locking, although those symptoms may represent a misinterpretation of extra-articular conditions such as snapping of the psoas tendon or of the tensor fascia lata.

The pain is usually aggravated by weight bearing, going upstairs, and prolonged seating with hip flexion and adduction as in limited seat space, such as a car seat.
Extra-articular pathology will cause pain mostly in the pubic area, lateral trochanter region, buttock region, or posterior thigh. Referred pain from spine or vascular claudication should be ruled out. Pelvic pathology and anterior abdominal wall hernia might cause pain in the groin region.
Physical examination starts with inspection of the patient gait while getting into the office. A limp, Trendelenburg lurch and poor trunk balance should be looked for[3]. Inspection may disclose pelvis malposition, joint contractures or limb inequality. The foot progression angle should be observed. The patient should sit for history taking. After history, the patient should lay supine on the examination table. Ligament laxity can be tested. Log roll the limb to elicit any pain secondary to intra-articular pathology by rotating the femoral head in the acetabulum. Bony prominences, muscles and tendons around the hip joint, along with, the sciatic nerve and bursa overlying the greater trochanter are then palpated. Anterior abdominal wall examination and groin hernia test should be done. The spine, sacroiliac joint and the knee should also be examined. A complete neurovascular assessment of the limb involved should then be performed. Ranges of motion should be done both actively and passively (Table 1).

Range of motion	Value
Flexion	110-120
Extension	10-15
Abduction	30-50
Adduction	20-30
External rotation at 90 degree	40-60
Internal rotation at 90 degree	30-40

Table 1. Hip range of motion

Special test:

- **Anterior labral stress test:** while the patient in supine position, takes the patients leg into flexion, adduction, and slight internal rotation to compress the anterior part of the labrum. A positive test has occurred if the pain has been reproduced and implies an anterior superior tear. Other clinical finding to look for would be crepitus, popping, clicking.
- **Posterior labral stress test:** patient lay in a prone position, and then the examiner will take the patients leg into passive hyperextension, abduction and external rotation. If this motion elicits the pain, a positive test has occurred secondary to posterior tear.
- **Anterior impingement test:** Passive combination of flexion, adduction and internal rotation will cause pain in the anterior groin, which may suggest the presence of FAI.
- **Posterior impingement test:** hyperextension and external rotation will cause posterior impingement and pain, although pain in this position might be secondary to instability.
- **Ober's test:** The patient is positioned in lateral decubitus with the affected side up. The examiner will stabilize the pelvis from the back and hold the leg in neutral rotation and abduction with the knee in 90 degrees of flexion. The hip is then extended and slowly adducted down towards the table. The knee will not reach the examination table because of restricted adduction due to the tight iliotibial band. Lateral knee pain might occur.

- **Snapping test:** Patient can be asked to reproduce the snapping. An audible snap tends to occur more frequently with internal coxa saltans (psoas snapping on the pubic eminence), and can be reproduced when the hip is actively extended from a flexed and abducted hip position. A palpable sapping on the lateral aspect of the hip suggests external coxa saltans (usually tight of thickened iliotibial band sliding over the greater trochanter). Patient can reproduce external snapping while performing cycling move in lateral decubitus. Palpation over the GT may cause tenderness.
- **The Trendelenburg test** should be performed to rule out gluteus medius weakness.
- **Thomas test:** The patient lay supine on the examination table and hold one knee in direction of his chest, while the other leg remains extended. Positive Thomas test occur when the patient cannot keep the opposing leg extended secondary to the hip fixed flexion contraction.

Imaging study: [4]

- *Anteroposterior (AP) pelvis view*: Standard pelvic view can be taken with the patient supine, or preferably standing. The coccyx should be centered 2-3 cm above the symphisis pubis. Both obturator foramens should look symmetrical.

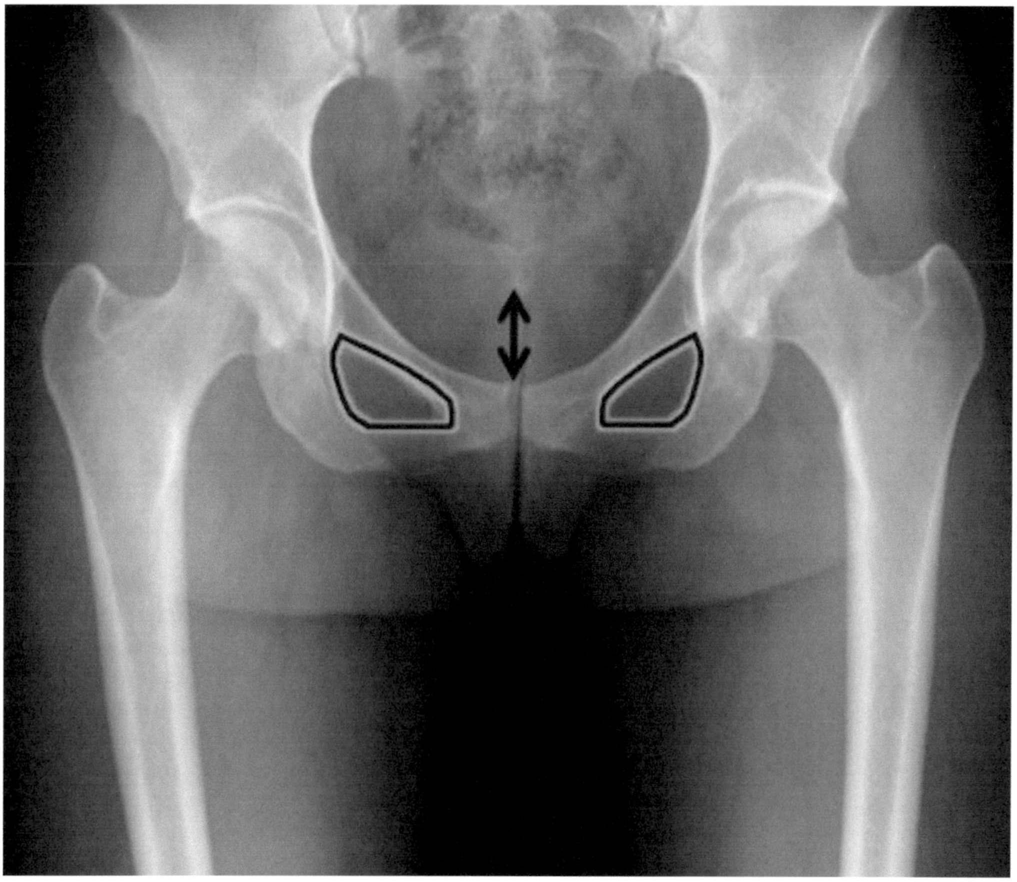

Fig. 1. AP pelvic view, centered view; symmetric obturator foramina, centered coccyx with 2-3 cm distance above the pubic symphisis.

- Lateral views of the hip:
    - *Frog leg lateral:* mostly a view of the proximal femur
    - *Cross table lateral:* view the acetabulum and proximal femur
    - *Dunn 45/90:* specific view of anterior femoral head-neck junction. This view can be taken with the hip at 45 or 90 degree of flexion.
    - *False profile:* for measuring anterior acetabular coverage

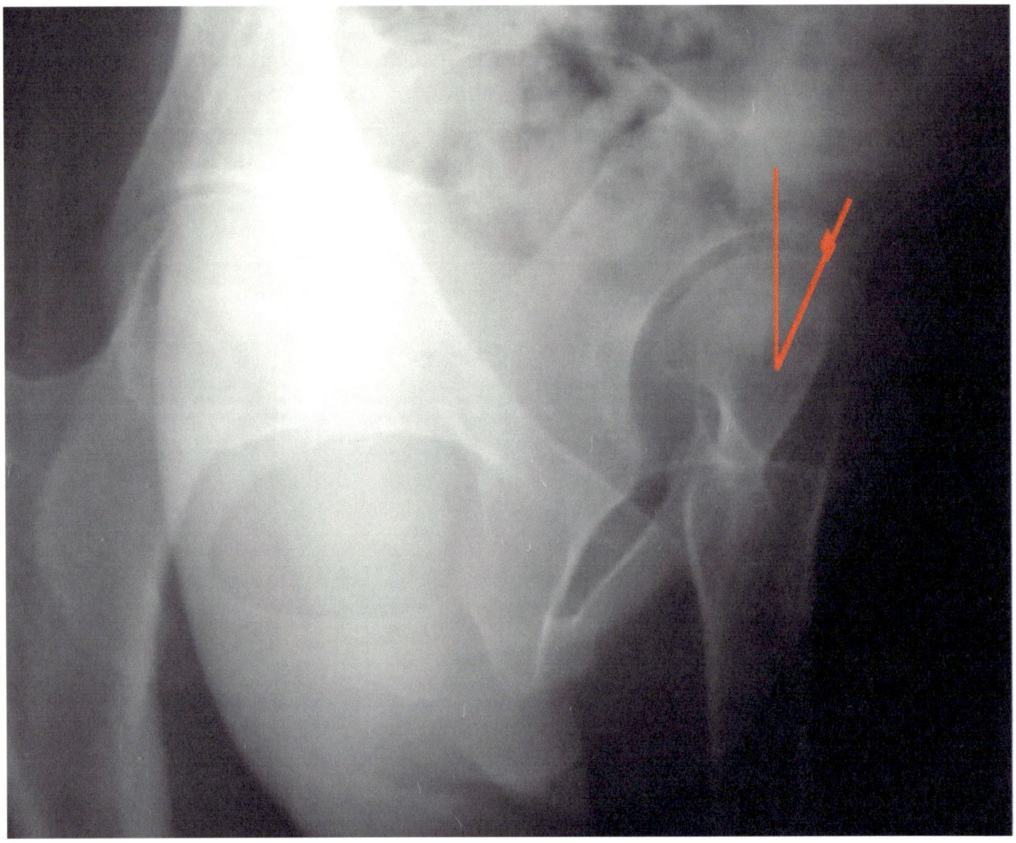

Fig. 2. False-profile view, the anterior centre-edge (VCA) angle quantifies the anterior cover of the femoral head, and angles of less than 20° are considered abnormal.

- *AP hip view*: the x-ray beam is centered on the hip joint. Not reliable for cross over sign.
- *Computer Tomography (CT) scans*: with 3-D reconstruction, can be more accurate for pre-operative impingement evaluation or other deformation of acetabulum or femur.
- *Magnetic resonance imaging (MRI) scan*: good diagnostic tool for both soft tissue and bone strucutre. Intra-articular contrast injection can be use for further evaluation of labrum. Alpha angle of Notzli was described on a specific MRI view, although it is currently measured on different radiographic modalities[5].
- *Ultrasound scan*: can provide dynamic evaluation. It can be used as therapeutic tool as well[6].
- *Bone scan*: usually non specific
- *Bursography*: can be used for snapping hip.

3. Hip arthroscopy

The first recorded attempt of arthroscopic visualization of the hip joint is attributed to Michael Burman in 1930. The limited indications of hip arthroscopy at that time and the anatomic constraints of the hip joint with suboptimal equipment design have limited the use of hip arthroscopy for long time. However with improved hip arthroscopy tools, the indications for hip arthroscopy continue to evolve. Currently, many clinical issues related to the hip joint and the surrounding tissue can be treated with hip arthroscopy. Degenerative hip conditions that can be treated with hip arthroscopy are listed in Table 2.

Degenerative Indications	Non-Degenerative indications
• Labral Lesions • Chondral injuries • FAI • Degenerative arthritis	• Loose bodies (traumatic or synovial chondomatosis) • Sepsis • Synovial disease • Instability • Coxa Sultan (extern or intern)

Table 2. Conditions treated with hip arthroscopy

3.1.1 Labral lesions

The etiology of labral tear is traumatic, degenerative, idiopathic or congenital. Labral pathology can also be classified based on location (anterior, superolateral, posterior). Anterior labral tears are the most common form in the western population, accounting for 90% of cases. Degenerative labral tears are more and more frequently felt to result from FAI and usually starts in the avascular (water-shield) white zone of the labral structure. In this zone, there is low chance of successful healing of the labral tear with conservative treatment. Labral tears may cause pain and microinstability of the hip joint. They also may increase friction within the joint and the strain within the articular cartilage; thereby possibly untreated lesion will result in accelerated degeneration of the joint. In FAI, persisting conflict between femoral neck and acetabulum will lead to chondral delamination and thinning, further the labral tear, paralabral cyst and ultimately, degenerative osteoarthritis

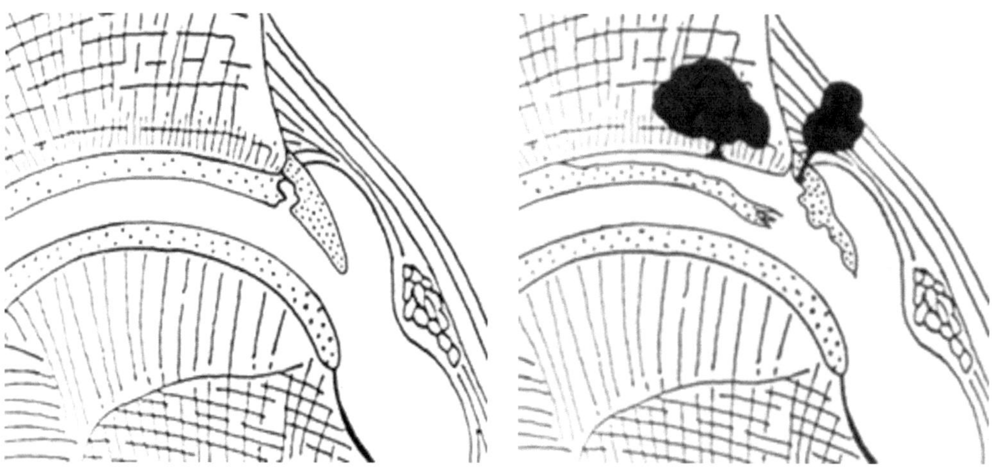

Fig. 3. Labral Tear begins at the articular labral junction, termed the *watershed region*. Progressive labral degenerations result in paralabral cysts and articular cartilage damage.

of the involved joint. With hip arthroscopy, the labrum can be debrided, resected, repaired or reconstructed.

3.1.2 Femoroacetabular impingement (FAI)

This is a descriptive diagnosis characterized by combined clinical features and pathomorphological findings that can result in degenerative changes. The patient's pathomorphology is characterized by either cam lesion, pincer lesion or a combination of both. Mechanical abutment of cam lesion commonly causes pathological changes starting with focal, deep chondral delamination in the anterolateral (superolateral) region of the acetabulum. Separation of the labrum-chondral junction will allow the synovial fluid to extravasate to the subchondral bone or para-labral region creating intra osseous or para-labral cyst (Figure 3). Leverage of head-cam lesion against the acetabulum with extreme range of motion can result in contre-coup lesion in posterinferior acetabulum [7]. Leading to global degenerative changes.

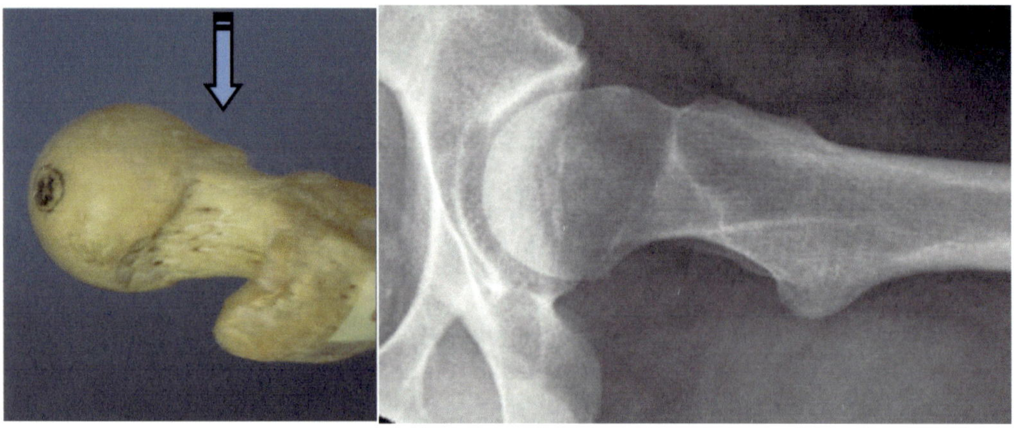

Fig. 4. Cam lesion as seen in skeletonized specimen and frog leg lateral view.

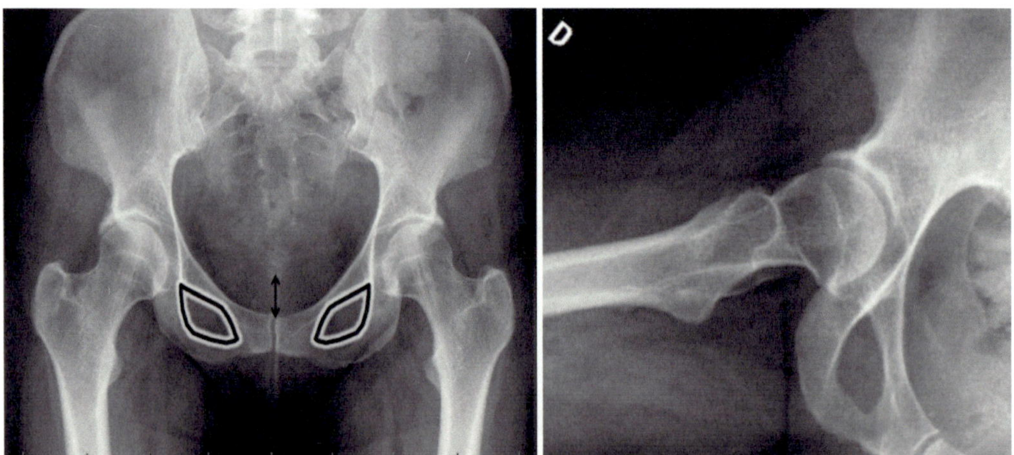

Fig. 5. Pincer Lesion, global over-coverage and labral calcification in 45 years old female. Notice the relatively minor degenerative changes on the anterior femoral head neck junction.

The pincer lesion will cause a crush-type injury of the labrum and progressive degenerative changes with minimal damage to the articular cartilage of the acetabulum.
Indication of hip arthroscopy in this setting is symptomatic FAI with concomitant labral and or cartilage lesion. The labrum is addressed as mentioned in the previous section, while the cartilage damage is addressed by debridement or micro fracture of the underlying subchondral bone. The osseous abnormalities are treated with an osteochondroplasty and acetabuloplasty as needed.

3.1.3 Degenerative arthritis

Arthroscopic intervention in early hip joint degeneration may relieve pain and others associated symptoms (i.e. catching, locking and range of motion limitation). However, as seen with knee arthroscopy, it provides little benefit on the long term and thus represents a limited indication for hip arthroscopy. Hip arthroscopy in this clinical scenario will provide limited role through removal of loose bodies, debridement of degenerative chondral or labral tears and subtotal synovectomy. Capsular release and osteophyte excision might improve the hip range of motion.
Before attempting hip arthroscopy for advance degenerative changes, patient needs to know the limitation of such procedure. The patient are less likely to benefit from hip arthroscopy when joint space is less than 50% of normal, with pain at rest, functionally depleting limitation of hip range of motion or pre-operative Harris Hip Score (HHS) of less than 60.

3.2 Surgical technique

Under general, spinal or combined anesthesia, the patient is positioned supine or in lateral decubitus according to the surgeon's preference. This section will only address the hip arthroscopy while the patient on supine position. A well-padded perineal post will be used to protect the pubis and provide counter traction force during distraction of the hip joint. The foot should also be well-padded befor connecting the foot attachments. Distraction of the hip joint is gently performed with the hip slightly flexed in neutral abduction and rotation until approximately 8 mm of joint space is achieved. Multiple portals can be used to visualize both central (articular surfaces) and peripheral (extra articular) compartments of the hip joint. Common portals used are anterior, anterolateral and posterolateral in relation to the Greater Trochanter (GT). Fluoroscopic views should be used during portal preparation to ensure enough joint distraction and to avoid labral penetration. The 70-degree lens is used most of the time. Labral tear, cartilage damage or over coverage can be treated as described above. Inspection of the peripheral compartment and excision of the cam lesion can be done without traction with the use of fluoroscopy x-ray to guide precise cam lesion excision. Dynamic assessment is helpful to assess the relief of FAI.

3.3 Postoperative rehabilitation

After arthroscopic osteochondroplasty and labral debridement, full weight bearing will be permitted, unless micro fractures were performed, in which case toe touch weight bearing is recommended for 6-8 weeks. Aggressive active-passive range of motion and proprioception exercise will be started early post operative. High impact sport is not allowed for 2 months post femoral neck osteoplasty.

3.4 Complications

Complications occur in 0.5% to 5% of patients and are most often related to the required distraction of the hip joint [8]. Sciatic, femoral or pudendal nerve palsy can result from prolonged traction time. Nerve injury tends to be transient neuropraxia, which completely resolve spontaneously in few weeks. A well-padded post should prevent perineal tear and pudendal nerve injury. Bleeding and lateral femoral cutaneous nerve injury can occur during portal placement. Postoperative persistent secondary to trochanteric bursitis, intra-articular capsular adhesion (especially between the capsule and repaired labrum, or between the capsule and anterior neck) may occur. Femoral neck fracture, avascular necrosis of the femoral head, and under or over resections of cam lesion can be a mode of failure. Instrumental breakage rarely happen, but sometimes requires open arthrotomy to remove the broken fragment. Incidence of deep venous thrombosis ranges from 0 to 3.7% in various retrospective clinical reports[9].

3.5 Results of arthroscopic FAI surgery

Hip arthroscopy for the treatment of FAI has only been used recently. Philippon et al studied 45 professional athletes at 1.6 years (6 months to 5.5 years) follow up. 93% of patients returned to professional competition, but only 78% remained active in professional sport at final follow up[10].

Sampson et al analyzed the results of 183 patients (194 hips) with positive impingement sign at preoperative assessment at maximum follow up of 29 months. 95% of the patients showed no sign of impingement at one year after surgery[11].

Byrd et al found an improvement of Harris Hip Score (HHS) from baseline of 20 points (range 17 to 60 point), which was reported in 83% of patients at 1 year follow up[12].

Another study reported by Philippon et al analyzed 112 patients at mean follow up of 2.3 years. The HHS improved from 58 to 84.3 in those patients with FAI associated with labral and chondral pathology. However, 8.9% of the patient underwent THA at mean follow up of 16 months[13].

4. Combined limited open arthrotomy and hip arthroscopy

Combined limited open arthrotomy and hip arthroscopy can be utilized to treat symptomatic anterolateral FAI: the hip arthroscopy will focus on any labral pathology and allow microfracturing for acetabular chondral damage. The limited arthrotomy approach will allow easy access to the pathologic part of the femoral head neck junction.

4.1 Surgical technique

Patient is positioned supine, exactly the same as described in previous section. After arthroscopic treatment of labral and chondral lesions, the traction is released. Anterior or anterolateral approach can be performed. We prefer a modified Watson-Jones approach, which allow better visualization of the anterolateral and posterolateral aspect of head neck junction. The 8-10 cm incision starts 2-3 cm distal and 2-3 cm lateral to the Anterior Superior Iliac Spine (ASIS) directed distally and laterally toward the anterior tip of GT. Subcutaneous dissection is carried down to the fascia lata. The interval between Tensor Fascia Lata (TFL) and Gluteus Medius (GM) muscles can be identified just anterior to the GT after incising the fascia. The GM is retracted posteriorly while the TFL is retracted anteromedialy. The rectus femoris tendon is identified and the hip joint capsule exposed. A T-shaped capsulotomy is performed with care to prevent injury of the labrum. Spiked tip retractors can be placed intracapsular anterior and posterior around the rim of the acetabulum which will allow safe dynamic assessment of the hip joint. We use a high-speed burr to resect the cam lesion on the anterolateral femoral neck then ensure effective resection by using intraoperative fluoroscopy and dynamic assessment of the hip joint. Removing all bone debris and minimizing muscle damage can play significant role in reducing the incidence of Heterotopic Ossification (HO). Capsular and fascia lata closure are performed at the end of the procedure.

4.2 Postoperative care

Weight bearing as tolerated is permitted early post operatively. Contact sport is not allowed for at least 2-3 months. Active and passive range of motion along with unrestricted strengthening is allowed. However, when rectus femoris tendon is violated, then restrictions will be applied on active straight leg raise (SLR) for 6 weeks. Subcutaneous low molecular weight heparin is given for 10 days.

4.3 Complications

1. Deep venous thromboses and thromboembolic disease.
2. Neurovascular injury.
3. Infection.
4. Femoral neck fracture.
5. HO.
6. Femoral head avascular necrosis (AVN)
7. Complications related to hip arthroscopy procedure.

4.4 Results

Lincoln et al reported a significant difference between the mean Harris hip score preoperatively and that at last follow-up (from 63.8 to 76.1) of 16 hips treated using a modified Heuter anterior approach combined with adjunctive hip arthroscopy.
Clohisy et al reported the results of combined arthroscopy and limited open osteochondroplasty for anterior FAI in 35 patients. HHS improved from 63.8 to 87.4 at minimum follow up of 2 years. No fracture of the femoral neck or AVN of the femoral head was reported[14].
Pierannunzii et al found that the mean HHS improved from 74.4 to 85.3 in 8 patients at mean follow up of 10 months[15].

5. Surgical dislocation of the hip joint

5.1 Indications

Surgical dislocation of the hip joint for the treatment of FAI is safe when performed with appropriate understanding of the vascular anatomy of the proximal femur. Surgical dislocation of the hip is considered the gold standard procedure for the treatment of FAI, despite the advance of hip arthroscopy technique and the encouraging results of the limited open surgical procedure. Surgical dislocation of the hip is especially indicated with global or posterior impingement requiring acetabular rim trimming, with severe deformity of the proximal femur or when chondral lesions of the femoral head have to be addressed. Patient with no more than mild arthrosis (Tonnis <=2) and age less than 50 years are considered the best candidates for such surgical intervention.

5.2 Contraindications

Advance arthrosis, is a contraindication for this procedure.

5.3 Surgical technique

The patient positioned in lateral decubitus under general or combined general and spinal anesthesia. The pelvis should be stabilized in proper orientation to allow proper evaluation of the acetabular version.

The incision is curvilinear, approximately 20-25 cm in length and centered over the GT curving slightly posteriorly at 20 degree angle. The fascia lata is incised and the interval between TFL and Gluteus Maximus (GMax) is developed to avoid violation of the GMax muscle fibers. The peritrochantric bursa is incised and retracted anteriorly. The greater trochanter, short external rotators, gluteus medius and vastus lateralis should be clearly visualized. The leg is positioned in 20-30 degrees of internal rotation and an oscillating saw is used to create a trigastrics sliding trochanteric osteotomy of 1-1.5cm thicknesses. Next the leg is repositioned in neutral rotation and the gluteus minimus is dissected off the hip capsule from posterior to anterior to allow full mobilization of the trochanteric fragment anteriorly for performing a safe Z-shape capsulotomy, the capsular incision starts at the anterior boarder of the GT and is directed proximally in line with the femoral neck with care

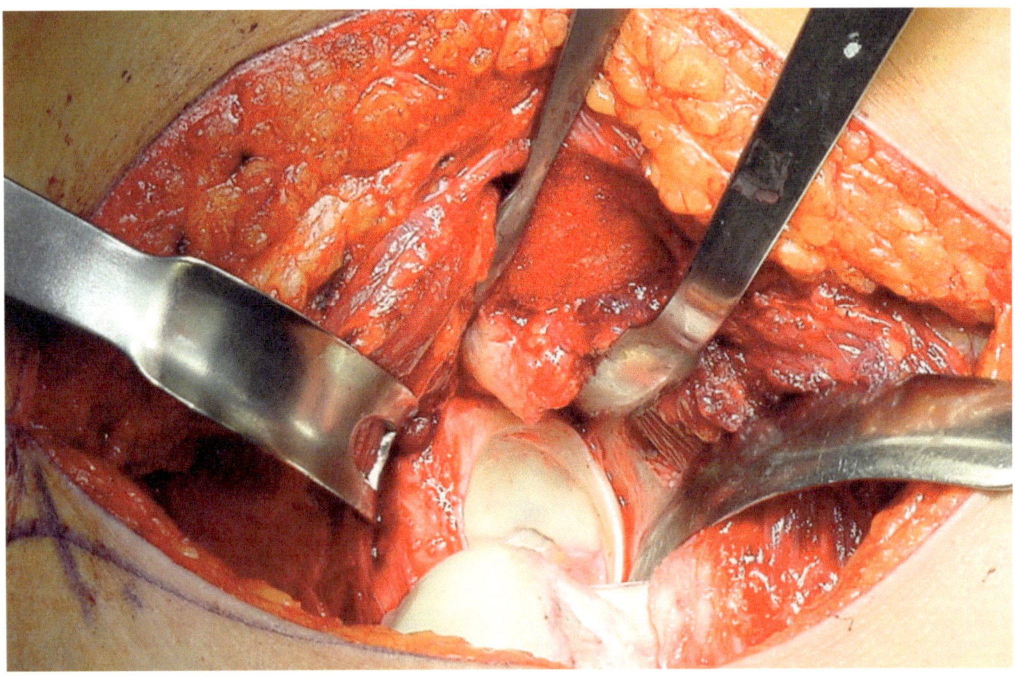

Fig. 6. 360 view provide inspection of the acetabulum, one retractor is impacted above the acetabulum. One retractor hooked on the anterior acetabular rim and a third retractor levers the neck against the incisura acetabuli.

not to injure the labrum. The proximal arm of the capsulotomy runs parallel to the acetabulum posteriorly toward the piriformis tendon, the closest the capsulotomy to the acetabular edge the less likely to risk injuring the lateral epiphyseal branches. The distal arm of the Z-shaped capsulotomy should not extend beyond the lesser trochanter. Distraction force with the use of bone hook with the hip in flexion and external rotation can help dislocating the femoral head. The ligamentum teres can prevent complete dislocation and a curved blunt tip long scissor should be used to cut the ligament if circumferential exposure of the femoral head is required. A straight spiked Hohmann retractor is placed anteriorly around the acetabular rim and a curved Hohmann is placed inferiorly under the transverse ligament to push the femoral head posteriorly. The leg is placed in a sterile bag anteriorly across the table. This will provide 360-degree acetabular exposure for cartilage defects treatment, acetabular rim trimming and labral re-fixation (Figure 6). To treat pathology on the femoral side, the retractors are removed and the head and neck are delivered back into the surgical wound for evaluation and treatment of any head cartilage defect and head-neck junction pathology (Figure 7).

When satisfactory treatment is completed, the femoral head is reduced and the capsule is closed with loose interrupted suture to prevent stretch of retinacular vessels. The greater trochanter fragment should be reduced and fixed with three 3.5mm screws. The fascia lata and overlying skin are closed in layers (Figure 8).

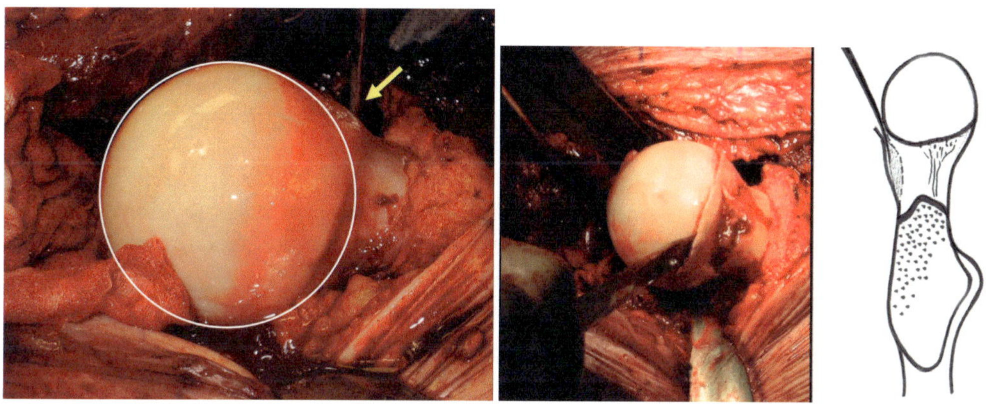

Fig. 7. The hip is flexed, externally rotated and distracted to dislocation of the femoral head. The cam lesion inspected and femoral neck osteoplasty is performed.

5.4 Postoperative care

Patient will be on DVT prophylaxis for 35 days and HO prophylaxis for 2 weeks (Celebrx 200mg twice a day). The patient will be allowed toe touch weight bearing for 6 weeks. Passive range of motion is allowed in all directions, however active abduction and deep flexion beyond 90 degree are not allowed for at least 6 weeks.

5.5 Complications

Complications of the surgical dislocation approach for patients who had had the procedure for multiple differential diagnoses (including Femoroacetabular impingement, Legg-Calve-Perthes disease in a skeletally mature hip, trauma, and deformity following a slipped capital

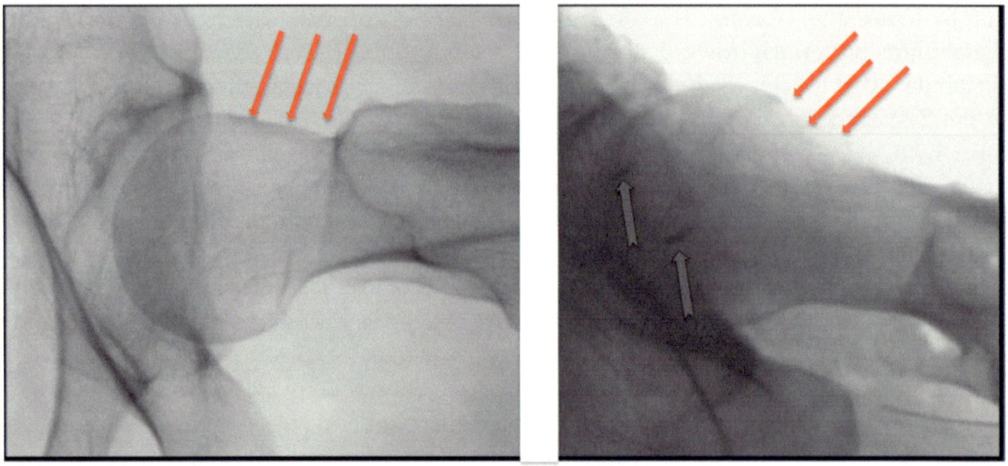

Fig. 8. Preoperative (left) and postoperative (right) lateral views of proximal femur and the acetabulum. Improved head neck offset after excision of the cam lesion. Notice the labral re-fixation after acetabuloplasty.

femoral epiphysis) were reported by different North American centers that participate in the ANCHOR (Academic Network for Conservational Hip Outcomes Research) group[16]. We listed all possible complications might be anticipated with this procedure, however ANCHOR have reported no cases of osteonecrosis, femoral neck fracture, or any complication leading to long-term morbidity, with the exception of the one sciatic nerve injury, which partially resolved.

1. DVT (0.5%)
2. Infection.
3. Neurovascular injury (permanent and complete major nerve palsy was not reported, however partial sciatic nerve palsy occur in one patient eventually recovered partially).
4. Heterotopic ossification (Brooke I & II 5.3%)[17].
5. Trochanteric fragment displacement and delay union (0.5% require no intervention), or nonunion (rate of 1.8 % that required refixation).
6. Femoral neck fracture
7. AVN
8. Hardware complications: breakage, irritation of surrounding soft tissue (trochanteric bursitis, psoas tendon when prominent medially).
9. Under-correction, or over correction of cam and pincer lesion.
10. Capsular adhesion.

5.6 Results

Retrospective reports demonstrate significant improvement in both radiographic and clinical functional scores.

Murphy et al reported on the surgical dislocation approach for FAI treatment in 23 patients with a mean follow up of 62 months. Preoperative hip scores of Merle d'Aubigné scale were average 13.2 (range, 11–15). THA was performed for 7 patients. Of the surviving 15 hips, the hip scores improved significantly to 16.9 ± 1.35 (range 13–18). No case of AVN was reported[18].

Likewise, Peters et al reported improvement in the mean Harris Hip Score from 70 points preoperatively to 87 points at the time of final follow-up in 29 patients [19].
Beaule et al reported the functional outcome of 34 patients (37 hip) following surgical dislocation to treat cam lesion with mean follow up period of 31.4 years. All activity and functional score demonstrated improved outcome (WOMAC score 61.2 to 81.4, UCLA activity scores 4.8 to 7.5, and mean SF-12 46.4 to 51.2). No osteonecrosis was reported and 9 patients required hardware removal [20].
Espinosa et al found less arthrosis at final follow up in 52 patients (60 hips) when labrum was refixed instead of removed after rim trimming for pincer type impingement. The recovery time and the final clinical and radiographic features favored labral re-fixation[21].
Beck et al reported the mid-term results of surgical dislocation of 19 hips and concluded that this procedure was not suitable for patient with advanced degenerative changes[22]. The same conclusion also reported by Murphy et al [18].

6. Periacetabular osteotomy

Developmental dysplasia of the hip can result in structural instability that exacerbates shearing forces across a limited acetabular cartilage surface area. Ultimately, the abnormal force distribution can result in rim failure and progressive degenerative hip disease[23].
The aim of periacetabular osteotomy is to change the acetabular cavity orientation, thus optimizing the joint mechanics through restoration of joint stability and transformation of *shearing forces* on an oblique acetabular roof to *compressive forces* on a reoriented horizontal acetabular roof.
It was found on long term radiographic follow up that patients with a Center Edge Angle (CEA) less than 16 degrees, acetabular index greater than 15 degrees and femoral head uncoverage more than 30% have higher incidence of osteoarthritis by age 60 [24].

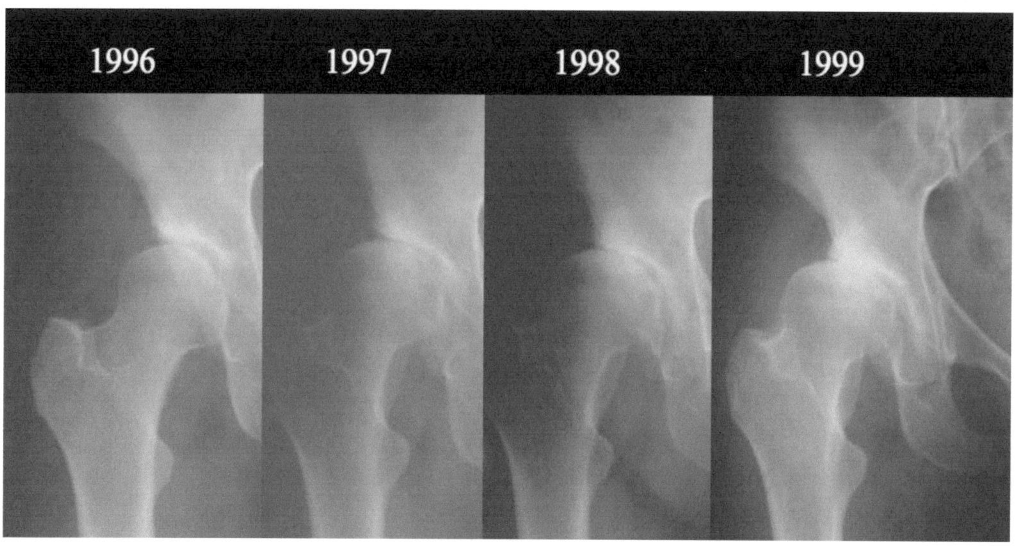

Fig. 9. Natural history of untreated acetabular dysplasia.

Various pelvic osteotomies were proposed to treat symptomatic hip dysplasia. Most of the techniques apply to the infant or adolescents. Salter innominate osteotomy has limited

degree of correction in adult hip dysplasia and it dose not solve hip-center lateralization because the acetabular fragment rotation is hinged on a fixed point (symphisis pubis). Double and triple osteotomy provides more freedom for rotation of the osteotomized fragment but since the acetabular fragment is still attached to the sacropelvic ligament, only limited correction angle is possible. This angle of correction can be improved through placing the osteotomy closer to the acetabulum. One disadvantage of this type of osteotomy is the size of acetabular fragment that can cause pelvic narrowing and might interfere with future child bearing in female patient. Spherical periacetabular osteotomy is a highly demanding surgical procedure; it can improve acetabular coverage but can't improve hip-center lateralization because the medial acetabular wall is intact. The osteotomy passes close to the acetabulum capsular attachment, which is considered to be an important source of blood supply to the acetabular bone. Performing a capsulotomy to evaluate intra-articular structure at the remaining time of the osteotomy will jeopardize the acetabular blood supply[25].
Reinhold Ganz initially described Bernese Periacetabular Osteotomy (PAO)[26]. It became widely recognized as an effective osteotomy for the treatment of acetabular dysplasia. Through improved geometric cut around the acetabulum, the polygonal shape acetabular fragment can be reoriented to achieve almost unlimited femoral head coverage and acetabular version as well as allowing control of medialization of the hip-center when needed. The vascular anatomy around the acetabulum is preserved, which allow safe capsulotomy for simultaneous evaluation and treatment of intra-articular pathology.

6.1 Indications

The clinical uses of Bernese PAO in adult patient are indicated in the presence of the following situations:

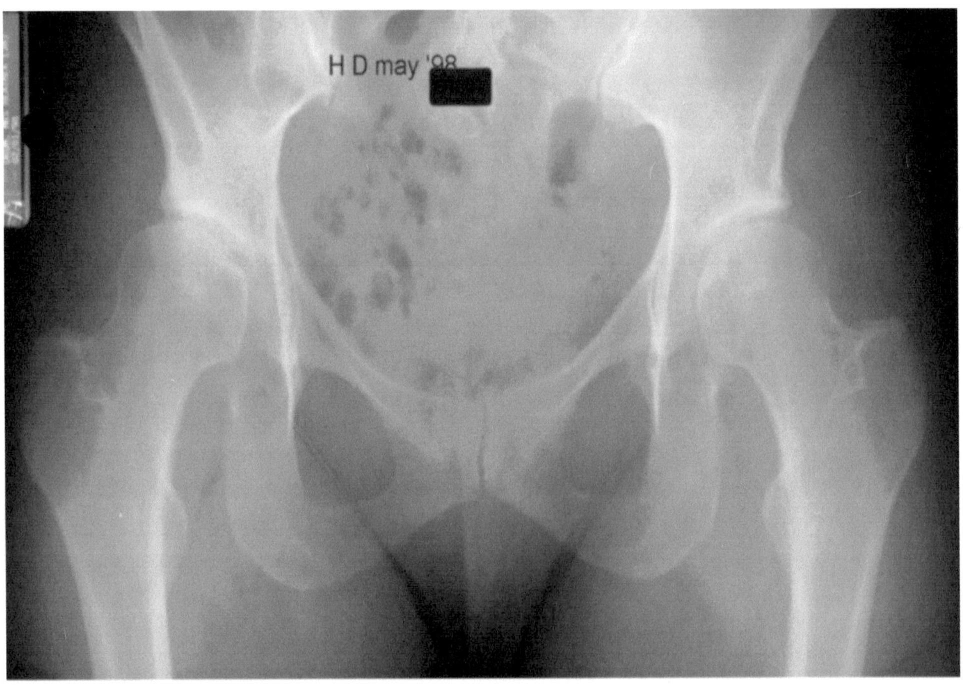

Fig. 10. Bilateral acetabular dysplasia in 17 years old patient.

1. Congruent and symptomatic early hip joint degenerative disease (Tonnis 1).
2. 20-30 degree of hip abduction range of motion.
3. Dysplastic acetabulum with
   a. CEA <20 degree
   b. Tonnis angle >10 degree
4. symptomatic acetabular retroversion without dysplasia can be an indication for PAO, it: Acetabular retroversion can be identified on a standard AP pelvis view (symmetrical obturator foramen and coccyx centered 2-3 cm above the symphisis pubis). The patient radiographic finding will be consistent with acetabulum retroversion if the hip center of rotation is lateral to posterior acetabular rim and the patient have both cross-over sign and ischeal spine sings[27, 28].

6.2 Contraindications

1. Open triradiate cartilage
2. Grade II Tonnis changes and more
3. Incongruent joint
4. Age over 40 has been associated with less favorable outcome in some studies[29, 30].

6.3 Surgical technique

Under general anesthesia, the patient is positioned supine and the limb on the dysplastic acetabulum side is prepped and draped free in sterile fashion. Antibiotics are given before incising the skin. A cell saver is used during this procedure.

A curvilinear incision is starting from the gluteal tubercle on the iliac crest and curved lateral to the ASIS distally for approximately 20 cm. Abdominal external oblique muscle is

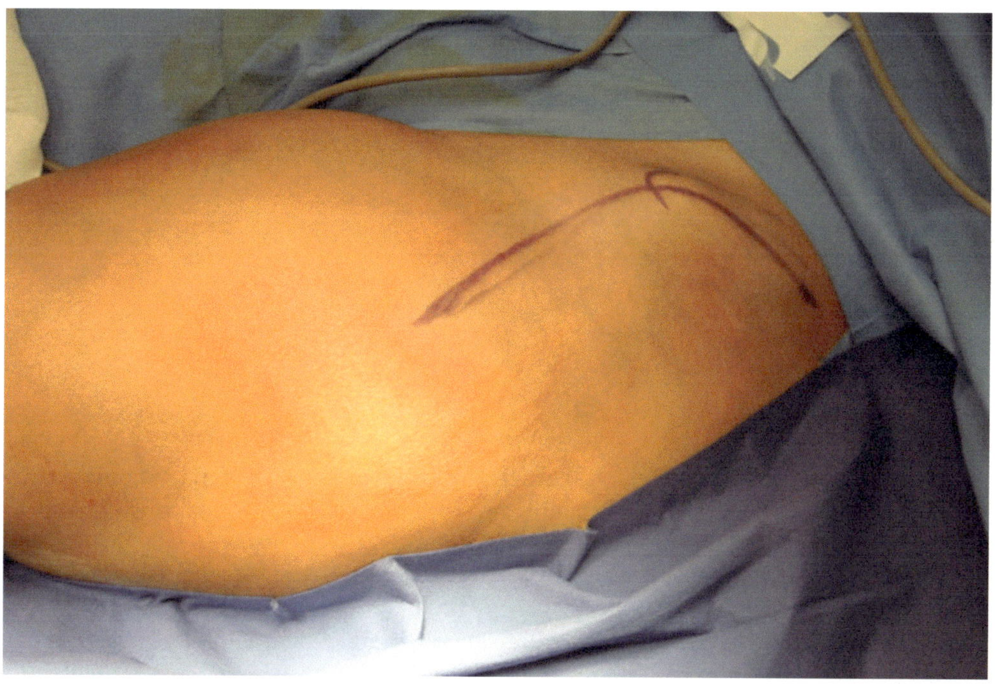

Fig. 11. Curvilinear incision for the anterior approach to perform PAO.

elevated off the internal iliac crest and the interval between TFL and the Sartorius is defined. The ASIS is osteotomized and retracted medially to expose the rectus femoris, which is released from the AIIS. The sartorius and rectus femoris are retracted medially and the TFL is retracted laterally. The ilocapsularis muscle is elevated off the anterior capsule. A spiked Hohmann retractor can be slid over the superior pubic ramus 1.5 cm medial to iliopectineal eminence and serves to retract the medial soft tissue including the psoas and the neurovascular bundle. The medial capsular tissue is freed of soft tissue attachment using long blunt and curved scissors. This provides a window to reach the ischeal tubercle and infracotyloid region, which is also freed of soft tissue attachments.
Four bone cuts are performed to create a polygonal acetabular fragment:

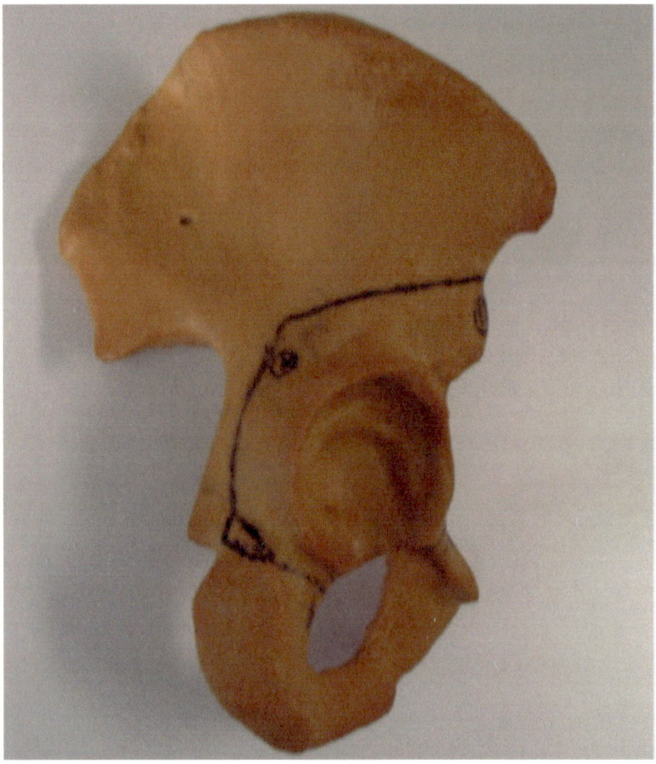

Fig. 12. Polygonal cuts around the acetabulum.

1. Partial ischeal cut using curved Ganz osteotome (avoid sciatic nerve injury by abducting the hip joint)
2. Superior pubic ramus cut using straight osteotome starting medial to iliopectineal eminence (avoid penetrating the joint by aiming 45 degrees medial, away from the acetabulum).
3. Iliac bone cut starting just distal to ASIS toward greater sciatic notch using oscillating saw.
4. The posterior column cut is one centimeter thick and done using both straight and curved osteotome starting off the third cut end with an angle of approximately120 degrees to join the first ischeal cut.

The acetabular fragment should be now free for re-orientation. We use two Schantz screws inserted in the acetabular fragment away from the zone of fixation to accomplish efficient orientation in both abduction and anteversion. Fluoroscopy is used to assess acetabulum version and orientation. The fragment can be allowed to rotate freely around the hip center of rotation. When the desired orientation is achieved, preliminary fixation is obtained with multiple Steinmann pins. True AP pelvic X-ray is done prior final fixation. Multiple screws are used to fix the acetabular fragment. The hip is then taken through full range of motion and if 90-degrees of flexion cannot be achieved, retroversion is corrected or a capsulotomy can be safely done to resolve any intra-articular pathology responsible for impingement.

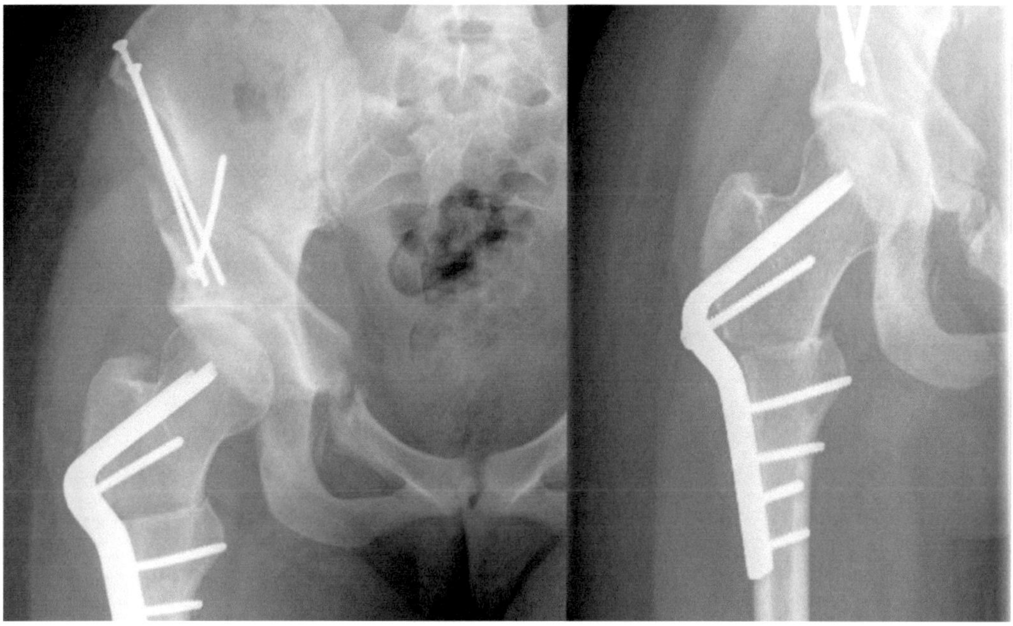

Fig. 13. Postoperative x-ray of the right hip for the same patient presented previously (figure 11) demonstrates combined PAO and proximal femoral osteotomy.

The rectus tendon is reattached to the AIIS using nonabsorbable suture transfixed through drill hole in the iliac bone. The ASIS is fixed with a screw or nonabsorbable suture drilled through the osteotomiesed fragment. A drain is left in place while closure is performed[31].

6.4 Postoperative care

Patients will be on DVT prophylaxis for 35 days. Non-weight bearing is indicated for 6 weeks, and then progressive weight bearing is started when radiographic evidence of healing of the osteotomy. Straight leg raising exercise is delayed for 6 weeks, and the hip joint can be taken through passive range of motion early postoperative.

6.5 Complications

Minor and major complications can occur when doing Bernese PAO. The complexity of the procedure combined with the surgeon learning curve can affect the overall outcome. It was observer that the major complication rate ranged from 6% to 37%[32]. There was a statistically significant decrease in major complications from 17% to 2.9% when comparing the first 35 cases with the second 35 cases of periacetabular osteotomy performed by one surgeon[33].

The complications reported in literatures include:

1. *General surgical complications:* such as bleeding, DVT, infection and HO
2. *Technique-related complication:* include nerve traction injury to the femoral nerve. Lateral cutaneous nerves of the thigh are involved commonly but usually recover. Sciatic nerve injury is rare. Femoral artery injury or femoral vein thrombosis can occur.
3. *Acetabular-fragment related complications:* include fracture through the posterior column, intra-articular extension of the osteotomy, under or over correction. Delayed union can happen, but nonunion of the acetabular fragment is rare; although nonunion of the superior pubic ramus osteotomy tends to occur more frequently.
4. *Hardware complications:* include joint penetration, fixation failure secondary to broken or migrated screw. Prominent screw can rub against the surrounding tissue leading to painful bursitis.

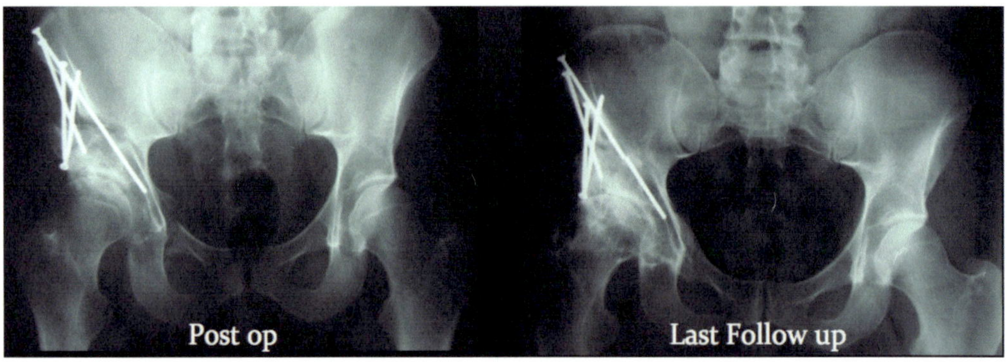

Fig. 14. Progressive degenerative changes lead to failure of PAO.

Ganz et al reported the need for removal of hardware in 17% and HO in 5%, however Trousdale et al reported 33% incidence of HO after PAO. The lateral femorocutaneous nerve is the most commonly injured (30%).[34-36]

6.6 Results

Clohisy et al has made a systematic review of the reported radiographic and clinical results of PAO based on the literatures published up to 2007 with certain inclusion criteria. There were 13 studies with a level of evidence that was generally low (IV). These data derived from various surgeons and institutions indicate PAO can reliably achieve deformity correction. All studies including clinical outcome analysis showed pain relief and improved hip function in the majority of patients at short to midterm follow up. In seven studies, there were correlated between suboptimal clinical results and advanced preoperative osteoarthritis. Failure of the osteotomy and the need to conversion to THA was noted in 0% to 17% of the cases [32].

7. Femoral osteotomy

Various proximal femoral osteotomies were described for different clinical indications. Intertrochanteric Osteotomy (ITO) may be used in adults, although the indications for ITO nowadays are more limited due to the improved outcome of THA. ITO may be useful to provide containment, congruency, coverage or rotational re-alignment of the hip joint through valgus, varus, flexion, extension, rotation or combination of all of these osteotomies. Post-traumatic deformity, rotational malalignment of the lower extremity, coxa valga, slipped capital femoral epiphysis and Legg-Calvé-Perthes disease are clinical conditions where ITO is commonly used.

7.1 Contraindications

1. Advanced degenerative changes
2. Inflammatory arthritis
3. The impossibility of obtaining a congruent joint on functional radiographic views
4. Limited joint range of motion with marked hip stiffness
5. Other relative contra-indications are advanced age, tobacco smoking and morbid obesity.

7.2 Surgical technique

The pre-requisite for a successfully executed ITO is proper pre-operative planning, adequate range of motion and appropriate choice of the fixation device.
A direct lateral approach to the femur is used. The planned osteotomy is performed under fluoroscopic assistance and defined with Steinman pins. A blade plate is used for fixation and the corresponding chisel is inserted in the desired position. The osteotomy is performed with an oscillating saw and can be fixed under compression with a blade plate or condylar plate.

7.3 Postoperative care

DVT prophylaxis is given for 2 weeks, and weight-bearing protection should de respected for 2 months. Passive and active ranges of motion are permitted.

7.4 Postoperative complications

In addition to common surgical complications, AVN and delayed union or non-union of the osteotomy can occur. Over correction or under correction can be a source of patient dissatisfaction. Hardware failure or soft tissue irritation might require removal after fracture healing.

7.5 Results

Multiple clinical studies on the use of proximal femoral osteotomy are reported in the literatures. Haverkamp et al reported the results of 276 patients that had ITO for various indications. The best clinical results at 10 years were achieved when the osteotomy was performed in young patient with posttraumatic deformity (90% success rate at 10 years). Arthritic changes in association with an idiopathic etiology had the worst results with only 50% success rate at final follow up[37].

8. Salvage procedure for degenerative hip joint pain

Salvage surgery, including the Chiari osteotomy and shelf procedures; do not provide coverage of the femoral head by a surface of hyaline cartilage. The hip capsule is interposed between newly formed acetabular roof and femoral head.

- *Chiari Pelvic Osteotomy:* Chiari medial displacement pelvic osteotomy may be used to treat degenerative hip pain in young patient with incongruent hip joint. The osteotomy is performed at 15 degrees superior inclination within the supracetabular iliac bone and the hip joint is displaced medially to improve superior coverage of the femoral head. Excessively low or too high osteotomy cut can give suboptimal clinical result. Sufficient acetabular fragment medial displacement is critical to provide enough femoral head coverage. The superior capsule is used as the articular surface under the displaced ilium. The posterinferior aspect of the hip is spared from disease, as seen on the false-profile roentgenogram. and a reconstructive osteotomy can be performed. Furthermore anterior coverage of the head is difficult to obtain with a medial displacement osteotomy. This procedure relies on fibrocartlage metaplasia of the capsule, results in lower functional outcome compared to other periacetabular osteotomies or THA. One advantage of this type of osteotomy is improving future acetabular component bone fixation[38].
- *Shelf Procedure:* Placing a bone graft in the superolateral region of the acetabulum as a shelf can provide containment and coverage of the femoral head, thus preventing lateral or upward migration of the femoral head. The shelf procedure provides greater lateral coverage but the original steep inclination of the acetabulum persists. The technique can be used as a supplemental procedure with other type of osteotomy and can be performed with a limited incision technique[39].

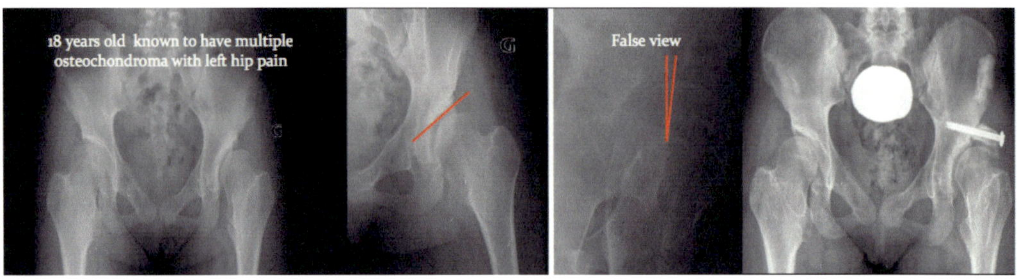

Fig. 15. Shelf procedure.

8.1 Hip fusion (arthrodesis)

Young patients with advanced unilateral degenerative hip changes, secondary to trauma or septic conditions are good candidate for hip fusion. Hip arthrodesis provides better clinical results in young (less than 35) active patient with normal contralateral hip, no pathology in the ipsilateral knee or lower spine and when the hip fusion technique preserves the abductor muscles integrity. Although a valuable option, it has many drawbacks including loss of motion, shortening of the extremity, increased expenditure of energy during walking, and increased stress on the low back and the ipsilateral knee[40].

Several techniques have been described. The femoral head and the acetabulum are denuded of cartilage and the hip is positioned in approximately 30 degrees of flexion, 0 to 5 degrees of adduction and 10 degrees of external rotation. The fixation can be intra articular (screws through the femoral head to the iliac bone), or extra articular (side plate, cobra plate, anterior plate). A trochanteric osteotomy is advisable to preserve the abductor function for future conversion of hip fusion to THA when side plate or cobra plate is used.

The reported clinical results of THA after hip fusion demonstrate a wide spectrum of clinical outcome. Hamadouche et al studies 45 THA performed after hip fusion at a mean follow up of 8.5 years. He reported 91% survival with walking improvement up to 2-3 years after surgery, however, 50% of patients required a cane for walking[41]. Joshi et al found that 79% of the patients had minimal pain with a 96% 10 years survival. The complications reported for the 208 fused hips converted to THA were 8 sciatic nerve and 7 femoral nerve palsies, 28 cases of HO, 5 dislocations and 3 infections[42].

9. Resection arthroplasty

Gathome Girdlestone described the surgical technique of resection arthroplasty of the hip joint to palliate hip condition secondary to chronic infection (i.e. tuberculosis hip infection). This procedure has been widely used to relive pain or to improve the hip range of motion in conditions such as advanced hip degeneration and chronic hip joint infection. Improvement in the treatment of infection, fracture fixation technique and the introduction of prosthetic hip replacement has significantly limited the role of hip resection arthroplasty. The current indications for resection arthroplasty are nonambulatory patient with significant cognitive or neuromuscular condition or patient with chronic prosthesis infection and significant comorbidity that cannot go through complex surgical procedure. After the Girdlestone procedure, patients have significant functional limitations secondary to weak abductor and limb length inequality[43].

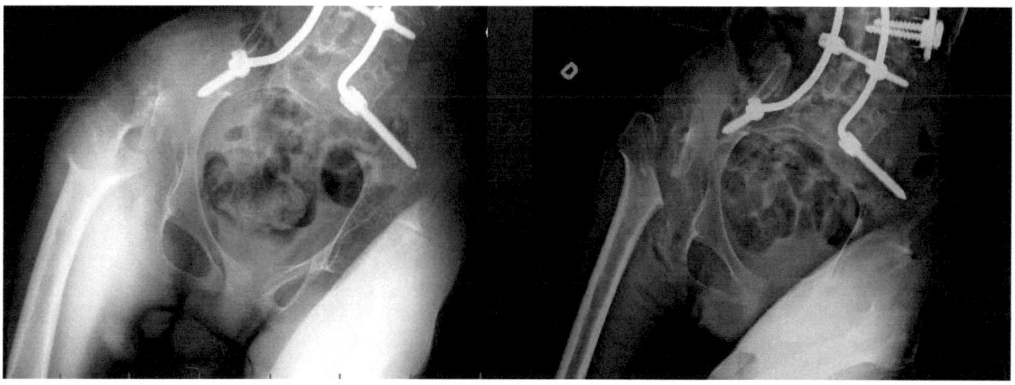

Fig. 16. 21 years old male patient (cerebral palsy patient), his health care provider notice increasing difficulty with perineal hygiene and increasing irritability when diaper changes are attempted. Intertrochanteric resection was performed to improve his hip range of motion and to alleviate his symptoms.

10. Summary

Non-arthroplasty surgical options for treating painful degenerative hip joint conditions are well established surgical procedures. Patient selection and proper preoperative evaluation is critical for successful long-term result. Understanding the indications and the contraindications as well as the limitations and the expected outcome of each procedure is critical during pre operative counseling of the patient about nonarthroplasty surgical option.

11. References

[1] Sochart, D.H. and M.L. Porter, *The long-term results of Charnley low-friction arthroplasty in young patients who have congenital dislocation, degenerative osteoarthrosis, or rheumatoid arthritis.* J Bone Joint Surg Am, 1997. 79(11): p. 1599-617.

[2] Dooley, P.J., *Femoroacetabular impingement syndrome: Nonarthritic hip pain in young adults.* Can Fam Physician, 2008. 54(1): p. 42-7.

[3] Van Iersel, M. and G. Mulley, *What is a waddling gait?* Disability & Rehabilitation, 2004. 26(11): p. 678-82.

[4] Clohisy, J.C., et al., *A systematic approach to the plain radiographic evaluation of the young adult hip.* J Bone Joint Surg Am, 2008. 90 Suppl 4: p. 47-66.

[5] Notzli, H.P., et al., The contour of the femoral head-neck junction as a predictor for the risk of anterior impingement. Journal of Bone & Joint Surgery - British Volume, 2002. 84(4): p. 556-60.

[6] De Pellegrin, M.P., W.G. Mackenzie, and H.T. Harcke, *Ultrasonographic evaluation of hip morphology in osteochondrodysplasias.* Journal of Pediatric Orthopedics, 2000. 20(5): p. 588-93.

[7] Beck, M., et al., Hip morphology influences the pattern of damage to the acetabular cartilage: femoroacetabular impingement as a cause of early osteoarthritis of the hip. Journal of Bone & Joint Surgery - British Volume, 2005. 87(7): p. 1012-8.

[8] McCarthy, J.C. and J.A. Lee, *Hip arthroscopy: indications, outcomes, and complications.* Instructional Course Lectures, 2006. 55: p. 301-8.

[9] Salvo, J.P., C.R. Troxell, and D.P. Duggan, *Incidence of venous thromboembolic disease following hip arthroscopy.* Orthopedics, 2010. 33(9): p. 664.

[10] Philippon, M., et al., Femoroacetabular impingement in 45 professional athletes: associated pathologies and return to sport following arthroscopic decompression. Knee Surg Sports Traumatol Arthrosc, 2007. 15(7): p. 908-14.

[11] Sampson, T.G., Arthroscopic treatment of femoroacetabular impingement: a proposed technique with clinical experience. Instr Course Lect, 2006. 55: p. 337-46.

[12] Byrd, J.W. and K.S. Jones, Arthroscopic femoroplasty in the management of cam-type femoroacetabular impingement. Clin Orthop Relat Res, 2009. 467(3): p. 739-46.

[13] Philippon, M.J., et al., Outcomes following hip arthroscopy for femoroacetabular impingement with associated chondrolabral dysfunction: minimum two-year follow-up. J Bone Joint Surg Br, 2009. 91(1): p. 16-23.

[14] Clohisy, J.C., et al., Combined hip arthroscopy and limited open osteochondroplasty for anterior femoroacetabular impingement. J Bone Joint Surg Am, 2010. 92(8): p. 1697-706.

[15] Pierannunzii, L. and M. d'Imporzano, Treatment of femoroacetabular impingement: a modified resection osteoplasty technique through an anterior approach. Orthopedics, 2007. 30(2): p. 96-102.

[16] Sink, E.L., et al., Multicenter Study of Complications Following Surgical Dislocation of the Hip. J Bone Joint Surg Am, 2011.

[17] Brooker, A.F., et al., Ectopic ossification following total hip replacement. Incidence and a method of classification. J Bone Joint Surg Am, 1973. 55(8): p. 1629-32.

[18] Murphy, S., et al., Debridement of the adult hip for femoroacetabular impingement: indications and preliminary clinical results. Clin Orthop Relat Res, 2004(429): p. 178-81.

[19] Peters, C.L. and J.A. Erickson, Treatment of femoro-acetabular impingement with surgical dislocation and debridement in young adults. J Bone Joint Surg Am, 2006. 88(8): p. 1735-41.
[20] Beaule, P.E., M.J. Le Duff, and E. Zaragoza, Quality of life following femoral head-neck osteochondroplasty for femoroacetabular impingement. J Bone Joint Surg Am, 2007. 89(4): p. 773-9.
[21] Espinosa, N., et al., Treatment of femoro-acetabular impingement: preliminary results of labral refixation. J Bone Joint Surg Am, 2006. 88(5): p. 925-35.
[22] Beck, M., et al., Anterior femoroacetabular impingement: part II. Midterm results of surgical treatment. Clin Orthop Relat Res, 2004(418): p. 67-73.
[23] Klaue, K., C.W. Durnin, and R. Ganz, *The acetabular rim syndrome. A clinical presentation of dysplasia of the hip.* Journal of Bone & Joint Surgery - British Volume, 1991. 73(3): p. 423-9.
[24] Murphy, S.B., R. Ganz, and M.E. Muller, *The prognosis in untreated dysplasia of the hip. A study of radiographic factors that predict the outcome.* Journal of Bone & Joint Surgery - American Volume, 1995. 77(7): p. 985-9.
[25] Schramm, M., et al., *The Wagner spherical osteotomy of the acetabulum. Surgical technique.* Journal of Bone & Joint Surgery - American Volume, 2004. 86-A Suppl 1: p. 73-80.
[26] Ganz, R., et al., A new periacetabular osteotomy for the treatment of hip dysplasias. Technique and preliminary results. Clin Orthop Relat Res, 1988(232): p. 26-36.
[27] Reynolds, D., J. Lucas, and K. Klaue, *Retroversion of the acetabulum. A cause of hip pain.* Journal of Bone & Joint Surgery - British Volume, 1999. 81(2): p. 281-8.
[28] Jamali, A.A., et al., Anteroposterior pelvic radiographs to assess acetabular retroversion: high validity of the "cross-over-sign". Journal of Orthopaedic Research, 2007. 25(6): p. 758-65.
[29] Matheney, T., et al., Intermediate to long-term results following the Bernese periacetabular osteotomy and predictors of clinical outcome. J Bone Joint Surg Am, 2009. 91(9): p. 2113-23.
[30] Garbuz, D.S., M.A. Awwad, and C.P. Duncan, *Periacetabular osteotomy and total hip arthroplasty in patients older than 40 years.* Journal of Arthroplasty, 2008. 23(7): p. 960-3.
[31] Matheney, T., et al., Intermediate to long-term results following the bernese periacetabular osteotomy and predictors of clinical outcome: surgical technique. J Bone Joint Surg Am, 2010. 92 Suppl 1 Pt 2: p. 115-29.
[32] Clohisy, J.C., et al., *Periacetabular osteotomy: a systematic literature review.* Clin Orthop Relat Res, 2009. 467(8): p. 2041-52.
[33] Davey, J.P. and R.F. Santore, *Complications of periacetabular osteotomy.* Clin Orthop Relat Res, 1999(363): p. 33-7.
[34] Ganz, R., et al., A new periacetabular osteotomy for the treatment of hip dysplasias. Technique and preliminary results. Clinical Orthopaedics & Related Research, 1988(232): p. 26-36.
[35] Trousdale, R.T., et al., Periacetabular and intertrochanteric osteotomy for the treatment of osteoarthrosis in dysplastic hips. J Bone Joint Surg Am, 1995. 77(1): p. 73-85.
[36] Peters, C.L., J.A. Erickson, and J.L. Hines, Early results of the Bernese periacetabular osteotomy: the learning curve at an academic medical center. J Bone Joint Surg Am, 2006. 88(9): p. 1920-6.

[37] Haverkamp, D. and R.K. Marti, Intertrochanteric osteotomy combined with acetabular shelfplasty in young patients with severe deformity of the femoral head and secondary osteoarthritis. A long-term follow-up study. J Bone Joint Surg Br, 2005. 87(1): p. 25-31.
[38] Chiari, K., *Medial displacement osteotomy of the pelvis.* Clin Orthop Relat Res, 1974(98): p. 55-71.
[39] Love, B.R., P.M. Stevens, and P.F. Williams, *A long-term review of shelf arthroplasty.* J Bone Joint Surg Br, 1980. 62(3): p. 321-5.
[40] Callaghan, J.J., R.A. Brand, and D.R. Pedersen, *Hip arthrodesis. A long-term follow-up.* Journal of Bone & Joint Surgery - American Volume, 1985. 67(9): p. 1328-35.
[41] Hamadouche, M., et al., Total hip arthroplasty for the treatment of ankylosed hips : a five to twenty-one-year follow-up study. J Bone Joint Surg Am, 2001. 83-A(7): p. 992-8.
[42] Joshi, A.B., et al., *Conversion of a fused hip to total hip arthroplasty.* J Bone Joint Surg Am, 2002. 84-A(8): p. 1335-41.
[43] Bittar, E.S. and W. Petty, *Girdlestone arthroplasty for infected total hip arthroplasty.* Clin Orthop Relat Res, 1982(170): p. 83-7.

2

Hip Arthroplasty

N. A. Sandiford[1], U. Alao[1], J. A. Skinner[2] and S. R. Samsani[3]
[1]*Specialist Registrar, Kent and Sussex Hospital, Mount Ephraim, Tunbridge Wells, Kent*
[2]*Consultant Orthopaedic surgeon Royal National Orthopaedic Hospital Brockley Hill, Stanmore*
[3]*Consultant Orthopaedic surgeon, Medway Maritime Hospital, Windmill Road, Gillingham, Kent*
United Kingdom

1. Introduction

1.1 History

Total Hip Arthroplasty (THA) has been hailed the 'The operation of the century.' (1) While the prevalence of coxarthrosis is relatively unchanged from ancient times, attempt at surgical treatment are relatively recent Themistocles Gluck is credited with performing the first hip arthroplasty in Germany in 1891. It was a hemi arthroplasty and he used an ivory femoral head. Early attempts at the turn of the 20th century focused on interpositional arthroplasty using a variety of tissues which included skin, fascia lata, and pig's bladder (1)! Also during this period Dr Ban saw, then chief of orthopaedics at the Mandalay General hospital in Burma, used hand made ivory components for patients with femoral neck fractures. He presented a report of his first 300 cases in 1969. His patients were aged between 24 and 87 years old. Eighty eight per cent returned to sports and bicycle riding within weeks post surgery.

The dawn of the modern era of hip arthroplasty was heralded by the vitallium mould design of Smith-Petersen. Wiles subsequently developed and inserted the first THA in 1938 in the UK.

The next most significant step was made by British surgeon Sir John Charnley. In the 1960's he introduced several pivotal concepts including the low friction arthroplasty, the use of polymethyl methacrylate cement as a grout and the use of high density polyethylene as a bearing surface. While several of Charnley's principles and techniques have evolved, the principles he proposed remain relatively unchallenged.

Arguably the most important modern advancement in arthroplasty surgery has been the establishment of joint registries. These provide invaluable data on survival, complications and can help to establish standards for practice. The Swedish joint registry is the most established of these. Much of the long term survival data for specific types of implants and fixation methods are extracted from this database. Registries are now in existence in most countries including the UK. The American Joint Replacement Registry (AJRR) is currently in the process of being formalised.

2. Indications

The main indication for total hip arthroplasty is pain secondary to primary or secondary osteoarthritis (2), and has remained largely unchanged for the past few decades. Results from the Swedish Registry show the mean age for THR was about 70 years old with a decrease in age seen in men while an increase was noted in women. Recent trends have seen a widening of the indications for performing total hip arthroplasty to include rheumatoid arthritis in cases of failed medical management. Such patients are often younger compared with elderly patients who commonly present with osteoarthritis and trauma (2). Other indications include avascular necrosis, metastatic disease and ankylosing spondylitis.

The use of total hip arthroplasty in treating femoral neck fractures has, and continues to generate controversy. There is a move towards basing the surgical management on patient-related, rather than diagnosis related approach as a reflection of this heterogeneous group of patients. For example, fit elderly patients with pre-existing symptomatic osteoarthritis who sustain a femoral neck fracture should be considered for total hip arthroplasty rather than internal fixation.

There are a number of studies that support this approach. Blomfeldt et al (3) conducted a randomised control trial comparing the outcome of patients with displaced neck of femur fractures, who are relatively fit, active and indecently mobile, treated with internal fixation or total hip arthroplasty. They treated one hundred and two patients with a mean age of eighty years. Forty nine patients where randomised to THR and fifty three underwent internal fixation. Their results showed similar mortality rate of 25% at four year follow-up but a better functional outcome, lower complication and re-operation rate in the total hip arthroplasty group compared to the internal fixation group. Another randomized prospective trial involving two hundred and seven patients by Keating et al (4), treated patients with internal fixation, hemiarthroplasty and total hip arthroplasty. Their results showed better functional outcome in the THA group in comparison to the other groups. Cost analysis also showed a higher rate for the internal fixation group due to higher re-operation rate but no difference between the THR group and hemiarthroplasty group.

3. Patient expectations

The widening indications for surgery have influenced the demographics of patients undergoing total hip arthroplasty and thus, their expectations. More and more young patients are being considered for total hip arthroplasty. These subgroups of patients generally tend to be very active and as result place more demands on the replaced hip. Even the modern day 'elderly' patient has higher expectations in comparison to previous decades as patients are offered surgery far earlier owing to improvement in technology and surgical technique. This emphasis on meeting patient's expectation and optimizing subsequent function has lead to objective scoring systems such as the Oxford Hip Score (OHS), Harris Hip Scores (HHS), the Western Ontario and McMaster University (WOMAC) scoring systems being developed and more recently in the UK patient related outcome measures. A study by Mancuso et al looking at the fulfilment of patient's expectation showed that only 43% patients (of 405) thought their pre-operative expectations where fulfilled fully. They showed that younger patients and those with a BMI of lower that 35kg/m^2 had a greater proportion of their expectations fulfilled (5).

The modern day THR, however, patient is more likely to be obese compared to previous generations and may develop early failure as a result. However, advances in implant design and tribology have increased the Orthopaedic Surgeon's armamentarium in facing these challenges.

4. Surgical technique

While the ideal approach for THA is as yet undecided, several approaches have been described and are used in routine practice. While no revolutionary changes have been made to the classically described techniques, significant refinements and advances have occurred particularly with the development of minimally invasive approaches for THA and the instruments to facilitate these approaches.

Previous techniques described include the lateral (Hardinge) (6), anterior (Smith-Petersen) (7), posterior (Moore or southern) and medial approaches (8), each with its unique risks and benefits. The approach most commonly used in the UK is the posterior (57%) followed by the anterolateral approach (37%) according to the United Kingdom National Joint Registry (UK NJR) (9). Personal communication with members of the British Hip Society has revealed that the posterior approach is favoured by the majority of specialist hip surgeons.

Results from the Swedish Arthroplasty Register (10) have suggested that the posterior approach is being performed less frequently (52% in 2008 vs 65% in 1992) likely due to an increased incidence of dislocation particularly with the minimally invasive posterior approach. The surgical approach used in our unit is the posterior approach which is described below after a description of the original procedure:

This approach, popularised by Moore, is also called the southern approach. It consists of a 10-15 cm incision centered on the posterior aspect of the greater trochanter. This is deepened through the fascia lata. The gluteus maximus is split along the line of the incision. This along with internal rotation of the hip allows visualisation of the common insertion of the short external rotators on the posterior aspect of the proximal femur. Also visible is a layer of fat which contains the sciatic nerve at its center. This must be protected. Internally rotating the hip moves this nerve out of the operative field.

Once the tendons are identified, stay sutures are placed in the tendons of the piriformis and obturator internus. These are then detached from the femur at their point of attachment. Deep to this layer is the posterior capsule. Once this is incised further internal rotation will lead to dislocation of the hip joint. Repair of the posterior structures is not routinely recommended with this description.

Early criticism of the posterior approach stemmed from several reports of higher dislocation rates in patients treated with this technique (11, 12). Many authors using this contemporary posterior approach have recorded very low dislocation rates and addition of posterior capsular repair has reduced the dislocation rates to <2% (13). Also when compared to the lateral approach, the incidence of postoperative abductor lurch is very low with posterior approach.

5. Dislocation rates

Despite early reports, studies over the last decade have shown that the incidence of dislocation decreases substantially if a posterior capsular repair is performed.

Masonis and Bourne (14) reviewed fourteen studies comprising 13,203 patients. Overall there was a six times increased rate of dislocation in patients treated with a posterior approach when compared to the trans trochanteric , anterolateral and direct lateral approaches. In the group which had a posterior approach dislocation rates among those patients who had a capsular repair was 2.03% compared to 3.95% in the group which had no repair performed. These results were pooled from multiple surgeons however and such heterogeneity has been associated with poor results, particularly among junior surgeons (15).

In a well designed single surgeon series Wilson et al (16) showed that dislocation rates reduced from 3.1% to 0.7% after a posterior repair was performed. Similar results have been reported by other authors (17, 18, 19) including Suh et al who reported that repair of the posterior structures reduced their dislocation rates in revision THA from 10% to 1.9% (13). These results are summarised in Table 1.

			Dislocation rates related to approach			
Authors	**Date**	**Number in study**	**Posterior**	**Anterolateral**	**Posterior with repair**	**Direct Lateral**
Palan et al	2009 (Prospective)	1089	2.3%	2.1%	_	_
Tsai et al	2008 (Retrospective)	204	6.38%	_	0%	_
Kwon et al	2006 (meta analysis)	_	4.46%	0.75	0.49%	0.43%
Wilson et al	2005 (Retrospective)	2213	3.9%	_	0.9%	_
Suh et al	2004 (Prospective)	346	6.4%	_	1%	_
Masonis and Bourne	2002 (Review)	13,203	3.95%	2.18	2.03	0.55

Table 1. Dislocation rates after the posterior approach- Summary of results

6. Our current technique (figures 1-5)

In our unit the posterior approach is used for both primary and revision THA. For primary THA a minimally invasive technique is routinely performed and is described below.

The patient is placed in a lateral decubitus position. The tip of the greater trochanter and the posterior boarder of the proximal femur are identified. A 10 to 12cm incision centered on the posterior one third of the tip of the greater trochanter is made which extends 5cm above and 5cm below this point. The incision proximal to the greater trochanter is angled backwards by 30 to 40 degrees. The incision is deepened to the level of the fascia lata which is also incised. The gluteus maximus is split along the line of the incision revealing the trochanteric bursa which is divided in line with the incision but preserved. Internal rotation of the hip at this stage brings the posterior aspect of the greater trochanter with its attached short external rotators into the operative field. At this stage we use a gauze swab to wipe the bursal tissue and fat off of the short external rotators (SER) attachment gently downward. This action exposes the tendons of short external rotators- from proximal to distal piriformis, superior gemellus, obturator internus, inferior gemellus and quadratus femoris- and moves the sciatic nerve away from the operative field. Next superior border piriformis tendon is identified and a curved retractor is placed under the gluteus minimus but above the superior border of piriformis tendon. Stay sutures are placed in the common tendon of the SER muscles and the underlying capsule (Figure 3). The short external rotators, along with posterior capsule, is then divided with diathermy at its point of attachment to the greater trochanter. Then posterior dislocation of the hip is performed by adduction, flexion and internal rotation of femur. Once the procedure is completed the short external rotators and the capsule is reattached via drill holes to the posterior part of greater trochanter.

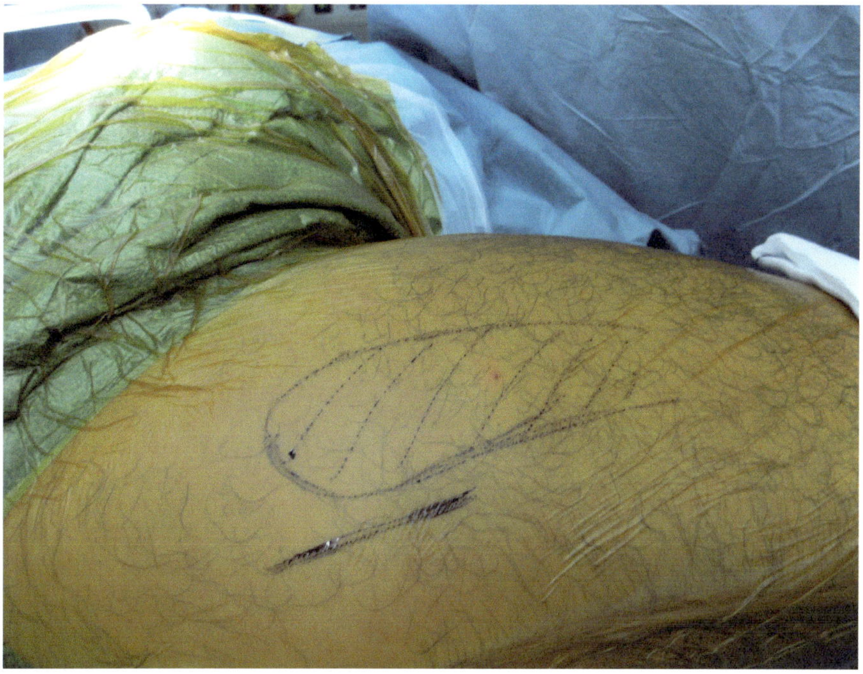

Fig. 1. Landmarks for the skin incision

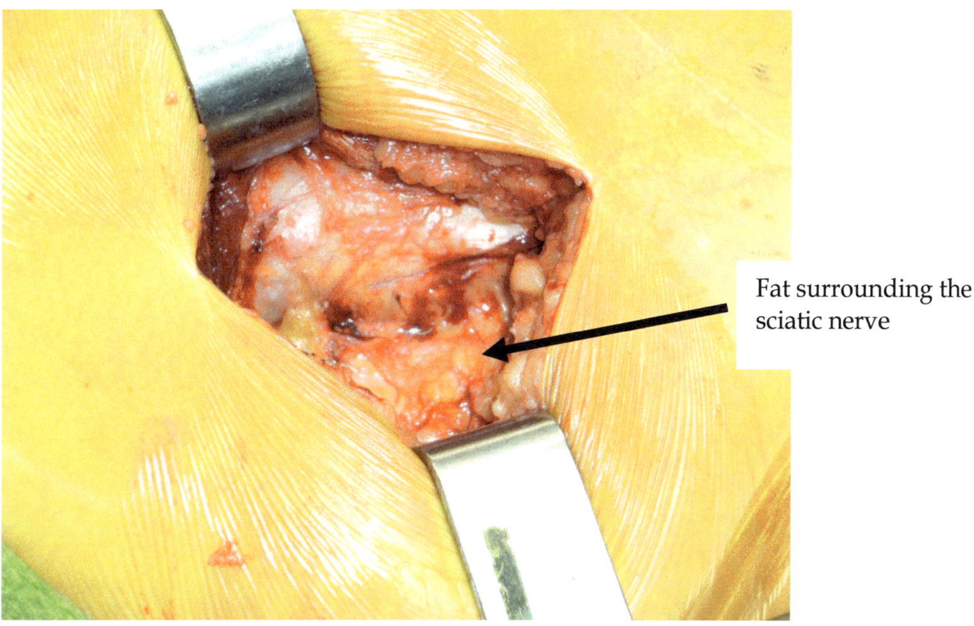

Fig. 2. Fat and bursa moved away from operative field. This protects the sciatic nerve.

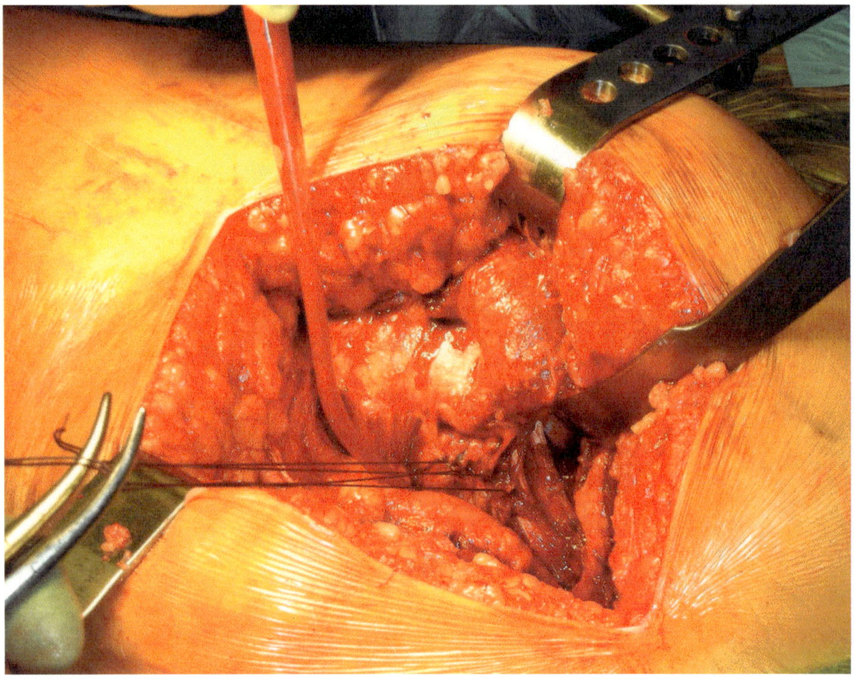

Fig. 3. Stay sutures in the short external rotator (SER) tendons

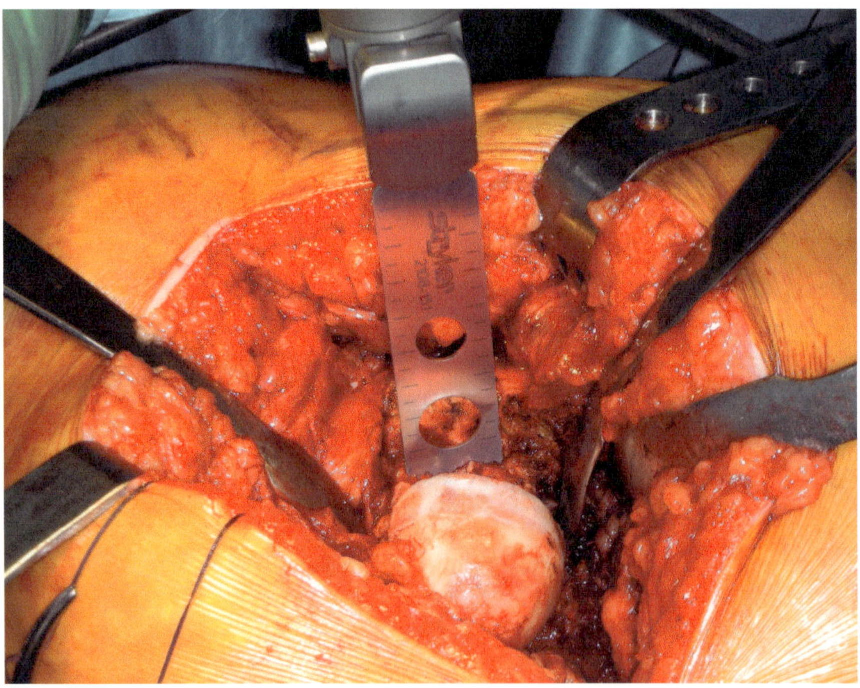

Fig. 4. Dislocated femoral head

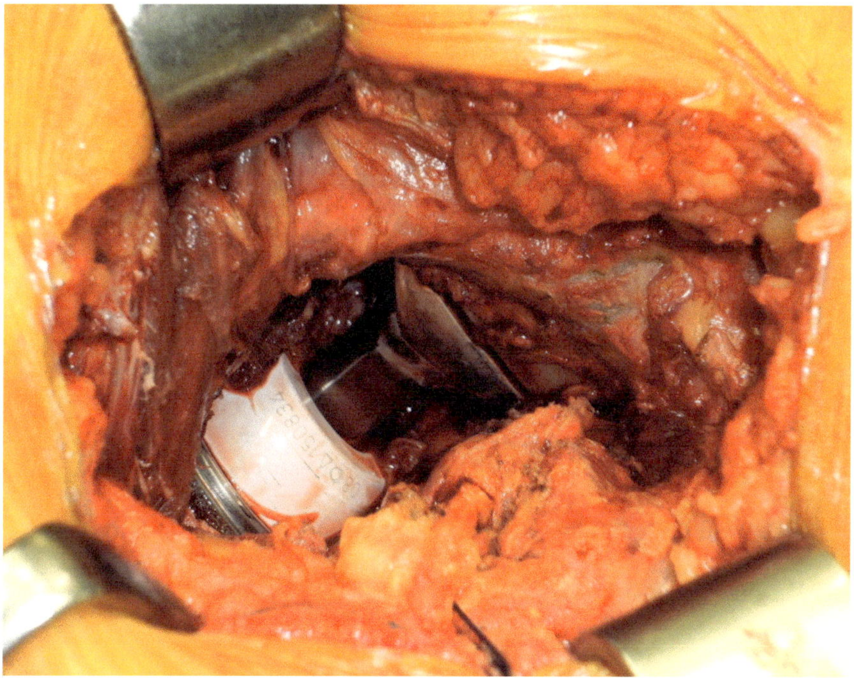

Fig. 5. Post reduction of THA

7. Minimally Invasive Surgical (MIS) approaches

Over the last decade minimally invasive techniques have drawn much attention. These methods represent a refinement rather than a revolution of standard approaches. They have been described for the anterior, posterior and lateral approaches. By definition a minimally invasive approach infers an incision length of ≤ 10cm.

Views and conclusions about MIS THA are conflicting but overall this is accepted as safe, but not better nor a replacement for established surgical approaches. This view is supported by level I evidence. In the UK the National Institute for Health and Clinical Evidence has recommended that the MIS posterior approach is safe but the Swedish Registry suggests that there is an increased incidence of dislocations with this approach which accounts for its decreasing use.

MIS THA has been extensively studied in the literature. Dorr et al (20) showed that while immediate post operative pain control and mobility were improved in the MIS group, there was no difference between this group and those in whom a conventional approach was used at 6 weeks and beyond. Recent level 1evidence (21) has revealed that when comparing the MIS anterolateral, classic posterior and MIS posterior approaches found similar results. This study also found that patients who had the posterior MIS approach had favourable outcomes when compared to the MIS anterolateral approach. Pagnano et al (22) also found that patients receiving the posterior MIS approach walked, achieved independence from assistive devices and returned to activities of daily living before those treated using a 2 incision approach.

While opinions on the clinical benefits of MIS THA seem to be in agreement, these differ on the overall benefits of this approach. Reininga et al (23) in their review, concluded that MIS

THA is a safe procedure although there is no firm evidence of functional benefit. Smith et al (24) reviewed 2849 hips, however, and found a significantly elevated risk of transient lateral femoral cutaneous nerve palsy in the group treated with the MIS technique, again with no functional benefits.

What has not been clarified in this area is the 'ideal' MIS approach, whether specialised instruments help, the group of patients best suited for this procedure and the learning curve for this technique.

8. Technology

A number of advances have been made since Sir John Charnley pioneered the Low Friction Arthroplasty in the 1960s. His design consisted of a stainless steel mono polar femoral stem and a polyethylene acetabular cup both fixed using polymethyl methaacyrlate bone cement. There are currently more than 100 hip stems and cups respectively submitted to the Orthopaedic Data Evaluation Panel (ODEP) for assessment, all of which has variable designs and choices of bearing surfaces.

The National Institute of Clinical Excellence (NICE) which issues guidance on selection of prosthesis advises that the best prosthesis should have a revision rate of 10% or less at ten years, demonstrable by long term viability studies. Cemented prosthesis has the longest viability studies but a number of uncemented prosthesis have passed the ten year mark with good results.

The trend is to use cemented prosthesis in elderly patients with poor bone quality, while uncemented stems are more commonly used in younger more active patients or those with good bone quality in general.

Well fixed cemented components depend primarily on two interfaces; implant cement interface and cement-bone interface. Adequate fixation of both interfaces is crucial to the long term survival of the prosthesis as the load is transmitted via the prosthesis to the cement-bone interface. Any weakness in either may lead to early failure. Considerable advancement has been made from the first generation cementing technique (finger packing, no cement gun, no cement restrictor or canal pressurization) to the third generation (elimination of air bubbles via vacuum preparation, stem centralizer and femoral canal pressurization) thus improving the stability of well fixed cemented implants. In addition, modern day cemented stems are modular, allowing for a range of femoral heads to be fixed for optimal soft tissue balancing and stability.

Uncemented implants coated with hydroxyapatite have either porous coated or grit-blasted surfaces and depend on 'biologic' fixation of bone by bony interdigitation into the stem. A well fixed uncemented stem requires cortical seating into the femoral canal. Some uncemented acetabular implants offer added security of screw fixation for improved stability.

9. Bearing surfaces

An ideal bearing surface has the following characteristics. (25)

1. low coefficient of friction
2. resistant to third body damage and wear
3. generates small amount of particles
4. has low cellular reaction to wear debris

A variety of significant advancements in bearing surfaces has been made since the dawn of modern era of hip arthroplasty. Figure 6 outlines the major advances.
Bearing surfaces can be split into two broad groups:
1. Hard on soft bearings
2. Hard on hard bearings

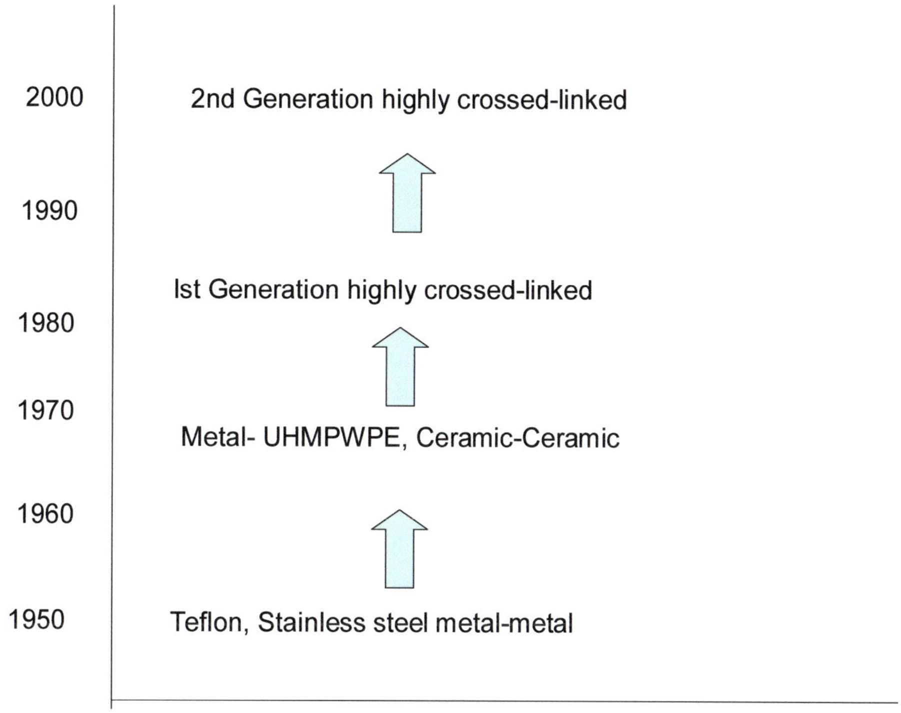

Fig. 6. Major advances in bearing surfaces.

10. Hard on soft bearings

The ultra high molecular weight polyethylene (UHMWPE) acetabular cup was introduced in 1962 coupled with metallic heads to form hard-on-soft bearing surface. UHMWPE consists of several long chains of monomer ethylene which serves to transfer load more effectively to the polymer backbone by strengthening intermolecular interactions. Early wear was a major problem with the early prostheses, particularly with larger bearing surfaces. The third body particle thus generated enters the effective joint space and stimulates a foreign body response resulting in osteolysis which is mainly mediated by macrophages (26). PE wear is related to three main factors; implant geometry and material properties, sterilization and shelf-life. Initially, it was widely accepted that the osteolysis was due to delayed reaction to bone cement (PMMA), this erroneous belief lead to the development of uncemented prosthesis such as the Austin Moore prosthesis. This change did not positively affect the wear profile of the PE cup.
One of the best advances to UHMPE liner use was the advent of highly crossed linked PE liner introduced in 1998. This is achieved by low dose gamma or electron beam radiation

and thermal treatment to increase their oxidation resistance. Its advantages include increasing resistance to abrasive and adhesive wear thereby improving bearing wear rates. Another example of a hard-on-soft surface is ceramic on PE but is not a widely used combination.

11. Hard on hard bearings

Wear-particle related osteolysis around THA components and subsequent failure rates lead to the development of other bearing surfaces such as metal-on-metal articulations. Cobalt-Chrome is the commonest metal alloy used. One of the main theoretical advantages of hard on hard bearing surfaces is reduction in osteolysis (27) by generating less wear particles. In addition, the particle size generated is also smaller (0.015-0.12um) compared to the particle size range (0.2-7um) that has been shown to trigger osteolysis. The first generation metal-on-metal hip arthroplasty showed a low rate of wear and long term results demonstrated that failure was due implant design rather than wear particles (28).

Other advantages of metal on metal surfaces include a higher scratch resistance and larger bearing components which increases the excursion distance, the distance needed to travel before the neck impinges and dislocate, due to the increase in head to neck ratio. This is particularly advantageous in revision surgery for dislocation.

Metal on metal bearings, however, are not completely biologically inert. A number of soft tissue reactions have limited its use. These include metallosis and aseptic lymphocytic vasculitis associated response (ALVAL). There is an increased risk for these adverse tissue reactions in females, smaller femoral head bearings and obesity (29).

Another type of hard on hard surfaces are ceramic bearings, first introduced in the mid 60s. They are harder than metal and have a lower wear rate especially when coupled with its self. In addition, the wear particles generated are biologically inert, eliminating the concerns of sift tissue reactions seen with metal on metal bearings. The main disadvantage, however, is its low resistance to fracture and squeaking, particularly seen in the taller, younger and heavier patients. Like polyethylene bearings, ceramic bearing surfaces have improved since the first generation implants which were more susceptible to fracture.

There are two types of ceramic bearings; alumina and zirconia. Zirconia femoral heads coupled with PE leads to accelerated wear and early failure and is thus not recommend coupling these two components.

12. Results

Total hip arthroplasty remains one of most successful operations in terms of cost effectiveness and symptom relief for patients.

The best prosthesis should have a demonstrable long survivorship and low revision rates. These attributes are best shown by National Joint Registries which not only provide early warning of failures but show cumulative experience of surgeons while eliminating potential bias by the innovator. The main goals of national joint registry is three fold; defining the epidemiology of a particular patient population, providing timely information about outcome and identifying risk factors for poor outcomes (30). The Swedish hip registry was the first national joint registry introduced in 1979. Its main goal was to describe the outcomes of primary hip replacements and to report complications. Since its inception, many other countries have started national joint registries. Many of these registries provide

the Orthopaedic community with the results of the oldest and newest prosthesis in the market while keeping track of modifications and innovations.
Charnley's cemented femoral stem has undergone a number of modifications since its inception, including changing from a monoblock to modular stem while retaining the stem geometry. The stem was later modified into the Elite-plus stem (Depuy, Warsaw, Indiana, USA) by undercutting the flange, reducing the diameter and addition of a stem centralizer.
Data for the Swedish hip registry shows favorable results for the original stems; the cohort operated on from 1979 to 1989 had a twenty-one-year survival rate of 81.7% based on 18,607 observations. The more recent cohort, (1990 to 2000), had a ten-year survival rate of 93% based on 20,162 observations (2). Similar results have been reproduced in other centres. Shculte et al showed 90% survivorship of the stem using revision as endpoint in 322 hips (31). The modern day Charnley Elite Plus stem also has favourable medium term results as shown in Kim YH et al prospective study in 194 young hips, with a mean age of 49.1 which demonstrated a 12 years survivorship of 99% using revision surgery as end point (32).
The Exeter femoral stem was introduced around the same time as the Charnley prosthesis and has also undergone a number of modifications since its inception. It is a double tapered, highly polished stem. The Swedish hip register showed a 7 year survival of 98.1% in 4,769 implants. While Carrington et al showed 100% and 90.4% for the femoral and acetabular components, respectively at 17 years using aseptic loosening as an endpoint (33).
Some uncemented femoral prosthesis, such has the Furlong hip replacement (Joint replacement Instrumentation limited, London. United Kingdom) also have favourable results. The Furlong stem is titanium, hydroxyapatite ceramic coated stem first introduced in 1985. Good short to medium term results has been reported in literature (34). The longest follow-up in literature is 21yrs which shows comparable results to previously mentioned cemented stems, 97.4% with revision for any reason as endpoint.
The Corail stem is another uncemented stem with long term results. First introduced in 1986, it is tapered HP coated stem made from titanium alloy. Since inception, it had been modified to a collarless stem and recently (2004) the neck was made slimmer and the taper shortened. The Norwegian Hip Registry shows 97% survivorship at 15 years using revision for any cause as endpoint (35).
These comparable results show that both cemented and uncemented stems can achieve good longevity. Its is likely that these results do not only reflect good implant design but also increased familiarity with use over the past number of years. Analysis of national hip registries show that most of the implants that fail to pass the 10 year mark or with survivorship of less that 90% tend to do so early (2 to 3 years) or at medium term (5-8 years).

13. Current controversies

A review of current orthopaedic literature would reveal many issues of debate and uncertainty. Two issues which currently attract much debate are those of Metal on Metal hip resurfacing (MoM HR) and the subject of thromboprophylaxis after THA. These are discussed below.

13.1 Metal on Metal hip resurfacing (MoM HR)

Resurfacing affected joint surfaces has always intuitively seemed to be correct when contemplating surgery for the arthritic hip joint. The Smith Peterson cup arthroplasty is considered by some the earliest attempt at surface replacement. Charnley in the early 1950's

performed surface replacements using thin shells of Teflon. Good function was briefly restored but severe osteolysis occurred in response to high Teflon wear.
The next main thrust came in 70's after THA with conventional stemmed components had been introduced and took the form of metal femoral components with high density polyethylene sockets. Memorable examples were the ICLH developed in UK by Freeman, Wagner contribution from Germany and the THARIES from the USA. Initial results were again spectacular but failure developed because of the large amounts of polyethylene debris.
The poor results of all these attempts led to the concept of resurfacing being abandoned. A British surgeon, Derek Mcminn, aware of how well metal on metal bearing surfaces had performed based on the results of late revision of both McKee Farrar , Stanmore and Ring hips replacements in Birmingham designed a new resurfacing with a metal on metal bearing surface with the metallurgy based on the results that had been learnt from these earlier metal on metal designs.
Contemporary MoM HR was thus pioneered in the UK by McMinn. Improved design, metallurgy and advances in engineering resulted in the design of the Birmingham Hip Resurfacing prosthesis. Original designs have been used in the UK since 1991 and approved by the United States Food and Drug Administration in 2006. Proposed advantages of this prosthesis include improved stability due to its large diameter, improved proprioception, improved range of motion and return to function, bone conservation and relative ease of revision. Early results have been encouraging but data from the UK National Joint Registry (NJR) suggest that MoM HR prostheses have relatively high early failure in certain groups and therefore revision rates. There have been concerns about increases blood levels of cobalt and chromium ions in patients with these prostheses in situ as well as the occurrence of periarticular destructive soft tissue lesions- so called pseudotumors.
Revision of failed MoM HR to stemmed modular MoM THA has also occurred with increasing frequency as a result of the proposed 'ease of revision.' These prostheses pose a new and unique issue to the arthroplasty community as there seems to be concerns with these components which are similar to those for MoM HR. Recent guidance from the British Hip Society (March 2011) has suggested that patients with these components be followed more closely than those with standard THA as the risk of adverse effects seem to be similar to hip resurfacing components. This is currently an area of intense controversy.

13.2 Throboprophylaxis after THA

This is the 2nd area of significant controversy with unique issues in the UK and USA. This issue creates such debate that we have presented a brief review of current evidence before discussing the controversy surrounding it.

13.3 Deep vein thrombosis (DVT) and Pulmonary embolism (PE) after THA

The incidence of radiologically detected DVT after lower limb arthroplasty surgery is 30-60% (for the entire limb) and 10- 20% for proximal segment veins. Symptomatic PE occurs in 1-2% of this group (36). The rate of fatal PE is 0.1-0.2% (37). Risk factors for DVT and PE include obesity, American Society of Anaesthesiologist's grade 3 or above, revision surgery, dementia and renal and cardiovascular disease.
A meta analysis of DVT prophylaxis regimens found that the rate of DVT's increased 2-3 fold if no thromboprophylaxis was used. The lowest rates of proximal DVT's occurred when warfarin and low molecular weight heparin (LMWH) were used. The incidence of symptomatic PE's was decreased by warfarin, pneumatic compression devices (PCD's) and

LMWH. The rate of fatal PE was unaffected. Major bleeding occurred in patients who received low dose heparin (38). This review concluded that warfarin was the best overall single agent.
When used as part of a multimodal approach aspirin has been found to have the same efficacy as warfarin (39). Multimodal approaches address each aspect of Virchow's Triad. It includes the use of regional anaesthesia, PCD's, chemical agents and early patient mobilisation. This approach has reduced the rate of asymptomatic and symptomatic DVT to 5.2% and 0.4% respectively (20). These authors found that patients on warfarin had a significantly increased incidence of wound haematomas compared to those on aspirin. Sharrock et al (40)reviewed >15000 patients and found a higher all cause mortality and increased incidence of non fatal PE's in those receiving contemporary potent anticoagulants (including LMWH, Fondaparinux and Rivaroxiban) and Warfarin than groups who received multimodal therapy.
This evidence seems to suggest that potent anticoagulants are not ideal in patients undergoing THA and conflicts with national guidance in the United Kingdom. It must be emphasized that patients should undergo pre operative assessment prior to a decision on the choice of thromboprophylaxis agent is made.

14. United Kingdom

A House of Commons Select Committee Report 2004- 2005 suggested that 2500 preventable deaths occurred annually as a result of deep venous thrombosis (DVT). It led to the publication of guidance by the National Institute for Health and Clinical Excellence (NICE) on thromboprophylaxis after THA in 2007. Challenges to these guidelines have arisen and include:

- The mortality figures stated in the parliamentary white paper have overestimated the number of deaths
- Using DVT as a surrogate end point for fatal PE has contributed to this inaccuracy
- Members of the guidance committee were linked to the pharmaceutical industry
- Recent evidence has suggested that since the implementation of these guidelines, both the amount and duration of pharmacological prophylaxis has increased along with the incidence of DVTs and their complications (41).

15. United States

In 2004, the American College of Chest Physicians (ACCP) made several recommendations for prevention of DVTs and pulmonary embolism which extended to include the orthopaedic community. The recommendations included aggressive prophylaxis regimens, but were based on the incidence of venographically detected DVTs and used this as a 'surrogate' for fatal pulmonary emboli. In their review process, the ACCP did not consider death and fatal PE as suitable end-points.
Subsequent to the implementation of their guidelines, several centres reported increases in their incidences of major complications, symptomatic DVT, PE, wound problems and re-operation rates, post THA (42).
These reports led to the development of separate guidelines by the American Academy of Orthopaedic Surgeons taskforce in 2006. This group shows prevention of symptomatic PE as

opposed to reduction of prevalence of DVT as their end-point. Their guidelines have been considered to be much more relevant, and safer, for orthopaedic patients.
This issue is still unresolved in both regions and continues to elicit debate.

16. Conclusion

In summary, total hip arthroplasty is a highly successful procedure in decreasing pain and improving activity across all age groups, genders and geographic regions. Patient expectations and demands have increase since the advent of the first generation THA but technological advancement is constantly trying to meet this demand. However, there will continue to be controversies regarding the 'ideal' prosthesis, bearing surface and method of fixation. Such controversies may encourage further technical and technological innovations as well as an improved understanding of peri-operative issues such as the optimal method of VTE prophylaxis.
Overall, THA will continue to be a highly successful procedure.

17. References

[1] Learmonth ID, Young C, Rorabeck C. The operation of the century: total hip replacement. Lancet. 2007 Oct 27; 370(9597):1508-19.
[2] Henrik Malchau, Peter Herberts, Thomas Eisler, Göran Garellick and Peter Söderman. The Swedish total hip replacement register. J Bone Joint Surg Am. 2002; 84:2-20.
[3] Blomfeldt R, Törnkvist H, Eriksson K, Söderqvist A, Ponzer S, Tidermark J. A randomised controlled trial comparing bipolar hemiarthroplasty with total hip replacement for displaced intracapsular fractures of the femoral neck in elderly patients. J Bone Joint Surg Br. 2007 Feb; 89(2):160-5.
[4] Keating JF, Grant A, Masson M, Scott NW, Forbes JF. Randomized comparison of reduction and fixation, bipolar hemiarthroplasty, and total hip arthroplasty. Treatment of displaced intracapsular hip fractures in healthy older patients. J Bone Joint Surg Am. 2006 Feb; 88(2):249-60.
[5] Mancuso CA, Jout J, Salvati EA , Sculco TP. Fulfilment of patient's expectation for total hip arthroplasty. J Bone Joint Surg Am. 2009; 91:2073-2078
[6] Hardinge K. The direct lateral approach to the hip. J Bone Joint Surg Br. 1982; 64(1):17-9
[7] SMITH-PETERSEN MN. Approach to and exposure of the hip joint for mold arthroplasty. J Bone Joint Surg Am. 1949 Jan; 31A (1):40-6.
[8] Hoppenfeld S, de Boer P. Surgical Exposures in Orthopaedics: The Anatomical Approach. 3rd Ed. Philadelphia, PA: Lippincott, Williams and Wilkins; 2003.
[9] http://www-new.njrcentre.org.uk/njrcentre/Default.aspx
[10] http://www.jru.orthop.gu.se/
[11] Mallory TH, Lombardi AV Jr, Fada RA, Herrington SM, Eberle RW. Dislocation after total hip arthroplasty using the anterolateral abductor split approach. Clin Orthop Relat Res. 1999 Jan; (358):166-72.
[12] Ritter MA, Harty LD, Keating ME, Faris PM, Meding JB. A clinical comparison of the anterolateral and posterolateral approaches to the hip. Clin Orthop Relat Res. 2001 Apr; (385): 95-9.

[13] Suh KT, Roh HL, Moon KP, Shin JK, Lee JS.Posterior approach with posterior soft tissue repair in revision total hip arthroplasty. J Arthroplasty. 2008 Dec; 23 (8):1197-203. Epub 2008 Mar 4.
[14] Masonis JL, Bourne RB. Surgical approach, abductor function, and total hip arthroplasty dislocation. Clin Orthop Relat Res. 2002 Dec;(405):46-53.
[15] Unwin AJ, Thomas M. Dislocation after hemiarthroplasty of the hip: a comparison of the dislocation rate after posterior and lateral approaches to the hip. Ann R Coll Surg Engl. 1994 Sep;76(5):327-9.
[16] R K Wilson; B Mohan; and D E Beverland. REPAIR OF THE SHORT EXTERNAL ROTATORS FOLLOWING POSTERIOR APPROACH TO TOTAL HIP REPLACEMENT AND ITS EFFECT ON DISLOCATION RATE. Journal of Bone and Joint Surgery - British Volume, Vol 87-B, Issue SUPP_III, 268.
[17] Kwon MS, Kuskowski M, Mulhall KJ, Macaulay W, Brown TE, Saleh KJ.Does surgical approach affect total hip arthroplasty dislocation rates? Clin Orthop Relat Res. 2006 Jun;447:34-8.
[18] Suh KT, Park BG, Choi YJ. A posterior approach to primary total hip arthroplasty with soft tissue repair. Clin Orthop Relat Res. 2004 Jan;(418):162-7.
[19] Van Stralen GM, Struben PJ, van Loon CJ. The incidence of dislocation after primary total hip arthroplasty using posterior approach with posterior soft-tissue repair. Arch Orthop Trauma Surg. 2003 Jun;123(5):219-22. Epub 2003 Apr 9.
[20] Dorr LD, Maheshwari AV, Long WT, Wan Z, Sirianni LE. Early pain relief and function after posterior minimally invasive and conventional total hip arthroplasty. A prospective, randomized, blinded study. J Bone Joint Surg Am. 2007 Jun;89(6):1153-60.
[21] Goosen JH, Kollen BJ, Castelein RM, Kuipers BM, Verheyen CC. Minimally invasive versus classic procedures in total hip arthroplasty: a double-blind randomized controlled trial. Clin Orthop Relat Res. 2011 Jan;469(1):200-8. Epub 2010 Mar 30.
[22] Pagnano MW, Trousdale RT, Meneghini RM, Hanssen AD. Slower recovery after two-incision than mini-posterior-incision total hip arthroplasty. Surgical technique. J Bone Joint Surg Am. 2009 Mar 1;91 Suppl 2 Pt 1:50-73.
[23] Reininga IH, Zijlstra W, Wagenmakers R, Boerboom AL, Huijbers BP, Groothoff JW, Bulstra SK, Stevens M. Minimally invasive and computer-navigated total hip arthroplasty: a qualitative and systematic review of the literature. BMC Musculoskelet Disord. 2010 May 17;11:92.
[24] Smith TO, Blake V, Hing CB. Minimally invasive versus conventional exposure for total hip arthroplasty: a systematic review and meta-analysis of clinical and radiological outcomes. Int Orthop. 2011 Feb;35(2):173-84. Epub 2010 Jun 18.
[25] Minakawa H, Stone MH, Wroblewski BM, et al. Quantification of third-body damage and its effect on UHMWPE wear with different types of femoral head. JBJS Br1998; 80-B: 894-9.
[26] YH Zhu, KY Chiu and WM Tang. Review Article: Polyethylene wear and osteolysis in total hip arthroplasty. Journal of Orthopaedic Surgery. Vol. 9 No. 1, June 200, 91-99.
[27] Michael H. Huo, Javad Parvizi, Nathan F. Gilbert. What's new in hip arthroplasty? J Bone Joint Surg Am. 2006; 88:2100-2113

[28] Schmalzried TP, Peters PC, Maurer BT, Bragdon CR, Harris WH. Long-duration metal-on-metal total hip arthroplasties with low wear of the articulating surfaces. J Arthroplasty 1996; 11:322-31.
[29] Ollivere B, Darrah C, Barker T, Nolan J, Porteous MJ. Early clinical failure of the Birmingham metal-on-metal hip resurfacing is associated with metallosis and soft tissue necrosis. J Bone Joint Surg *[Br]* 2009; 91-B: 1025-30.
[30] William J. Maloney National Joint Replacement Registries: Has the Time Come? J Bone Joint Surg Am. 2001; 83:1582-1585.
[31] KR Schulte, JJ Callaghan, SS Kelley and RC Johnston. The outcome of Charnley total hip arthroplasty with cement after a minimum twenty-year follow-up. The results of one surgeon. J Bone Joint Surg Am. 1993; 75:961-975.
[32] Kim YH, Kim JS, Yoon SH. Long-term survivorship of the Charnley Elite Plus femoral component in young patients. J Bone Joint Surg [Br] 2007; 89-B: 449-54.
[33] N. C. Carrington, R. J. Sierra, G. A. Gie, M. J. W. Hubble, A. J. Timperley, J. R. Howell. The Exeter Universal cemented femoral component at 15 to 17 years, an update of the first 325 hips. J Bone Joint Surg *[Br]* 2009; 91-B: 730-7.
[34] Singh S, Trikha SP, Edge AJ. Hydroxyapatite ceramic-coated femoral stems in young patients, a prospective 10 year study. J Bone Joint Surg [Br] 2004; 86-B: 1118-23.
[35] Hallan G, Lie SA, Furnes O, Engesaeter LB, Vollset SE, Havelin LI. Medium- and long-term performance of 11 516 uncemented primary femoral stems from the Norwegian arthroplasty register. J Bone Joint Surg [Br] 2007;89-B:1574-80.
[36] Gillespie W, Murray D, Gregg PJ, Warwick D. Risks and benefits of prophylaxis against venous thromboembolism in orthopaedic surgery. J Bone Joint Surg Br. 2000 May;82(4):475-9.
[37] Murray DW, Britton AR, Bulstrode CJ. Thromboprophylaxis and death after total hip replacement. J Bone Joint Surg Br. 1996 Nov;78(6):863-70.
[38] . Freedman KB, Brookenthal KR, Fitzgerald RH Jr, Williams S, Lonner JH. Ameta-analysis of thromboembolic prophylaxis following elective total hip arthroplasty. J Bone Joint Surg Am. 2000 Jul;82-A(7):929-38.
[39] Beksaç B, González Della Valle A, Anderson J, Sharrock NE, Sculco TP, Salvato EA. Symptomatic thromboembolism after one-stage bilateral THA with a multimodal prophylaxis protocol. Clin Orthop Relat Res. 2007 Oct;463:114-9.
[40] Sharrock NE, Gonzalez Della Valle A, Go G, Lyman S, Salvati EA. Potent anticoagulants are associated with a higher all-cause mortality rate after hip and knee arthroplasty. Clin Orthop Relat Res. 2008 Mar;466(3):714-21.
[41] Jameson SS, Bottle A, Malviya A, Muller SD, Reed MR. The impact of national guidelines for the prophylaxis of venous thromboembolism on the complications of arthroplasty of the lower limb. J Bone Joint Surg Br. 2010 Jan;92(1):123-9
[42] Burnett RS, Clohisy JC, Wright RW, McDonald DJ, Shively RA, Givens SA, Barrack RL. Failure of the American College of Chest Physicians-1A protocol for lovenox in clinical outcomes for thromboembolic prophylaxis. J Arthroplasty. 2007 Apr; 22(3):317-24.

3

Hip Fracture in the Elderly: Partial or Total Arthroplasty?

Samo K. Fokter[1] and Nina Fokter[2]
[1]Celje General and Teaching Hospital
[2]Maribor University Clinical Centre
Slovenia

1. Introduction

The growing number of femoral neck fractures will have a large impact on health economics of developed countries in the coming decades. Great numbers of patients are already hospitalised yearly due to femoral neck fractures. These numbers are expected to augment importantly in the future years as the life expectancy and osteoporosis incidence increase in the ageing population. In the past, conservation of femoral head was supposed to be the ideal treatment for dislocated femoral neck fractures. However, conservation of femoral head with internal fixation has shown a high incidence of aseptic necrosis and non-union. Therefore, this treatment is now mostly applied to younger patients without osteoporosis and arthritis. In this chapter we review the topic of management of displaced femoral neck fractures in the elderly from a historical, surgical, and economical perspective. The emphasis is placed on the treatment rationale, surgical technique, and long-term clinical results. The authors' preferred choice of treatment of these sometimes difficult cases is also presented and illustrated.

2. Internal fixation or arthroplasty?

Therapeutic approaches for treatment of elderly patients with dislocated femoral neck fractures (Garden III-IV) include internal fixation of bone fragments, hemiarthroplasty or total hip arthroplasty (THA), and there is still no consensus about the optimal treatment. In a large multicentre prospective randomised study Rogmark et al. compared the results of internal fixation and hip arthroplasty in patients older than 70 years with a 2-year follow-up (Rogmark et al., 2002). They found 43% of treatment failures in the internal fixation group and only 6% of treatment failures in the arthroplasty group.
Bhandari et al. performed a meta-analysis of 14 prospective randomised studies comparing internal fixation with arthroplasty and discovered that 17% of patients could have been spared a revision surgery had they been treated with arthroplasty instead of internal fixation (Bhandari et al., 2003). Similar findings were described by Keating et al. in a study of patients older than 60 years with femoral neck fracture (Keating et al., 2006). At 2-year follow-up, 39% of the patients treated with internal fixation needed a secondary surgical procedure, whereas secondary surgery was required only in 5% of the patients treated with hemiarthroplasty and in 9% of the patients treated with THA. The complication rate can

certainly be lowered by fast diagnostic procedures and a shorter time in bed waiting for the surgery. Internal fixation with femoral head preservation should be performed in the first 6 hours after the injury or only exceptionally in the first 24 hours. In older injuries hip arthroplasty should be performed (Sendtner et al., 2010). The bone healing potential is especially low in older patients (Figure 1).

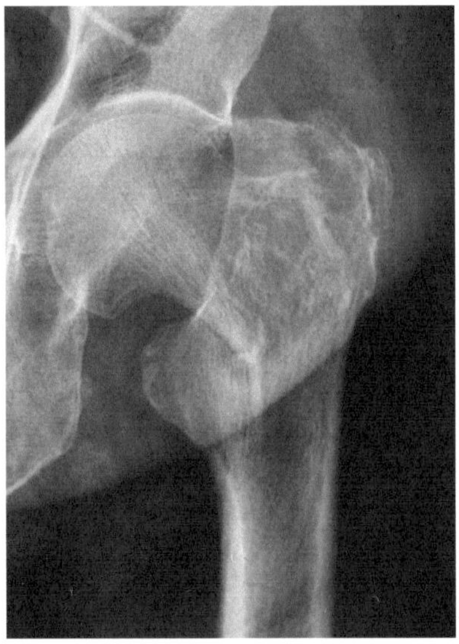

Fig. 1A. Proximal femoral fracture in a 74-year old female osteoporotic patient.

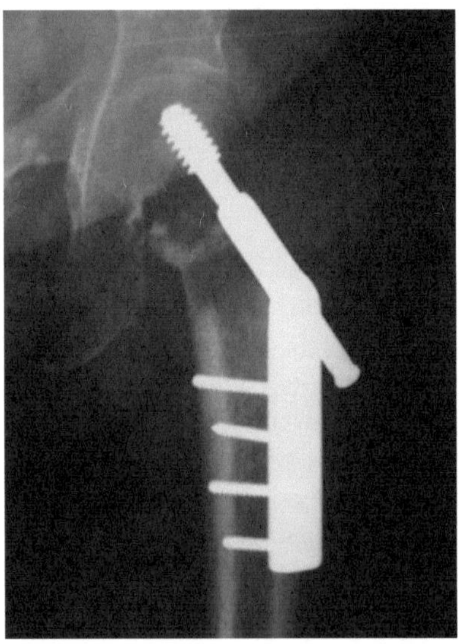

Fig. 1B. No signs of bony healing 6 months after open reduction and internal fixation with a dynamic hip screw (DHS) device. The patient is unable to walk.

In case we do not decide for preservation of the femoral head the remaining treatment options are unipolar hemiarthroplasty, bipolar hemiarthroplasty and THA.

3. Hemiarthroplasty

While hemiarthroplasty avoids the known risks of internal fixation, it brings other risks of its own: infection, stem loosening, dislocation, and groin pain as an effect of acetabular protrusion (Figure 2) or cartilage erosion (the so-called endoprosthetic arthritis).

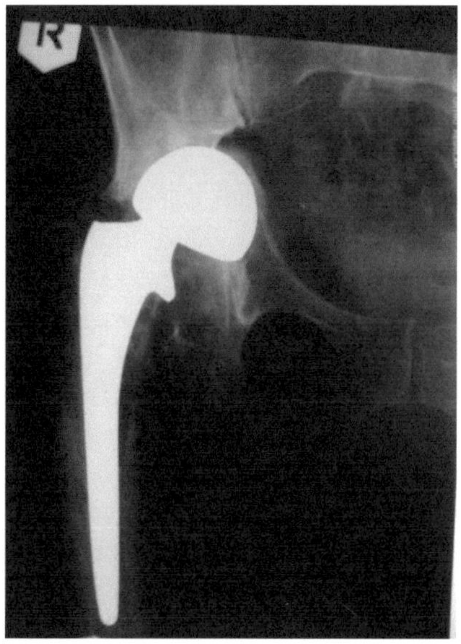

Fig. 2A. Acetabular fracture in a 64-year old patient 5 years after bipolar hemiarthroplasty for right femoral neck fracture.

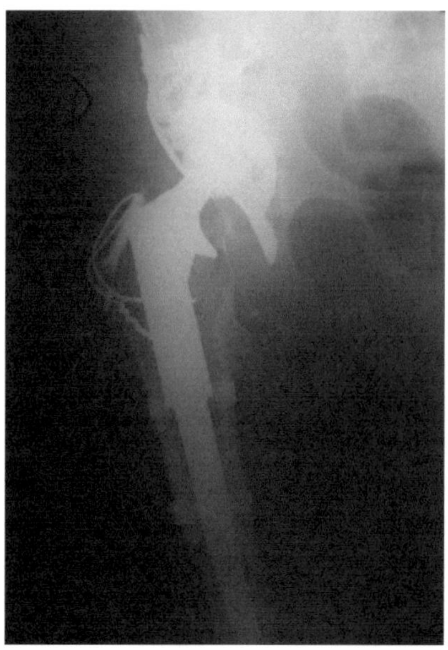

Fig. 2B. The same patient after revision total hip arthroplasty with insertion of a Bursch-Schneider acetabular supportive ring.

Unipolar hemiarthroplasty has been in use for more than half a century. The short-term results of this treatment are usually good, with rare infections and dislocations. However, the rates of mid- and long-term complications (5 to >20 years postoperatively) are high due to acetabular cartilage erosion. The cartilage defect causes pain and is the main reason for conversion to THA. Kofoed and Kofod found that as much as 55% of patients living alone needed conversion to THA two years after unipolar arthroplasty for femoral neck fracture (Kofoed & Kofod, 1983). The factors accelerating acetabular cartilage erosion are young age, high activity level and the length of follow-up (Macaulay et al., 2006).

The aim of introducing bipolar hemiarthroplasty in the 1970s was to prevent the development of endoprosthetic arthritis. Some motion is carried out among the components of the prosthesis, which theoretically diminishes acetabular wear. However, the functional importance of the prosthesis-prosthesis motion remains unclear. In a prospective randomised study of 115 patients over the age of 65 years with dislocated femoral neck fracture treated with either unipolar or bipolar hemiarthroplasty, Raija et al. found no statistical difference between the groups in quality of life and functional outcome at one year follow-up (Raija et al., 2003). Cornell et al. compared the results of treatment of 47 patients with an average age of 77 years. They noted better hip rotation and abduction and higher walking speed in the group treated with bipolar hemiarthroplasty compared to the group treated with unipolar hemiarthroplasty. On the other hand, they found no statistical difference in postoperative complication rates, lengths of hospitalisation and functional outcomes between the two groups (Cornell et al., 1998). Similar conclusions were reached by Parker and Gurusamy who compared the results of prospective randomised trials including a total of 857 patients (Parker & Gurusamy, 2004). The research showed an absence of significant differences between unipolar and bipolar hemiarthroplasty concerning hip dislocation, acetabular cartilage erosion, infection, reoperation rate and deep vein thrombosis at an average follow-up of 2 years.

Unipolar hemiarthroplasty is generally recommended for elderly, less active patients with a shorter life expectancy. These are the patients with the least benefit from the potential advantages of the more expensive bipolar hemiarthroplasty. Some authors advise against bipolar hemiarthroplasty in the elderly because of its higher price, long-term complications due to polyethylene wear, and higher rates of hip dislocations requiring an open reposition (Giliberty, 1983).

4. Total hip arthroplasty

In the past, THA was used in elderly patients with femoral neck fractures only in cases of coexisting acetabular disease. In 2004 Healy and Iorio proved that elderly patients treated with THA for displaced femoral neck fractures achieved a more independent living, a longer interval to reoperation or death, and better cost effectiveness than patients treated with internal fixation or hemiarthroplasty (Healy & Iorio, 2004).

Older studies have reported a higher incidence of hip dislocations after THA for femoral neck fractures compared to elective THA for acetabular cartilage disease. The reason for the higher dislocation rate was supposed to be the greater range of motion in patients with a fractured femoral neck. However, more recent studies have not confirmed the supposed differences concerning perioperative morbidity, functional outcome, and radiological signs of loosening (Abboud et al., 2004). Enocson et al. nevertheless recommended a careful choice of surgical approach in order to minimise the risk of dislocation (Enocson et al., 2009). In a prospective cohort study including 698 patients treated with THA for displaced femoral neck fracture or its complications, the least dislocations were noted in the anterolateral approach group (2%), while the dislocation rate in the posterolateral approach group was six times higher (13%). An additional reduction of dislocation risk in THA inserted via posterior approach can be achieved with the use of cemented dual articulation acetabular component (Tarasevicius et al., 2010).

Longer-term results of THA for femoral neck fracture were published by Lee et al. (Lee et al., 1998). They reported on treatment of 126 patients with an average age of 75 years and a 9-year follow-up. 10% of the patients had one or more postoperative dislocations, but 99% had mild or no pain and 69% reached their preoperative level of function or better. The study showed a higher complication rate in THA than is usual for hemiarthroplasty, but on the other hand revealed good clinical results and long-term prosthesis survival.

Total hip arthroplasty is a durable treatment option for femoral neck fractures in the elderly and gives a good functional outcome, but comes with the price of a higher complication rate, such as dislocation or postoperative delirium (Gallo et al., 2010). Surgical technique adapted to osteoporotic bone and careful implant selection regarding fixation influence the success of treatment for femoral neck fractures (Figure 3). The risk of dislocation depends on the surgical approach, the reconstruction of hip biomechanics, the head size and offset, the quality of capsular closure, and the experience of the surgeon (Ames et al., 2010; Leighton et al., 2007; Rutz et al., 2010).

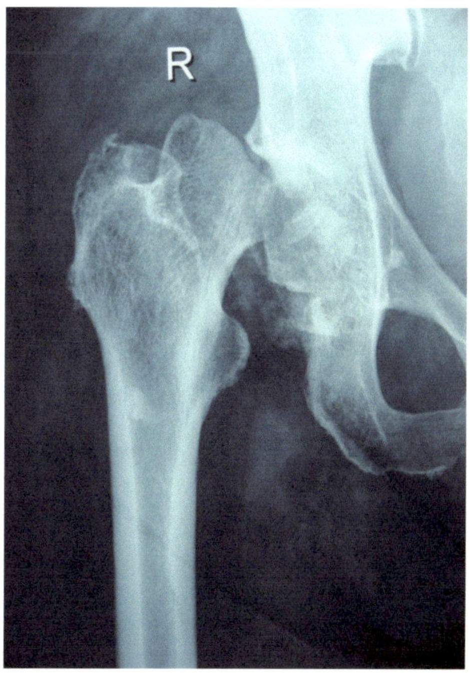

Fig. 3A. Subcapital fracture in a 71-year old female patient with osteoporosis.

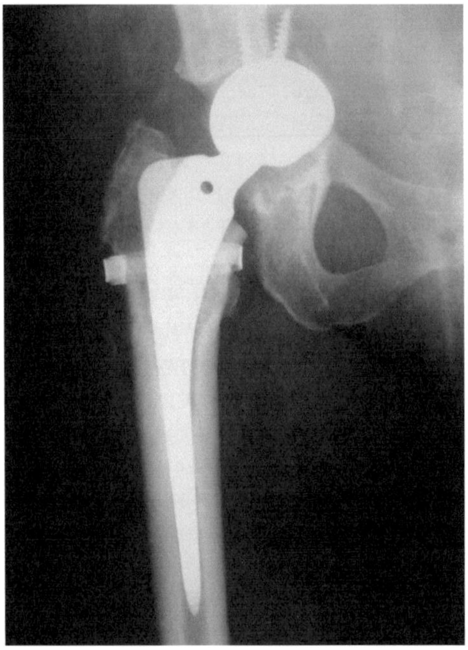

Fig. 3B. Acetabular fracture and intrapelvic cup (press-fit type) migration noted 6 weeks after primary uncemented THA in the same patient. Note that intraoperative femoral shaft fracture also occurred and was treated with a cerclage belt.

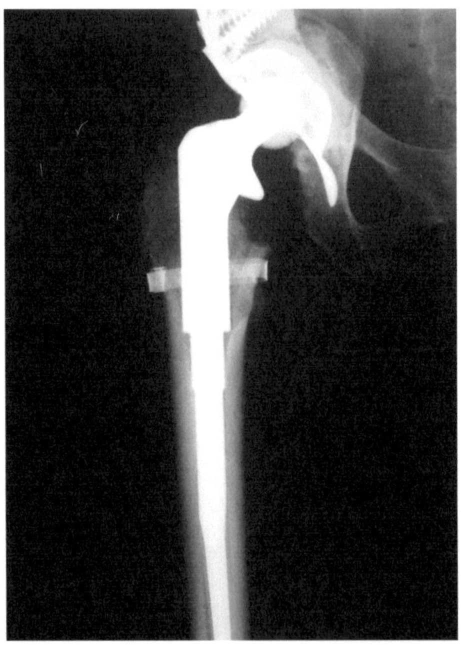

Fig. 3C. The same patient after revision THA with modular femoral stem and a Bursch-Schneider acetabular supportive ring.

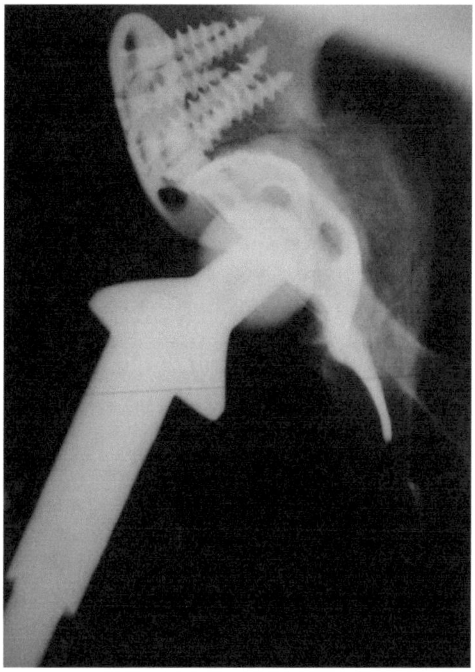

Fig. 3D. The same patient after revision THA on lateral radiograph. Note massive autologous bone grafts under the Bursch-Schneider ring.

5. Cemented or cementless hip arthroplasty?

There is still a lively ongoing debate in the orthopaedic community as to which method of fixation of the implant is superior to the other. Although the development of total hip replacement began with cementless THA in the late fifties, cemented THA has been more popular after Charnley's systematic promotion of low friction arthroplasty, which included fixation with bone cement (Charnley, 1961). Nevertheless, cementless THA rapidly gained acceptance during the 1980s when materials that allowed bone ingrowth became available. A meta-analysis comparing the survival rate of cemented and cementless THA reported that cemented THA was slightly superior (Morsched et al., 2007). However, the difference between the groups was no longer significant when revision surgery of the cup or the stem was regarded as treatment failure. At present, it is not possible to ascertain the superiority of any of the two options. In the authors' institutions, cemented type of fixation is used in the majority of fracture cases.

Figved et al. recently raised the question whether a specific type of fixation should be used for the treatment of displaced femoral neck fractures (Figved et al., 2009). In the randomized, controlled trial in patients 70 years and older comparing a cemented implant with hydroxyapatite-coated uncemented implant, both with a bipolar head, the mean Harris hip score showed equivalence between the groups after 3 months and 12 months. The complication and mortality rates were similar in both groups. However, the duration of surgery was 12.4 minutes shorter and the mean intraoperative blood loss was 89 mL less in the cementless group.

6. Hemiarthroplasty or total hip arthroplasty?

Rogmark et al. tried to evaluate which patients to treat with THA and which with hemiarthroplasty in the course of surgical treatment of femoral neck fractures (Rogmark et al., 2002). In the multicentre prospective randomised trial comparing internal fixation to arthroplasty, they divided the arthroplasty group to hemiarthroplasty and THA according to the scoring system for patients with femoral neck fracture (Table 1). Patients with a score of 15 or more were treated with THA and the others with hemiarthroplasty. The scoring system favoured THA in younger (age 70-80 years), alert patients who were capable of independent walking before the injury. The authors noted no significant difference between the THA and hemiarthroplasty groups. The overall dislocation rate was 8%. They concluded that the good functional outcome and the relatively low incidence of dislocations proved the value of their scoring system for choosing the appropriate patients for each treatment option.

Patient Variables	Points*
Age	
70 to 80 years	5
> 80 years	2
Habitat	
Own home	5
Sheltered home	2
Walking aids	
One cane or none	5
Canes, walking frame	2
Mental status	
Alert	5
Slight confusion	2

*A total score ≥15 points indicates treatment required with total hip arthroplasty.

Table 1. Rogmark preoperative scoring system for patients with femoral neck fractures (Rogmark et al., 2002).

Hopley et al. recently published a systematic review comparing THA with hemiarthroplasty considering reoperation rates, mortality, complications, functional outcome and quality of life (Hopley et al., 2010). They identified 3821 references, inspected 202 papers and included 15 papers with a total of 1890 patients. The meta-analysis showed that THA carried a lower risk of reoperation than hemiarthroplasty. THA also showed better ratings in the Harris hip score than hemiarthroplasty. However, the rates of dislocation (relative risk 1.48; 95% confidence interval 0.89 to 2.46) and general complications (relative risk 1.14, 95% confidence interval 0.87 to 1.48) were slightly higher for THA.

Arthroplasty is thus indicated in most patients over the age of 65 years with femoral neck fractures. Hemiarthroplasty is indicated in institutionalised patients and patients with comorbidities who are not expected to live longer than 6 or 7 years. Studies show a high reoperation rate in patients living longer than 6 to 7 years after hemiarthroplasty. THA is indicated in active patients with little or no comorbidities as it represents the most successful treatment in terms of pain relief and is also cost effective (Kyle, 2010). Recent advances in the materials and technology of THA components allowing the use of larger femoral heads, as well as better surgical techniques have made THA safer and less prone to dislocation and other mechanical complications. Economical analyses demonstrate that due to the costs of complications THA is more cost effective than internal fixation or hemiarthroplasty in patients surviving 2 years or longer after their initial femoral neck fracture. An increasing number of authors therefore believe that THA should be granted a larger role in the treatment of displaced femoral neck fractures than it has had in the past (Schmidt et al., 2009).

7. Cost

We live in a time of global recession and information about the cost of treatment is unfortunately not unimportant. Iorio et al. calculated the costs of treatment of femoral neck fractures in the elderly during a 2-year postoperative period (Iorio et al., 2001). Surgical treatment methods included reduction with internal fixation, unipolar hemiarthroplasty, bipolar hemiarthroplasty, and THA. The analysis included the costs of hospitalisation, rehabilitation, and probability-adjusted costs of revision. The calculated total cost of cemented THA was 20,670 US dollars, hybrid THA 21,066 US dollars, bipolar hemiarthroplasty 22,043 US dollars, unipolar hemiarthroplasty 21,597 US dollars, and internal fixation 24,606 US dollars. The authors concluded that taking into account complication rates, mortality, revision surgeries and functional outcome, THA is the most cost effective treatment option for femoral neck fractures in the elderly.
The current costs of treatment for femoral neck fractures in the elderly in Northern Europe have been analysed by Frihagen et al. (Frihagen et al., 2010). They randomised 222 patients with an average age of 83 years to internal fixation or hemiarthroplasty. The patients were followed for 2 years. The analysis included costs of hospitalisation, rehabilitation, community-based care, and nursing home use. Primary hospital treatment was less expensive in the group treated with internal fixation (9,044 euros) than in the hemiarthroplasty group (11,887 euros). The relation changed when they included all hospital costs (rehabilitation, revision surgeries, formal and informal contact with the hospital): 21,709 euros for internal fixation and 19,976 euros for hemiarthroplasty. When all costs of the 2-year treatment were included (with community-based care and nursing home), internal fixation was much more expensive (47,186 euros) than hemiarthroplasty (38,615 euros).

8. Summary

Strong evidence exists in favour of primary arthroplasty over internal fixation for displaced femoral neck fractures in the elderly. Hemiarthroplasty is indicated for institutionalised patients, and patients with comorbidities who are not expected to live longer than a few years. THA is definitely indicated for patients with concurrent degenerative or rheumatic arthritis. Besides, evidence is accumulating that THA may be more effective than hemiarthroplasty in terms of pain relief and functional outcome in younger, more active patients with intact acetabulum and longer life expectancy. Regarding costs to the society, hemiarthroplasty is more favourable than internal fixation on the short term, and THA is more favourable than hemiarthroplasty on the medium term. Considering the growing life expectancy, primary THA should be chosen more often for the treatment of displaced femoral neck fractures even in the elderly.

9. References

Abboud, J. A., Patel, R. V., Booth Jr, R. E. & Nasarian, D. G. (2004). Outcomes of total hip arthroplasty are similar for patients with displaced femoral neck fractures and osteoarthritis. *Clinical Orthopaedics and Related Research*, Vol.421, No.4, (April 2004), pp. 151-154

Ames, J. B., Lurie, J. D., Tomek, I. M., Zhou, W. & Koval, K. J. (2010) Does surgeon volume for total hip arthroplasty affect outcomes after hemiarthroplasty for femoral neck fracture? *The American Journal of Orthopedics (Belle Mead),* Vol.39, No.8, (August 2010), pp. E84-89

Bhandari, M., Devereaux, P. J., Swiontkowski, M. F., Tornetta 3rd, P., Obremskey, W., Koval, K. J., Nork, S., Sprague, S., Schemitsch, E. H. & Guyatt, G. H. (2003) Internal fixation compared with arthroplasty for displaced fractures of the femoral neck: A meta-analysis. *Journal of Bone and Joint Surgery, American Volume,* Vol.85, No.9, (September 2003), pp. 1673-1681

Charnley, J. (1961) Arthroplasty of the hip: A new operation. *Lancet,* Vol.277, No.7187, (May 1961), pp. 1129-1132

Cornell, C. N., Levine, D., O'Doherty, J. & Lyden, J. (1998) Unipolar versus bipolar hemiarthroplasty for the treatment of femoral neck fractures in the elderly. *Clinical Orthopaedics and Related Research,* Vol.348, No.3, (March 1998), pp. 67-71

Enocson, A., Hedbeck, C. J., Tidermark, J., Pettersson, H., Ponzer, S. & Lapidus, L. J. (2009) Dislocation of total hip replacement in patients with fractures of the femoral neck: A prospective cohort study of 713 consecutive hips. *Acta Ortopaedica,* Vol.80, No.2, (April 2009), pp. 184-189, ISSN 1745-3674

Figved, W., Opland, V., Frihagen, F., Jervidalo, T., Madsen, J. E. & Nordsletten, L. (2009) Cemented versus uncemented hemiarthroplasty for displaced femoral neck fractures. *Clinical Orthopaedics and Related Research,* Vol.467, No.9, (September 2009), pp. 2426-2435

Frihagen, F., Waaler, G. M., Madsen, J. E., Nordsletten, L., Aspaas, S. & Aas, E. (2010) The cost of hemiarthroplasty to that of internal fixation for femoral neck fractures. *Acta Orthopaedica,* Vol.81, No.4, (August 2010), pp. 446-452

Gallo, J., Cechova, I. & Zapletalova, J. (2010) Early complications associated with total hip arthroplasty due to femoral neck fracture. *Acta Chirurgiae Orthopaedicae et Traumatologiae Cechoslovaca,* Vol.77, No.5, (October 2010), pp. 389-394

Giliberty, R. P. (1983) Hemiarthroplasty of the hip using low-friction bipolar endoprosthesis. *Clinical Orthopaedics and Related Research,* Vol.175, No.5, (May 1983), pp. 86-92

Healy, W. L. & Iorio, R. (2004) Total hip arthroplasty: Optimal treatment for displaced femoral neck fractures in elderly patients. *Clinical Orthopaedics and Related Research,* Vol.429, No.12, (December 2004), pp. 43-48

Hopley, C., Stengel, D., Ekkernkamp, A. & Wich, M. (2010) Primary total hip arthroplasty versus hemiarthroplasty for displaced intracapsular hip fractures in older patients: Systematic review. *British Medical Journal,* No.340, (June 2010), c2332

Iorio, R., Healy, W. L., Lemos, D. W., Appleby, D., Luzzhesi, C. A. & Saleh, K. J. (2001) Displaced femoral neck fractures in the elderly: Outcomes and cost effectiveness. *Clinical Orthopaedics and Related Research,* Vol.383, No.2, (February 2001), pp. 229-242

Keating, J. F., Grant, A., Masson, M., Scott, N. W. & Forbes, J. F. (2006) Randomized comparison of reduction and fixation, bipolar hemiarthroplasty, and total hip arthroplasty: Treatment of displaced intracapsular hip fractures in healthy older patients. *Journal of Bone and Joint Surgery, American Volume,* Vol.88, No.2, (February 2006), pp. 249-60

Kofoed, H. & Kofod, J. (1983) Moore prosthesis in the treatment of fresh femoral neck fractures: A critical review with special attention to secondary acetabular degeneration. *Injury,* Vol.14, No.6, (May 1983), pp. 531-540

Kyle, R. F. (2010) Subcapital fractures: In the bucket or on top of the neck? *Orthopedics,* Vol.33, No.9, (September 2010), p.644

Lee, B. P., Berry, D. J., Harmsen, W. S. & Sim, F. H. (1998) Total hip arthroplasty for the treatment of an acute fracture of the femoral neck: Long-term results. *Journal of Bone and Joint Surgery, American Volume,* Vol.80, No.1, (January 1998), pp. 70-75

Leighton, R. K., Schmidt, A. H., Collier, P. & Trask, K. (2007) Advances in the treatment of intracapsular hip fractures in the elderly. *Injury,* Vol.38, No.S3, (September 2007), pp.S24-S34

Macaulay, W., Pagnotto, M. R., Iorio, R., Mont, M. A. & Saleh, K. J. (2006) Displaced femoral neck fractures in the elderly: hemiarthroplasty versus total hip arthroplasty. *Journal of the American Academy of Orthopaedic Surgeons,* Vol.14, No.5, (May 2006), pp. 287-293

Morsched, S., Bozic, K. J., Ries, M. D., Malchau, H. & Colford Jr., J. M. (2007) Comparison of cemented and uncemented fixation in total hip replacement: a meta-analysis. *Acta Orthopaedica,* Vol.78, No.3, (June 2007), pp. 315-326

Parker, M. J. & Gurusamy, K. (2004) Arthroplasties (with and without bone cement) for proximal femoral fractures in adults. *Cochrane Database of Systematic Reviews,* Vol.2, CD001706

Raia, F. J., Chapman, C. B., Herrera, M., Schweppe, M. W., Michelsen, C. B. & Rosenwasser, M. P. (2003) Unipolar or bipolar hemiarthroplasty for femoral neck fractures in the elderly? *Clinical Orthopaedics and Related Research,* Vol.414, No.9, (September 2003), pp. 259-265

Rogmark, C., Carlsson, A., Johnell, O. & Sernbo, I. (2002) A prospective randomised trial of internal fixation versus arthroplasty for displaced fractures of the neck of the femur: Functional outcomes for 450 patients at two years. *Journal of Bone and Joint Surgery, British Volume,* Vol.84, No.2, (March 2002), pp. 183-188

Rutz, E., Leumann, A., Rutz, D., Schaefer, D. & Walderrabano, W. (2010) Total hip arthroplasty for fractures of the proximal femur in older patients. *Hip International,* Vol.20, No.2, (April-June 2010), pp. 215-220

Schmidt, A. H., Leighton, R., Parvizi, J., Sems, A. & Berry, D. J. (2009) Optimal arthroplasty for femoral neck fractures: Is total hip arthroplasty the answer? *Journal of Orthopaedic Trauma,* Vol.23, No.6, (July 2009), pp. 428-433

Sendtner, E., Renkawitz, T., Kramny, P., Wenzl, M. & Grifka, J. (2010) Fractured neck of femur - internal fixation versus arthroplasty. *Deutsches Aerzteblatt International,* Vol.107, No.23, (June 2010), pp.401-407

Tarasevicius, S., Busevicius, M., Robertson, O. & Wingstrand, H. (2010) Dual mobility cup reduces dislocation rate after arthroplasty for femoral neck fracture. *BMC Musculoskeletal Disorders,* Vol.6, No.11, (August 2010), pp. 175-178

4

Why Minimally Invasive Surgery in Hip Arthroplasty?

Antonio Silvestre, Fernando Almeida, Pablo Renovell,
Raúl López, Laura Pino and Luis Puertes
School of Medicine Valencia/Hospital Clínico Valencia
Spain

1. Introduction

Hip replacement surgery is a successful procedure since its commencement. Special attention to minimally invasive access in hip reconstruction has been paid by orthopedic community, implant manufactures, mass media and patients for the last ten years. Nowadays though there is controversy about clinical effectiveness and cost-effectiveness of minimally invasive surgery (MIS) approaches (De Verteuil et al., 2008), many surgeons are using MIS for hip replacement. MIS means tissue sparing, gentle maneuvers, concern about muscles, sheaths, insertions, bone and of course the skin, in a word "preserve tissues". These techniques have supposed an effort for the surgeons to place hip prosthesis with the accuracy of standard reproducible approaches and with a similar rate of complications.

We went through the boom of minimally invasive prosthetic surgery in our Institution seven years ago. Encouraging results obtained by other authors drove us to cadaveric and laboratory training before using this technique in patients.

In the beginning we started with the mini-posterior approach as posterior access to the hip was the most commonly used in our Hospital. We thought benefits for the patients could be obtain from reducing surgical access in terms of accelerated rehabilitation program, analgesic control, blood loss, hospital stay and economic impact, without consequences in long-term results. Good outcomes shown in this paper strengthen our daily work. Four years later in an attempt to reduce posterior dislocation rate after hip prosthesis (around 4.5% in our media and up to 10% in some reports) according to our principle of "preserve tissues", we started using the direct anterior approach with a fracture table (AMIS) in order to perform a muscle sparing procedure that showed a lower posterior dislocation rate than the mini-posterior and standard posterior approaches.

This practice leads us to this restrospective paper that compares our results among these approaches.

2. Material and methods

We evaluated 199 hips (187 patients) which received reconstructive surgery in our Institution. Surgery was performed by three senior surgeons of our Hospital since May 2004 until December 2009. We selected only patients with analogous demographic data and surgeries done by these three senior physicians to homogenize results and implants. No hip fracture was

included in this series and diagnosis was primary osteoarthritis in 118 hips and secondary osteoarthritis due to osteonecrosis in 31 hips, rheumatoid arthritis in 26 hips, Perthes disease in 11 hips, mild hip dysplasia in 12 hips and pigmented villonodular synovitis in one hip. The exclusion criteria were severe DDH (different implants are needed) and history of previous surgery on the operated hip that affects functional recovery after hip surgery.
Patients were distributed in three groups according to the surgery performed. Group A included 92 patients (99 hips) who received hip prosthesis through a standard postero-lateral approach. Group B included 46 patients (49 hips) who were operated by a posterior mini invasive access and group C was formed by 49 patients (51 hips) who received a direct anterior approach with the help of a fracture table. Group B and C were performed by the two senior surgeons who got cadaver and laboratory training before clinical use of this technique in patients. Demographic data are shown in table 1.
Implants used in all cases were versafit cup CC and quadra system stem (cementless implants in 73 hips and hybrid hip in 11 hips) [Medacta® International SA; Italy] and bihapro cup and 3-V cementless system stem or PMB cemented system stem (cementless in 98 hips and hybrid in 17 cases) [Biomet; Warsaw, IN]. Bearing surfaces were choose depending on the age of the patients, as we prefer ceramic on ceramic bearing surface for young active patients (under 65 years of age) and metal or ceramic on PE for older people.

	GROUP A	GROUP B	GROUP C
Number of hips	99 (92 patients)	49 (46 patients)	51 (49 patients)
Age	66.19±10.99	66.32±11.72	65.19±13.19
Sex (M/F)	53/39	25/21	29/20
Body Weight (Kg)	81.5±1.7	76±1.9	77.2±1.2
Height (cm)	163.5±2.3	163.4±1.8	162.7±0.7
Body mass index (Kg/m²)	30.6±1.3	27.8±1.6	29.3±1.1
Preoperative diagnosis			
Osteoarthritis	60	28	32
Osteonecrosis	12	8	11
RA	14	6	4
Perthes	6	3	2
Hip displasia	7	4	1
Pigmented villonodular synovitis			1
Preoperative HSS	57.010 (SD 4.09)	57.959 (SD 6.26)	56.606 (SD 6.16)

Table 1. Demographic data of the patients

Institutional approval was obtained from the Hospital for the new techniques. Learning curve affected results in the beginning of the procedure and fluoroscopy was used during the beginning of these series to aid in implant position and anatomic referencing.
No great changes were adopted for the mini invasive posterior access, as patient position is similar to the conventional posterolateral approach. A more straight oblique and proximal incision was employed for the mini-posterior access. Specific devices designed for the different approaches were used in order to get proper placement of the implants. The cup was inserted in 40-45° abduction angle in the different groups but a bigger anteversion angle was applied to the acetabulum in the posterior approaches to avoid posterior dislocation of the hip. Femoral reaming, broaching and stem implantation were resumed in the mini-

posterior access as in conventional postero-lateral approach with the aid of some devices developed to bring up proximal femur into the incision.

Our operative technique for direct anterior approach (AMIS) was the same that described F. Laude (Laude, 2006). Patients were placed in supine position on an orthopaedic table with the foot of the operated leg secured in a traction device (Medacta®). The operation table was positioned in horizontal condition to the floor and the pelvis was checked to be set in neutral angle tilting angle. Towel pads were placed under the buttock to stabilize pelvic movement and to bring up proximal femur into the incision during flexion and adduction of the leg. The cup was inserted in 40-45° inclination angle by referring alignment rod to the interconnecting line of bilateral ASIS and 10° anteversion angle by referring the rod to the operation table. Controls by image intensifier were used during first cases to estimate inclination and anteversion angle. After cup placement, traction and gentle external rotation was applied to the operated leg. The supero-lateral capsule and the pubo-femoral ligament were released for appropriate femoral exposure and preparation. Femoral reaming, broaching and stem implantation were performed after verifying the direction of the femoral axis and anterior bow of the femur.

Full weight bearing was allowed from the second-third postoperative day depending on laboratory results and need of red cell transfusion, except in complicated cases. Walking with a walker or crutches was started from the second day after surgery. Patients were permitted to go up and down the stair using handrail from the fifth day after surgery. Using a cane or a walker was based on patient's ability. Physical theraphists instructed gait training and ambulation during patient's hospital stay. Patients left the hospital when they get sufficient hip function for their activity of daily living.

Operative time (skin incision to skin closure) and intraoperative and postoperative blood loss volume were evaluated as indices of operative invasion. Intraoperative blood loss volume was estimated by using the volume in the suction device adding up the weight of compresses used during surgery. Postoperative blood loss volume was measured by drain output postoperatively, which was removed 48 h after surgery. Laboratory tests were used to determine haemoglobin concentration and haematocrit (HCT) 36-48 h after surgery to get a more real scene of the patient's hemodynamic status.

Standard protocol during the time of this study for all the patients was low molecular-weight heparin for 28 days postoperatively. Elastic stocking was applied to both legs for intraoperative deep venous thrombosis until first outpatient visit. Ultrasound was obtained only in patients with symptoms of deep vein thrombosis. Cefazolin (Kefol®) two grams were given intravenously an hour before surgery, followed by 1 gr/8h for two days after surgery. Analgesic drugs were given during hospital stay but no morphic therapy was used in the immediate postoperatory.

Patients were assessed preoperatively and postoperatively at 6 weeks, 3 months and annually thereafter with clinical evaluation including gait, need for assistance devices, ROM and visual analog pain score. Standard radiographs of the operated hip were taken at 6 weeks, 3 months and at annual review. Radiological assessment was performed by measuring cup inclination, cup anteversion angle and positioning of cup within the safe zone of Lewinnek (Lewinnek et al., 1978). Stem alignment of varus or valgus positioning of less than 3° was considered neutral position on AP X-ray. Hip function was assessed clinically using the Harris Hip Score at 6 weeks, 3 months, and annually. Data are collected pre and postoperatively from patient questionnaires and from an independent senior orthopaedic surgeon (R.L.) assessment at each visit. All known complications were captured and collected for descriptive study.

Differences in laboratory levels, drain output measures, length of hospital stay, visual analog pain score and gait parameters between groups were examined using an unpaired Student's t-test with the aid of SPS-15. The significance level was set at $P<.05$ for all analysis.

3. Results

Three groups were established depend on the access employed to the hip joint. Underlying diagnosis was ortheoarthritis and osteonecrosis in 74.87% of cases.
Mean operative time was longer in first cases after introduction of the new techniques (mini posterior and AMIS) due to our learning curve, but this rate returns to equivalent operative time value as the standard postero-lateral approach after our fifteen surgeries. Hip access has no significant difference in surgery time [P= 0.44]. The average blood loss during the surgery was 162.4±57.7 ml for group A, 149.4±57.3 ml for group B and 141.5±54.2 ml for group C as meticulous hemostasis was applied in all cases and a sealer device was used in the last group. Measurement of blood loss in drain output shows a significant difference between group C and A [P=0.04] but no between group B and A. The overall risk of red cell transfusion was bigger in group A that in the rest of groups. Average length of the hospital stay that shows significant differences between minimally invasive procedures and standard access of the hip [P=0.023] could be explained by other facts as introduction of accelerate rehabilitation programmes linked to the new techniques. However, absence of skilled nursing or extended-care facilities affects patients discharge to home in our environment. Other indices of operative invasion, hip stability and walking ability are reported in table 2.
Five posterior hip dislocations were observed in group A and two in group B. No hip dislocation has been assessed in group C.
Analyzing hip recovery we checked that time required to single-leg stance for more than 5 seconds was 21.3 days in group A (range 12-76 days), 20.9 (range 10-75 days) and 17.1 days (range 5-75 days) in group C. There were no significant differences in the single-leg stance between anterior and posterior approaches. However this competence depends on patient's age, therapist's cooperation and previous functional status. Positive Trendelenburg's sign was identified in mostly all the patients before surgery, but at six weeks it was recognized in only 3.92 % of hips in group C. Negative Trendelenburg's sign was acquired in this group at 17.3 days (range 5-75 days). There were significant differences between anterior and posterior approaches [P=0.048].
In our series required time up to walking by two canes or a walker was 3.494±1.163 for group A, 2.571±0.912 for group B and 2.262±0.68 for group C. No significant differences have been found among the different approaches. Patients from group C were able to walk by a single cane more than 250 meters at 15.0 days (range 3-35 days) and fifty-six percent of these patients were capable to walk without the use of assistive walking aids at three weeks postoperatively. On the opposite patients from group A and B were able to walk by a single cane more than 250 meters at 19.4 days (range 5-41 days). There were significant differences between posterior and anterior access to the hip [P= 0.039] (table 3).
Harris hip score results are shown in table 2, but no significant differences were observed among the three groups. Visual analog pain score after surgery improved to 3.030±0.984 in group A, 2.489±0.71 in group B and 2.213±0.798 in group C. Significant differences were detected when comparing group C with the others groups [P<0.05] (table 3). Three patients (two in group A and one in group C) developed inguinal pain three months after surgery. An infiltration of the ileopectineus bursa resolved their symptoms.
Ninety-six cups (96.07%) had been implanted within the safe zone of the Lewinnek method in this series (Lewinnek et al., 1978). Less anteversion angle was applied to the cups in the

anterior approach to avoid anterior dislocation. On the other hand anteversion angle was bigger in group A and B (posterior access) to prevent from posterior dislocation of the hip. Stem alignment in anteroposterior radiograph was 178.56±0.97 in group A, 179.23±1.13 in group B and 179.85±1.94 in group C with no cases or varus o valgus position (more than 3° in the A-P X-ray).

	GROUP A	GROUP B	GROUP C
Operative time(minutes)	**79.25±18.90**	**84.61±16.47**	**87.24±30.51**
Blood loss (drain ouput)	**624.64±10.62 ml**	**595.91±13.21 ml**	**579.01±14.91**
Need transfusión	**22.77%**	**16.21%**	**14.75%**
Preoperative Hb	**13.45±1.32 g/dl**	**13.58±1.07 g/dl**	**13.38±1.39 g/dl**
Postoperative Hb	**8.89±0.69 g/dl**	**9.3±0.78 g/dl**	**9.76±1.16 g/dl**
Preoperative HTO	**39.35±3.64**	**39.61±3.13**	**39.06±4.14**
Postoperative HTO	**26.51±2.14**	**27.96±2.40**	**28.38±3.12**
Lenght of hospital stay after surgery	**7.35±2.04 days (84.8%)**	**6±1.81 days (83.6%)**	**4.78±1.23 days (83.6%)**
Presence of Trendelenburg's sign			
1 week	**87 hips (87.87%)**	**43 hips (87.75%)**	**41 hips (80.39%)**
3 weeks	**44 hips (44.44%)**	**21 hips (42.85%)**	**14 hips (27.65%)**
6 weeks	**13 hips (13.13%)**	**6 hips (12.24%)**	**2 hips (3.92%)**
Average time to single-leg stance > 5''	**21.3 days**	**20.9 days**	**17.1 days**
No assistive walking aids (3 weeks)	**47 hips (47.47%)**	**24 hips (48.97%)**	**29 hips (56.82%)**
HHS			
6 weeks	**72.61±3.23**	**73.74±3.23**	**79.27±7.45**
3 months	**83.82±4.20**	**84.91±4.96**	**88.08±6.09**
1 year	**90.74±6.16**	**91.15±6.04**	**91.34±6.07**

Table 2. Indices of operative invasion, hip stability and walking ability

Intraoperative and postoperative complications are shown in Table 4. Main surgical complications were observed in our learning curve (15 first cases) of the minimally invasive techniques as we think these are demanding procedures which require experience in hip surgery. Intraoperative complications were detected and settled during surgery. Proximal femoral perforations identified during broaching and reaming the femur in the AMIS procedure (group C) did not alter the procedure. Periprosthetic fractures were fixed with cerclage cable fixation and major throchanteric fractures require cerclage cable fixation in posterior approaches (group A and B) but no fixation was used in the anterior access (group C). A femoral shaft fracture was confirmed during preparation for the insertion of the stem in group C; enlarging of the exposure in zigzag way allowed us to reduce and fixed the fracture with a femoral plate with screws and cables. The case requiring acute revision was cup dislodgment checked with X-ray control that needed re-operation two days after first surgery.
Deep infections needed two-stage revision of the hips; the average interval between first-stage resection and reimplantation was 5.2 months. On the other hand superficial wound infections were resolved by superficial debridement and irrigation with wound closure. Lateral femoral cutaneous nerve paresthesias verified in group C improved six months after

surgery. The cases of clinically evident deep-vein thrombosis were treated with pharmacologycal therapy. A young patient of group C died two days after surgery due to a fatal embolism. All cases of length leg discrepancy were less than 1 cm and well tolerated by the patients, so we do not include as complications.

	Hb decrease	HTO decrease	Blood loss (drain output)	Lenght of hospital stay	Visual analog score	Walk by a single cane 250 m
Group B-A	P= 0.058	P= 0.2	P> 0.05	P= 0.02	P> 0.05	P> 0.05
Group C-A	P= 0.0001	P= 0.08	P= 0.04	P= 0.02	P=0.02	P= 0.03
Group C-B	P= 0.0001	P= 0.3	P= 0.33	P= 0.007	P= 0.008	P= 0.03

Table 3. Comparative of some results between groups (P values)

	Group A Cases (number) and treatment	Group B Cases (number) and treatment	Group C Cases (number) and treatment
Femoral shaft fracture	0	0	1 *Femoral plate (screws and cable fixation)*
Periprosthetic fracture	2 *Cerclage cable fixation*	2 *Cerclage cable fixation*	1 *Cerclage cable fixation*
Proximal femoral perforation	0	3 *No treatment*	2 *No treatment*
Major throchanteric fracture	3 *Cerclage cable fixation*	3 *Cerclage cable fixation*	4 *No treatment*
Cup dislodgment	0	0	1 Acute revision
Posterior dislocation	5 *Closed reduction*	2 *Closed reduction*	0
Deep infection	4 *Two-stage revision*	2 *Two-stage revision*	0
Superficial infection	5 *Debridement*	2 *Debridement*	2 *Debridement*
Nonfatal DVT	6 *Pharmacologycal therapy*	3 *Pharmacologycal therapy*	2 *Pharmacologycal therapy*
Stem subsidence	2 *Well tolerated*	0	1 *Well tolerated*
Paresthesias of the lateral aspect of the thigh	0	0	4
Fatal embolism. RIP	0	0	1

Table 4. Complications in our series

4. Discussion

Access to hip joint for placing a THA has been gained by different approaches along history. Each one has advantages and disadvantages but nevertheless we can assume total hip replacement is a successful procedure. Different viewpoints and discussions persist nowadays regarding fixation procedures, gliding couples and materials. In this context appeared years ago the concept of "minimally invasive surgery" that must be distinguished from less invasive surgery (Judet, 2006). This background supposed a breeding soil to show immeasurable advantages of these techniques. Plenty of reports were published describing its benefits in terms of economy, accelerated rehabilitation and comfort for the patients. These encouraging results explained the anxiety of the people about this useful surgery. However time has put these procedures in his place (Goosen et al., 2011; Maffiuletti et al., 2009; Nakata et al., 2009; Pospischill et al., 2010; Roy et al., 2010; Sugano et al., 2009). However there are some evidences of benefits reported by minimally invasive procedures (Berend et al., 2009; Duwelius & Dorr, 2008; Khan et al., 2006; Lamontagne et al., 2011; Matziolis et al., 2011; Müller et al., 2011; Nakata et al., 2009; Stehlík et al., 2008; Varela et al., 2010). We believe that with a good selection of the patients and after an education and training schedule these techniques are safe and reproducible.

Muscle damage and blood loss was two our main concerns in hip surgery. We have not established a pre-donation autologous blood protocol at our Institution and economic analysis of this practice was no cost-benefit in our environment. In order to lessen red cell transfusion we start the mini-posterior approach delighted with encouraging reports from other authors (Khan et al., 2006; Mazoochian et al., 2009; Sculco & Boettner, 2006). Though we reduced red cell transfusion with our mini-posterior access (group B) compare to the standard approach (group A) 16.32% vs 22.77% no significant differences were found in blood loss in the drain output, haemoglobin and HTO decrease [P>0.05].

It is believed that muscle protection enables the patient to start the rehabilitation program earlier and to reduce the length of his/her hospital stay (Goosen et al., 2011; Nakata et al., 2009; Palieri et al., 2011; Stehlík et al., 2008; Varela et al.,2010). Our plan was to minimize injure to muscles and/or bone to accelerate rehabilitation but we were not so worried about short scars. We had no doubt in enlarging the incision if it was required during our performances to be confident with the stem or cup position or to avoid damaging soft tissues. After introduction of the mini-posterior approach (group B) decrease in length hospital stay was observed with significant differences to standard access (group A) [P= 0.02], but usually when new techniques are introduced more attention is paid to questions as rehabilitation programmes and shortening hospital stay. We have also found in our series an improving in HHS and visual analog score for the first three months, however without significant differences with the standard approach.

Once the two of our main concerns were improved, we focused our attention in posterior dislocation. The posterior approach, the most commonly used at our Institution and all around the world has a high hip dislocation rate, up to 10 % in some reports (around 4.5% in our media) (Berry et al., 2004; Heithoff et al., 2001; Khan et al., 2006; Peters et al., 2007). In an attempt to prevent dislocations (none in group C in this series), being respectful with soft tissues we looked for news approaches as the AMIS, three and a half years ago. We believe this direct anterior approach, classically known as "Smith-Peterson" but initially described by the German surgeon Carl Hueter, provides an excellent exposure of the hip, is a muscle sparing procedure and has a lower dislocation rate than the posterior approach (Matta et al.,

2005; Siguier et al., 2004). We have no great experience with the antero-lateral approach but even though its dislocation rate is low, we have found more limping after THA in patients with the lateral approach.
As well as lessening the rate of posterior hip dislocations this technique allows a proper exposure of the acetabulum (Mast & Laude 2011) and it is widely accepted. In the current literature few reports have compared the extent and location of muscle damage between posterior and the direct anterior approaches (Nakata et al., 2009; Meneghini et al., 2005). Only Meneghini and colleagues reported a comparative cadaveric study about muscle damage evaluation with both approaches (Meneghini et al., 2005). He concluded that main differences related to injured muscle were in the gluteus minimus, being less harmful the anterior approach (8.5% vs 18%). Another comparative study shows that more patients could walk without assistive devices 3 weeks after surgery with the anterior direct approach (34%) than with the posterior one (Nakata et al., 2009). For that reasons, we started using the AMIS approach that let us get access to the hip through an inter-muscular (sartorius muscle and tensor fascia lata muscle) and inter-nervous (femoral nerve and superior gluteal nerve) portal. The anterior approach, which remains as the standard approach to the hip in paediatric orthopaedic surgery (Berger et al., 2004) regained popularity in adult procedures with the outbreak of the minimally invasive surgeries.
The principal advantage of this portal is that even an extensile exposure was required the gluteal muscles were keep intact. We agree with the idea that "minimally invasive surgery" does not imply short scars but require paying attention to soft tissues (Barton & Kim, 2009; Sculco, 2004; Waldman, 2003; Wojciechowski et al., 2007). Injuries to a muscle or its attachments impair muscle propioception and reduce its strength. Preventing muscle or attachments injure helps restoring normal muscular tension and improve stabilization of the hip joint.
Haemoglobin decreases after anterior minimally invasive procedure shows significant differences comparing this group with the mini posterior and standard approach [P= 0.0001], but no significant results were obtained with HTO. Blood loss in the drain output also reflects significant differences making the comparison to standard approach (group A) [P= 0.04] but not with the mini-posterior access (group B) [P= 0.33]. The reduction in blood loss was attributed to meticulous care with haemostasis to avoid wound hematomas as the only layer was closed was the sheath of the TFL (Morris et al., 2010), however most of the bleeding in hip replacement depends on bone bed not on the size of the wound. It is admitted that wound hematoma formation may be greater in the direct anterior approach as the incision is anterior and there is less inherent pressure on the wound that may aid in hemostasis. We believe that meticulous haemostasis is required to obtain a good view of the joint, so we prefer to use bipolar sealer to avoid bleeding (Morris et al., 2010). These details allow us to control blood loss, give us a neat exposure of the hip joint and let us take anatomic references for accurate component placement.
We found an improvement in HHS (Klausmeier et al., 2010; Lugade et al., 2010; Matziolis et al., 2011) and Trendelenburg's test (Nakata et al., 2009) with the AMIS. Visual analog pain score also improved with significant differences related to group A and B [P= 0.02 and P= 0.008]. Walking ability and length of hospital stay show significant differences comparing results to group A and B [P< 0.05] (Berend et al., 2009; Khan et al., 2006; Lamontagne et al., 2011; Maffiuletti et al., 2009; Morris et al. 2010; Nakata et al., 2009; Seng et al. 2009). Patients in group C were in hospital for a mean 4.78 days with the majority discharged to home (83.6%). Lower blood loss and muscle sparing that allowed the patients an accelerated

program of rehabilitation made them more confident after surgery to start walking, sitting or getting out of bed. Our patients used assistive devices as crutches or walkers during their hospital stay.

The concept of tissue sparing surgery has been an important fact in surgical techniques for the last ten years. It includes reduced incisions with small scars, but the real point toward these procedures attempt is preserving soft tissues. These techniques are as much careful as possible with muscles, sheaths, insertions, bone and of course the skin. They suppose new exposure techniques and of course new instruments to place the same prosthesis with the accuracy of the standard approaches and with few complications. Manufactures, tribologists and engineers have done a great effort to make possible these techniques but some of the advantages found in the current paper in terms of patient comfort, anaesthetic parameters, related costs, length of hospital stay, analgesic use, blood loss and patient rehabilitation explain the enthusiasm of orthopaedic surgeons in these procedures. According to the classification of Duncan in 2006, based on approach to the skin, number of skin incisions and technique of dissection the anterior direct approach is an "intermuscular approach" meanwhile the lateral and posterior approaches, with a standard or mini-incision, are classified as "transmuscular approaches" as they include and invasive operating step with muscle and tendon sectioning. Only the double access can be considered as a tissue sparing surgery but sometimes requires new design for the implants and prolonged used of an x-ray C-arm to check component placement. Besides these facts, cadaveric studies suggest greater muscle damage occurs with the two-incision technique than with the direct anterior approach (Mardones et al., 2005; Meneghini et al., 2005).

Zati (Zati et al., 1997) and He (He et al., 1988) concluded that, in early post-operative time, the afferent nerves to the muscle are more important than hip capsule receptors. Accepting that hypothesis tendon sectioning should be avoid because this gesture can affect sensomotory capacity of the joint so rehabilitation programme will be longer and worse functional scores will be obtain. This could explain better early functional outcome scores and visual analog score pain in the anterior direct approach compared to posterior procedures.

Every time a new procedure is established, great concern about possible complications arises in surgeons' mind. Minimally invasive approaches are related to longer surgery time and recommended in selected patients (Vail & Callaghan, 2007). However, a learning curve is necessary to take a new surgical access into practice. We have checked longer operating time in group B and C particularly in our first cases, but not significant differences were found [P= 0.44].

D'Arrigo (D'Arrigo et al., 2009) reported the rate of complications is not reduced along a geometric pattern during the learning curve of the anterior minimally invasive surgery, whereas surgical time was significantly correlated with this learning curve, so longer time was required in their first ten cases than in the rest. The idea of preserving muscles and tendons and absence of own experience in this approach made us to be carefully with the method of dissection, lengthening surgery time. All that measures applied in the present report have given 6-week HHS and visual analog pain scores significantly better than in posterior approaches (standard and mini-incision). This experience agrees the reports of Kim (Kim, 2006) and Ogonda (Ogonda et al., 2005) as mini-incision posterior approach implies direct muscle transection and remarks the difference between a small-incision and a tissue sparing surgery.

Minimally invasive techniques require some training and experience in hip surgery, especially for cup placement and femoral exposure. We verified our complications with the use of these techniques and how complications rate changed over time related to surgeons' experience. Of course this is a descriptive not comparative study within all surgeries done by a reduced group of surgeons, so complication rates may not be widespread.

Intraoperative major trochanteric fractures seen in our series related to femoral exposure didn't need fixation in group C as abductor mechanism was not damage. No restrictions were placed on patients postoperatively and no loss of strength, disturbance of gait or pain was notice with these trochanteric avulsions at latest follow-up. Better understanding of the tension applied on the femur and improving in our superior capsular release during exposure resolved this problem. Beside these facts, the stem we have used in group C and some hips of group B (quadra, Medacta®, IT) has a wide proximal section that requires invasion of the inner part of the major trochanter and places it at risk of fracture. On the opposite major throchanteric fractures of group A and B were fixed with cerclage band and gait restrictions were used though not affecting outcomes.

Proximal femoral perforations due to hard reaming of the proximal femur, mainly in muscular male patients with a short varus femoral neck, were our more frequent obstacle to get an accurate stem placement with minimally invasive procedures, mainly in AMIS group. Sariali (Sariali et al., 2008) reported 7 falses reamings of the proximal femur, all noted intra-operatively and without consequences. We noticed this complication in difficult femoral exposures that did not let external rotation and lateral displacement of the proximal femur. All femoral perforations occurred in our learning curve in muscle male patients with severe flexion contractures and have been avoided by improving our technique during femoral broaching. A more horizontal insertion angle of the starting broach is required in these cases for femoral reaming. Careful exposure of the proximal femur and enough releasing of the posterior capsule and pubo-femoral ligament must be done to move the femur in front of the incision.

Periprosthetic fracture and femoral shaft fracture happened after adjusting the bigger stem to a Dorr type C femur and they were detected and resolved intraoperative. We don't agree the idea of higher prevalence of varus stem in minimally invasive procedures (Bernasek et al., 2010) as we have not found outliers in our series (Hart et al., 2005). Cup placement in anterior hip access is another challenge to surgeons familiarized with posterior incision as the pelvis tilt in fracture table. Cup dislodgment reported was a mistake of the surgeon and not a real complication of the technique as he felt self-confident with the acetabulum purchase without testing the grip of the cup.

Rapid early return to function related to minimally invasive surgery (Duwelius & Dorr, 2008; Khan et al., 2006; Seng et al., 2009) has been reported in many papers but these techniques have shown increase complications, especially with the two-incision technique (Desser et al., 2010; Pagnano et al., 2005; Tanavalee et al., 2006). Mini-posterior and direct anterior approach report show rapid recovery function for patients (Duwelius & Dorr, 2008; Klausmeier et al., 2010; Lin et al., 2007; Mardones et al., 2005; Procyk, 2007; Stehlík et al., 2008) but these were limited to the early experience of a few surgeons.

Medical complications encountered in our series were similar to other large series of THAs (Clohisy & Harris, 1999; Duwellius et al., 2007). Paresthesias of the lateral aspect of the thigh (group C) were observed in four cases as we place the incision two finger breadths lateral from ASIS to avoid injuring of the lateral femoral cutaneous nerve.

We can conclude that minimally invasive procedures confer rapid functional recovery of the hip (Bhandari et al., 2009; Fink et al., 2010; Lin et al., 2007; Matta et al., 2005; Pospischill et al., 2010; Varela et al., 2010) and our data suggest that after an education and training schedule for hip experienced surgeons, they could be a safe and reproducible technique. Efforts should focus on how to prevent complications particularly during the learning curve. Moreover, a new spatial guidance for cup and stem placement in anterior hip access should be assumed by surgeons used to lateral and posterior approaches.

5. References

Barton C, Kim PR. Complications of the direct anterior approach for total hip arthroplasty. Orthop Clin North Am 2009; 40 (3): 371- 5

Berend KR, Lombardi AV Jr., Seng BE, Adams JB. Enhanced early outcomes with the anterior supine intermuscular approach in primary total hip arthroplasty. J Bone Joint Surg Am 2009; 91 Suppl 6: 107-20

Berger R, Jacobs JJ, Meneghini RM et al. Rapid rehabilitation and recovery with minimally invasive total hip arthroplasty. Clin Orthop Relat Res 2004; 429: 239-47

Bernasek TL, Lee WS, Lee HJ, Lee JS, Kim KH, Yang JJ. Minimally invasive primary THA: anterolateral intermuscular approach versus lateral transmuscular approach. Arch Orthop Trauma Surg. 2010 Nov; 130(11): 1349-54. Epub 2010 Jan 13

Berry DJ, von Knoch M, Schleck CD, et al. The cumulative long-term risk of dislocation after primary Charnley total hip arthroplasty. J Bone Joint Surg 2004; 86A (1): 9-14

Bhandari M, Matta JM, Dodgin D, Clark C, Kregor P, Bradley G, Little L. Outcomes following the single incision anterior approach to total hip arthroplasty: a multicenter observational study. Orthop Clin North Am. 2009; 40: 329-42

Clohisy JC, Harris WH. The Harris-Galante porous coated acetabular component with screw fixation: an average ten-year follow-up study. J Bone Joint Sur Am 1999; 81: 66-73

D'Arrigo C, Speranza A, Monaco E, Carcangiu A, Ferretti A. Learning curve in tissue sparing total hip replacement: comparison between different approaches. J Orthopaed Traumatol (2009) 10:47–54

De Verteuil R, Imamura M, Zhu S, Glazener C, Fraser C, Munro N, Hutchison J, Grant A, Coyle D, Coyle K, Vale L. A systematic review of the clinical effectiveness and cost-effectiveness and economic modelling of minimal incision total hip replacement approaches in the management of arthritic disease of the hip. Health Technol Assess. 2008 Jun; 12(26): iii-iv, ix-223.

Desser DR, Mitrick MF, Ulrich SD, Delanois RE, Mont MA. Total hip arthroplasty: comparion of two-incision and standart techniques at an AOA-accredited community hospital. J Am Osteopath Assoc. 2010; 110 (1): 12-5

Duncan CP (2006) Minimally invasive or limited incision hip replacement classification. In: Proceedings, MIS meet CAOS symposium, Scottsdale, pp 26–28

Duwelius PJ, Dorr LD. Minimally invasive total hip arthroplasty: an overview of the results. Instr Course Lect. 2008; 57: 215-22

Duwellius PJ, Burkhart RL, Hayhurst JO, Moller H, Butler JB. Comparison of the 2-incision and mini-incision posterior total hip arthroplasty technique: a retrospective match-pair controlled study. J Arthroplasty 2007; 22: 48-56

Fink B, Mittelstaedt A, Schulz MS, Sebena P, Singer J. Comparison of a minimally invasive posterior approach and the standard posterior approach for total hip arthroplasty A prospective and comparative study. J Orthop Surg Res. 2010 Jul 27; 5: 46

Goosen JH, Kollen BJ, Castelein RM, Kuipers BM, Verheyen CC. Minimally invasive versus classic procedures in total hip arthroplasty: a double-blind randomized controlled trial. Clin Orthop Relat Res. 2011 Jan; 469(1): 200-8. Epub 2010 Mar 30

Hart R, Stipcák V, Janecek M, Visna P. Component position following total hip arthroplasty through a miniinvasive posterolateral approach. Acta Orthop Belg. 2005 Feb; 71(1): 60-4

He XH, Tay SS, Ling EA (1988) Sensory nerve endings in monkey hip joint capsule: a morphological investigation. Clin Anat 11(2): 81–85

Heithoff BE, Callaghan JJ, Goetz DD, et al. Dislocation after total hip arthroplasty: a single surgeon's experience. Orthop Clin North Am 2001; 32(4): 587-91

Judet T. Revolution, progression or illusion. Does minimally invasive surgery exist for hip arthroplasty. Interact Surg; 2006; 1: 3-4

Khan RJ, Fick D, Khoo P, Yao F, Nivbrant B, Wood D. Less invasive total hip arthroplasty: description of a new technique. J Arthroplasty 2006 Oct; 21(7): 1038-46

Kim YH. Comparison of primary total hip arthroplasties performed with a minimally invasive technique or standart technique. J Arthroplasty 2006; 21: 1092-8

Klausmeier V, Lugade V, Jewett BA, Collis DK, Chou LS. Is there faster recovery with an anterior or anterolateral THA? A pilot study. Clin Orthop Relat Res. 2010 Feb; 468(2): 533-41. Epub 2009 Sep 10

Lamontagne M, Varin D, Beaulé PE. Does the anterior approach for total hip arthroplasty better restore stair climbing gait mechanics? J Orthop Res 2011 Mar 15. doi: 10.1002/jor.21392. [Epub ahead of print]

Laude F. Total hip arthroplasty through an anterior Hueter minimally invasive approach. Interact Surg 2006; 1: 5-11

Lewinnek GE, Lewis JL, Tarr R, t al. Dislocations after total hip-replacement arthroplasties. J Bone Jt Surg 1978; 60A: 217-20

Lin DH, Jan MH, Liu TK, Lin YF, Hou SM. Effects of anterolateral minimally invasive surgery in total hip arthroplasty on hip muscle strength, walking speed, and functional score. J Arthroplasty. 2007 Dec; 22(8): 1187-92

Lugade V, Wu A, Jewett B, Collis D, Chou LS. Gait asymmetry following an anterior and anterolateral approach to total hip arthroplasty. Clin Biomech (Bristol, Avon). 2010 Aug;25(7): 675-80. Epub 2010 Jun 9

Maffiuletti NA, Impellizzeri FM, Widler K, Bizzini M, Kain MS, Munzinger U, Leunig M. Spatiotemporal parameters of gait after total hip replacement: anterior versus posterior approach. Orthop Clin North Am. 2009 Jul; 40(3): 407-15

Mardones R, Pagnano MW, Nemarish JP, et al. Muscle damage after total hip arthroplasty done with two-incision and mini-posterior techniques. Clin Orthop 2005; 441: 63-7

Mast NH, Laude F. Revision total hip arthroplasty performed through the Hueter interval. J Bone Joint Surg Am. 2011 May;93 Suppl 2:143-8

Matta JM, Shahrdar C, Ferguson T. Single-incision anterior approach for total hip arthroplasty on an orthopaedic fracture table. Clin Orthop Relat Res 2005; 441: 115-24

Matziolis D, Wassilew G, Strube P, Matziolis G, Perka C. Differences in muscle trauma quantifiable in the laboratory between the minimally invasive anterolateral and transgluteal approach. Arch Orthop Trauma Surg. 2011 May; 131(5): 651-5. Epub 2010 Oct 17

Mazoochian F, Weber P, Schramm S, Utzschneider S, Fottner A, Jansson V. Minimally invasive total hip arthroplasty: a randomized controlled prospective trial. Arch Orthop Trauma Surg. 2009 Dec; 129(12): 1633-9. Epub 2009 May 8

Meneghini RM, Pagnanno MW, Trousdale RT, et al. Muscle damage during MIS total hip arthroplasty: Smith-Petersen versus posterior approach. Clin Orthop Relat Res 2005; 453: 292-8

Morris MJ, Berend KR, Lombardi AV Jr. Hemostasis in anterior supine intermuscular total hip arthroplasty: pilot study comparing standart electrocautery and a bipolar sealer. Surg Technol Int 2010; 20: 352-6

Müller M, Tohtz S, Dewey M, Springer I, Perka C. Muscle trauma in primary total hip arthroplasty depending on age, BMI, and surgical approach : Minimally invasive anterolateral versus modified direct lateral approach. Orthopade. 2011 Mar; 40(3): 217-223

Nakata K, Nishikawa M, Yamamoto K, Hirota S, Yoshikawa H. A clinical comparative study of the direct anterior with mini-posterior approach: two consecutive series. J Arthroplasty 2009 Aug; 24(5): 698-704. Epub 2008 Jun 13

Ogonda L, Wilson R, Archibold P, et al. A minimally-incision technique in total hip arthroplasty does not improve early postoperative outcomes. J Bone Joint Surg Am 2005; 87: 701-10

Pagnano MW, Leone J, Lewallen DG, Hanssen AD. Two-incision THA had modest outcomes and some substantial complications. Clin Orthop Relat Res 2005; 441: 86-90

Palieri G, Vetrano M, Mangone M, Cereti M, Bemporad J, Roselli G, D'Arrigo C, Speranza A, Vulpiani MC, Ferretti A. Surgical access and damage extent after total hip arthroplasty influence early gait pattern and guide rehabilitation treatment. Eur J Phys Rehabil Med. 2011 Mar; 47(1): 9-17. Epub 2010 Oct 8

Peters CL, McPherson E, Jackson JD, et al. Reduction in early dislocation rate with large-diameter femoral heads un primary total hip arthroplasty. J Arthroplasty 2007; 22 (6 Suppl-2) 140-4

Pospischill M, Kranzl A, Attwenger B, Knahr K. Minimally invasive compared with traditional transgluteal approach for total hip arthroplasty: a comparative gait analysis. J Bone Joint Surg Am. 2010 Feb; 92(2): 328-37

Procyk S. Initial results with a mini-posterior approach for total hip arthroplasty. Int Orthop. 2007 Aug; 31 Suppl 1: S17-20

Roy L, Laflamme GY, Carrier M, Kim PR, Leduc S. A randomised clinical trial comparing minimally invasive surgery to conventional approach for endoprosthesis in elderly patients with hip fractures. Injury. 2010 Apr; 41(4): 365-9. Epub 2009 Nov 1

Sariali E, Leonard P, Marnoudy P. Dislocation after total hip arthroplasty using Hueter anterior approach. J Arhroplasty 2008; 23: 266-72

Sculco TP, Boettner F. Minimally invasive total hip arthroplasty: the posterior approach. Instr Course Lect. 2006; 55: 205-14

Sculco TP. Minimally invasive total hip arthroplasty. In the affirmative. J Arthroplasty 2004; 19 (4 Suppl 1): 78-80

Seng BE, Berend KR, Ajluni AF, Lombardi AV Jr. Anterior-supine minimally invasive total hip arthroplasty: defining the learning curve. Orthop Clin North Am. 2009 Jul; 40(3): 343-50

Siguier T, Siguier M, Brumpt B. Mini-incision anterior approach does not increase dislocation rate: a study of 1307 total hip replacement. Clin Orthop Relat Res 2004; 426: 164-73

Stehlík J, Musil D, Held M, Stárek M. Minimally invasive total hip replacement--one-year results. Acta Chir Orthop Traumatol Cech. 2008 Aug; 75(4): 262-70

Sugano N, Takao M, Sakai T, Nishii T, Miki H, Nakamura N. Comparison of mini-incision total hip arthroplasty through an anterior approach and a posterior approach using navigation. Orthop Clin North Am. 2009 Jul; 40(3): 365-70

Tanavalee A, Jaruwannapong S, Yuktanandana P, Itiravivong P. Early outcomes following minimally invasive total hip arthroplasty using a two-incision approach versus a mini-posterior approach. Hip Int 2006; 16 Suppl 4: 17-22

Vail TP, Callaghan JJ. Minimal incision total hip arthroplasty. J Am Acad Orthop Surg. 2007 Dec; 15(12): 707-15

Varela Egocheaga JR, Suárez-Suárez MÁ, Fernández-Villán M, González-Sastre V, Varela-Gómez JR, Murcia-Mazón A. Minimally invasive posterior approach in total hip arthroplasty. Prospective randomised trial. An Sist Sanit Navar. 2010 May-Aug; 33(2): 133-43

Waldman BJ. Advancements in minimally invasive total hip arthroplasty. Orthopaedics 2003; 26 (8 Suppl): s 833-6

Wojciechowski O, Kusz D. Kopec K et al. Minimally invasive approaches in total hip arthroplasty. Orthop Traumatol Rehabil 2007; 9(1): 1-7

Zati A, Degli Espoosti S, Spagnoletti C et al (1997) Does total hip arthroplasty mean sensorial and proprioceptive lesion? A clinical study. Chir Organi Mov 82(3): 239–247

5

Minimally Invasive Total Hip Arthroplasty

Mel S. Lee
College of Medicine, Chang Gung University,
Department of Orthopedic Surgery, Chang Gung Memorial Hospital at Linkou
Taiwan

1. Introduction

Total hip arthroplasty (THA) is one of the most reliable procedures that can provide short-term high clinical success rates and long-term durable outcome. The surgery has been developed for more than 40 years and most of the clinical practices are standardized for the patient care. In the past, THA had been done by making a wound about 25 cm in length. Many surgeons believed that big wounds should be the standard approach for THA because the surgery is a big surgery and could only be reliably done with big wounds. In recent 10 years, this concept of "big surgery-big wound" has been challenged in many fields of surgery. Taking the arthroscopic ligament reconstruction surgery or laparoscopic cholecystectomy surgery as the examples, many surgical procedures can now be safely and adequately performed by the minimally invasive (MIS) approaches. Although impossibly be done by an arthroscopy, the surgical approaches for THA have been adopting the concept of MIS and modified by many surgeons. However, the definition of a MIS-THA is not as straightforward as the words meanings. Based on the incision length, it is generally agreed upon that an incision less than 10 cm can be defined as MIS-THA. However the MIS can also be interpreted as less soft tissue trauma or less bone tissue trauma when doing the THA. The incision wound length then is not necessarily equal to the extent of tissue injury during the procedure. To date, the MIS-THA can be divided into two categories. One decreases the wound and muscle cutting and emphasizes the tissue repair through either a lateral or a posterior route. [1-4] The other spares muscle sectioning during the procedure through one [5,6], two [1,7-11], or multiple [12] incisions. The abridged incision methods minimize the incision length and can be extensile if difficulties are encountered during THA. The muscle sparing methods use tissue intervals for surgery but could be difficult if complications happened intraoperatively. In the literature, the complication rates are significantly higher in inexperienced, low-volume surgeons in the "learning curve" period for the muscle sparing techniques. [13] THA, however, is a reliable procedure and its clinical results should not be compromised by the surgical approaches. For those surgeons who start to learn the procedure, standard surgical approach with bigger wounds is strongly recommended.
In the learning curve period of the MIS-THA, the incision should start from a standard length and then gradually reduces its size as the experiences accumulated. To master the MIS-THA surgical techniques, surgeons also need to familiar with the anatomy and different surgical approaches for THA. [14]

2. Surgical approaches for total hip arthroplasty

For the surgical approaches, THA can be done by different routes. Each approach has its potential advantages and limitations. Followings are the commonly used approaches for THA.

2.1 The transtrochanteric approach

The transtrochanteric approach osteotomizes the greater trochanter and retracts it along with the gluteal medius and minimus anteriorly to facilitate exposure. It is nowadays seldom performed on primary cases and is performed selectively on revision cases, secondary reconstruction after hip fractures, and for distal transfer of the greater trochanter. The transtrochanteric approach is originally done at the level between the insertion of hip abductors and the origin of the vastus lateralis. It is however associated with complications such as nonunion or proximal migration of the greater trochanter that often result in weakness of the abductors with marked limping gait or even instability of the THA. To avoid proximal migration of the greater trochanter and enhance the union rates, both the insertion of gluteal muscles and the origin of the vastus lateralis can be preserved on the greater trochanter as a whole construct and be slide anteriorly during the procedure. The trochanteric slide or flip approach prevents untoward proximal migration of the greater trochanter and enhances the fixation stability of the trochanter. [15] The trochanteric slide technique can be further modified by extending the osteotomy to the lateral cortex of the proximal femur to facilitate implant or cement removal in complex cases. [16]

2.2 The transgluteal approach (direct lateral)

The transgluteal approach splits the gluteal medius along its muscle fibers and cut about one third or half of the gluteal medius from its musculotendinous insertion on the trochanter. **(Figure 1)** The muscle is retracted ventrally and the underlying gluteal minimus

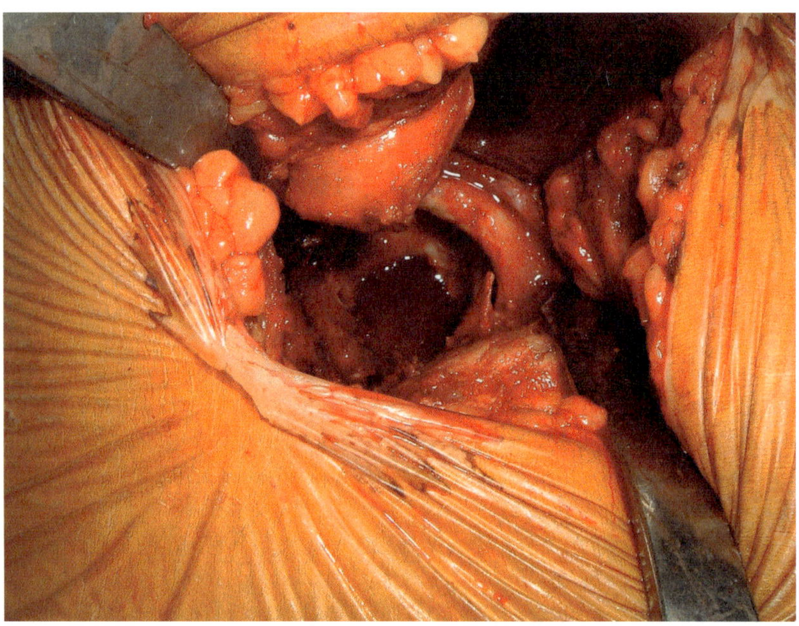

Fig. 1. The direct lateral approach detaches 1/3 of the gluteal medius from the greater trochanter to facilitate anterior dislocation of the hip joint.

and the joint capsule are then incised in a T-manner to facilitate anterior dislocation of the hip. In standard lateral approach of Hardinge [17], part of the vastus muscle can be incised to help the exposure. In modified method, the origins of the vastus muscle can be spared to decrease the tissue trauma. Possible risks of the approach involve an injury to the muscular braches of the superior gluteal nerve or direct injury to the muscle fibers by compression or retraction during surgery. This will result in damage to the gluteal muscles or muscular insufficiency and is associated with higher chance of Trendelenburg sign **(Figure 2)** postoperatively. [18]

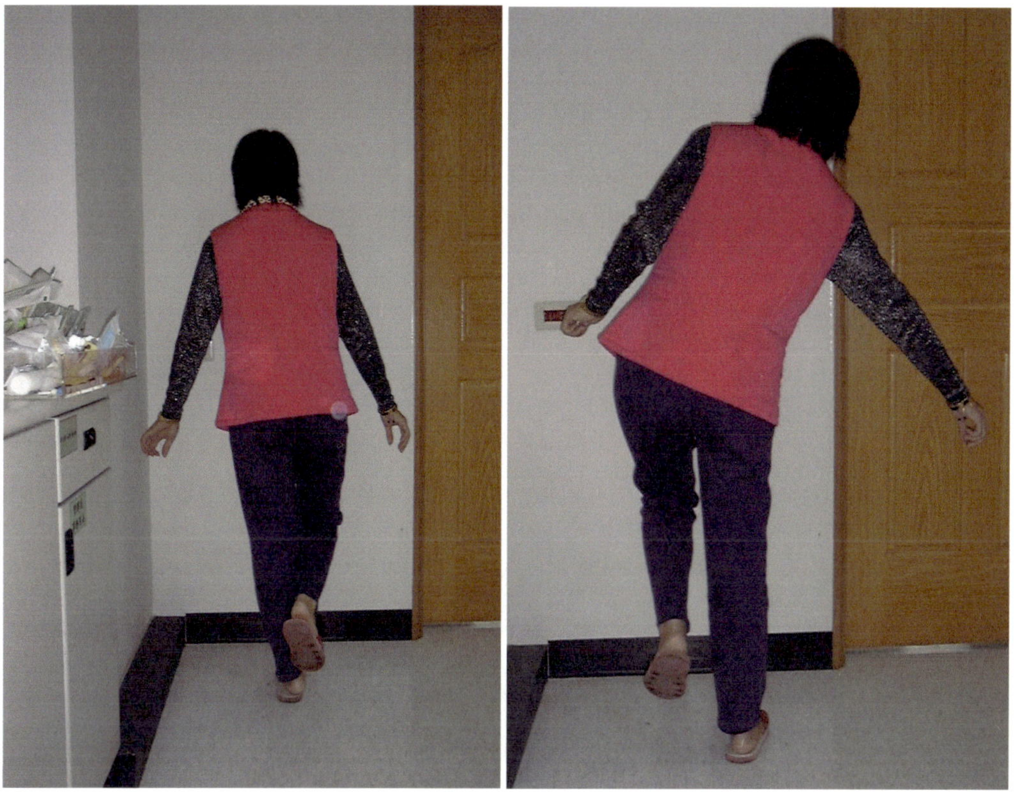

Fig. 2. The patient with abductors weakness. (A) When standing on the sound leg, the pelvis can be kept level and will not drop. (B) When standing on the affected leg, patient will compensatory list to the affected side to avoid pelvis dropping. (Duchenne sign)

2.3 The posterolateral approach

The posterolateral approach is probably the most popular surgical approach for THA for many orthopedic surgeons. Skin incision is made along the posterior border of the proximal femur centered on the top of the greater trochanter. The muscle part of the gluteal maximus is split along its fibers. The short external rotators and the posterior joint capsule are detached from the posterior border of the femur. The hip is dislocated posteriorly by internally rotation, flexion, and adduction. Cares should be taken to identify and protect the sciatic nerve during the procedure. After the THA, a secure and tight repair of the posterior capsule should be performed to decrease the dislocation rates. [3,4]

2.4 The anterolateral approach

Between the anatomical interval of the gluteal medius and tensor fascia latae superficially, the so-called Watson-Jones interval, the anterior hip joint capsule can be exposed by retracting the rectus femoris medially and the gluteal muscles laterally. During the exposure of the anterior femoral neck, the assistant can gradually rotate the leg in externally rotated position. Usually the neck should be cut in place because the complete anterior dislocation of the hip is difficult. The acetabulum is exposed by placing two retractors, one on the front to protect the rectus femoris and one on the back to push the femur posteriorly. The femur is exposed by placing the limb in hyperextension, adduction, and 90° external rotation. One retractor is placed behind the greater trochanter to protect the gluteus medius. One retractor is placed below the proximal medial neck to leverage the proximal femur for canal preparation. [5] Because only the fasica layers were split without detaching muscles from the hip, special retractors are often needed to facilitate exposure and dislocation of the hip.

2.5 The anterior approach

The direct anterior approach is usually performed with the patient in the supine position. [6] Dissection is in the Smith-Peterson interval between the fascia of the Sartorius muscle and the fascia of the tensor fascia lata muscle. The skin incision begins from a point distal to the anterior superior iliac spine and extends obliquely in the direction of the tensor fascia lata. By blunt dissection, the Sartorius muscle can be retracted medially and the muscle belly of the fascia lata can be retracted laterally. At this point, the underlying fascia between the rectus femoris and the inferior fasica layer of the tensor fascia lata can be exposed. In this layer, the ascending branches of the lateral femoral circumflex vessels can be identified and ligated. A Cobra retractor is put around the anterior inferior femoral neck above the capsule to elevate the reflected head of rectus femoris. Another Hohmann retractor is put around the posterior femoral neck and the posterior acetabulum to retract the gluteal muscles behind. Sometimes part of the reflected head of the rectus femoris need to be released to help the exposure. The anterior hip capsule can then be incised or excised. The retractors can then be put intra-articularly while cutting the femoral neck. For the aceabular preparation, visualization of the bony landmarks can be done by putting a Hohmann retractor under the posterior rim of acetabulum to push the proximal femur posteriorly and by another retractor on the medial wall of the acetabulum above the pubic bone. For femoral preparation, the leg needs to be positioned in hyperextension, adduction and external rotation. The posterior medial capsule along with the short external rotator muscles are released in a stepwise manner. The leg is put in the "figure of 4" position and a blunt Cobra retractor can be put behind the greater trochanter to gradually elevate the proximal femur.

2.6 The combined approach

By combining the above surgical routes, THA can also be done by the double incision methods [1,7-11] or the triple incision method [12]. The double incision method is a modified method of the direct anterior approach by Berger and Mears. [14] Patient is put in the supine position and the hip joint is approached via the Smith-Peterson interval. [7,8] The anterior skin incision is made along the long axis of the femoral neck. The fascia and muscle over the hip joint are split without cutting into their attachment. Two Hohmann retractors, one medial and one lateral to the femoral neck, are used to retract the gluteal medius laterally and the rectus femoris medially. The femoral neck needs to be cut in situ because dislocation of the hip joint is almost impossible by such a limited dissection. Usually the femoral neck needs to be doubly cut at the head-neck junction and at the standard neck cut level. After removing the bone block of the femoral neck, a space is created for the ease of femoral head retrieval. The acetabulum is prepared as the standard direct anterior approach. Another incision is made posterior to the greater trochanter. The fascia and muscles of the gluteal maximus are split in line with its muscle fibers. Similar to the technique of femoral intramedullary nailing, the femoral canal is prepared by sequential enlargement with reamers. Under the fluoroscopic guidance, both the acetabular and the femoral component can be implanted in predetermined position.

We and others have modified the two-incision technique by putting the patient in the lateral decubitus position [9-11]. The anterior skin incision is made perpendicular to the long axis of the femoral neck about 3 to 4 finger-breadth distal to the ilioinguinal line. **(Figure 3)** The hip joint is approached through the Smith-Peterson interval. Double neck cutting to the hip joint is also needed. While the anterior skin incision is made along the intertrochanteric line, the greater trochanter and the proximal femur can be visualized more easily by gentle retraction of the gluteus medius and tensor fascia lata. By this modification, the process of femoral canal preparation can be safely done under direct vision without the help of the fluoroscopic monitoring. [9-11,19]

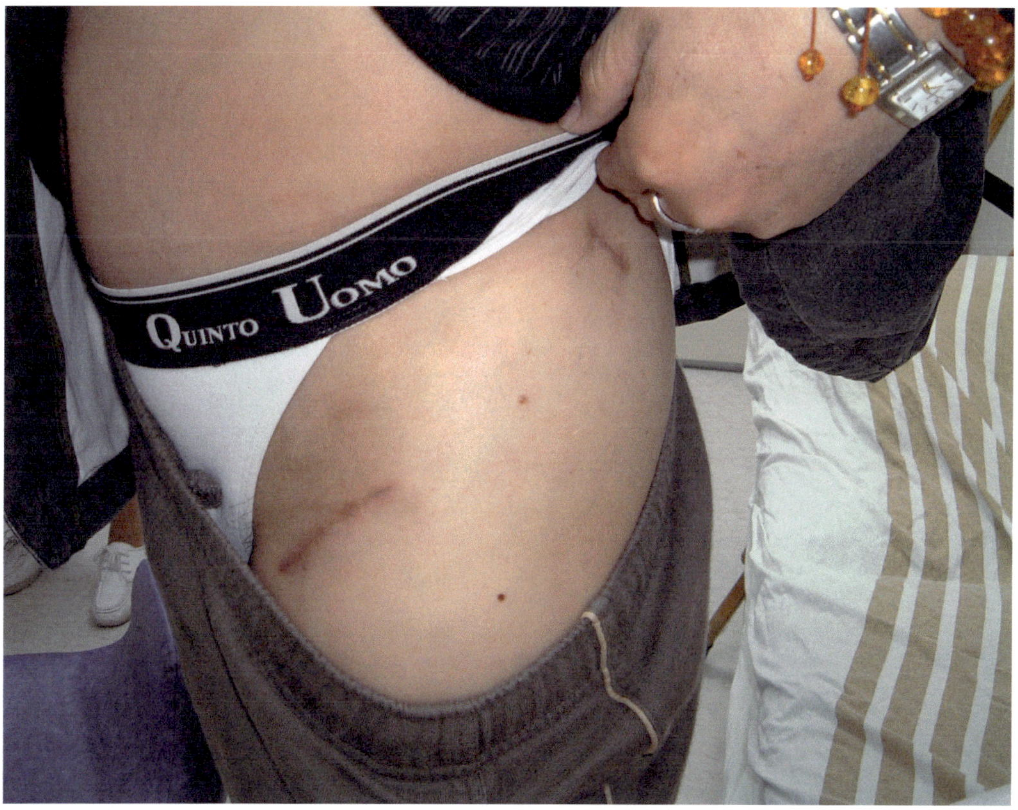

Fig. 3. Skin incision of the modified two-incision method.

The triple incision method is similar to the double incision method. It can be done with the patient in the supine or in the lateral decubitus position. Basically the incisions for the acetabulum and the femur exposure are not different from the original 2-incision method and the tissue intervals used for surgery are the same. The third incision is only needed in some heavy muscular or obese cases whereas the appropriate handling of the surgical instruments to the desirable position cannot be done. [12]

2.7 The omega approach

The approach is a lateral approach to the hip joint with the patient in the supine or lateral position. [20] Skin incision is centered over the greater trochanter. The fascia lata and gluteus maximus are split in the line of the skin incision. An aponeurotic flap including the gluteus medius and the vastus lateralis is elevated subperiosteally. The dissection starts proximally in the plane between the tendons of gluteus medius and piriformis. The attachments of gluteus medius and gluteus minimus from the greater trochanter are mobilized by sharp dissection. The dissection continues distally to involve the anterior border of the vastus lateralis as a single continuous strip of tissue. The shape of the incision resembles the Greek letter omega. Care should be taken to create the "osteoaponeurotic" flap as a whole construct. The entire muscle flap of gluteus medius, minimus, and vastus lateralis is mobilized off the anterior capsule of the hip. The hip capsule is incised in a T-shape manner. Subsequent repair of the osteoaponeurotic flap can be augmented by interrupted non-absorbable sutures by passing the sutures through holes drilled in the bone.

2.8 Patient positioning and special operation table

MIS-THA can be done with the patient in the supine or lateral position depending on the surgeon's preference. As a general rule, if the THA is performed from the anterior route, a supine position will be more intuitive. If the THA is performed from the lateral or posterolateral route, a lateral position should be easier for the surgeon. The patient positioning is important in performing the THA because the implant positions are often determined intraoperatively with the reference to the patient's position, bony anatomy, and the environmental setting. In MIS-THA, it is even more important because the bony anatomy and landmarks are sometimes less visualized. The proper patient positioning is also necessary during the THA because the operated leg needs to be manipulated in different directions and positions to facilitate hip dislocation, bone preparation, and check for the leg length equality.

In the supine position, a sandbag or an inflatable pillow can be put beneath the buttock to help the hyperextension of the hip. The foot-piece of the operative table on the operated side can be lowered and the leg can be put in a "figure of 4" position in hyperextension, adduction, and external rotation. The proximal femur then can be more easily accessed from the anterior wound. [21]

In the lateral position, the positions and directions of the operated leg depend on the surgical approaches for the femur preparation. With the posterolateral approach, the leg needs to be adducted, internally rotated, and flexed. With the transgluteal approach or omega approach, the leg needs to be adducted, externally rotated, and flexed. Both the posterolateral and the transgluteal approach can be done on a standard operation table. An operation table with the foot-piece that can be removed or lowered is required for the anterolateral (Watson-Jones) approach because during the femur preparation the leg needs to be adducted, externally rotated, and hyper-extended. **(Figure 4)** If the operation table is not available, the patient needs to be put toward the side of the table to facilitate the hip extension postion.

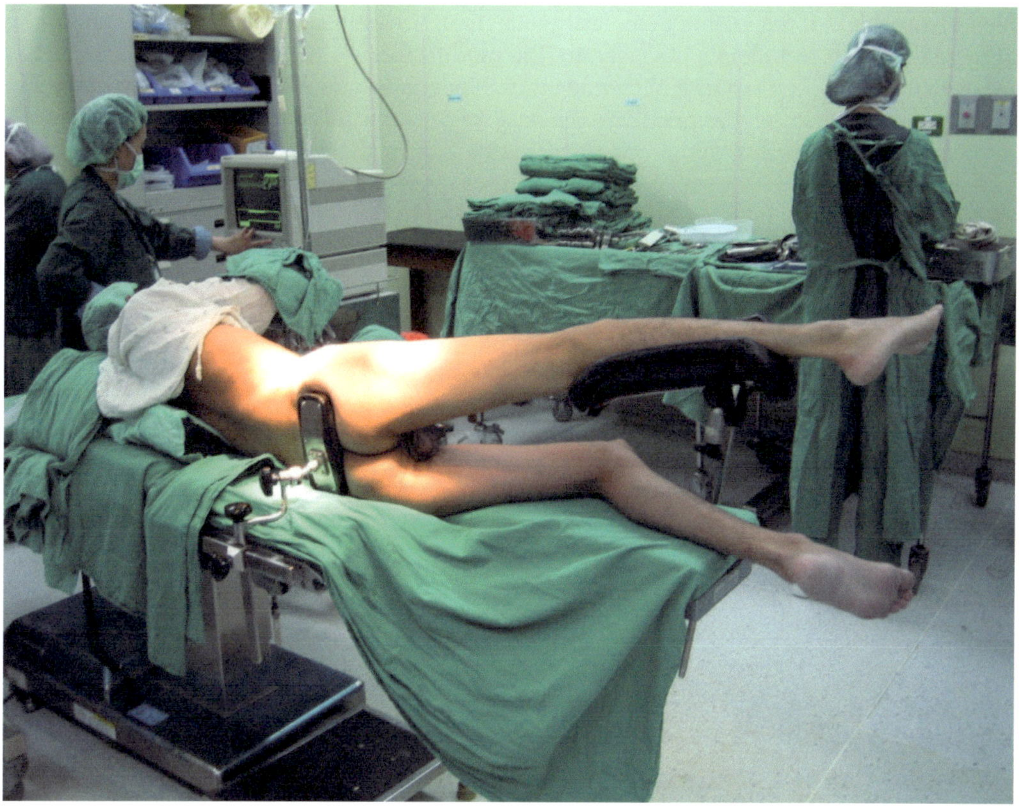

Fig. 4. The special operation table for modified Watson-Jones approach.

Matta et al. has described a unique method of THA using direct anterior approach to the hip. [22] The patient is put on a fracture table that the leg can be pulled by traction in extension and external rotation position. Fluoroscopy can be used during the procedure to control the leg length. However the technique needs a well organized surgical team to adjust the traction and fluoroscopy. Some rare complications such as the ankle fracture or calcaneal fracture have been reported.

2.9 MIS-THA

For many years, THA through a reduced wound has been performed in patients on a selective base by many surgeons. However in the past decade, the issue about MIS-THA has provoked great attention and controversy among the society and the publicity. The two-incision technique was publicized by Berger et al. in the Rush-Presbyterian University Hospital. [7,8] In the following years, many studies including prospective randomized trial, large cohort study, case control study, clinical series, and expert opinions about a variety of MIS-THA are reported. As described previously, the MIS-THA can be divided into two categories. The first is the abridged incision MIS-THA and the second is the muscle-sparing MIS-THA.

2.10 Abridged incision MIS-THA

Because the major difference between the abridged incision techniques and the conventional techniques is the length of incision, the abridged incision techniques are now more popular and acceptable to the orthopaedic surgeons than the muscle-sparing techniques. The abridged incision techniques basically are the modification of the conventional approaches by reducing the skin incision and creating a mobile window for surgical field visualization. Special instruments are designed for the ease of surgery **(Figure 5)** For the transgluteal approach to the hip joint, about one third to one half of the musculotendinous portion of gluteus medius and minimus are detached from the greater trochanter to facilitate anterior dislocation of the hip joint. Care should be taken not to damage the superior gluteal nerve by overstretching the muscle fibers. For the posterlateral MIS approach to the hip joint, the piriformis tendon or part of the quadratus femoris tendon can be preserved. The hip is dislocated posteriorly by internal rotation, adduction, and flexion. Emphasis has also been on the secure repair of the posterior capsule and the short external rotators after prosthesis implantation. By this modification, this approach proves to be a reliable and safe procedure and the dislocation rates are significantly decreased. [3,4]

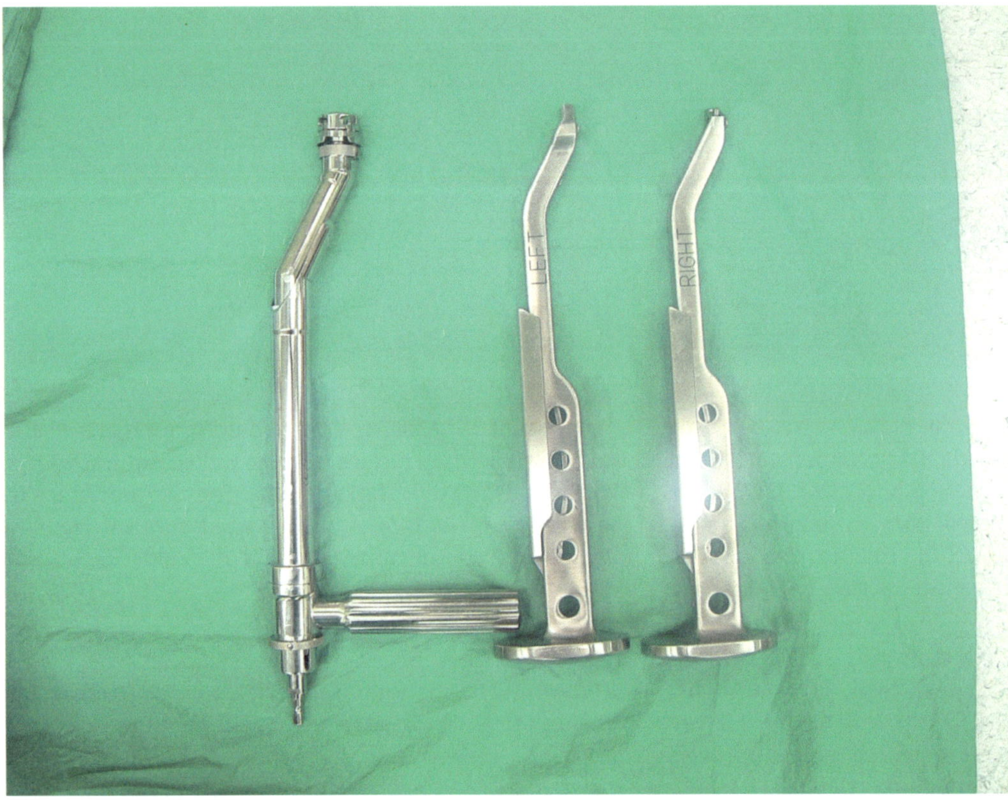

Fig. 5. Dog-legged instruments can be used to avoid skin and soft tissue impingement during MIS surgery.

2.11 Muscle-sparing MIS-THA

The muscle-sparing MIS-THA uses tissue intervals and avoids muscle sectioning for prosthesis implantation. Single-incision or multi-incision muscle-sparing MIS techniques have been described in the literatures. The single-incision techniques include the anterolateral (modified Watson-Jones) approach [5] and the direct anterior approach (Smith-

Peterson) [6,21,22]. The multiple-incision techniques include the two-incision approach [7-11] or the three-incision approach [12]. Although the muscle sparing MIS-THA techniques are also the modification of the classic anterior or anterolateral approach to the hip joint, these techniques are greatly different from the classic ones in terms of the skin incision and tissue dissection. Because the muscles around the hip joint are not cut or detached, dislocation of the hip for the ease of surgical exposure is difficult. Usually a double cut to the femoral neck is needed with one cut over the head-neck junction and the other cut at the desired position above the lesser trochanter.

In MIS direct anterior approach, both acetabular cup and femoral stem can be implanted in a single incision with the patients in the supine position. The single-incision techniques use the Smith-Peterson interval and can be facilitated by using a fracture table or by lowering the leg to hyperextend the hips. [6,21,22]

In the multi-incision techniques, the acetabular cup and femoral stem are separately implanted through different incisions depending on the musculatures and sizes of the patients. Patients can also be placed in supine or lateral position. Intraoperative fluoroscopy is usually advised because direct visualization of the femur during stem implantation is difficult. Under the fluoroscopic guidance, the procedure is very similar to the closed femoral intramedullary nailing technique. [7,8] However by modifying the direction of the skin incisions and position of the patients, the procedure could be done without intraoperative fluoroscopy because direct visualization of the proximal femur is possible. [1,9,10]

The muscle-sparing techniques are less popular than the abridged incision or the conventional techniques. The techniques are challenging and need a steeper learning curve because the surgical anatomy and surgical landmarks are less apprehensible among most surgeons and their surgical team members as well. Special instruments, operation table, or additional training are highly demanded to facilitate and to safe-guard the procedures.

2.12 Clinical results of the MIS-THA

The increasing popularity of MIS-THA has led to some debates regarding to the safety and clinical results for the "new technologies". Although a decade has been passed, the follow-up length is still inadequate and good quality randomized control studies are not enough to make a conclusion.

For the evaluation of abridged incision posterior approach, Ogonda had performed a randomized control trial by comparing the standard approach with the MIS-THA approach among different groups of surgeons. Ogonda et al. found the MIS-THA using mini-posterior approach was safe and reliable but provided no extra-benefit as compared to the standard posterior approach in terms of the functional outcomes and the ambulatory ability. [23,24] Kim reported on 60 simultaneous bilateral THA in 30 patients, with each patients serving as his or her own control. [25] The only difference between the MIS-THA and the standard THA was less blood loss in the MIS group. Dorr et al. had combined the imageless navigation system with the mini-posterior MIS-THA technique. They found the MIS-THA using the mini-posterior approach had shortened hospital stays, earlier mobility, less pain, and higher satisfaction in the early postoperative period. [3] The higher satisfaction among the patients with the MIS-THA is associated with the successful implementation of patient education and rehabilitation program. In the high motivated patients, the psychologic expectation and the physical recovery are more realistic. [26]

The muscle-sparing approaches include the direct anterior, the two- , or the three-incision techniques. Theoretically the muscle sparing techniques should have more rapid functional recovery because the muscles around the hip joint are not violated. As a matter of fact, the muscle sparing techniques are more difficult than the conventional or the abridged incision techniques. Pagnano et al. reported that the muscle-sparing two-incision technique had modest outcomes and substantial complications. [27] By using cadaver studies, they also found evidences of more muscles damage with the two-incision technique than the mini-posterior technique. [28] Others had reported some unusual catastrophic complications and heterotopic ossification by using the muscle-sparing technique. [29,30] As a contrast, high satisfaction and rapid recovery were consistently found in patients treated by experienced surgeons. [7,8,31] Duwelius et al. had compared the two-incision technique with the posterior MIS technique by using historical match-pair control cases and found that the mini-posterior technique had less blood loss and shorter operation time and the two-incision technique had better functional recovery and shorter hospital stays. [31] We had modified the two-incision technique by setting the patient in the lateral position and changed the orientation of the skin incision to facilitate the surgical exposure of the proximal femur. When compared with the standard transgluteal approach, the modified two-incision technique was proven to be safe and had comparable hospital courses and operative results. [1] Using dynamometer to check the muscular torques preoperatively and postoperatively, it was reported that the muscular recovery of the hip flexors were earlier in the postoperative period than the hip extensors by using the modified two-incision technique. [10]

The single-incision muscle-sparing MIS-THA are less reported in the literature except those from the technique developers. [5,6,21,22] Laffosse et al. had compared the anterolateral mini-invasive technique with the posterior mini-invasive approach and reported that both techniques had comparable surgical results and similar implant positioning. [32] Hu et al. had performed a prospective study on 20 patients who had two-incision THA on one hip and modified Watson-Jones THA on the other. [33] It was noted that in the early postoperative period, more patients would prefer the two-incision side to the modified Watson-Jones side. Taking the similarity of the two muscle-sparing techniques in regards to the anterior approach to the hip joint, it was postulated that the manipulation of the leg into hyperextension, external rotation, and adduction in the modified Watson-Jones technique could be the potential reason for the differences in patient's preference. We had used the modified Watson-Jones MIS-THA in more than 400 cases and had perceived similar clinical outcomes as compared with other MIS techniques. However it is usually recommended that special surgical tools, operation table, and a coordinated surgical team are the keys to success. [5,32,33]

2.13 Navigation & MIS-THA

By decreasing the surgical wound, it is difficult to visualize the surgical field in the MIS-THA. This surgical exposure is even more limited for the muscle-sparing MIS techniques. Without the help of the visualization of the surgical landmarks during operation, the operation becomes a blind method and is highly dependent on the surgeon's experiences and skillfulness. To safeguard the surgical results and to overcome the difficulty, fluoroscopy is used during the operation to provide real-time image for the verification of the implant positioning. [7,8,13,14] Fluoroscopy can also be combined with the navigation system to verify the size and position of the implants intraoperatively. By implementing the computer tomography-based or imageless navigation system with the MIS techniques, the positioning of the acetabular component could be improved by reducing the outliers with more consistent results. [3,34-36] We had adopted an imageless navigation system to the modified two-incision MIS-THA and compared the results with the use of intraoperative fluoroscopy. It was found the imageless navigation system could be a reliable tool for the cup placement as compared to intraoperative fluoroscopy. [9] However the navigation technology for the femoral component implantation is still unsatisfactory. So the navigation system cannot substitute the fluoroscopy for the original combined incision muscle-sparing MIS-THA. As described above, we had modified the two-incision technique by changing the incision direction and the patient positioning. [1,9,10] Similar to the technique described by Irving, the modified technique of two-incision THA can be safely done without the use of fluoroscopy or navigation system. [11] It is noteworthy to emphasize that the use of intraoperative fluoroscopy is not a guarantee to the safety of operation. A hairline fracture which may occur during press-fit of the implant cannot be detected by a fluoroscopy. [19] Such fracture can only be recognized by direct visualization. To overcome this difficulty, a fully porous coated stem is recommended for the muscle-sparing MIS techniques. [7,8,13,14]

2.14 Safety and complications of MIS-THA

It is assumed that the complication rates of the MIS-THA would not be lower than the conventional THA and it could be even higher if they were done by inexperienced hands especially by using the muscle-sparing techniques. The enthusiasm for the MIS-THA has declined recently because some complications have alarmed surgeons to practice more cautiously with the new MIS techniques. [13,27,29,30] The MIS-THAs, especially the multi-incision muscle-sparing techniques, are considered as unsafe with no proven benefits in clinical recovery or muscle damages. [27,28] The complications associated with the two-incision technique included higher incidence of proximal femoral fractures (2.8%) and partial, temporary injures to the lateral femoral cutaneous nerve in the so called "learning curve". [13]

However these reported complications are still not enough to conclude the MIS-THAs, muscle-sparing techniques in particular, are unsafe and associated with more complications. In the literature, the complication rates in conventional posterior or posterior mini-THA were not different with equal rates of infection, dislocation, or peroneal nerve palsy. [3,25,37,38] Ogonda et al. performed a prospectively randomized study on 219 hips by assigning them to conventional posterior or mini-posterior group. [23] The conventional group had 2 mortalities and 1 deep venous thrombosis while the mini-posterior group had 1 infection and 1 dislocation. No mortality were found in the mini-posterior group. In another study comparing conventional and mini-posterior groups, there were even higher complication rates in the conventional group. [39] By reviewing a limited number of patients retrospectively, there were higher rates of complications in the two-incision group as compared with the posterior approach group. [27,31] The two-incision group had higher complication rates (14% versus 5%) that included 4 calcar fractures, 1 dislocation, and 2 femoral nerve palsy in the 80 two-incision cases and 4 calcar fractures and 2 dislocations in the 120 posterior cases. [27] In a study of 134 hips in 125 patients by using a modified two-incision technique, there was neither major complications nor perioperative mortality. [40] Linear fractures of the femoral calcar occurred in 6 hips. Transient paresthesia of the lateral femoral cutaneous nerve was seen in 2 patients.

According to the clinical reports in the literature, the MIS-THA is associated with difficulties in the surgical techniques and should be apprehended by the surgeons to prevent complications.

2.15 Coordinating the MIS-THA team

The reasons to use the MIS techniques are to avoid unnecessary tissue destruction, to decrease tissue trauma, to increase patient's satisfaction, and to improve the clinical outcomes. However it is not enough to fulfill the goals for the early recovery by the improvement in the surgical technique alone. The surgical team, the nursing team, the physical therapy team, and the anesthesia team need to be coordinated. The multidisciplinary implementation of clinical pathway, more efficient physical therapy protocols, better anesthesia, effective postoperative pain management, and education programs are equally important as the improvement in the surgical techniques. In the author's institute, the average hospital stay after a THA is about 4 days. When the length of stay shortens, all treatments need to be accelerated without compromising the contents and qualities of medical care. In an interesting study, patients' satisfactions for a MIS-THA were highly related to the psychologic reasons. [26] Those patients who share the decision-making processes before choosing the MIS-THA will more likely take responsibility for their outcomes and cope with the treatment team.

For the improvement in the surgical techniques, it is recommended that the surgeon, the assistants, and the nursing staffs should take a training course before start. Because the adoption of a new technology needs a process of learning curve, it is also recommended that the inexperienced surgeons should work with a supervisor for about 20 cases to familiar with all the procedures. The assistants should know their roles and the steps of surgery to streamline the surgical procedures. For the MIS approach, the visualization of the surgical field is difficult for the operating surgeon. It is sometimes impossible for the assistants to see the surgical field. If the assistants can not apprehend their roles and try enthusiastically to see every anatomic detail, the difficulty for the surgeon is increased. The surgical team should use the concept of "mobile window" by moving the retractors back and forth to check the surgical anatomy one at a time. As the treatment team becomes more organized, it is more efficient to provide better quality of care and meet the interest of better patients' satisfaction.

3. Conclusion

Although the risks and benefits of MIS-THA are still inconclusive in the literature, nowadays almost all surgeons claim that they adopt some forms of MIS approach into their practice and patient care. [41-47] The reasons include the pressure from the peer groups, the patients' needs, the research and academic interests, the industrial promotion, and the surgeons' self-expectation. Information for the MIS-THA on the internet and other sources impose the MIS-THA as a metaphor of high-tech, quick-recovery, full-function, and better-satisfaction. As the conventional THA has been developed for more than 50 years and has been one of the most reliable and safe procedure in medicine, we should cautiously adopt the MIS techniques into our practice without any compromising to the gold standards of a successful THA. The fixation, the implant position, the alignment, the choice of the bearing surface, and the recreation of the normal biomechanics are the fundamental parts for long term success. The abridged incision techniques can have smaller wounds but the surgeon should not limit the incision length because most the studies indicated there were no difference in the surgical results and the clinical outcomes. For the muscle-sparing techniques, the complications are sometimes catastrophic and unacceptable in inexperienced hands in the learning curve period. The surgeons should take a cautious start by joining expert teams or taking training courses. In conclusion, the concept of MIS-THA has changed the perspectives of patient care in the hip surgery. Increasing awareness of the patients has changed the pattern of orthopedic practice. Orthopedic surgeons should take the full responsibility and master their most familiar and comfortable technique of THA. They should also adopt the MIS-THA into their practice, in the best interests of the patients, to provide long-lasting clinical outcomes and minimize trauma to the patients.

4. References

[1] Chen DW, Hu CC, Chang YH, Yang WE, Lee MS. Comparison of clinical outcome in primary total hip arthroplasty by conventional anterolateral transgluteal or 2-incision approach. J Arthroplast 2009;24:528-532.

[2] Sculco TP, Jordan LC. The mini-incision approach to total hip arthroplasty. Instr Course Lect 2004;53:141-147.

[3] Dorr LD, Maheshwari AV, Long WT, Wan Z, Sirianni LE. Early pain relief and function after posterior minimally invasive and conventional total hip arthroplasty. A prospective, randomized, blinded study. J Bone Joint Surg Am 2007;89:1153-1160.

[4] Swanson TV. Early results of 1000 consecutive, posterior, single-incision minimally invasive surgery total hip arthroplasties. J Arthroplast 2005;20:Suppl 26-32.

[5] Bertin KC, Röttinger H. Anterolateral mini-incision hip replacement surgery. A modified Watson-Jones approach. Clin Orthop 2004;429:248-255.

[6] Lovell TP. Single-incision direct anterior approach for total hip arthroplasty using a standard operating table. J Arthroplast 2008;23:S64-S68.

[7] Berger RA. Total hip arthroplasty using the minimally invasive two-incision approach. Clin Orthop 2003;417:232-241.

[8] Berger RA, Jacobs JJ, Meneghini RM, Valle CD, Paprosky W, Rosenberg AG. Rapid rehabilitation and recovery with minimally invasive total hip arthroplasty. Clin Orthop 2004;429:239-247.

[9] Lee MS, Kuo CH, Senan V, Chen WJ, Chen LH, Ueng SWN. Two-incision total hip replacement: Intraoperative fluoroscopy versus imageless navigation. Hip International 2006;16 (Suppl): S35-S41.

[10] Chou SW, Ueng SWN, Lee MS. Muscular recovery of hip flexors and extensors after two-incision total hip arthroplasty. Chang Gung Med J 2008;31(6):576-582.

[11] Irving JF. Direct two-incision total hip replacement without fluoroscopy. Orthop Clin N Am 2004;35:173-181.

[12] Kennon RE, Keggi JM, Wetmore RS, Zatorski LE, Huo MH. Keggi KJ. Total hip arthroplasty through a minimally invasive anterior surgical approach. J Bone Joint Surg Am 2003;85(Suppl 4): 39-48.

[13] Archibeck MJ, White RE Jr. Learning curve for the two-incision total hip replacement. Clin Orthop 2004;429:232-238.

[14] Berry DJ, Berger RA, Callaghan JJ, Dorr LD, Duwelius PJ, Hartzband MA, Lieberman JR, Mears DC. American orthopaedic association symposium: minimally invasive total hip arthroplasty: development, early results, and a critical analysis. J Bone Joint Surg Am 2003;85: 2235-2246.

[15] Solberg BD, Moon CN, Franco DP. Use of a trochanteric flip osteotomy improves outcomes in Pipkin IV fractures. Clin Orthop 2009;467:929-933.

[16] Mardones R, Gonazalez C, Cabanela ME, Trousdale RT, Berry DJ. Extended femoral osteotomy for revision of hip arthroplasty. Results and complications. J Arthroplast 2005;20:79-83.

[17] Hardinge K. The direct lateral approach to the hip. J Bone Joint Surg Br. 1982;64:17-19.

[18] Picado CH, Garcia FL, Marques W, Jr. Damage to the superior gluteal nerve after direct lateral approach to the hip. Clin Orthop 2007;455:209-211.

[19] Hu CC, Yang WE, Chang YH, Chen DWC, Ueng SWN, Lee MS. Fluoroscopy can not recognize intraoperative fracture in patients receiving two-incision total hip arthroplasty. J Arthoplast 2008;23:1031-1036.

[20] Learmonth ID, Allen PE. The omega lateral approach to the hip. J Bone Joint Surg 1996;78-B:559-561.

[21] Bohler N, Hipmair G. The minimal invasive surgery anterior approach with supine patient positioning: a step-wise introduction of technique. Hip International 2006;16(Suppl4):48-53.

[22] Matta J, Shahrdar C, Ferfuson T. Single-incision anterior approach for total hip arthroplasty on an orthoaedic table. Clin Orthop 2005;441:115-124.

[23] Ogonda L, Wilson R, Archbold P, Lawlor M, Humphreys P, O'Brien S, Beverland D. A minimal-incision technique in total hip arthroplasty does not improve early postoperative outcomes. A prospective, randomized, controlled trial. J Bone Joint Surg Am 2005;87(4):701-710.

[24] Bennett D, Ogonda L, Elliott D, Humphreys L, Lawlor M, Beverland D. Comparison of immediate postoperative walking ability in patients receiving minimally invasive and standard-incision hip arthroplasty. A prospective blinded study. J Arthoplasty 2007;22:490-495.

[25] Kim YH. Comparison of primary total hip arthroplasties performed with a minimally invasive technique or a standard technique. A prospective and randomized study. J Arthroplasty 2006;21:1092-1098.

[26] Dorr LD, Thomas D, Long WT, Polatin PB, Sirianni LE. Psychologic reasons for patients preferring minimally invasive total hip arthroplasty. Clin Orthop 2007;458:94-100.

[27] Pagnano MW, Leone J, Lewallen DG, Hanssen AD. Two-incision THA had modest outcomes and some substantial complications. Clin Orthop 2005;441:86-90.

[28] Mardones R, Pagnano MW, Nemanich JP, Trousdale RT. Muscle damage after total hip arthroplasty done with the two-incision and mini-posterior techniques. Clin Orthop 2005;441;63-67.

[29] Fehring TK, Mason JB. Catastrophic complications of minimally invasive hip surgery. A series of three cases. J Bone Joint Surg Am 2005;87:711-714.

[30] Feinblatt JS, Berend KR, Lombardi AV Jr. Severe symptomatic heterotopic ossification and dislocation: a complication after two-incision minimally invasive total hip arthroplasty. J Arthroplasty 2005;20(6):802-806.

[31] Duwelius PJ, Burkhart RL, Hayhurst JO, Moller H, Butler JBV. Comparison of the 2-incision and mini-incision posterior total hip arthroplasty technique. A retrospective match-pair control technique. J Arthroplast 2007;22:48-56.

[32] Laffosse JM, Accadbled F, Molinier F, Chiron P, Hocine B, Puget J. Anterolateral mini-invasive versus posterior mini-invasive approach for primary total hip replacement. Comparison of exposure and implant positioning. Arch Orthop Trauma Surg 2008;128(4):363-369.

[33] Hu CC, Chern JS, Hsieh PH, Shih CH, Ueng SWN, Lee MS. Two-incision versus modified Watson-Jones total hip arthroplasty in the same patient - a prospective study on clinical outcomes and patient's preference. Chang Gung Med J 2011 (In Press).

[34] Wixson RL, MacDonald MA. Total hip arthroplasty through a minimal posterior approach using imageless computer-assisted hip navigation. J Arthroplasty 2005;20,Suppl 3:51-56.

[35] Parratte S, Argenson JA. Validation and usefulness of a computer-assisted cup-positioning system in total hip arthroplasty. A prospective, randomized, control study. J Bone Joint Surg Am 2007;89:494-499.

[36] Haaker RGA, Tiedjen K, Ottersbach A, Rubenthaler F, Stockheim M, Stiehl JB. Comparison of conventional versus computer-navigated acetabular component insertion. J Arthroplast 2007;22:151-159.

[37] Geubbels ELPE, Wille JC, Nagelkerke NJD, Vandenbroucke-Grauls CMJE, Grobbee DE, de Boer AS. Hospital-related determinants for surgical-site infection following hip arthroplasty. Infect Control Hosp Epidemiol 2005;26:435-441.

[38] Ridgeway S, Wilson J, Charlet A, Kafatos G, Pearson A, Coello R. Infection of the surgical site after arthroplasty of the hip. J Bone Joint Surg Br 2005;87 (6):844-50.

[39] Khan RJK, Fick D, Khoo P, Yao F, Nivbrant B, Wood D. Less invasive total hip arthroplasty: description of a new technique. J Arthroplast 2006; 21:1038-1046.

[40] Lu ML, Chou SW, Yang WE, Senan V, Hsieh PH, Shih HN, Lee MS. Hospital course and early clinical outcomes of two-incision total hip arthroplasty. Chang Gung Med J 2007;30(6):513-520.

[41] Wright JM, Crockett HC, Delgado S, Lyman S, Madsen M, Sculco TP. Mini-incision for total hip arthroplasty. A prospective, controlled investigation with 5-year follow-up evaluation. J Arthroplasty 2004;19(5):538-545.

[42] Siguier T, Siguier M, Brumpt B. Mini-incision anterior approach does not increase dislocation rate. A study of 1037 total hip replacements. Clin Orthop 2004;426:164-173.

[43] de Beer J, Petruccelli D, Zalzal P, Winemaker MJ. Single incision minimally invasive total hip arthroplasty: length doesn't matter. J Arthroplasty 2004;19(8):945-950.

[44] Howell JR, Masri BA, Duncan CP. Minimally invasive versus standard incision anterolateral hip replacement: a comparative study. Orthop Clin North Am 2004;35(2):153-162.

[45] Asayama I, Kinsey TL, Mahoney OM. Two-year experience using a limited-incision direct lateral approach in total hip arthroplasty. J Arthroplast 2006;21:1083-1091.
[46] Meneghini RM, Smits SA. Early discharge and recovery with three minimally invasive total hip arthroplasty approaches. Clin Orthop 2009;467:1431-1437.
[47] Labovitch RS, Bozic KJ, Hansen E. An evaluation of information available on the internet regarding minimally invasive hip arthroplasty. J Arthroplast 2006;21:1-5.

6

The Effect of Drainage After Hip Arthroplasty

Andrej Strahovnik and Samo K. Fokter
General and Teaching Hospital Celje
Slovenia

1. Introduction

Closed suction drainage is a routinely used method in all fields of surgery. The idea to drain a wound is quite old. Supposedly, Hippocrates had already used a wooden tube to drain the operative wound (Levy, 1984). In orthopaedic surgery, Waugh and Stinchfield were the first who popularized the method of draining. Their preference to draining was based on their retrospective study, where they observed the incidence of wound infection after various orthopaedic procedures (Waugh & Stinchfield, 1961). The group of 100 patients with closed suction drainage was compared with a similar group (identical procedure, same comorbidities and the same surgeon) of 100 patients without the drainage. Wound infection occurred in 1% of patients with closed suction drainage and in 3% of patients without the drainage. They also noted that the post-operative rehabilitation was quicker if they drained the operated joint after an arthroplasty. Even though the difference in incidence of wound infection was not statistically significant, they concluded that a more benign postoperative course can be expected if the drains are used.

After that, the use of drains quickly spread in all areas of orthopaedic surgery. It seemed logical to drain the operative wound. Exposed intramedullary canal and trabecular bone make it difficult to create a perfect hemostasis. A hematoma inevitably forms which increases the pressure on the surrounding tissues. Increased pressure impairs blood flow and healing of the operative wound. Additionally, a hematoma is also a good culture medium for bacteria (Cheung et al., 2008; Parvizi et al., 2007). The function of phagocytic cells to eliminate these bacteria in hematoma is weakened. The first reason for this weakened elimination is that phagocytic cells have a hardened access to the bacteria in the hematoma. Secondly, due to the low level of opsonic proteins in hematoma, the destruction capacity of phagocytic cells is damaged (Alexander et al., 1976). Therefore, in order to prevent the infection of the surgical wound, it appears logical to drain the wound to avoid or at least reduce the formation of hematoma.

New studies have emerged at the end of the 20th century. These studies have questioned the logical mechanism of drainage and the use of drainage in hip arthroplasty. There are several potential adverse effects from draining. Drain tubes may become contaminated and allow a retrograde migration of the skin bacteria around the wound. In addition, drains may be inadvertently sutured to surrounding tissues and are difficult to remove post-operatively. Furthermore, drains may increase the amount of blood loss and increase the need for transfusion. The findings from these new studies have convinced many surgeons to change their routine and re-think the need for drainage in total hip arthroplasty.

2. Literature search methods

All randomized controlled trials that compared closed suction drainage to no-drainage after elective hip arthroplasty were searched. Additionally, studies that could provide further information on relevant aspects of drainage (eg. relative amount of drainage in the first 24 hours, hematoma size estimation using one or two drain tubes, bacterial growth on suction drain tips, etc.) were included. Trials involving other than elective hip arthroplasty (arthroplasty for fracture treatment) were excluded. The following search terms were used in Pubmed database: "drainage hip arthroplasty", "drains hip arthroplasty", "serous drainage hip arthroplasty". Two authors independently examined all articles that were obtained with this search strategy. Articles were assessed for relevance and handpicked. Differences between authors were resolved by discussion.

The selection procedure resulted in 6 studies directly comparing the use of closed suction drainage to un-drained wound closure (Murphy & Scott, 1993; Kim et al., 1998; Widman et al., 2002; Della Valle et al., 2004; Johansson et al., 2005; Walmsley et al., 2005). The basic information about the studies is depicted in Table 1.

Study	Drained group (hips, n)	Un-drained group (hips, n)	Number of drains (n)	Time of drain removal (h)	Follow-up
Murphy & Scott, 1993	20	20	2	24	10 days
Kim et al., 1998	48	48	2	24	1 year
Widman et al., 2002	10	12	2	24	NA*
Della Valle et al., 2004	53	51	2	next morning	3 months
Johansson et al., 2005	54	51	NA	NA	2 months
Walmsley et al., 2005	282	295	1	24	3 years

* data not available

Table 1. Studies with a direct comparison of drained group to un-drained group.

Seven studies, which in addition to groups with and without closed suction drainage after hip arthroplasty, compared groups with different interventions (eg. additional group after knee arthroplasty; two drained groups, one with 24-hour drainage, the other with 48-hour drainage; two drained groups, one with autologous blood transfusion drain, one with conventional closed suction drainage) were also included in a review (Beer et al., 1991; Ritter et al., 1994; Ovadia et al., 1997; Niskanen et al., 2000; Kumar et al., 2007; Strahovnik et al., 2010; Cheung et al., 2010). Characteristics of those studies are presented in Table 2.

Three more studies were included with relevant data on infection of the surgical wound, one study with data on hematoma size and two studies on the prolonged serous secretion from the surgical wound (Willett et al., 1988; Sørensen & Sørensen, 1991; Overgaard et al., 1993; Parrini et al., 1988; Wood et al., 2007; Patel et al., 2007).

Study	Drained group (hips, n)	Un-drained group (hips, n)	Additional intervention - arm
Beer at al., 1991	12	12	two knee groups
Ritter at al., 1994	78	62	two knee groups
Ovadia et al., 1997	18	12	two knee groups
Niskanen et al., 2000	27	31	two knee groups
Kumar et al., 2007	19	15	two knee groups
Strahovnik et al., 2010	46	42	group with 48h drainage
Cheung et al., 2010	52	48	group with autologous transfusion drain

Table 2. Studies with additional research arm(s).

Different aspects of wound healing with or without drainage after hip arthroplasty were reviewed and compared among the selected studies. The effectivenes of drainage with regard to those aspects is discussed under the following heading. Drainage also has an unwanted side effect that was not present in the un-drained groups, which is reported in a later heading as a complication.

3. Effectiveness of drainage in total hip arthroplasty

The impact of drainage on the bacterial growth and wound infection was regarded as the most important outcome. The drainage influence on the size of hematoma, the healing of the surgical wound, the need for transfusion and hospital stay were also reported in most of the studies.

3.1 Bacterial growth and wound infection

No significant difference in the occurrence of wound infection was found in the studies that were directly comparing patients whose wounds were drained and patients with un-drained wounds. If infection was present, it was regarded as superficial in the majority of cases. Deep wound infection was very rare or none. Results are summarized in Table 3.

Other studies that were comparing groups with additional intervention, as well as drainage and no-drainage groups after hip arthroplasty, also could not show any differences in wound infection.

Altogether, there were 30 out of 719 patients with wound infection (superficial and deep) in the drained groups, and 27 out of 699 patients in the no-drained groups (relative risk 1.08; 95% confidence interval 0.65 - 1.80).

Wound infection is a serious complication after elective hip arthroplasty. It should be regarded as the most important reported outcome. The problem is that the occurrence of wound infection, either superficial or deep, is very low. In order to achieve the required power and still get a clinically significant difference between groups, a large number of patients would need to be included in a study. In a hypothetical scenario, where we would have, for example, a 6% incidence of wound infection in the drained group, and a 3% incidence in the no-drained group (no published study reported such a big difference), and

the power of a study 0.8, we would need at least 312 patients to achieve a significant difference with probability less than 0.05.
The only single study that included a sufficient number of patients was from Walmsley et al. They found the rate of superficial infection 2.9% in the drained group and 4.8% in the un-drained group. The rate of deep wound infection was 0.4% in the drained group and 0.7% in the un-drained group. The differences in the incidence of wound infection were not statistically significant. The only existent meta-analysis on hip arthroplasty managed to pool 711 patients with drained wounds and 704 patients with un-drained wounds (Parker et al., 2008). The pooled results indicated that there was no significant difference between the wounds treated with a drain and those treated without a drain with respect to the occurrence of wound infection.

Study	Wound infection - deep&superficial (n/N)		Deep wound infection (n)	
	Drained group	Un-drained group	Drained group	Un-drained group
Beer et al., 1991	0/12	0/12	0	0
Murphy & Scott, 1993	1/20	0/20	NA	NA
Ritter et al., 1994	0/78	0/62	0	0
Ovadia et al., 1997	0/18	0/12	0	0
Kim et al., 1998	0/48	0/48	NA	NA
Niskanen et al., 2000	1/27	1/31	0	0
Widman et al., 2002	1/10	1/12	1	1
Della Valle et al., 2004	2/53	0/51	0	0
Johansson et al., 2005	3/54	2/51	0	0
Walmsley et al., 2005	19/282	23/295	1	2
Kumar et al., 2007	0/19	0/15	0	0
Strahovnik et al., 2010	1/46	0/42	0	0
Cheung et al., 2010	2/52	0/48	0	0

Table 3. Incidence of wound infection.

Another problem with reporting incidence of wound infection is limited follow-up. Many studies followed patients only until first clinical control. This may have resulted in an underreporting of not only the infection rate but of several other outcomes as well (eg. re-operation rate).
We can conclude that drainage does not have a clinically relevant effect on wound infection after hip arthroplasty.

3.1.1 Connection between wound infection and duration of drainage

The supposedly beneficial effect of drainage on the bacterial growth in the drained hematoma was actually one of the first assumptions to become questioned. Willett et al. performed a study with 120 patients after hip arthroplasty (Willett et al., 1988). They implied a connection between wound infection and the duration of drainage. Even though the correlation did not reach the statistical significance, the authors recommended removal of drains 24 hours after the operation. Drainage after 24 hours did not reduce the size of hematoma, but it did increase the chance of bacterial infection.

Similarly, Sørensen and Sørensen also investigated the relation between bacterial growth and duration of drainage (Sørensen & Sørensen, 1991). They prospectively followed 489 patients after various orthopaedic operations. They showed that signs of wound infection and drain tip cultures were significantly more often positive, if the drainage lasted more than 6 days. The explanation they offered was that the drain allows the bacteria on the skin around the wound to retrogradely migrate.

On the other hand, another study between drain tip cultures and the duration of drainage did not show any statistically significant correlation (Overgaard et al., 1993). The authors commented that this unexpected lack of correlation might be explained with a relatively short duration of drainage in their study (maximum 3 days). They also noticed that most of the drainage occurred within first 12 hours, and hence also recommended to remove the drains rather sooner than later.

Additional studies on relationship between the duration of drainage and bacterial infection were performed (Drinkwater & Neil, 1995; Erceg & Becić K, 2008; Rowe et al., 1993). A general consensus was gradually formed that the optimal time to remove the drains in hip arthroplasty would be 24 hours after the operation. Drainage after first 24 hours does not evacuate significant amount of blood and only increases the chance of bacterial retrograde migration.

3.2 Hematoma size

Several studies evaluated the size of hematoma after hip arthroplasty (Murphy & Scott, 1993; Kim et al., 1998; Widman et al., 2002). Hematoma size can be evaluated using different methods, but none of them is very accurate. Most of the studies used a formula which uses pre-operative and post-operative hematocrit values to calculate hidden blood loss (hematoma). In some studies an ultrasound examination of the thigh was used, in order to measure the thickness of blood mantle around the prosthesis. Other methods have also been used, such as a scintigraphy with labeled erythrocytes or a simple tape measurement of the thigh circumference.

In one study a calculated hidden loss in the wound was compared between a group with drainage and a group without the drainage (Murphy & Scott, 1993). Hematoma in the drained group was not smaller. The authors explained this unexpected result with a tamponade effect mechanism. The tamponade effect refers to the fact that the bleeding in the wound continues until the pressure in the wound increases. In order to achieve the critical pressure, enough bleeding must occur to fill out the space (dead space) around the prosthesis. Since the tissues around the hip prosthesis are relatively rigid and immobile, the suction from the drain does not reduce the space around prosthesis (dead space). In other words, regardless the wound is drained or not, enough bleeding into the wound must occur to create the tamponade effect. Furthermore, a drain enlarges the dead space for the amount of space of a drain tube and a drain device. Therefore, even more blood must be lost to achieve the tamponade effect, if a drain is used. Paradoxically, drains therefore increase the blood loss after the operation.

Widman et al. used a more objective method of determining the hematoma size (Widman et al., 2002). They used a scintigraphy with labeled erythrocytes to compare a group of patients with two-drain drainage to a group of patients without the drainage. The hematoma size was quantitatively measured using SPECT (single photon emission computed tomography). Even though a smaller hematoma was found when two drains were used, the difference

between patients with drained wounds and patients with un-drained wounds was not statistically significant. Patients with drainage also lost more blood and more often required blood transfusion in the postoperative period. The authors´ interpretation was consistent with a tamponade effect theory.
On the other hand, Kim et al. routinely used ultrasound to assess the size of wound hematoma on the sixth or seventh day after the surgery (Kim et al., 1998). The wound hematoma was classified as none, small or large, according to the thickness of the hypoechogenic density along the region of the wound. Thirteen drained wounds (27.1%) and 26 non-drained wounds (54.2%) had large hematomas; large hematomas were significantly more often present in patients without the drainage. In addition, 13 wounds with closed suction drainage (27.1%) and 4 wounds without the drainage (8.3%) did not have hematomas, which was also statistically significant difference. The possible explanation the authors offered was that the use of suction drains may not evacuate hematomas completely in the hip joint, and that small hematomas re-accumulate in the hip joint after the drain is removed.
Another study examined the hematoma size using an ultra-sonographic evaluation (Parrini et al., 1988). Within 82 patients after total hip arthroplasty, a comparison between patients with two drains and patients with one drain was made. A hematoma in the wound was always present, regardless to the number of drains. However, the authors did found the hematoma to be significantly smaller in patients, where two drains were used instead of one.
We also performed a study where we compared 3 groups: a group without drainage, a group with 24-hour drainage and a group with 48-hour drainage. A semi-quantitative estimation of the wound hematoma size was performed with measurements of the operated thigh circumference. Measurements of the thigh circumference were routinely performed before and after elective total hip arthroplasty. In the un-drained group, the change of thigh circumference significantly increased in the post-operative period, when compared with the change in both drained groups. Most of the increase of thigh circumference occurred within first 48 hours after the procedure. Our results were consistent with findings of both previous studies. The use of drainage slightly decreases hematoma size in the post-operative period. However, the drains do not evacuate hematomas completely, and hematomas re-accumulate to a certain extent after the drains are removed.

3.3 Healing of the surgical wound

There are few studies thoroughly describing wound healing parameters, such as bruising of the wound area and persistent drainage from the wound. No study reported any serious healing complications (eg. necrosis of the skin around the wound). Most of the studies described healing as uneventful in either drained or un-drained groups and did not notice any difference.

3.3.1 Bruising of the wound area

There is only one study reporting bruising around the wound area after hip arthroplasty. Kim et.al measured the area of bluish discoloration around the wound site. The ecchymosis was present in 11 hips from the un-drained group, as opposed to 3 hips from the drained group ($p<0.05$). They recommended the routine use of suction drains after primary total hip arthroplasty to reduce ecchymosis around the wound. Other studies did not specifically report the bruising around the wound area.

3.3.2 Persistent drainage from the wound site

There are two types of prolonged drainage in hip arthroplasty. The first type occurs in the surgical wound and can happen whether the wound is drained or not. The second type of drainage occurs only in drained wounds, at the drain site after the drain is removed.

The drainage from the surgical wound usually starts on the first post-operative day and rarely lasts for more than a couple of days. The drainage is usually bloody. This type of drainage is more frequent if the wound is not drained. Kim et al. found persistent drainage from the surgical wound in 3 of 48 wounds with suction drains and 11 of 48 wounds without suction drains. Other studies do not specifically report the drainage from the wound site.

Sometimes a later secretion from the surgical wound develops which is serous in nature and may last longer. This type of serous secretion has been linked to the development of superficial surgical site infection and deep wound infection (Saleh et al., 2002). Serous secretion allows an open communication between the deep layers of the surgical wound and the skin. The longer this communication exists, the more chance there is for migration of bacteria from the skin.

Two studies have analyzed risk factors that predispose to the longer duration of prolonged serous secretion from the wound site. Wood et al. associated time to dryness of the surgical wound with: wound length, body mass index (BMI) and estimated volume of blood in the dissected tissues (Wood et al., 2007). Patel et al. found that prolonged wound drainage correlated with: morbid obesity (BMI $\geq 40 kg/m^2$), increased volume of drain output and use of low-molecular-weight heparin (Patel et al., 2007). In both studies, the length of hospital stay was significantly increased in patients with prolonged drainage. Patel et al. also stated that each day of prolonged wound drainage increased the risk of wound infection by 42% following a total hip arthroplasty.

3.3.3 Re-operation for wound healing complication

There was no statistically significant difference in the re-operation rate between the groups (Table 4).

Study	Drained group (n/N)	Un-drained group (n/N)
Kim et al., 1998	0/48	0/48
Della Valle et al., 2004	1/53	0/51
Johansson et al., 2005	0/54	0/51
Walmsley et al., 2005	1/282	0/295
Strahovnik et al., 2010	1/46	0/42
Cheung et al., 2010	0/52	0/48

Table 4. Re-operation due to wound healing complications.

3.4 Post-operative range of hip motion

There was only one study numerically reporting post-operative range of motion. Kim et al. reported no extension lag in either group at the 2-month follow-up. Mean flexion reached 90° in the drained group and 95° in the group without drainage.

3.4.1 Need for re-enforcement of the dressing

Since more patients without closed suction drainage have a persistent drainage from the surgical wound, more wounds need to be re-enforced in the early post-operative period.

Several studies have reported a greater need for re-enforcement of the dressing in the un-drained groups (Table 5). Two of them have found a statistically significant difference between drained and un-drained groups (Kim et al. 1998; Strahovnik et al., 2010).

Study	Drained group (n/N)	Un-drained group (n/N)
Kim et al., 1998	3/48	11/48
Niskanen et al., 2000	1/27	4/31
Della Valle et al., 2004	6/53	10/ 51
Strahovnik et al., 2010	2/46	20/42

Table 5. Studies with reported need for re-enforcement of the dressing.

3.5 Need for blood transfusion

The majority of included studies evaluated the need for transfusion. The need for transfusion is an easily measured parameter and could be one of the most important evidences of the tamponade effect theory. One point needs to be addressed with regard to the transfusion needs as an outcome measure. Different transfusion triggers were used in analyzed studies. Some authors used an absolute hemoglobin cutoff point, with values bellow that point necessitating a blood transfusion. Others used various recommended algorithms or they simply treated each patient and their requirements for allogeneic blood on an individual basis. In some studies the transfusion algorithm was not well described. This heterogeneity of transfusion policies could not be eliminated in the analysis. Different transfusion triggers among and even within the studies reduce the reliability of the need for transfusion as an outcome measure.

There is a trend in the need for more blood transfusion if drains are used in total hip arthroplasty. Many studies showed the increased need for transfusion in patients with drained wounds but only studies by Walmsley et al., Strahovnik et al. and Cheung et al. showed that the need for transfusion was significantly more often required in patients with drainage (Table 6).

Study	Patients transfused		p
	Drained group (n/N)	Un-drained group (n/N)	
Ovadia et al., 1997	9/18	2/12	0.06
Widman et al., 2002	9/10	6/12	0.07
Della Valle et al. 2004	21/53	18/51	0.7
Johansson et al. 2005	36/54	28/51	0.3
Walmsley et al., 2005	93/282	78/295	0.042
Kumar et al., 2007	13/19	10/15	0.13
Strahovnik et al., 2010	22/46	30/42	0.024
Cheung et al., 2010	19/52	6/48	0.02

Table 6. Incidence of transfusion needed in drained and un-drained groups.

For included studies in Table 6, the relative risk for transfusion in patients with closed suction drainage opposed to patients without drainage was 1.23 (95% confidence interval 1.05 - 1.44). Accordingly, more units of red cell concentrates were given to patients in the drained groups (Table 7). However, when there was a need for blood transfusion, patients received approximately the same amount of red cell concentrates, regardless of the fact whether the wound was drained or not.

Study	Units of blood given (n)/number of patients)	
	Drained group	Un-drained group
Ovadia et al., 1997	13U/9	3U/2
Johanson et al., 2005	110U/36	69U/28
Cheung et al., 2010	36U/19	11U/6

Table 7. Number of units of red cell concentrates given.

Results are consistent with the tamponade effect theory. Drains evacuate the blood that would otherwise be required to achieve the sufficient intra-wound pressure in order to stop the bleeding. The more blood is evacuated, the greater the need for transfusion.

3.6 Hospital stay

With the exception of studies by Cheung et al. and Della Valle et al., which reported a significant difference between the drained and un-drained group, other studies did not found any differences in hospital stay after hip arthroplasty. Drainage does not seem to directly affect the duration of hospitalization. Mean values of hospital stay ranged from 5 to 10 days in both of groups (Table 8). Within the two studies with statistically significant difference in hospital stay, only the difference of one day could be regarded as clinically relevant. Authors interpreted that this difference in length of stay is most likely a reflection of the greater amount of time it took for the drained wounds to become dry. However, wound-healing disturbances in the drained group might have been related to an allogeneic transfusion (in this particular study, the transfusion rates were much higher in patients with closed suction drainage), and not to drain usage per se.

Study	Drained group (days)	Un-drained group (days)	p
Ovadia et al., 1997	10	8.3	0.06
Della Valle et al., 2004	5.1	4.7	0.01
Walmsley et al., 2005	10	10	NA
Kumar et al., 2007	8.9	8.4	0.32
Strahovnik et al., 2010	7	7	0.55
Cheung et al., 2010	7	6	0.03

Table 8. Average hospitalization time.

Namely, there seems to be a relation between allogeneic transfusion and disturbances in wound healing, which in turn affects the hospital stay. The mechanism by which wound-healing disturbances and length of hospital stay are related are still unclear (Weber et al., 2005). First possible explanation is a direct effect of tissue hypoxia as a consequence of decreased values of hemoglobin in the post-operative period. However, in a clinical study, the anemia was present in groups without closed suction drains as well and did not affect wound healing. This effect seems, therefore, unlikely. The alternative explanation might be the immuno-modulatory effect of allogeneic blood. Experimental studies have shown that the immuno-modulatory effects of allogeneic blood transfusion might lead to a decrease in proangiogenic factors that are essential for wound healing (eg. interleukin 8). Allogeneic blood tranfusion might therefore induce a small but significant delay in wound healing. Since drainage seems to affect the transfusion rates, it might also indirectly influence the hospital stay.

3.7 Cost analysis

Three studies analyzed the costs of drainage in total hip arthroplasty. The savings of the cost of closed suction units (hemovacs) was reported if drains were omitted in hip arthroplasty (Ritter et al., 1994; Kim et al., 1998). Della Valle et al. stated that the additional sum could be saved due to a shorter hospital stay in patients without closed suction drainage.

4. Complications of drainage

The unwanted side effects, which occur only in patients where closed suction drainage was used, are described here. The possible deleterious effects of drains on wound infection, need for transfusion and hospital stay were already discussed in the previous section.

4.1 Prolonged drainage from the drain site

Prolonged drainage from the wound is the second type of prolonged drainage in hip arthroplasty. This type of persistent, prolonged drainage occurs on the drain site after the drain is removed. It is more frequent (up to 50% of patients with drainage) and usually more persistent.

Our own study showed that prolonged secretion from the drain site typically started on the third post-operative day and lasted for four days on the average. Prolonged secretion rarely lasted more than 14 days. In addition, the incidence and duration of prolonged serous secretion were comparable between the group with 24-hour drainage and the group with 48-hour drainage. The greatest proportion of patients with active secretion in both groups was present on the 5th post-operative day (Figure 1).

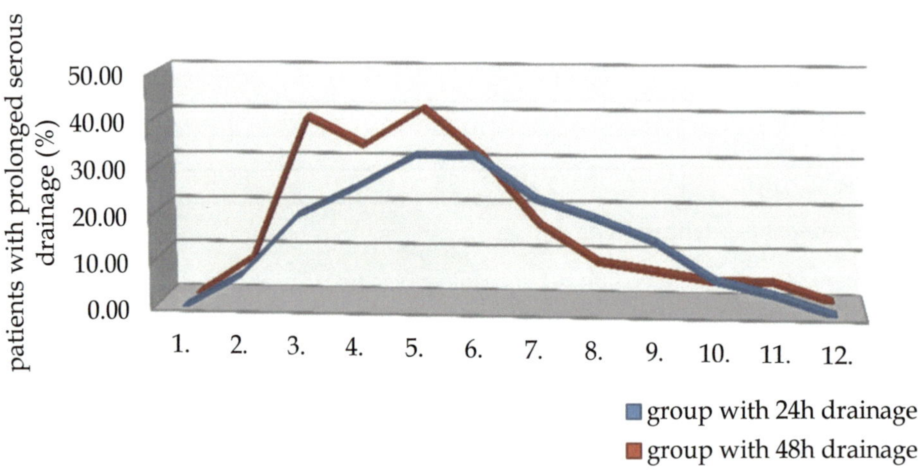

Fig. 1. Proportion of patients with active secretion from the drain site in groups with drainage.

Division of prolonged drainage on the drainage from the wound site and the drainage from the drain site is arbitrary. The cause of drainage is the same regardless on the location. The drainage is linked to a hematoma that develops around the prosthesis. At first, the drainage is bloody, but later turns to serous fluid as the red cells in hematoma sediment. Since the hematoma in the wound is always present whether the drain is present or not, prolonged drainage is always possible. In the un-drained wounds, the drainage can occur through the incision plane, especially if the fascia was not meticulously sutured. In case of a drained wound, the hematoma drains through the drain tube. After the drains are removed, the hematoma may drain through the un-healed drain canal (Figure 2). The drainage stops with the healing of the canal.

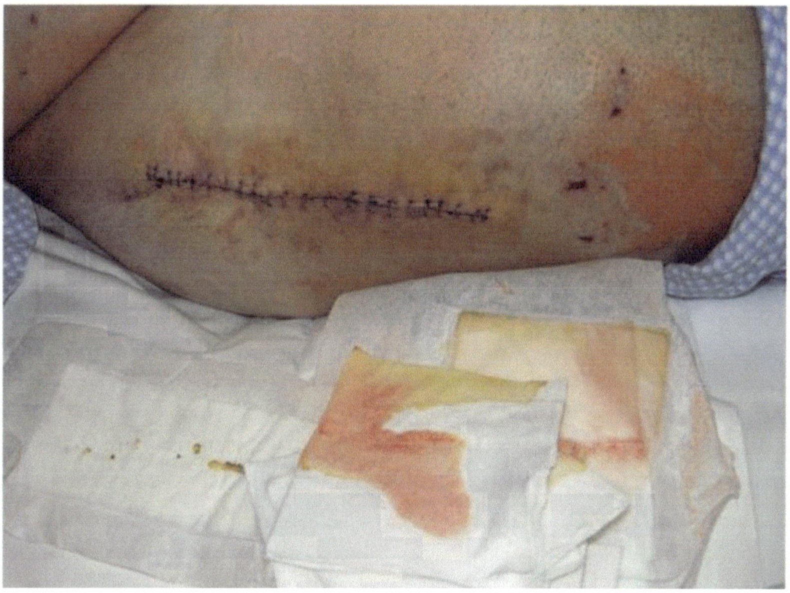

Fig. 2. Wound with prolonged serous secretion through an un-healed drain canal.

In conclusion, late secretion from the drain site is frequent and usually spontaneously resolves within 3 to 4 days. Longer secretion, especially longer than 14 days, predisposes to the development of wound infection. Careful observation, supervised regular changing of the dressings and even revision surgery may be necessary to stop the secretion in persistent cases.

5. Additional methods to influence the drainage

Several additional methods can be applied to decrease the bleeding and hence drainage from the surgical wound. The use of hypotensive anesthesia is well established in orthopaedic surgery. A thorough hemostasis at the end of the procedure is also a prerequisite in hip arthroplasty. Some advocate the use of pneumatic wound compression as a method of reducing post-operative bleeding.

Recently, pharmacological strategies have become of interest to decrease excessive blood lost. An intravenous administration of tranexamic acid before hip arthroplasty significantly decreased peri-operative bleeding (Ekbäck et al., 2000; Singh et al., 2010). Tranexamic acid seems to be a cost-effective and safe mean of minimizing blood loss and reduction in hemoglobin concentrations as well as the need for allogeneic blood transfusion, without increasing the risk of thromboembolic events.

6. Conclusion

Common practice of draining has recently become questioned in orthopaedic surgery. Many randomized trials have been performed, trying to provide a definite answer about the efficacy of draining. Even though the number of trials on the topic is considerable, very few have good methodology which would allow us to draw reliable conclusions. The majority of studies were underpowered for accurate assessment of most important outcomes (eg. wound infection, re-operation rate). Many of them also had a short follow-up period, which allows underreporting of important medical events.

Having already realized the drawbacks of studies in the literature, Parker et al. carried out a meta-analysis. However, due to enormous variety of methods in the orthopaedic community, it is very hard to find studies with homogeneous group of patients. The common denominator of selected studies in their meta-analysis as well as in this review was an elective total hip arthroplasty. Numerous other parameters that could affect the outcomes could not be controlled. For example, even though patients underwent the same procedure, the surgical approach was not uniform in the included studies. Patients varied also in several other parameters: diagnosis, number of drains placed, location of drains, duration of drainage, type of prosthesis, use of thromboprophylaxis, compression of the thigh, trigger for transfusion, post-operative rehabilitation regime, patient's discharge trigger and follow-up period. All these parameters were not uniform or were not even reported.

An evaluation of most of the reported outcomes was given in our review. Since a simple division into pro draining and con draining could not be made for the majority of the observed outcomes, we summarized our conclusions about outcomes as a degree of certainty with regard to the evidence available. Our conclusions are presented in Table 9.

outcome	in favor of		draining	in disfavor of	
	definite evidence	some evidence	undecided	some evidence	definite evidence
Wound infection			X		
Hematoma formation			X		
Bruising of the wound		X			
Drainage from wound		X			
Re-operation			X		
Rehabilitation			X		
Need for re-enforcement		X			
Need for transfusion				X	
Hospital stay				X	
Cost					X
Drainage from drain site					X

Table 9. List of outcomes and categorization in terms of pro et contra draining.

In conclusion, randomized studies have shown that closed suction drainage is not necessary in total hip arthroplasty and may be, in some aspects, even deleterious. However, due to the heterogeneity of practice, every surgeon must combine his own routine with the decision to drain.

7. References

Alexander JW, Korelitz J, Alexander NS. (1976). Prevention of wound infections. A case for closed suction drainage to remove wound fluids deficient in opsonic proteins. *Am J Surg,* Vol. 132, No. 1, (July 1976), pp. 59-63, ISSN 0002-9610

Beer KJ, Lombardi AV, Mallory TH, Vaughn BK. (1991). The efficacy of suction drains after routine total joint arthroplasty. *J Bone Joint Surg Am,* Vol. 73, No. 4, (April 1991), pp. 584-586, ISSN 0021-9355

Cheung EV, Sperling JW, Cofield RH. (2008). Infection associated with hematoma formation after shoulder arthroplasty. *Clin Orthop Relat Res,* Vol. 466, No. 6, (June 2008), pp. 1363-1367, ISSN 0009-921X

Cheung G, Carmont MR, Bing AJ,Kuiper JH, Alcock RJ, Graham NM. (2010). No drain, autologous transfusion drain or suction drain? A randomised prospective study in total hip replacement surgery of 168 patients. *Acta Orthop Belg,* Vol. 76, No. 5, (October 2010), pp. 619-627, ISSN 0001-6462

Della Valle AG, Slullitel G, Vestri R, Comba F, Buttaro M, Piccaluga F. (2004). No need for routine closed suction drainage in elective arthroplasty of the hip. A prospective randomized trial in 104 operations. *Acta Orthop Scand,* Vol. 75, No. 1, (February 2004), pp. 30-33, ISSN 0001-6470

Drinkwater CJ, Neil MJ. (1995). Optimal timing of wound drain removal following total joint arthroplasty. *J Arthroplasty,* Vol. 10, No. 2, (April 1995), pp. 185-189, ISSN 0883-5403

Ekbäck G, Axelsson K, Ryttberg L, Edlund B, Kjellberg J, Weckstrom J et al. (2000). Tranexamic acid reduces blood loss in total hip replacement surgery. *Anest Analg,* Vol. 91, No. 5, (November 2000), pp. 1124-1130, ISSN 0003-2999

Erceg M, Becić K. (2008). Postoperative closed suction drainage following hip and knee aloarthroplasty: drain removal after 24 or after 48 hours? *Lijec Vjesn,* Vol. 130, No. 5-6, (May-June 2008), pp. 133-135, ISSN 0024-3477

Johansson T, Engquist M, Pettersson LG, Lisander B. (2005). Blood loss after total hip replacement: a prospective randomized study between wound compression and drainage. *J Arthroplasty,* Vol. 20, No. 8, (December 2005), pp. 967-971, ISSN 0883-5403

Kim YH, Cho SH, Kim RS. (1998). Drainage versus nondrainage in simultaneous bilateral total hip arthroplasties. *J Arthroplasty,* Vol. 13, No. 2, (February 1998), pp. 156-161, ISSN 0883-5403

Kumar S, Penematsa S, Parekh S. (2007). Are drains required following a routine primary total joint arthroplasty? *Int Orthop,* Vol. 31, No. 5, (October 2007), pp. 593-596, ISSN 0341-2695

Levy, M. (1984). Intraperitoneal drainage. *Am J Surg,* Vol. 147, No. 3, (March 1984), pp. 309-314, ISSN 0002-9610

Murphy JP, Scott JE. (1993). The effectiveness od suction drainage in total hip arthroplasty. *J R Soc Med,* Vol. 86, No. 7, (July 1993), pp. 388-389, ISSN 0141-0768

Niskanen RO, Korkala OL, Haapala J, Kuokkanen HO, Kaukonen JP, Salo SA. (2000). Drainage is of no use in primary uncomplicated cemented hip and knee arthroplasty for osteoarthritis. A prospective randomized study. *J Arthroplasty,* Vol. 15, No. 5, (August 2000), pp. 567-569, ISSN 0883-5403

Ovadia D, Luger E, Menachem A, Dekel S. (1997). Efficacy of closed wound drainage after total joint arthroplasty. A prospective randomized study. *J Arthroplasty,* Vol. 12, No. 3, (April 1997), pp. 317-321, ISSN 0883-5403

Overgaard S, Thomsen NB, Kulinski B, Mossing NB. (1993). Closed suction drainage after hip arthroplasty. Prospective study of bacterial contamination in 81 cases. *Acta Orthop Scand,* Vol. 64, No. 4, (August 1993), pp. 417-420, ISSN 0001-6470

Parrini L, Baratelli M, Parrini M. (1988). Ultrasound examination of haematomas after total hip replacement. *Int Orthop,* Vol. 12, No. 1, pp. 79-82, ISSN 0341-2695

Parvizi J, Ghanem E, Joshi A, Sharkey PF, Hozack WJ, Rothman RH. (2007). Does "excessive" anticoagulation predispose to periprosthetic infection? *J Arthroplasty,* Vol. 22, No. 6 Suppl 2, (September 2007), pp. 24-28, ISSN 0883-5403

Patel VP, Walsh M, Sehgal B, Preston C, DeWal H, Cesare PE. (2007). Factors associated with prolonged wound drainage after primary total hip and knee arthroplasty. *J Bone Joint Surg Am,* Vol. 89, No. 1, (January 2007), pp. 33-38, ISSN 0021-9355

Ritter MA, Keating M, Faris PM. (1994). Closed wound drainage in total hip or total knee replacement. A prospective, randomized study. *J Bone J Surg Am,* Vol. 76, No. 1, (January 1994), pp. 35-38, ISSN 0021-9355

Rowe SM, Yoon TR, Kim YS, Lee GH. (1993). Hemovac drainage after hip arthroplasty. *Int Orthop,* Vol. 17, No. 4, pp. 238-240, ISSN 0341-2695

Saleh K, Olson M, Resig S, Bershadsky B, Kuskowski M, Gioe T, et al. (2002). Predictors of wound infection in hip and knee joint replacement: results from a 20 year surveillance program. *J Orthop Res,* Vol. 20, No. 3, (May 2002), pp. 506-515, ISSN 0736-0266

Singh J, Ballal MS, Mitchell P, Denn PG. (2010). Effects of tranexamic acid on blood loss during total hip arthroplasty. *J Orthop* Surg (Hong Kong), Vol. 18, No. 3, (December 2010), pp. 282-286, ISSN 1022-5536

Sørensen AI, Sørensen TS. (1991). Bacterial growth on suction drain tips. *Acta Orthop Scand,* Vol. 62, No. 5, (October 1991), pp. 451-454, ISSN 0001-6470

Strahovnik A, Fokter SK, Kotnik M. (2010). Comparison of drainage techniques on prolonged serous drainage after total hip arthroplasty. *J Arthroplasty,* Vol. 25, No. 2, (February 2010), pp. 244-248, ISSN 0883-5403

Walmsley PJ, Kelly MB, Hill RF, Brenkel I. (2005). A prospective, randomised, controlled trial of the use o drains in total hip arthroplasty. *J Bone J Surg Br,* Vol. 87, No. 10, (October 2005), pp. 1397-1401, ISSN 0301-620X

Waugh TR, Stinchfield FE. (1961). Suction drainage of orthopaedic wounds. *J Bone Joint Surg Am,* Vol. 43, (October 1961), pp. 939-946, ISSN 0021-9355

Weber EW, Slappendel R, Prins MH, van der Schaaf DB, Durieux ME, Strumper D. (2005). Perioperative blood transfusions and delayed wound healing after hip replacement surgery: Effects on duration of hospitalization. *Anesth Analg,* Vol. 100, No. 5, (May 2005), pp. 1416-1421, ISSN 0003-2999

Widman J, Jacobsson H, Larsson SA, Isacson J. (2002). No effect of drains on the postoperative hematoma volume in hip replacement surgery. A randomized study using scintigraphy. *Acta Orthop Scand,* Vol. 73, No. 6, (December 2002), pp. 625-629, ISSN 0001-6470

Willett KM, Simmons CD, Bentley G. (1988). The effect of suction drains after total hip replacement. *J Bone Joint Surg Br,* Vol. 70. No. 4, (August 1988), pp. 607-610, ISSN 0301-620X

Wood JJ, Bevis PM, Bannister GC. (2007). Wound oozing after total hip arthroplasty. *Ann R Coll Surg Eng,* Vol. 89, No. 2, (March 2007), pp. 140-142, ISSN 0035-8843

7

Rehabilitation of Patients Following Arthroplasty of the Hip and Knee

Magdalena Wilk-Frańczuk
Frycz-Modrzewski Cracow University,
Cracow Rehabilitation Center, Scanmed St. Rafael Hospital, Cracow
Poland

1. Introduction

Arthroplasty (Latin arthroplastica) with endoprosthesis is a reconstructive procedure whose purpose is to restore the damaged joint by creating a substitute joint with actions similar to those of the physiological joint. The term "arthroplasty" is used interchangeably in the literature with "total joint replacement" or "alloplasty."

There are several indications for arthroplasty, especially involving the large joints of the lower limbs, such as hip or knee, which are exposed to significant loads. Total joint replacement is mainly applied to joints damaged by a disease process (e.g. osteoarthritis). Arthroplasties are performed in people of all ages; however, elderly patients make up the majority. Primarily cemented or uncemented prostheses are implanted, rarely the so-called hybrid type, where only one element is embedded in bone cement. Regardless of the type of prosthesis, however, or its construction, the operated joint, or the surgical approaches used, as well as the patient's age, Body Mass Index (BMI), or general state of health, each patient needs an adequate rehabilitation protocol. This protocol should be instituted before surgery, or immediately after if the operation is performed on an emergency basis.

Since the application of the first prosthesis, there has been continuous progress in this field. This applies to the materials and design of the prostheses, the surgical techniques used, and post-operative rehabilitation. The largest differences relate to the point at which physiotherapy begins and (and perhaps most importantly) when the patient stands up and full weight is put on the joint. The physician, usually the orthopedic surgeon who performed the operation, makes the decision to implement rehabilitation. But the decision as to when to stand the patient up and the assessment of the load capacity of the operated limb also belong to physiotherapist.

Close interdisciplinary cooperation is always of great importance for the patient, in this case the patient after arthroplasty, who often requires an individual rehabilitation program (Grotle et al., 2010). This individualization involves some modifications of the general scheme of rehabilitation developed and used in orthopedic and rehabilitation centers. After standard operations, the early full loading of the operated limb gives much better post-operative results, and the patient regains functional capacity sooner. Outcome assessment should be monitored. Studies have used different research methods, including the functional evaluation of patients using different scales, such as the Harris scale, a 100-point scale that assesses the quality of life especially of older patients, as well as the impact of various factors such as BMI on the healing process (Cichy et al., 2008; Dudda et al., 2010; Starowicz et al., 2005). In addition to standard physiotherapy assessment instruments, methods based on computer analysis use dedicated equipment and computer programs (e.g. stabilometry platforms, sEMG, strain gauge tests, photoelastic tests, pedobarography, and thermal tests – Burnfield et al., 2010; Cichy & Wilk, 2006; Cichy et al., 2008; Maguire et al., 2010; Wilk et al., 2004, 2008). This allows for more objective results, and also leads to the formulation of new ideas for modifying and optimizing patient rehabilitation programs.

2. Rehabilitation after hip arthroplasty

Arthroplasty with prosthesis, or total hip replacement with an artificial joint to replace the one that has been destroyed, has ushered in a new era in the treatment of degenerative arthritis. The occurrence of osteoarthritis seems to be a consequence of the European style of civilization, as it almost does not occur in India, Mexico, South America, Africa, or the Far East (except for Japan and Australia). In Poland, according to epidemiological studies by various authors, osteoarthritis affects approximately 10 to 20% of the population, and therefore between 4 and 8 million people, including approximately 4% between 18 and 34 years of age and up to 85% of people over the age of 75. From the clinical point of view, and in terms of frequency, osteoarthritis of the hip occupies a prominent place next to osteoarthritis of the knee and spinal joints. It is characterized by localized pain in the groin area, on the front or side of the thigh, and is often associated with radiating pain around the knee. These symptoms appear and worsen after exercise, or a longer walk, but often also occur at rest and at night. There is stiffness in the morning or after prolonged immobilization of the joint, and the dysfunction is often associated with swelling, limited range of motion, muscle weakness, and radiographic changes.

The etiology of osteoarthritis of the hip is easy to determine if the patient has a congenital or acquired defect during development, such as hip dysplasia, Perthes disease, or deformity of the femoral head. Some other factors that are easy to determine are adverse biochemical changes occurring in articular cartilage, or a dislocation or fracture within the joint in the past. Frequently, however, the cause of the disease remains difficult to establish, because degenerative-deforming hip joint diseases are not an homogeneous disease entity, but a complex of lesions arising as a result of different causal factors. Given the diversity of these factors, degenerative-deforming changes of the hip joints can be divided into two basic groups: - primary (idiopathic) coxarthrosis and secondary coxarthrosis. The first group includes patients diagnosed on the basis of clinical examinations, along with radiological and laboratory tests. and cannot be said to prove the root cause of the disease. The second group are patients with, for example, congenital or acquired hip disorders.

The diagnostic criteria for primary hip osteoarthritis adopted and published in 2000 by the American College of Rheumatology include pain in the joint and at least two of the three following symptoms: ESR <20 mm after 1 hour; edge or central osteophytes detected radiographically; joint space stenosis (Moody, 2000).

The degenerative process is irreversible. However, appropriately individualized and systematic conservative treatment helps to reduce pain, maintain range of motion, and increase muscle strength, thereby reducing disability and slowing the progression of the disease. This treatment involves the use of NSAIDs and analgesics, and an appropriate rehabilitation program, which consists of physical treatments, kinesitherapy, and if necessary the selection of appropriate auxiliary orthopedic equipment (canes, crutches, walkers). Possible supplements include occupational therapy and education involving the patients and their families, to make them familiar with the specific nature of the disease, ongoing conservative treatment, prevention, and surgical options.

Unfortunately, conservative treatment of osteoarthritis only slows the progress of the disease, and is therefore associated with the slow deterioration of the patients' overall efficiency and their ability to perform activities of daily living, such as walking, washing, performing physiological functions without assistance, dressing, preparing meals, etc. That is why a person who has severe pain while walking, even when at rest, and significant motor deficits, even with small radiographic changes, requires surgical treatment. The method of choice is the replacement of the overused or damaged joint with an artificial one. In the overwhelming number of cases this concerns older patients (over 65 years of age), especially women (at a ratio of 3:1). Hip prosthesis implantation in these patients has now become standard procedure in Poland and worldwide.

The creator of replacement arthroplasty is considered historically to be Themistocles Gluck, who in 1891 developed and implanted the first artificial ball-and-socket joint. Further studies were focused on finding new materials for the implants, new models and surgical techniques. The most significant development of hip joint replacement began in the 1960s and continues until today. The founder of modern total joint replacement is J. Charnley, who made the first implantation of a hip prosthesis with a polyethylene acetabulum. Since 1951, polymethylmethacrylate has been used as bone cement for fixing cemented prostheses. However, a fundamental feature of this cement is its "aging," as evidenced by the occurrence of cracking and irritation due to reactive granulation tissue, which separates the cement from the bone, leading to loosening of the prosthesis. The development of technology and operating methods did not produce improved rehabilitation until the 1980s. In general, cemented prostheses are used to treat older patients, for whom early mobilization is important with full weight bearing during ambulation with both lower limbs. This is important because of age-related, physiological changes in motor coordination and muscle strength and to prevent complications from the respiratory and circulatory systems.

The first cementless prosthesis was applied in the 1980s. These prostheses are designed for young people with the potential for regeneration and osteogenesis of the bone, and good structural conditions of the acetabulum and femur. The construction of cementless endoprostheses is intended to match the material to the biological and strength features of the bone. The fastening elements of cementless prostheses are the result of many studies, which have recently led to the creation of threaded or press-fitted cups. The construction and method of mounting screwed-in and press-fitted prostheses produces good stabilization and the ability to distribute forces evenly over the entire length of the stem and acetabular surface, which also allows for quick loading of the limb.

The further development of arthroplasty depends primarily on interdisciplinary cooperation with physicians,engineers, and physiotherapists. The introduction of the implant to the bone always changes the distribution of internal stresses. Biomechanical studies (Będziński & Ścigała, 2000) on the effects of various types of endoprosthesis stems on the strain in the shaft of the femur showed non-physiological stress distribution and deformation of bone tissue in the case of long stems. Recently short-stemmed prostheses allow for a more favorable distribution of bone strain and smaller overloads in some areas within the femur when loading the lower limb. Evaluation of the results of surgical treatment and rehabilitation with the use of short-stem endoprosthesis shows a subjective reduction in pain intensity and less time to stand up and learn to walk, which is beneficial for speeding up the healing process and returning the patient to independent performance of activities of daily life after 4 - 8 weeks. This is also a financial issue (shorter hospital stay, no need for third party assistance, etc.).

Development of the stem design for the hip prosthesis has been moving in the direction of shorter and smaller stems, in which the stress distribution between implant-bone will allow the most accurate reproduction of physiological conditions. New solutions in hip surface replacement are also used for this purpose. In addition, the way of thinking has changed in favor of implanting a greater number of cementless prostheses in the elderly, whenever proper bone structure allows for such a possibility.

The criteria for evaluating treatment outcomes using endoprosthesis are the same for all stypes, and include the assessment of prosthesis stabilization, subjective sensations of pain, and functional capacity, as affected by muscle strength and range of motion. Muscle strength, an important factor for functional capabilities, depends partly on individual and hereditary characteristics, such as the cross section of the muscle and its structure, but primarily on the level of physical activity (Wilk et al., 2004; Wilk & Frańczuk, 2003, 2005a; Wilk-Frańczuk et al., 2011). The latter develops and takes shape during normal human development. Rapid increases in muscle strength begin in boys at age 13-14 and lasts until age 19-20. In later years (after age 30) it remains constant, then decreases. In girls, the stabilization of muscle strength occurs after puberty. As a result of the processes of human aging, physical capacity gradually decreases. Between the ages of 20 and 30 years, skeletal muscles make up about 45% of the human body, but after 70 years of age, only 27%. The decrease in muscle strength (about 1% per year) as a result of the process of aging is caused primarily by progressive muscle atrophy and changes occurring in peripheral nerves. This leads to limitations, and even loss of locomotion, which is a serious problem because it leads to a decrease in the cardio-pulmonary exercise capacity of the patient and the development of metabolic diseases. In the United States, research on the effects of rehabilitation combined with strength training for older people found that even at the age of 90 it is possible to increase isometric force, slow down significantly the loss of muscle mass, and enhance locomotor capabilities.

In the case of hip arthroplasty with a prosthesis, functional outcome seems to be the most convincing parameter of assessment, hence early and appropriate rehabilitation is very important to obtain the best functional outcome, as we have emphasized above. Arthroplasty, by eliminating pain and increasing the range of motion in the joint that is reduced by osteoarthritis, allows training to be intensified, which increases muscle mass and strength. Thus the patient gets, in addition to pain relief, the possibility of recovering locomotion, and thereby obtains greater functional efficiency and an important factor contributing to a higher quality of life (QOL). Patient assessment from this point of view is rare in the literature, where most of the authors work on a variety of point-scales, taking into account the local and overall efficiency of the patient, and in some cases also the radiological picture. For many years the basic, relatively simple method of evaluating the functional status of the patient after surgery arthroplasty was the Charnley or Harris test. This assessment is still widely used as an additional outcome measure. The value of the Harris scale (Harris Hip Score) has been well documented in the literature (the scale has been in use since 1969). It also features very reproducible results, and the evaluation includes the assessment ofQOL parameters. The Harris scale assesses the following groups of parameters: pain (intensity, medications used); gait (limping, use of crutches or canes, walking distance); performance of daily activities (climbing stairs, sitting, tying shoes); ability to use public transport; hip range of motion (detailed ranges); presence or absence of deformities (contractures or shortening of the limb).

The end result of the evaluation of individual parameters is a sub-point value, all of which when added give the total score on a scale from 0 to 100 points.

A number of other scales have been developed for the clinical evaluation of patients with osteoarthritis of the hip, before and after surgery. Currently in use, in addition to the aforementioned Harris scale, are the Merle d'Aubigne-Postel scale, the Bellamy scale, the WOMAC scale (Western Ontario and McMasters Universities Questionnaire), whose particular advantage is allowing the patient to make a self-assessment, the JOA scale (Japanese Orthopaedic Association), the Wolfe scale, and the Lequesne scale.

Technological progress has made it possible to develop more objective methods for assessing the results of arthroplasty. These include the assessment of gait parameters. The basic parameters initially used to evaluate gait basic included gait speed, step frequency, and step length, measured by means of micro switches attached to the patient's shoes. In subsequent years there has been a new method to identify and assess the symmetry of the lower limbs and gait cycle phases using miniature accelerometers. There is also a more thorough analysis of gait using a series of images made with the patient walking, at a frequency from 300 to 1200 shots per minute, or even something as unusual as the method developed by Bergman's team, based on the implantation of a prosthesis fitted with a telemetry transmitter. Another contemporary method is to measure ground reaction forces during gait using dynamographic platforms. These allow us to measure ground reaction forces in all directions and linear momentum, and therefore to assess the accuracy of limb loading when walking. Currently, the latest optical electronic devices have been used to develop gait analysis systems for registering the movement trajectory of markers placed on the patient, often with the addition of integrated graphics platforms, known as dynamographic platforms. There are also other devices, such as, for example, gas meters for measuring oxygen and carbon dioxide in exhaled air, and electromyography.

Such tests allow us to collect a large amount of information; however, they are feasible only in specialized laboratories and report only the overall efficiency of the system. Assessment by these means is incomplete and does not affect measurements of range of motion in the operated joint and the pelvic girdle muscle forces responsible for individual movements. Such studies may be more useful for assessing the efficiency of locomotion, and indirectly serve to evaluate the use of implants, but they do not return function and muscle strength. Recently, encouraging results of functional assessment of muscles and ranges of motion after implantation of prostheses in the operated limb have been obtained using the technique of wireless surface electromyography - sEMG (Maguire et al., 2010).

There is no generally accepted rehabilitation protocol for patients after total hip replacement with cemented or cementless prosthesis. The differences relate to both the methods of rehabilitation and the date of commencement of full loading of the operated joint (Iyengar et al., 2007; Wilk & Frańczuk, 2005a). A constant search for optimal solutions is therefore necessary. Rehabilitation after cemented hip arthroplasty starts from the first day after surgery with the introduction of breathing exercises. The second day begins with isometric exercises, passive-active exercises of the operated limb, active exercises of the unaffected limb and upper limbs. On the third day we begin to stand the patients up and teach them to walk with crutches or a walker with no weight bearing. What is most preferred, however, is for the patient to behave consistently with the features of normal gait - the operated foot is put on the ground with no weight bearing. At the end of the first week after the operation, gradual loading of the operated limb begins, starting with 20-30% of body weight. A weight training floor is most often used to teach the patient the proper balance of body weight. Full weight bearing is applied after the stitches have been removed.

In the case of cementless hip arthroplasty, all motor activity is often delayed. Exercises usually begin on the first day, but the patient stands for the first time on the 5th to 14th day after surgery, and partial loading of the operated limb starts 4-6 weeks after surgery, with full weight bearing after 3-4 months. Some authors recommend no weight bearing for up to 6 months, although others support full weight bearing as soon as possible (2-3 days after surgery), especially when screwed-in implants have been used (e.g. Zweymüller-Stemcup). In general, in the first weeks after arthroplasty the appropriate positioning of the operated limb is recommended - slight adduction, 5 degree hip and knee flexion, neutral rotation position. Excessive abduction, internal rotation and crossing the legs are contraindicated.

Based on many years of research and observation, I believe that after the standard procedure, when the prosthesis is properly implanted, the rehabilitation protocol for both cemented and cementless prostheses should be the same, and include early loading of the operated limb (Cichy et al., 2008; Wilk & Frańczuk, 2003, 2004). This does not apply to non-standard patients (extra implants strengthening the acetabulum, bone grafts, proximal femur fracture fixation, etc.). Limb loading in these cases is delayed; the patients usually walk with crutches till the bone is healed, and after that gradual weight bearing is introduced. It is best to start learning before surgery.

It has been shown that in the first period after surgery the greatest impact on the progress of rehabilitation results from: minimally invasive surgery within the interval between the tensor fasciae latae, rectus femoris and sartorius muscles, or within the interval between the tensor fasciae latae and gluteus medius muscles; epidural analgesia in the first 24 hours after surgery; the use of Continuous Passive Motion (CPM) in the first days after surgery.

In contrast to arthroplasty performed with minimally invasive approaches, the other operating approaches require a delay in the entire rehabilitation process, mainly related to standing the patient up and teaching ambulation, even by a few weeks, because premature active rehabilitation in the first weeks after surgery can lead to dislocation of the implant (Dudda et al., 2008). The type of implanted prosthesis may also affect postoperative functionality.

A common problem after total hip replacement is a subjective sense of unequal length of the legs. If there is no actual reduction in the relative limb length, one should take into account the possibility of pelvic positioning dysfunction, which can be expressed by the asymmetry of iliac spine positioning (anterior superior and posterior superior). Asymmetrical muscle tone can be the cause of this.

About 1100 hip and knee replacements per year are done in our center (the Cracow Rehabilitation Center). Lateral or antero-lateral approaches are routinely used for hip replacement, and the anterior approach with ischemia for knee replacement. The mean operating time for this type of treatment varies between 45 and 60 minutes, with spinal anesthesia, and the patients are subjected to a constant process of rehabilitation. Before the operation the patients are informed about the stages of rehabilitation that will follow, and learn to walk on crutches with different loads on the lower limbs, which increases their conscious and active participation in the treatment process.

On the first post-operative day CPM is introduced, which improves the limb blood supply, accelerates the absorption of the hematoma, reduces the hypertonicity of periarticular tissues, and allows the patient to get rid of the anxiety associated with the movement of the operated joint. In subsequent days, exercises are gradually introduced, applying the principles of individualization and gradation of difficulty. On the third day, walking re-education begins, with gradually increasing weight bearing and the use of appropriate orthopedic aids (walker, crutches). Due to the fact that arthroplasty is most often related to a chronic degenerative process, which also causes major progressive pathological changes in connective tissue and contributes to a significant reduction in patient activity, special attention is paid to the restoration of normal movement patterns. It is also essential to learn to maintain and control proper posture, which may be disturbed due to the abnormal movement patterns both before and after surgery (e.g. due to the constant need to relieve one leg, abnormal movement with the use of one crutch).

One of the characteristic features of degenerative joint diseases is that only a relatively small percentage of the patients who present for treatment (8-10%) are vocationally active. Many studies have shown that once patients have been relieved of their pain symptoms, they are more willing to exercise and become physically active. It is also important to draw attention to the analysis of treatment outcomes in the first period after surgery. This period is especially important, since exercises can be intensified immediately after surgery, and it is during this period that CPM can be applied most effectively. In any event, the impact of the latter is not perceptible at a later stage. Early rehabilitation (especially CPM), commenced immediately after surgery, along with appropriate pharmacotherapy and the application of elastic pressure stockings on the lower limbs, also helps to prevent such complications as pneumonia, venous embolisms or thrombosis. This is consistent with the observations of other authors. The results of studies on muscle strength suggest that muscle strength begins to recover about 3 months after surgery, while an appropriate program of rehabilitation can lead to increased muscle strength within 6 months. This observation is confirmed by the analysis of range of motion. When functionality is evaluated according to the Merle D'Aubigne functional scale, published research results indicate that a distinct majority of patients recover good functionality in the operated limb after six months. These results are similar to those obtained in respect to muscle strength, although they do not in fact show the dynamics of change in respect to either muscle strength or range of motion.

In the prevention of disorders of posture, those patients who will have to use elbow crutches for a longer period of time are advised to use two crutches rather than one, which affects the symmetry of body work during ambulation. Approximately one week after surgery, the patient learns to walk up and down stairs, initially leading with the non-operated limb while going up, and with the operated limb while going down. Throughout the period of treatment we adapt the rehabilitation program to the individual patient, and where indicated we use other physiotherapeutic methods (e.g. physical agents).

The rehabilitation applied initially in the orthopedic department should be continued later at home, with the cooperation of the family, or, if that is not possible, in a medical rehabilitation unit (Iyengar et al., 2007). The lack of appropriate rehabilitation in this early period can often seriously undermine the effects of the surgeon's efforts. In the later, post-discharge period, our patients are often advised to try Nordic Walking.

3. Rehabilitation after arthroplasty of the knee

From the clinical point of view, as previously stated, gonarthrosis, along with coxarthrosis and spondylarthrosis, is among the most significant joint pathologies. When the changes are significant, gonarthrosis can be handicapping, while pain occurs with even minor deviations from the physiological norm. In most cases the causes of the disease are difficult to determine, since degenerative and deformative changes do not constitute a unified nosological entity, but rather a syndrome of pathological changes caused by the operation of various etiological factors. Research has shown that gonarthrosis does not affect only the elderly, since degenerative changes in the knee also occur in much younger persons. Among the generally recognized risk factors are the following: abnormalities in joint structure; biomechanical disturbances; overloading of the joint; microlesions; obesity.

Gonarthrosis can also be caused by deformities (varus more often than valgus), which cause one of the joint components to be overloaded. Conservative treatment consists in rehabilitation and pharmacotherapy, while patients are advised to adopt a conservative lifestyle and lose weight. The degenerative process that has begun is slowed down under the influence of conservative treatment, but even so the changes tend to progress. As in the case of hip arthroplasty, the appearance of severe pain that occurs both during ambulation and at rest, along with restricted range of motion in the knees, eventually leads to a significant degree of disability. In that situation, the treatment of choice is surgery, involving the replacement of the damaged joint with an artificial one.

The physiological exhaustion of tissue that is characteristic of aging, especially in the weight-bearing joints, is one of the most commonly cited causes of primary degenerative disease of the largest joint in the human body, the knee. The external loads on this joint that result from the forces of gravity and ground reaction are to a large extent dependent on body mass. The load on the joint in standing position constitutes approximately 43% of body weight (Kabsch & Bober, 2001). During ambulation, the pressure on the joint surfaces changes depending on the gait phase: the greatest load occurs at the beginning of the support phase. These parameters can also change in the event of varus or valgus deformations of the joint, which amplify the pressure on the most heavily loaded parts of the joint. Biomechanical research has produced different models of knee joint loading (the Maquet model, the Denham model), taking account of assymetrical loads on joint surfaces in the case of varus or valgus deformities of the lower joints. Indeed, such deformities are among the indications for surgical treatment. When the angle of deviation is not too great, correctional popliteal osteotomy of the tibia is applied. Deformities that produce a greater angle of deviation require arthroplasty with endoprosthesis, especially when they are accompanied by deformities of the joint surfaces.

As in the case of the hip joint, the increased number of knee arthroplasties performed in the last decade has produced a search for new solutions in surgery and rehabilitation. The first knee endoprostheses were implanted in the 1950s, when a leading role in their development was played by Smith-Petersen, Waldius, and Campbell, among others. These prostheses had a hinge construction, which often caused early loosening. In the 1960s and 70s, new types of prosthesis were introduced. In 1971, the Canadian surgeon Frank H. Gunston, who was cooperating at that time with Sir John Charnley on a new type of hip prosthesis (consisting of a metal femoral part mounted on bone cement and a polyethylene acetabulum), developed a polycentric knee prosthesis, based on their joint research. Since that time there has been constant progress, thanks to research on improving the construction of the prosthesis in such a way as to reproduce most accurately the movement of a natural joint, and on the application of construction materials that are as biocompatibile as possible. Many prosthesis models have been designed, two of which are currently most often used: mobile-bearing and fixed-bearing, posterior stabilized with a pin to replace the functions of the posterior cruciate ligament. Among these designs there are many types of prostheses that can be adapted to the individual patient, including, for example, unicompartmental prostheses (Zeni & Snyder-Mackler, 2010).

Both types of prosthesis, mobile-bearing and fixed-bearing, have their adherents. In the case of mobile-bearing prostheses, what is emphasized is the possibility to achieve a greater range of flexion in the knee joint and a physiological gait. Fixed-bearing prostheses, in turn, provide greater possibilities to correct deformities in the knee joint, but they can also cause shearing forces to develop, which can lead to loosening of the joint. However, it is often emphasized in the literature that the frequency of occurrence of loosening in both types of prosthesis is comparable. On the other hand, in the case of the knee joint, the implantation of a prothesis with a modeling system that uses an MRI of the lower limb reduces bleeding (since it is then unnecessary to open the medullary canal), shortens operating time, and, as indicated by preliminary studies, makes it possible to obtain better outcomes, in terms of a quicker recovery of full functionality of the operated limb.

Progress and the development of knee arthroplasty with endoprosthesis has made it necessary to adapt rehabilitation procedures, so as to obtain the best possible outcome for the patient. There are many different factors, before, during, and after surgery, that can affect the treatment outcome; the primary goal of the surgery itself is to reduce pain and increase the range of motion in the limb affected by pathological changes. These two effects, in turn, are intended to promote recovery of normal gait, thereby allowing the patient to regain functional independence and normal activity in daily life, which is a major factor in QOL. It should be obvious, then, that proper rehabilitation, adapted to the individual needs and capabilities of the patient and to contemporary standards of practice, plays a very significant role in outcome. In publications from as late as the mid-1990s, there are still descriptions of post-operative rehabilitation that began on the 2nd or 3rd day after surgery with kinesitherapy (active-passive and passive exercises), becoming gradually more intensive over the next several days. It was only on the 8th day after surgery that the patient was encouraged to sit on the edge of the bed, and on the 10th day that the first attempt was made to stand the patient up, followed by ambulation training from the 12th to the 14th day (Nolewajek et al., 2008), who studied the risk factors for deep vein thrombosis in the lower limbs in patients after total knee arthroplasty, found that the time when the patient first stands up is of major importance in the prevention of embolic or thrombotic complications, alongside age, obesity, and duration of surgery. Rehabilitation after arthroplasty of the knee is oriented primarily towards allowing the patient to return to normal activities of daily living and functional independence as soon as possible.

An appropriate program of rehabilitation is thus an essential element in treatment, to prepare the patient for surgery and after surgery, with the goal of standing the patient up as soon as possible, teaching ambulation, and recovering as much functionality as possible. The rehabilitation process is often lengthy, and the patient's physical fitness before surgery is of no small importance. Currently, given the necessity to adapt the rehabilitation program to each individual patient, rehabilitation begins on the 1st or 2nd day post-operatively, with respiratory exercises and isometrics, accompanied by active-passive and active exercises.

The patient stands for the first time on the 2nd or 3rd day post-operatively, initially with a high walking platform, followed by ambulation training with elbow crutches. On the 7th to 9th day post-operatively the patient begins to learn how to walk up and down stairs, and then, depending on the patient's fitness and gait mechanics with crutches, two-beat ambulation with a single elbow crutch on the arm contralateral to the operated knee. It is essential, however, to pay attention to the patient's body posture in motion, and if asymmetrical shoulder positioning is observed during ambulation with one crutch, then the use of two crutches is recommended. Just as in the case of hip replacement surgery, this prevents the patient from becoming accustomed to an abnormal pattern of motion.

The rehabilitation of patients after total knee arthroplasty is a complex task for the physiotherapist. An important goal is to achieve full extension of the joint and the greatest possible flexion. This task is rendered all the more difficult by the fact that practically every patient has pain symptoms that hinder or prevent intensive kinesitherapy. Pain reduction, then, can be regarded as the first goal of rehabilitation. An analysis of the impact of low temperatures on the human body leads to the conclusion that its analgesic effect is the one felt most quickly. In the research group, this effect was noted in all patients. The analgesic effect has been observed by many authors, in respect to different joints (knee, hip). The research performed first by our group on the application of local cryotherapy in the treatment of painful shoulder syndrome has shown that this method makes a major contribution to eliminating pain, which makes it possible to implement therapeutic exercises at an early stage. Under the influence of pain, a vicious circle often forms: pain causes a limited range of mobility in the joint, which leads to increased muscle tension and further limitation of motion, steadily increasing the level of pain.

The implementation of a systematic rehabilitation program for patients after total knee arthroplasty, both cemented and cementless, not only produces good outcomes, but also, as in the case of other surgical procedures, prevents complications. Among the rehabilitation techniques used with knee arthroplasty patients there are some special methods, such as CPM, biological feedback devices, or physicotherapy, especially local cryotherapy (Wilk & Frańczuk, 2004, 2005a, 2005b). Disturbances of proprioception after surgery render it necessary to include exercises in a closed kinematic chain and exercises to correct equilibrium in the later stage of the rehabilitation program.

Stabilometric platforms or parapodiums are very useful for evaluating equilibrium in patients recovering from total knee arthroplasty. These devices, in addition to teaching various activities, often connected with biofeedback, can also provide an objective evaluation of treatment outcome. The application of rotors with computer analysis of training supports the proper training of the symmetrical work of the lower limbs after total knee arthroplasty.

4. Rehabilitation after arthroplasty of the hip or knee in older patients

The increasing percentage of older persons in the general population is making it essential to search diligently for ways to preserve a level of fitness that would allow functional independence to be preserved, even in advanced old age (Marks, 2010). At present the maximum duration of human life is estimated at 110-120 years (though there are persons who live longer, and there are frequent news reports about persons who are older yet), but this pertains to persons characterized by exceptional genetic traits, and is also conditioned by biological and environmental conditions. An example of this problem might be the more than 100,000 centenarians living in Japan, as compared to some African countries, where the average life expectancy does not exceed 50 years. Still, given the increasing life expectancy, the literature increasingly divides the older population into three separate age brackets: the "young-old" (65-74), the "old old" (75-84), and the "oldest old" (over 85) (Evgeniadis et al., 2008; Wilk-Frańczuk et al., 2011; Wright et al., 2011). This increasing life span, undoubtedly related to the progress of civilization, including advances in medicine, means that more and more people are reaching the age of 65 in much better health than was the case in previous generations. Women continue to make up a majority of the older population, since their life expectancy is several years longer on the average than that of men. However, research performed with a group of 94 centenarians showed that the men in this group, though they made up only 12% of the whole group, were in better physical condition and generally led a more active life.

In spite of the fact that a constantly growing number of older persons are fitter and more active than before, still, the progress of involutionary processes in physiological aging causes limitations and poses numerous problems, especially after age 75. The frequent co-occurrence of several pathological processes with the physiological changes of normal aging often makes diagnosis and treatment difficult. The problems are compounded by deteriorating sensory perception and frequent depressive episodes, which renders it necessary to make medical personnel aware of the differences in the course of disease and associated treatment in the elderly patient.

One of the basic goals of treatment is to make it possible for the older person to return to independence in activities of daily living. This is conditional upon good health, and fundamentally affects the quality of life. The period during which the patient is dependent upon someone else should be as short as possible, and the family's support should be oriented towards motivating the patient to return to health. The primary means to achieving the greatest possible functionality and maintaining it throughout the lifespan is comprehensive rehabilitation, understood both as the sum of all its components, and as a model of procedure. The individualization of this process is particularly essential in older patients, especially in respect to the possibility of conducting parts of the rehabilitation program in the patient's home or in the form of ambulatory rehabilitation. This reduces the appearance of cognitive and emotional disturbances associated with the stress that is caused by being away from home, in an unfamiliar place. Older patients are often reluctant to agree to hospitalization, since for them the hospital is associated with serious illness and death. In situations where a hospital stay is inevitable, for example when surgery is necessary, its duration should be as brief as possible.

Currently, modern rehabilitation is creating conditions for standing the patients up and teaching them to walk as early as possible. In older persons with deformative and degenerative changes, eliminating pain and increasing locomotor capacity, in terms of gait ergonomics and efficiency, is of crucial importance to quality of life. One of the factors that has the most influence on the whole course of rehabilitation is the possibility of full weight bearing on the operated limb at the earliest possible moment. Another factor that reduces the number of potential fatal post-operative complications has been the introduction, since the beginning of this century, of preventive measures against thrombotic and embolic complications, not only in the form of low molecular weight heparin, but also thanks to changes in the philosophy of rehabilitation and a more active approach to elderly patients. This pertains not only to patients in orthopedic and traumatological wards, but also others, for example, patients in cardiological units after a heart attack. A more active and earlier rehabilitation based on early standing and the application of modern physiotherapeutic methods, such as CPM and other forms of kinesitherapy, has become something like a natural supplement to surgery. Of particular significance in this group of patients are the following: comprehensive, interdisciplinary preparation for surgery; rehabilitation that begins even before the operation; weight-bearing on the operated limb as soon as possible after surgery (Wilk & Frańczuk, 2004).

All of these factors contribute significantly to enabling the older patient to recover functionality, reducing the period of dependence on others, and improving the quality of life. The individualization of treatment, in turn, involves taking into account all dysfunctions and the level of mental and physical fitness, as well as the patient's involvement in planning rehabilitation. Currently, due to changes in both orthopedic procedures and rehabilitation, the mortality rate in this patient group is not high (several percent), and is more dependent on concomitant disorders in elderly patients, such as diabetes and other diseases, or dementia, which can hinder cooperation with medical personnel, or the medical history, than on the arthroplasty itself. This is also indicated by the results in hip arthroplasty that are now being achieved even in patients over 85 , the "oldest old". The final outcome of rehabilitation in these patients has not been observed to be significantly different from those of patients in other age brackets.

The rehabilitation program is always adapted to the current condition and subjective well-being of the patients, as well as their individual physical capacities. Before arthroplasty there are active, assisted, isometric, and respiratory exercises, along with positions and exercises to prevent edema. The patients are informed about what will happen after surgery, how soon they will stand and learn to walk, and about increasing weight-bearing on the operated lower limb with a walker and elbow crutches. All patients receive pharmacotherapy to prevent thrombosis for 14 days after surgery, while still hospitalized, using low molecular weight heparin administered subcutaneously (which is also continued after discharge, for an average of about 6 weeks). Elastic stockings are used in the perioperative period, and epidural anesthetics are also administered for a period of 48 hours after surgery. Rehabilitation commences on the first day after surgery, using respiratory exercises, which are continued as long as the patient remains on the ward. Next, on the second and third days, there are isometric and active-passive exercises for the operated limb, as well as CPM using electrical rail devices, such as the Artromot, Physiotek, or Canwell machines (extension and flexion of the hip with simultaneous flexion of the knee, and with the last-mentioned device, the ankle joint as well). The range of flexion in the hip joint is gradually increased to the extent possible given the patient's capacity. During this same period the patient gradually begins to stand, beginning with sitting on the edge of the bed, then standing beside the bed with a walker and learning to walk. As muscle function is recovered in the lower limb, the program is expanded to include assisted and active exercises, the walking distance is increased, and more weight is placed on the operated limb. On the 11th or 12th day after surgery, the first attempts are made to walk up and down stairs. There are two rehabilitation sessions daily (with CPM for 120-180 minutes a day), and after discharge the patient is instructed as to how to proceed further.

An important new direction for research in this area is the evaluation of posture stability, equilibrium, and displacing the center of gravity. For this purpose it is possible to use both clinical tests and appropriate devices, which often allow for a graphic display of the results. One example of this type of apparatus is the static-dynamic parapodium, to which a special computer program can be added, both to make a graphic representation of the results of rehabilitation and to provide exercises for the patient. Such devices can also be used to evaluate the risk of falls in those cases where the risk is greatest, i.e. with elderly patients. Thus the results of these tests can also have an indirect effect on the prevention of fractures (Wilk & Frańczuk, 2003; Wilk-Frańczuk et al., 2010).

As previously mentioned, the dysfunctional changes that occur with older patients co-occur with the physiological processes of aging. We are often dealing with the simultaneous appearance of different diseases associated with this period of life and those that occur in other age groups as well, which in the elderly may or may not show characteristic features. This co-occurrence of pathological changes often leads to handicap, which is especially true of disorders of the musculo-skeletal system, such as degenerative changes, rheumatoid arthritis, or osteoporotic fractures, as well as disorders of perception (Piva et al., 2011). That is why rehabilitation begins before the planned surgery, which makes it possible to prepare the patient and minimize anxiety about life after the surgery, through conscious planning of activities and the repetition of previously learned and already familiar patterns of motion. The changes occurring in old age, along with pathological changes that impair perception and the posture control system, lead to disregulation of stability, and often, as a result, to falls, which are the major internal cause of injuries and fractures in older persons (the external causes include environmental and situational factors). In as many as half of these patients, repeat injuries occur.

This problem also affects persons who have undergone arthroplasty, for whom the consequences of an injury are particularly dangerous due to their impact on the implant. Various parameters are used in tests involving the evaluation of equilibrium and stability in older persons, including especially the Tinetti test, the Duncan test, the Berg scale, or the Romberg maneuver. Nevertheless, for purposes of prevention in elderly patients it is essential to use methods and exercises aimed at improving equilibrium. The rehabilitation program should also include exercises to increase muscle strength in the upper limbs, especially the shoulders. This is very important for the patient's locomotion during the early post-operative period, when the patient is forced to move about on crutches. As in other age groups, walking on crutches should be symmetrical, preferably two-beat with symmetrical work of the upper limbs. Family support is also particularly important, oriented towards motivating the patient to take an active role in the process of treatment and supporting the patient's desire to recover fitness and health, and to continue rehabilitation later, at home (Iyengar et al., 2007).

5. Reeducation and methods of evaluating and testing gait

Walking is the most important means of human locomotion, and the inability to walk has a significant negative impact on QOL (Starowicz et al., 2005). Walking can be defined as a rhythmic, alternating movement of the lower limbs, combined with displacement of the trunk and concomitant movements of the upper limbs. During normal gait one lower limb is always in contact with the ground through the foot; what differentiates walking from running, then, is that in the former there is a phase of double support, which in running is replaced by a phase of flight.

Walking requires the simultaneous participation of all the joints in the lower limb in an extraordinarily complex movement chain. In addition, movements in the spinal joints, including the cervical segment, are of great importance, as are the alternating movements of the upper limbs. The involvement of all parts of the body in the mechanism of walking requires a well-coordinated, complicated control mechanism in the nervous system, which explains why walking is not possible immediately after birth, when the nervous system is not yet fully developed. Normal, physiological walking as a means of locomotion is extraordinarily energy efficient, which is why even slight disturbances increase the energy cost and reduce effectiveness. There are two phases in walking on a level surface when the energy cost is high. The first of these is when walking begins, when it is necessary to overcome inertia in order to displace body mass forward, and the second is stopping, when it is necessary to inhibit the movement of the limbs and trunk.

The kinematic pattern of normal gait is very similar in everyone. This is especially true of the movements that take place in all the joints involved in walking in the sagittal plane (e.g. in some people we can see greater deviations of the center of gravity while walking). The forces at work while walking result from the actions of muscles that evoke acceleration and slowing of the appropriate parts of the body, along with gravity and momentum. Walking is often described as an alternating process of losing and regaining equilibrium. Taking a step is associated with throwing the foot forward and displacing the body's center of gravity forward, which produces a loss of equilibrium. The forces of gravity and forward momentum cause a resultant continuation of the movement that has just begun. The fall is avoided by the reflex strategy of regaining equilibrium, i.e. the reaction of putting the foot on the floor, which is associated with the return of the center of gravity into the projection area of the rectangle of support. If walking is to be continued, the center of gravity must once again be displaced forward. During the next step, propulsion results from a much weaker contraction of the flexors in the calf of the leg, thanks to the momentum gained in the preceding step; then the body moves forward, and the next reflex step occurs. This mechanism is continued for as long as desired, and the momentum achieved allows for energy conservation as soon as an even cadence of successive steps is achieved.

The movement pattern in the hip joint is much less complex during walking than in the knee or ankle joints. In the entire walk cycle, the hip joint has one extension phase and one flexion stage, whereas the knee and ankle joints each perform two phases of each type in one cycle. However, while in the knee and ankle joints the range of motion involves only the sagittal plane (flexion and extension), the proper participation of the hip joint in walking requires a free range of motion in all three planes, since abduction, adduction, and rotation are elements of gait markers, i.e. factors contributing to the reduction of displacing the center of gravity. The limitation of abduction, adduction, and rotation results in the disruption of this mechanism, which is why the range of flexion and extension in the hip joint can often be preserved even when walking is impaired. When the heel strikes the ground, the hip joint is in light flexion, while the gluteus maximus and the posterior thigh muscles immediately contract, in order to initiate extension of the hip joint. The knee joint is in full extension or about 5° of flexion, while the posterior group of thigh muscles control the flexion of the knee that follows after the heel hits the ground. The upper ankle joint is in almost full dorsal flexion. When the body mass is shifted onto that limb, the group of hip adductors begins to act, followed almost immediately by the hip abductors, stabilizing the pelvis relative to the thigh. At the same time, the gluteus maximus tenses, extending the hip and stopping the internal rotation of the thigh. During the support phase, extension begins in the hip joint, as a result of the action of the extensor muscles; the knee joint increases its flexion in order to minimize the impact of the heel striking the ground and the vertical displacement of the center of gravity, which occurs when the weight of the body is displaced forward above the limb stabilized on the ground.

The flexion of the knee in the support phase is one of the classic gait markers, and can assume a value up to 30°. In the ankle joint, there is a controlled plantar flexion for safe release of the foot onto the ground. The contraction of the quadriceps softens the impact of the heel on the ground and controls the momentum of the body, now pushing the knee forward. In the support phase, the activity of the muscles virtually stops, with the exception of the calf muscles. This group begins to act during this phase, achieving its greatest activity just before the heel is lifted from the ground. The phase of taking the heel off the ground follows, as a result of propulsion and displacement of the center of gravity to the anterior part of the foot after full dorsal flexion of the foot has been obtained. Towards the end of this phase the contraction of the flexors of the foot adds the movement component necessary to push off from the ground. Then the hip adductors begin again, and the cycle starts all over.

The rehabilitation of arthroplasty patients should always be connected with reeducation in walking, preceded by a thorough evaluation of its mechanisms and existing disturbances of motion in the joints, and the activity of the particular muscles. The high degree of complication of the act of walking requires that it be divided into components for the sake of analysis. Some of the terminology pertains to the duration of particular phenomena, some to the spatial positions, the values of forces, and the distances covered by particular parts of the body (e.g. length of stride, length of the walk cycle, the walk cycle, its phases, speed, cadence, and gait markers). Gait disturbances can be viewed in both temporal and spatial relations, which is why a complete analysis must include both of these aspects. A complete gait analysis consists of the following: testing the force of pressure on the ground; a three-dimensional video record of the movement of the patient's anthropometric points; electromyographic tests of the activity of the muscles that participate in walking (Cichy & Wilk, 2006; Cichy et al., 2008; Giaquinto et al., 2007).

The application of all three of these elements gives the most complete picture of gait disturbances. Degenerative disease of both the hip joint and the knee joint significantly impairs the efficiency of gait, leading to a progressive deterioration of the quality of life.

Several specific groups of gait disorders can be noted in patients with osteoarthritis. These result from the major symptoms of osteoarthritis. The most striking change is slow gait, involving the ineffective use of momentum and greater fluctuations in the center of gravity in the sagittal plane. Pain in one of the lower limbs and reduced range of motion in the hip joint, in turn, result in gait impairment in the isometric aspect. So-called unisometric gait is present, and is characterized by impaired coordination, reduced duration of the support phase, shortening of stride length, shortening of the length of the affected limb and longer duration of the gait cycle. The most severe variant occurs when one of the lower limbs (mostly the affected one) is dragged forward, and only the healthy one is pushed forward. In pathological gait associated with osteoarthritis, deterioration of the isochronous aspect is also observed, which leads to to the formation of the so-called antalgic gait. The patient then prolongs the healthy limb support phase, in order to prepare the affected limb for contact with the ground, then "jumps" over the diseased limb and tries to put the healthy limb back on the ground. The impaired coordination of upper limb movements is associated with impaired balance and an asymmetrical loading pattern in both lower limbs.

The gait disturbances described above usually present simultaneously. Asymmetry of gait in patients with osteoarthritis of the hip has been noted (Cichy & Wilk, 2006). The asymmetry of the load on the lower limbs in a static test (while standing) is not detectable in

patients, if shortening of the affected limb is not above 2 centimeters. When stride length is observed, changes have been detected in patients with osteoarthritis of the hip compared to a similar age group of the healthy population.
Gait re-education follows the principle of gradation of difficulty, and the program should also include improvement of balance and stability, so it is important to ensure patient safety (prevention of falls). Various methods are used to work with the patient, such as PNF, sensorimotor training, and hydrokinesitherapy. The rehabilitation program usually begins with exercises designed to achieve the correct loading of the lower limbs and gait pattern. Gradation is usually obtained by increasing the time of exercises, the number of repetitions, the distance, or by changing environmental conditions, such as walking on uneven ground, or walking outside the building. It is also important to introduce to the therapy elements of ordinary life, such as moving objects, and so called double tasks, which are intended to distract the patient who is focused on walking (simultaneous conversation, counting, observation, etc.).

6. Some special methods used in rehabilitation after total joint replacement

6.1 Continuous passive motion

Continuous Passive Motion (CPM) is one of many methods of rehabilitation after total joint replacement, which is the modern continuation of the G.J. Zander method, formerly known as mechanotherapy or the Zander method. One of the proponents and supporters of mechanotherapy is R.B. Salter, professor of orthopedic surgery in Toronto, who developed a method of continuous passive motion based on mechanical devices. From 1970 to 1986, Salter conducted research on the negative influence of immobilization on the joints, proving the beneficial effect of intermittent motion, and then continuous motion. In 1978 he constructed the first mechanical CPM device for patients after surgery in the extremities (fractures, arthroplasties). They were used immediately after surgery for a week. Some of the observed benefits include milder and fewer postoperative complications, improved blood supply to the extremities, faster wound healing, and the positive attitude of patients towards new therapies, which is also important. Studies conducted by American physicians from 1981 to 1984 confirmed these earlier observations, and also proved that the time of hospitalization of patients with CPM therapy was shorter compared to the control group, which used traditional rehabilitation. A number of devices have been constructed for CPM, including American devices, called Auto-Flex, the Toronto Medical Corporation's CPM, the German Artromot, and the Chinese or Italian Physiotek or Canwell. They allow the performance of physiological motions in the joints in a certain direction (depending on the device) and predetermined range of motion. At the same time it is possible to adjust the size of the leverage individually to the patient's posture, so that movements are performed in accordance with the joint axes. The authors of studies of the impact of CPM on the musculo-skeletal system draw attention to improved metabolism within the exercised joints, accelerated wound healing, decreasing periarticular soft tissue tension, more rapid absorption of the intra-articular hematoma, better blood supply to the limb, increased strength in the ligaments, and the antiedema and antithrombotic effects and lack of pain during exercise, thus hastening patient recovery (O'Driscoll & Giori, 2000).

6.2 Devices with biofeedback

One of the methods currently used in rehabilitation after total hip and knee replacement is the use of devices with biological feedback (biofeedback). These include visual feedback (in the form of images, charts, colors), auditory (sounds of changing intensity), thermal and strength biofeedback. The patient, thanks to the information obtained about how to perform a specific task (depending on the device used) can constantly and actively alter the force required for its implementation, or the method, or the direction, for example, so as to achieve the desired level of accuracy. Treatment with biofeedback is especially helpful in patients with locomotor pathology, which results in disorders in the control of movements, the formation of abnormal movement patterns or problems with balance. Among pathological process of this type, degenerative arthritis of the lower limbs and its surgical treatment can undoubtedly be included, since these disorders lead to disturbances in the normal gait model. Gradual progressive restriction of motion and increasing pain often cause severe impairment of both the mechanics and efficiency of gait. It is not uncommon for patients who have had degenerative arthritis for many years to move with crutches or a cane, and their gait causes pain and becomes increasingly more tiring. Arthroplasty and the postoperative period are also associated with different types of gait disorders, which may also lead to a shift in the center of gravity, which in turn causes an overload of other structures of the musculoskeletal system. Incorrect motor habits often become fixed. It is important, then, after arthroplasty, either hip or knee, for the rehabilitation program to include gait re-education, which can be supported by exercises using biofeedback to restore normal movement patterns (Kuczma et al., 2007; Rasch et al., 2010; Wilk-Frańczuk et al., 2010).

Many types of devices using biological feedback are currently available. Among these are static-dynamic parapodia, which, through dedicated computer software, use mostly video and audio feedback. This allows for balance exercises involving, for example, appropriate balancing and moving the center of gravity, with a visual record of the results. Through these exercises the patient learns to consciously control a particular function in a manner adequate to received visual and auditory information. Parapodia are also used to achieve a passive standing position from sitting in a wheelchair or a chair, while enabling the patient to control the speed of standing up. Another type of device is a gyro, some of which are controlled by computer-aided motion with the possibility of using an electric motor drive. They allow for exercises against active or passive resistance, with a capacity for resistance grading. Visual feedback of speed and asymmetry of the lower limbs are used for this purpose. These rotors are used, among other things, for gait re-education, in order to mitigate the consequences of limitations of physical activity in people with weak muscle strength and spasms. After each exercise the computer built into the device displays an analysis of the training just completed.

Studies on the suitability of equipment using biofeedback show that they allow for the confirmation of function improvement, control of distribution of weight, and stronger patient motivation to take on new tasks related to functional improvement.

6.3 Cryotherapy

Cryotherapy, or surface application of cryogenic temperatures to trigger the body's physiological response to cold, can be applied in various forms. It is primarily local cryotherapy that is used, by means of a device that employs liquid nitrogen, carbon dioxide or chilled air. Another form of cryotherapy, general cryotherapy, involves subjecting the

patient's whole body to the effects of low temperatures (-110°C - -160°C) in a cryochamber. In the case of local cryotherapy, the lowest temperatures (measured at the outlet of the nozzle) are obtained by using liquid nitrogen.
Cryotherapy is used in many diseases, including ankylosing spondylitis, rheumatoid arthritis (RA), degenerative joint disease, overstrain and traumatic diseases of the musculoskeletal system, or in persistent pain syndromes. Many authors have shown a positive effect on pain reduction, an anti-inflammatory effect, an antiedema effect, and reduced muscle tension. Low temperatures, thanks to the body's physiological reactions, also make it possible to intensify kinesitherapy. In most patients, the use of topical cooling at very low temperatures results in subjectively pleasurable sensations. This is mainly due to the abolition of pain, enabling intensive exercise, which leads in turn to improved joint mobility sufficient to perform basic activities free of pain. Local cryotherapy treatment implemented in the rehabilitation protocol reduces pain in all patients after total knee replacement, reduces or eliminates edema of the operated lower extremity, and by its analgesic and antiedema effect improves gait efficiency and esthetics. Cryotherapy treatment in the vicinity of the knee allows the cooling of this area of the body by about 10°C, followed by the application of kinesitherapy to speed up warming of the tissues, so that after about 15 minutes the temperature approaches the baseline temperature. Patients with no kinesitherapy after local cryotherapy around the knee note slower warming of the same area (Wilk et al., 2008). The observed effect of faster return of temperature to the baseline value may be due to the so-called after-effect phenomenon, consisting in the fact that intra-articular temperature is close to skin temperature and, unlike the muscles, under the influence of the cessation of cooling is not further reduced. Thus cryotherapy treatments performed on joints require direct kinesitherapy afterwards in order to make proper use the effect of cryotherapy, as was confirmed in the study (Wilk & Frańczuk, 2005b; Wilk et al., 2008).

7. References

Będziński, R. & Ścigała, K. (2000). Biomechanika stawu biodrowego i kolanowego. In. Biocybernetyka i Inżynieria Biomedyczna 2000. Tom 5. Nałęcz M. (Ed.), pp.113-158. EXIT ISSN 83-87674-67-2, Warszawa, Poland

Burnfield, J.M., Shu, Y., Buster, T. & Taylor, A. (2010). Similarity of Joint Kinematics and Muscle Demands Between Eliptical Training and Walking: Implication for Practice. *Physical Therapy*, Vol.90, No. 2, pp. 289-305, p-ISSN 0031-9023, e-ISSN 1538-6724

Cichy, B. & Wilk, M. (2006) Gait analysis in osteoarthritis of the hip. *Medical Science Monit*or, Vol. 12, No. 12, pp. 507-513. p-ISSN 1234-1010, e-ISSN 1634-3750

Cichy, B., Wilk, M. & Śliwiński, Z. (2008). Changes in gait parameters in total hip arthroplasty patients before and after surgery. *Medical Science Monit*or, Vol. 14, No. 3, pp. 159-169, p-ISSN 1234-1010, e-ISSN 1634-3750

Dudda, M., Gueleryuez, A., Gautier, E., Busato, A. & Roeder, C. (2010). Risk factors for early dislocation after total hip arthroplasty: a matched case-control study. *Journal of Orthopaedic Surgery, Vol.* 18, No. 2, pp. 179-183, ISSN 1022-5536

Evgeniadis, G., Beneka, A., Malliou, P., Mavromoustakos, S. & Godolias, G. (2008). Effects of pre- or postoperative therapeutic exercise on the quality of life, before and after total knee arthroplasty for osteoarthritis. *Journal of Back and Musculoskeletal Rehabilitation*, No. 21, pp. 161–169, ISSN 1053-8127

Giaquinto, S., Ciotola, E., Margutti, F. & Valentini, F. (2007). Gait during hydrokinesitherapy following total hip arthroplasty. *Disability and Rehabilitation*, Vol. 29, No. 9, pp. 743 - 749, ISSN 0963-8288

Grotle, M., Garratt, A.M., Klokkerud, M., Løchting, I., Uhlig, T. & Hagen, T.B. (2010). What's in Team Rehabilitation Care After Arthroplasty for Osteoarthritis? Results From a Multicenter, Longitudinal Study Assessing Structure, Process, and Outcome. *Physical Therapy*, Vol. 90, No. 1, pp. 121-131, p-ISSN 0031-9023, e-ISSN 1538-6724

Iyengar, K.P., Nadkarni, J.B., Ivanovic, N. & Mahale, A. (2007). Targeted early rehabilitation at home after total hip and knee joint replacement: Does it work?. *Disability and Rehabilitation*, Vol. 29, No. 6, pp. 495-502, ISSN 0963-8288

Kabsch, A. & Bober, T. (2001). Selected issues in the biomechanics of the knee joint. *Polish Journal of Physiotherapy*, Vol. 1, No. 2, pp. 179-182, ISSN 1642-0136

Kuczma, W., Srokowska, A., Owczarzak, M., Hoffman, J., Hagner, W. & Srokowski, G. (2007). The Phenomenon of Biofeedback in Neurological Rehabilitation Traded on "Balance Trainer". *Acta Balneologica*, Vol. 49, No. 2, pp. 79-85, ISSN 0005-4202

Maguire, C., Sieben, J.M., Frank, M., & Romkes, J. (2010). Hip abductor control in walking following stroke - the immediate effect of canes, taping and TheraTogs on gait. *Clinical Rehabilitation*, No. 24, pp. 37–45, p-ISSN 0269-2155, e-ISSN 1477-0873

Marks, R. (2010). Disabling hip osteoarthritis: gender, body mass, health and functional status correlates. *Health*, Vol. 7, No. 2, pp. 696-704, ISSN 1949-4998

Moody, J. (2000). Recommendations for the medical management of osteoarthritis of the hip and knee . 2000 Update American College of Rheumatology Subcommittee on Osteoarthritis Guidelines. *Arthritis & Rheumatism*, No .43, pp. 1905-1915, ISSN 0004-3591

Nolewajka, M., Gaździk, Sz.& Wieczorek, P. (2008). DVT risk factors after Total hip or knee replacement. *Journal of Orthoppaedics Trauma Surgery and Related Research*, Vol. 3, No. 11, pp. 17-30, ISSN 1897-2276

O'Driscoll, S.W. & Giori, N.J. (2000). Continuous passive motion (CPM): Theory and principles of clinical application. *Journal Res. & Dev*, Vol. 37, No. 2, pp. 179-188.

Piva, S.R., Teixeira, P.E.P., Almeida, G.J.M., Gil, A.B., DiGioia, III A.M., Levison, T.J. & Fitzgerald G.K. (2011). Contribution of Hip Abductor Strength to Physical Function in Patients With Total Knee Arthroplasty. *Physical Therapy*, Vol. 91, No.2, pp. 225-233. p-ISSN 0031-9023, e-ISSN 1538-6724

Rasch, A., Dalén, N. & Berg, H.E. (2010). Muscle strength, gait, and balance in 20 patients with hip osteoarthritis followed for 2 years after THA. *Acta Orthopaedica*, Vol. 81, No. 2, pp. 183–188, ISSN 1745-3674

Starowicz, A., Szwarczyk, W., Wilk, M. & Frańczuk, B. (2005). The evaluation of quality of life among patients after total hip replacement. *Polish Journal of Physiotherapy*, Vol. 5, No. 3, pp. 313-322, ISSN 1642-0136

Wilk, M. & Frańczuk, B. (2003). Analysis of changes in the strenght of muscles acting on the hip joint in patients recovering from hip arthroplasty. *Polish Journal of Physiotherapy*, Vol. 3, No. 4, pp. 309-315, ISSN 1642-0136

Wilk, M. & Frańczuk, B. (2004). Evaluating changes in the range of movement in the hip joint in patients with degenerative changes, before and after total hip replacement. *Ortopedia Traumatologia Rehabilitacja*, Vol. 6, No. 3, pp. 342-349, ISSN 1509-3492

Wilk, M. & Frańczuk, B. (2005a). Rehabilitation of patients after hip arthroplasty using Continuous Passive Motion. *Polish Journal of Physiotherapy,* Vol. 5, No. 1, pp. 8-14, ISSN 1642-0136

Wilk, M. & Frańczuk, B. (2005b). Local cryotherapy in patients recovering from total knee replacement. *Polish Journal of Physiotherapy,* Vol. 5, No. 3, pp. 329-333, ISSN 1642-0136

Wilk, M., Frańczuk, B., Trąbka, R. & Szwarczyk, W. (2004). Outcome of early rehabilitation with continuous passive motion for patients recovering from surgical reconstruction of the knee due to degenerative changes. A preliminary report. *Polish Journal of Physiotherapy,* Vol. 4, No. 2, pp. 163-166, ISSN 1642-0136

Wilk, M., Trąbka, R. & Śliwiński, Z. (2008). Changes in knee joint thermograms following local cryotherapy combined with various physiotherapy regimens. *Polish Journal of Physiotherapy,* Vol. 8, No 3, pp. 267-271, ISSN 1642-0136

Wilk-Frańczuk, M., Tomaszewski, W., Zemła, J., Noga, H. & Czamara, A. (2011). Analysis of rehabilitation procedure following arthroplasty of the knee with the use of complete endoprosthesis. *Medical Science Monit*or, Vol. 17, No. 3, pp. 165-168, p-ISSN 1234-1010, e-ISSN 1634-3750

Wilk-Frańczuk, M., Zemła, J. & Śliwiński, Z. (2010). The application of biofeedback exercises in patients following arthroplasty of the knee with the use of total endoprothesis. *Medical Science Monit*or, Vol. 16, No. 9, pp. 423-426, p-ISSN 1234-1010, e-ISSN 1634-3750

Wright, A.A., Cook, C.E., Flynn, T.W., Baxter, G.D. & Abbott, J.H. (2011). Predictors of Response to Physical Therapy Intervention in Patients With Primary Hip Osteoarthritis. *Physical Therapy,* Vol. 91, No. 4, pp. 510-524, p-ISSN 0031-9023, e-ISSN 1538-6724

Zeni, Jr J.A. & Snyder-Mackler, L. (2010). Early Postoperative Measures Predict 1- and 2-Year Outcomes After Unilateral Total Knee Arthroplasty: Importance of Contralateral Limb Strength. *Physical Therapy,* Vol. 90, No. 1, pp. 43-54, p-ISSN 0031-9023, e-ISSN 1538-6724

8

Methods for Optimising Patient Function After Total Hip Arthroplasty

Tosan Okoro[1,2], Andrew Lemmey[1],
Peter Maddison[1,2] and John G. Andrew[2]
[1]*Bangor University,*
[2]*Ysbyty Gwynedd, Betsi Cadwaladr University Health Board, Bangor*
United Kingdom

1. Introduction

Symptomatic hip osteoarthritis occurs in 3% of the elderly (Felson 2004) and is associated with poor general health status (Dawson et al. 2004). Treatment strategies for hip pain have traditionally involved conservative measures (analgesia, exercise, education, weight reduction) and surgical intervention (joint replacement) is the most effective treatment for end stage disease (Birrell et al. 2000, Di Domenica et al. 2005).

According to the National joint registry, the number of primary total hip replacements (THR) in England and Wales in 2008/2009 totalled 77608, which is a steady rise from the amount reported in 2007/2008 (73632) and 2006/2007 (51981) (National Joint Registry for England and Wales 2010). The average age of patients undergoing a primary total hip replacement is 66.7 years (SD 13.1) with females slightly older than males (average 68.4 years (SD12.4) vs. 65.8 years (SD 12.24) respectively) (National Joint Registry for England and Wales 2010).

As technology and surgical techniques for total hip replacement (THR) improve, patient expectations have also increased, including for an early return to normal physical function and activities (Wang, Gilbey & Ackland 2002). A reduced time between surgery and mobilisation has been found to have an influence in reducing length of stay and increasing patient satisfaction (Husted et al. 2008). This is particularly important due to the introduction of initiatives such as integrated care pathways, which have rapidly reduced the length of hospital stay following joint replacement with inpatient physiotherapy time also reduced (National Audit Office 2003). The median length of stay for THR patients according to data collated from a total of 125 acute trusts in England (2004-2005) was 7 days (interquartile range IQR 5-10) (Wilson et al. 2008).

Whilst THR generally resolves pain, function usually remains substantially sub-optimal. At 24 months following total joint arthroplasty, patients with low pre-operative function are five times more likely to require assistance from another person for their activities of daily living compared to those with high preoperative function (relative risk 5.2, 95% CI 1.9-14.6; (Fortin et al. 2002)). This protracted disability has detrimental economic, social and health consequences. Optimising function after surgery is therefore an important component of rehabilitation.

2. Predictors of outcome following total hip replacement

A recent prospective multivariate regression analysis of factors affecting outcome after THR has shown that the most important factor to influence outcome is the preoperative Western Ontario and McMaster Universities Osteoarthritis (WOMAC) physical function (PF) score (Wang et al. 2009). WOMAC is one of the most widely used disease-specific outcome instruments in people with osteoarthritis. The study by Wang et al identified three independent variables; pre-operative WOMAC PF score, gender and the presence of co morbidities as significantly affecting the WOMAC PF score at 1 year post-operatively. Previous studies have hypothesised that high preoperative functional status has a positive effect on outcome whilst others have suggested that it leaves little room for improvement in functional status (Montin et al. 2008, Roder et al. 2007, Young et al. 1998). Patients with better preoperative functional scores are likely to have higher postoperative scores, whereas patients with poorer preoperative scores are likely to experience greater improvements in function (Wang et al. 2009). Greater improvement in functional outcome are observed in male vs. female patients and this could be due to the fact that women are more likely than men to seek THR at the more advanced stages of their disease (Katz et al. 1994).

Patients with preoperative co morbidities are more likely to have a poorer short-term outcome in terms of physical function and this recent finding by Wang et al is consistent in the literature (Lubbeke et al. 2007, Roder et al. 2003, Wood, McLauchlan 2006). Patients with significant preoperative co morbidities have more inpatient complications such as hypotension, neuropathy, thromboembolic events, septicaemia, cardiac arrest, myocardial infarction, respiratory failure, and renal failure after THR than those who do not (Imamura & Black 1998). Patients with hip osteoarthritis with musculoskeletal co morbidities such as low back pain and osteoarthritis of the non-operated hip, have less long term functional improvement after THR (Nilsdotter et al. 2003). A combination of more pain pre-operatively, higher age and postoperative low back pain predicts a worse outcome after THR in WOMAC PF after 3.6 years of follow-up (Nilsdotter et al. 2003). Function and pain in patients with lower preoperative physical function does not to improve postoperatively to the level achieved by those with higher preoperative function (Fortin et al. 1999).

Old age predicts a poor postoperative outcome after THR and this is consistent with the impression that older people with self reported conditions restricting mobility in addition to arthritic pain in the hip or knee are at higher risk of psychological distress and physical dysfunction (Nilsdotter et al. 2003, Hopman-Rock et al. 1997).

3. Muscle strength and its relation to function after total hip replacement

The most common preoperative complaints by patients who elect to have THR are pain and loss of mobility (Trudelle-Jackson, Smith 2004). It therefore follows that the most commonly reported outcomes of THR in the literature relate to pain relief and restoration of mobility (Trudelle-Jackson, Smith 2004). Outcome studies of pain reduction and range of motion restoration, usually conducted 3 to 6 months after THR, indicate an overall satisfaction by patients and physicians (Barber et al. 1996). Outcome studies performed at least 1 year after THR reveal that impairments and functional limitations persist in the absence of pain. Impairments that persist at least 1 year after THR include decreased muscle strength and postural stability on the side of the replaced hip (Trudelle-Jackson et al. 2002). There are reported deficits in muscle strength of the involved hip after THR of 10-21% when compared to the uninvolved hip at 1 year post-surgery (Trudelle-Jackson et al. 2002, Shih et al. 1994). The atrophic changes that occur about the hip persist up to 2 years following THR and this is evidenced by increased fat infiltration (Rasch et al. 2009). There is a suggestion by the authors that earlier operation may prevent the development of these changes and that fatty infiltration may be reversed by intensive rehabilitation (Rasch et al. 2009).

Frail elderly persons with sarcopenia (degenerative loss of skeletal muscle mass and strength associated with aging) often undergo musculoskeletal-related surgery, and the hospitalisation-associated immobilisation further compromises the skeletal system, with potentially grave consequences (Suetta et al. 2004). Many elderly patients fail to regain their preoperative level of function and self-care (Sashika et al. 1996).

Immobilisation due to major surgery and hospitalisation can cause a severe decline in muscle mass, muscle strength and muscle function (Bloomfield 1997, Covinsky et al. 2003, Hill et al. 1993). Muscle strength declines 4% per day during the first week of immobilisation, making it very important that physical training is commenced as soon as possible after surgery (Wigerstad-Lossing et al. 1988).

Physical training can improve strength and functional performance in healthy elderly and frail nursing home residents (Harridge et al. 1999, Lexell et al. 1995). Supervised progressive resistance training (PRT) in the early post-operative phase has been shown to be effective in restoring muscle mass, contractile rate of force development, and functional performance than rehabilitation regimes based on functional exercises and electrical stimulation (Suetta et al. 2004). Strength training that is initiated 6 to 8 weeks or more than 6 months after hip surgery also significantly increases muscle strength (Sashika et al. 1996, Hauer et al. 2002). Recent studies suggest this is feasible in a supervised facility and that it offers an effective way of increasing maximal muscle strength in elderly postoperative patients with significant gains in muscle fibre size and pennation angle that resemble those typically seen in young healthy individuals (Suetta et al. 2008).

Gait dysfunctions and asymmetries, both pre-and post-THR surgery, are also evident in patients with unilateral hip osteoarthritis (Madsen et al. 2004). This is inherently dangerous because it is well known that gait dysfunctions or lower limb muscular weakness heighten the risk of falls especially when negotiating uneven terrain such as a step or a chair (Madsen et al. 2004). Dysfunction can also lead to reduced mobility, living independence, and physical activity levels (Galea et al. 2008)

4. Impact of aging on muscle

Aging and disuse are two of the main conditions leading to skeletal muscle atrophy in humans (Suetta et al. 2008). In both conditions, the loss of muscle mass leads to a decrease in muscle force production, and there may also be a significant additional contribution from changes in muscle architecture (Narici et al, 2005). The loss of muscle mass with aging accelerates from the sixth decade onward, partly owing to a decreased number of muscle fibres and also as the result of general muscle fibre atrophy (Lexell et al, 1991). Cross sectional studies indicate that type II fibres are more vulnerable to the aging process than type I fibres (Lexell et al, 1991) but other studies have found more marked type I atrophy (Frontera et al, 2000). Muscle mass has been estimated to decrease by 30% during the life span (Lexell et al, 1995) and maximal muscle strength is reduced as a result of aging by~1.5% per year from the sixth decade onwards (Skelton et al. 1994). Muscle strength has also been shown to decrease approximately 50% from age 30 to 80 (Sinaki 2004). Marked alterations in muscle architecture potentially contribute to loss of muscle strength (Narici et al, 2005) and muscle fibre pennation angle reduction of 10-13% in old compared to young individuals suggests this (Narici et al, 2003).

5. Exercise regimes for improving function

One hour of physical training twice a week increases the muscle strength in the quadriceps muscle by 21% and grip strength by 14% with not more than eight weeks of physical training (Heislein et al, 1994). Similarly, low to moderate physical activity during 16 weeks of physical training is associated with a 30-100% increase in muscle strength in both men and women while the bone mass (BM) at best increases by 3% (Ryan et al. 1994). There are reports that muscle strength increases by up to 200% even in octogenarians, a much larger increase than the 2-20% increases in muscle volume or the 1-2% increases in BM with a similar training program (Daley & Spinks 2000, Fiatarone et al. 1994, Lexell 1999, Province et al. 1995).

Women above age 60 who exercise with aerobics twice per week improve their balance, co-ordination and muscle strength (Lord et al. 1995). The muscle strength in the quadriceps muscle improved by 29% and the sway of the body was reduced by 6%, while the BM was unchanged during the intervention year. The most commonly used rehabilitation regimes for elderly individuals are based on functional types of exercises without external loading (Suetta et al. 2008), although this type of intervention does not prevent further muscle atrophy (Reardon et al. 2001). Resistance training is an effective method to induce muscle hypertrophy and increase muscle strength and functional performance in the elderly (Harridge et al 1999) and using it in the postoperative phase has been shown to be an effective method to restore muscle function in this group of patients (Hauer et al. 2002).

Progressive resistance training (PRT) by definition elicits positive health and performance adaptations by challenging the skeletal muscles with loads that can be lifted repetitively to the onset of neuromuscular fatigue, the point at which appropriate technique can no longer be maintained (American College of Sports Medicine, 1998). PRT sessions are optimal when followed by periods of recovery ranging from 48 to 72 h to allow for physiological super compensation (i.e. positive adaptation) (Cheema et al. 2007). To facilitate continued adaptation, training intensity (i.e. load) and volume (i.e. number of sets) are progressively increased, and exercises are adjusted as indicated throughout the training regimen, to attenuate the onset of a plateau in physiological adaptation. Once the physiological plateau has been reached, health and performance are maintained with continued training, which may involve periodical manipulations of the PRT variables, including training frequency, training intensity (load), training volume (sets), types of exercises, and time under tension per repetition (Cheema et al. 2007).

PRT is a well-established and safe exercise modality for individuals of all ages and fitness levels, including those afflicted with severe chronic illnesses (Fiatarone et al. 1994, Cheema et al. 2007). It is particularly efficacious for adult and elderly cohorts given its efficacy in counteracting sarcopenia, abating osteoporosis and helping reverse the physiological and functional impairments that accrue with age (Fiatarone et al. 1994).

6. The evidence for pre-operative exercise regimes

Appropriate exercise offers many benefits in treating the patient with osteoarthritis (Macera et al. 2003). Stronger, better-conditioned periarticular muscles, tendons, and ligaments have advantageous biomechanical effects on attenuating joint forces during movement (Felson et al. 2000). In more severe disease, which often leads to reduced mobility and disuse atrophy,

exercise can improve pain, muscle strength, cardiovascular fitness, self-efficacy, and function (van Baar et al. 1999).
Exercise is a cornerstone of rehabilitation following total joint arthroplasty and other surgical procedures (Eyigor et al. 2004). Using exercise in the pre-operative period has variable benefit. An improvement has been demonstrated in the preoperative functional status after a 6 week presurgical exercise program (water and land based strength training activities) in patients awaiting total hip and knee arthroplasty in comparison to patients having routine rehabilitation but this effect is not maintained after 8 and 26 weeks of follow up (Rooks et al. 2006). This fits in with a previous study by Wijgman et al (Wijgman et al. 1994), which reported that preoperative physical therapy and instruction were not useful for patients before total hip arthoplasty. In their sample of 31 patients, few differences were observed between the patients and control subjects on measures such as the visual analogue pain scale and the Harris hip score (Wijgman et al. 1994). More recent work by Gocen et al (Gocen et al. 2004) also showed that instruction and pre-operative physiotherapy is of no benefit in terms of improving outcome (measured with the Harris Hip Score and Visual analogue scale) after THR surgery.
A systematic review by Ackerman and Bennell (Ackerman & Bennell 2004) found that only two randomised controlled trials involving patients undergoing THR surgery demonstrated a benefit of performing pre-operative exercise. Both Wang et al (Wang, Gilbey & Ackland 2002) and Gilbey et al (Gilbey et al. 2003) used pre-operative stationary bikes, resistance training of the lower limb and hydrotherapy with post-operative hydrotherapy, progressive strengthening exercises and aerobic activity. Wang et al (Wang, Gilbey & Ackland 2002) reported a significantly higher mean gait velocity for the exercise group from three to 24 weeks post-operatively, and a greater mean distance walked by the exercise group at 24 weeks post-operatively. Gilbey et al (Gilbey et al. 2003) found that the exercise group experienced significantly larger gains in hip strength, WOMAC scores, and hip ROM from three to 24 weeks post-operatively. The systematic review concluded that the major limitation of these studies was the addition of an intensive post-operative exercise program for the intervention group only, so it is impossible to determine which of the pre-operative regimes was responsible for the improvements seen. There is therefore a lack of conclusive evidence to justify the use of pre-operative regimes to optimise function after THR surgery.

7. The evidence for post-operative home or centre-based exercise regimes to improve function

Early targeted rehabilitation has been shown to reduce hospital length of stay without an increase in complication rates after THR (Iyengar et al. 2007). Exercise programs beyond the normal postoperative rehabilitation period have been shown to reduce pain and leg stiffness, improve physical function and lessen the chance of accidental falls in THR patients (Gilbey et al. 2003). A disadvantage of these programs is the need for patients to exercise under the supervision of professional staff at a hospital or rehabilitation centre (Galea et al. 2008). This makes program delivery expensive due to the high costs associated with supervision, treatment and transport (Galea et al. 2008). In addition, some THR patients are excluded because difficulties with mobility and transport to a centre exclude participation (Marottoli et al, 1992). Studies comparing home- and centre-based rehabilitation programs for THR patients have found no difference in WOMAC scores, complication rates and patient satisfaction after 3 and 12 months of follow up (Mahomed et al. 2008).

An important factor in both home and centre based regimes is the use of PRT. A systematic review performed by the author (manuscript submitted for publication) on level 1 evidence-(randomised controlled trials) for regimes for rehabilitation after THR found the use of PRT to be predictive of functional benefit, when measured either using objective measures such as muscle strength or subjective functional measures such as the WOMAC. These centre-based interventions (Hesse et al, 2003; Husby et al, 2009; Jesudason et al, 2002; Liebs et al, 2010; Suetta et al, 2004) were performed in the early period (<1 month following surgery) and the home-based interventions (Jan et al, 2004; Trudelle-Jackson et al 2004) were performed late (>1 month following surgery).

A limitation of the home-based interventions assessed in the literature is that follow-up does not extend beyond the end of the exercise interventions periods. Thus, it is not clear whether the benefits evident at the end of the exercise intervention are maintained in the longer term. The other obvious shortcoming is the lateness of the intervention in the home setting and consequently the failure to ameliorate or prevent the exacerbated loss of muscle and function after surgery. A recent systematic review by Di Monaco et al (Di Monaco et al. 2009) suggests that the difficulties in THR rehabilitation research are that there is a lack of multicentre clinical trials with large sample sizes to inform the design of optimal physical exercise programs.

8. Motivators and barriers to improving function through exercise

Routine physical exercise improves one's general physical health (Wang et al. 2002) decreases the risk of medical conditions such as coronary artery disease, diabetes, osteoporosis and hypertension (Bouchard & Despres 1995); reduces mental health concerns such as depression (Newson & Kemps 2007); and can prevent falls (Barnett et al. 2003). Recent research also suggests that physical exercise plays a role in the maintenance of cognitive vitality in older age (Colcombe et al. 2004).

A recent study has shown that specific motivators and barriers to exercise differ with age, education, gender, psychological and physical well-being and current level of exercise (Newson & Kemps 2007). People over the age of 75 are more likely to be motivated to exercise purely to maintain an active lifestyle than those aged 63 to 74 years, and medical problems are more likely to prevent them from engaging in exercise compared than their younger counterparts (Newson & Kemps 2007). Men were found to be more likely than women to be motivated to exercise for the challenging nature of exercise. On the other hand, women are more likely than men to report health concerns as a reason to exercise, and they are more likely to blame a lack of exercise facilities and exercise specific knowledge as factors to prevent them from exercising (Newson & Kemps 2007).

High-level exercisers find the challenge to exercise to be more of a motivator than their low level counterparts, who reported health concerns to be a more important motivator. Low-level exercisers also noted a concern that factors associated with exercise and a lack of facilities and knowledge about exercise prevented them from exercising (Newson & Kemps 2007). The authors conclude that intervention programs for older adults need to take into account the specific contextual factors of the individual. The average age of patients undergoing THR surgery in the UK is 66.7 years (National Joint Registry for England and Wales 2010). According to Newson et al, these patients (63-74 years old) view keeping their fitness (feel-good nature of exercise, enjoyment) as the most important motivator whilst the most significant barrier is situational i.e. having no one to exercise with, disliking exercising alone and adverse weather conditions.

9. Outcome measures for assessing function

The need for THR is predicted to grow by 174% between 2005 and 2030 (Kurtz et al. 2007). It is therefore important that patient outcomes after surgery are continuously monitored and reviewed, to improve practise and optimise outcomes after surgery (Wylde et al. 2009). Central to assessing the effectiveness of hip replacement in a clinical setting is choosing the appropriate outcome measure (Wylde et al. 2009). In orthopaedics, outcomes after surgery can be assessed using five different methods, namely radiographic analysis, implant survivorship analysis, surgeon-based outcome measures, performance-related assessment and patient reported outcome questionnaires (Wylde et al. 2009).

Performance related assessment involves assessing the individual as they perform a specific task that is evaluated in a standardised manner using predetermined criteria (Wylde et al. 2009). A recent review (Terwee et al. 2006) has found that 26 performance measures have been used to assess function in patients with lower limb arthritis or joint replacement including walking, stair-climbing and chair tests. A moderate correlation has been reported between the results of patient self-reported functional ability and performance measures (Stratford et al. 2003; Terwee et al. 2006). This could be because performance related tests may not reflect the true demands and exertions associated with activities of daily living (Wylde et al. 2009). Other limitations include the fact that they are time consuming and only consider physical function whilst neglecting other important domains of outcome such as pain, quality of life and general well-being (Terwee et al. 2006).

Generic Health	Disease specific	Joint-specific
Assess subjective general health status with comparisons across different disease states and treatment options e.g. SF36. Assesses 8 dimensions of health related quality of life (HRQoL): Bodily pain, physical role functioning, physical role limitations, general health, vitality, social role functioning, emotional role limitations and mental health.	Focus solely on symptom and disabilities relating to particular condition but are not particular to the joint of assessment. e.g. for Rheumatoid arthritis AIMS (Arthritis Impact Measurement Scale) which has 9 component scales which assess mobility, physical activity, social activity, social role, activities of daily living, pain, dexterity, anxiety and depression. For Osteoarthritis, Western Ontario and McMaster University Osteoarthritis index (WOMAC) which is a 24 item measure of pain, stiffness and function.	Specific to the joint of assessment and attempt to exclude the influence of co morbidities E.g. Oxford Hip score which is a short 12 item questionnaire specifically developed to assess functional ability and pain in patients undergoing hip replacement. The questionnaire displays good psychometric properties and has a larger effect size than other tools such as the SF36.

Table 1. Types of Patient Reported Outcome Measures (PROMs) (Bellamy et al. 1988; Brazier et al. 1992; Dawson et al. 1998; Jenkinson & Layte 1997; Meenan et al. 1980; Salaffi et al. 2005; Ware et al. 1992, 1996)

Surgeon based assessment tools such as the Harris Hip Score assume concordance between the view of patients and clinicians, which is an erroneous assumption across all healthcare settings (Wylde et al. 2009). Within Orthopaedics, a lack of correlation has been demonstrated between surgeon and patient ratings of pain, function and satisfaction after joint replacement (Anderson et al. 1996; Bullens et al. 2001).Whereas surgeons may judge the success of joint replacement on the range of motion, alignment and stability, patients may evaluate outcome in terms of vitality and ability to return to leisure activities (Wylde et al. 2009). This inconsistency between patient and clinician ratings of health has guided the development of rigorous validated patient-reported outcome measures (Wylde et al. 2009).

Patient reported outcome measures (PROMs) are advantageous because they are a cost-effective, efficient and minimally intrusive method of collecting data on patients (Wylde et al. 2009). PROMS can be grouped into generic health, disease specific and joint specific (Table 1). A limitation of all PROMs is the issue of recall bias towards patients reporting the most severe and recent pain they have experienced (Jensen et al. 2008).

10. Areas that remain to be explored

Total hip replacement surgery provides good relief for patients' pain but fails to fully restore physical function. The impairment of muscle function that occurs in relation to aging is exacerbated by the impact of surgery and subsequent immobilisation. Pre-operative regimes to improve functional outcome have not been shown to be beneficial. Post-operative regimes on the other hand, if including PRT, appear to have a significant benefit on patient function following THR regardless of the timing of the intervention. Centre-based regimes are plagued with issues of high transport and supervision costs. Early home based PRT studies that are effective and safe; with adequate follow-up after THR surgery would potentially improve outcomes after THR at an affordable cost, and appear an important area for future research.

11. Acknowledgements

I would like to dedicate this chapter to Iyé, Roli and Edosa- the rocks on which I build my world. I would also like to thank the North Wales Research Committee for their support.

12. References

"American College of Sports Medicine Position Stand. The recommended quantity and quality of exercise for developing and maintaining cardiorespiratory and muscular fitness, and flexibility in healthy adults", 1998, Medicine and science in sports and exercise, vol. 30, no. 6, pp. 975-991.

Ackerman, I.N. & Bennell, K.L. 2004, "Does pre-operative physiotherapy improve outcomes from lower limb joint replacement surgery? A systematic review", The Australian journal of physiotherapy, vol. 50, no. 1, pp. 25-30.

Anderson, J.G., Wixson, R.L., Tsai, D., Stulberg, S.D. & Chang, R.W. 1996, "Functional outcome and patient satisfaction in total knee patients over the age of 75", *The Journal of arthroplasty,* vol. 11, no. 7, pp. 831-840.

Barber, T.C., Roger, D.J., Goodman, S.B. & Schurman, D.J. 1996, "Early outcome of total hip arthroplasty using the direct

lateral vs the posterior surgical approach", Orthopedics, vol. 19, no. 10, pp. 873-875.

Barnett, A., Smith, B., Lord, S.R., Williams, M. & Baumand, A. 2003, "Community-based group exercise improves balance and reduces falls in at-risk older people: a randomised controlled trial", Age and Ageing, vol. 32, no. 4, pp. 407-414.

Bellamy, N., Buchanan, W.W., Goldsmith, C.H., Campbell, J. & Stitt, L.W. 1988, "Validation study of WOMAC: a health status instrument for measuring clinically important patient relevant outcomes to antirheumatic drug therapy in patients with osteoarthritis of the hip or knee", *The Journal of rheumatology,* vol. 15, no. 12, pp. 1833-1840.

Birrell, F., Croft, P., Cooper, C., Hosie, G., Macfarlane, G.J. & Silman, A. 2000, "Radiographic change is common in new presenters in primary care with hip pain. PCR Hip Study Group", Rheumatology (Oxford, England), vol. 39, no. 7, pp. 772-775.

Bloomfield, S.A. 1997, "Changes in musculoskeletal structure and function with prolonged bed rest", Medicine and science in sports and exercise, vol. 29, no. 2, pp. 197-206.

Bouchard, C. & Despres, J.P. 1995, "Physical activity and health: atherosclerotic, metabolic, and hypertensive diseases", Research quarterly for exercise and sport, vol. 66, no. 4, pp. 268-275.

Bullens, P.H., van Loon, C.J., de Waal Malefijt, M.C., Laan, R.F. & Veth, R.P. 2001, "Patient satisfaction after total knee arthroplasty: a comparison between subjective and objective outcome assessments", *The Journal of arthroplasty,* vol. 16, no. 6, pp. 740-747.

Cheema, B., Abas, H., Smith, B., O'Sullivan, A., Chan, M., Patwardhan, A., Kelly, J., Gillin, A., Pang, G., Lloyd, B. & Singh, M.F. 2007, "Progressive exercise for anabolism in kidney disease (PEAK): a randomized, controlled trial of resistance training during hemodialysis", Journal of the American Society of Nephrology : JASN, vol. 18, no. 5, pp. 1594-1601.

Colcombe, S.J., Kramer, A.F., McAuley, E., Erickson, K.I. & Scalf, P. 2004, "Neurocognitive aging and cardiovascular fitness: recent findings and future directions", Journal of molecular neuroscience : MN, vol. 24, no. 1, pp. 9-14.

Covinsky, K.E., Palmer, R.M., Fortinsky, R.H., Counsell, S.R., Stewart, A.L., Kresevic, D., Burant, C.J. & Landefeld, C.S. 2003, "Loss of independence in activities of daily living in older adults hospitalized with medical illnesses: increased vulnerability with age", Journal of the American Geriatrics Society, vol. 51, no. 4, pp. 451-458.

Daley, M.J. & Spinks, W.L. 2000, "Exercise, mobility and aging", Sports medicine (Auckland, N.Z.), vol. 29, no. 1, pp. 1-12.

Dawson, J., Fitzpatrick, R., Murray, D. & Carr, A. 1998, "Questionnaire on the perceptions of patients about total knee replacement", *The Journal of bone and joint surgery.British volume,* vol. 80, no. 1, pp. 63-69.

Dawson, J., Linsell, L., Zondervan, K., Rose, P., Randall, T., Carr, A. & Fitzpatrick, R. 2004, "Epidemiology of hip and knee pain and its impact on overall health status in older adults", Rheumatology (Oxford, England), vol. 43, no. 4, pp. 497-504.

Di Domenica, F., Sarzi-Puttini, P., Cazzola, M., Atzeni, F., Cappadonia, C., Caserta, A., Galletti, R., Volonte, L. & Mele, G. 2005, "Physical and rehabilitative approaches in osteoarthritis", Seminars in arthritis and rheumatism, vol. 34, no. 6 Suppl 2, pp. 62-69.

Di Monaco, M., Vallero, F., Tappero, R. & Cavanna, A. 2009, "Rehabilitation after total hip arthroplasty: a systematic review of controlled trials on physical exercise programs", European journal of physical and rehabilitation medicine, vol. 45, no. 3, pp. 303-317.

Eyigor, S., Hepguler, S. & Capaci, K. 2004, "A comparison of muscle training methods in patients with knee osteoarthritis", Clinical rheumatology, vol. 23, no. 2, pp. 109-115.

Felson, D.T., Lawrence, R.C., Dieppe, P.A., Hirsch, R., Helmick, C.G., Jordan, J.M., Kington, R.S., Lane, N.E., Nevitt, M.C., Zhang, Y., Sowers, M., McAlindon, T., Spector, T.D., Poole, A.R., Yanovski, S.Z., Ateshian, G., Sharma, L., Buckwalter, J.A., Brandt, K.D. & Fries, J.F. 2000, "Osteoarthritis: new insights. Part 1: the disease and its risk factors", Annals of Internal Medicine, vol. 133, no. 8, pp. 635-646.

Fiatarone, M.A., O'Neill, E.F., Ryan, N.D., Clements, K.M., Solares, G.R., Nelson, M.E., Roberts, S.B., Kehayias, J.J., Lipsitz, L.A. & Evans, W.J. 1994, "Exercise training and nutritional supplementation for physical frailty in very elderly people", The New England journal of medicine, vol. 330, no. 25, pp. 1769-1775.

Fortin, P.R., Clarke, A.E., Joseph, L., Liang, M.H., Tanzer, M., Ferland, D., Phillips, C., Partridge, A.J., Belisle, P., Fossel, A.H., Mahomed, N., Sledge, C.B. & Katz, J.N. 1999, "Outcomes of total hip and knee replacement: preoperative functional status predicts outcomes at six months after surgery", Arthritis and Rheumatism, vol. 42, no. 8, pp. 1722-1728.

Fortin, P.R., Penrod, J.R., Clarke, A.E., St-Pierre, Y., Joseph, L., Belisle, P., Liang, M.H., Ferland, D., Phillips, C.B., Mahomed, N., Tanzer, M., Sledge, C., Fossel, A.H. & Katz, J.N. 2002, "Timing of total joint replacement affects clinical outcomes among patients with osteoarthritis of the hip or knee", Arthritis and Rheumatism, vol. 46, no. 12, pp. 3327-3330.

Frontera, W.R., Hughes, V.A., Fielding, R.A., Fiatarone, M.A., Evans, W.J. & Roubenoff, R. 2000, "Aging of skeletal muscle: a 12-yr longitudinal study", Journal of applied physiology (Bethesda, Md.: 1985), vol. 88, no. 4, pp. 1321-1326.

Galea, M.P., Levinger, P., Lythgo, N., Cimoli, C., Weller, R., Tully, E., McMeeken, J. & Westh, R. 2008, "A targeted home- and center-based exercise program for people after total hip replacement: a randomized clinical trial", Archives of Physical Medicine and Rehabilitation, vol. 89, no. 8, pp. 1442-1447.

Gilbey, H.J., Ackland, T.R., Wang, A.W., Morton, A.R., Trouchet, T. & Tapper, J. 2003, "Exercise improves early functional recovery after total hip arthroplasty", Clinical orthopaedics and related research, vol. (408), no. 408, pp. 193-200.

Gocen, Z., Sen, A., Unver, B., Karatosun, V. & Gunal, I. 2004, "The effect of preoperative physiotherapy and education on the outcome of total hip replacement: a prospective randomized controlled trial", Clinical rehabilitation, vol. 18, no. 4, pp. 353-358.

Harridge, S.D., Kryger, A. & Stensgaard, A. 1999, "Knee extensor strength, activation, and size in very elderly people following strength training", Muscle & nerve, vol. 22, no. 7, pp. 831-839.

Hauer, K., Specht, N., Schuler, M., Bartsch, P. & Oster, P. 2002, "Intensive physical training in geriatric patients after severe falls and hip surgery", Age and Ageing, vol. 31, no. 1, pp. 49-57.

Heislein, D.M., Harris, B.A. & Jette, A.M. 1994, "A strength training program for postmenopausal women: a pilot study", Archives of Physical Medicine and Rehabilitation, vol. 75, no. 2, pp. 198-204.

Hesse, S., Werner, C., Seibel, H., von Frankenberg, S., Kappel, E.M., Kirker, S. & Kading, M. 2003, "Treadmill training with partial body-weight support after total hip arthroplasty: a randomized controlled trial", Archives of Physical Medicine and Rehabilitation, vol. 84, no. 12, pp. 1767-1773.

Hill, G.L., Douglas, R.G. & Schroeder, D. 1993, "Metabolic basis for the management of patients undergoing major surgery", World journal of surgery, vol. 17, no. 2, pp. 146-153.

Hopman-Rock, M., Odding, E., Hofman, A., Kraaimaat, F.W. & Bijlsma, J.W. 1997, "Differences in health status of older adults with pain in the hip or knee only and with additional mobility restricting conditions", The Journal of rheumatology, vol. 24, no. 12, pp. 2416-2423.

Husby, V.S., Helgerud, J., Bjorgen, S., Husby, O.S., Benum, P. & Hoff, J. 2009, "Early maximal strength training is an efficient treatment for patients operated with total hip arthroplasty", Archives of Physical Medicine and Rehabilitation, vol. 90, no. 10, pp. 1658-1667.

Husted, H., Holm, G. & Jacobsen, S. 2008, "Predictors of length of stay and patient satisfaction after hip and knee replacement surgery: fast-track experience in 712 patients", Acta orthopaedica, vol. 79, no. 2, pp. 168-173.

Imamura, K. & Black, N. 1998, "Does comorbidity affect the outcome of surgery? Total hip replacement in the UK and Japan", International journal for quality in health care : journal of the International Society for Quality in Health Care / ISQua, vol. 10, no. 2, pp. 113-123.

Iyengar, K.P., Nadkarni, J.B., Ivanovic, N. & Mahale, A. 2007, "Targeted early rehabilitation at home after total hip and knee joint replacement: Does it work?", Disability and rehabilitation, vol. 29, no. 6, pp. 495-502.

Jan, M.H., Hung, J.Y., Lin, J.C., Wang, S.F., Liu, T.K. & Tang, P.F. 2004, "Effects of a home program on strength, walking speed, and function after total hip replacement", Archives of Physical Medicine and Rehabilitation, vol. 85, no. 12, pp. 1943-1951.

Jenkinson, C. & Layte, R. 1997, "Development and testing of the UK SF-12 (short form health survey)", *Journal of health services research & policy,* vol. 2, no. 1, pp. 14-18.

Jesudason, C. & Stiller, K. 2002, "Are bed exercises necessary following hip arthroplasty?", The Australian journal of physiotherapy, vol. 48, no. 2, pp. 73-81.

Katz, J.N., Wright, E.A., Guadagnoli, E., Liang, M.H., Karlson, E.W. & Cleary, P.D. 1994, "Differences between men and women undergoing major orthopedic surgery for degenerative arthritis", Arthritis and Rheumatism, vol. 37, no. 5, pp. 687-694.

Kurtz, S., Ong, K., Lau, E., Mowat, F. & Halpern, M. 2007, "Projections of primary and revision hip and knee arthroplasty in the United States from 2005 to 2030", *The Journal of bone and joint surgery.American volume,* vol. 89, no. 4, pp. 780-785.

Lexell, J. 1999, "Effects of strength and endurance training on skeletal muscles in the elderly. New muscles for old!", Lakartidningen, vol. 96, no. 3, pp. 207-209.

Lexell, J. 1995, "Human aging, muscle mass, and fiber type composition", The journals of gerontology.Series A, Biological sciences and medical sciences, vol. 50 Spec No, pp. 11-16.

Lexell, J., Downham, D.Y., Larsson, Y., Bruhn, E. & Morsing, B. 1995, "Heavy-resistance training in older Scandinavian men and women: short- and long-term effects on arm and leg muscles", Scandinavian journal of medicine & science in sports, vol. 5, no. 6, pp. 329-341.

Lexell, J. & Taylor, C.C. 1991, "Variability in muscle fibre areas in whole human quadriceps muscle: effects of increasing age", Journal of anatomy, vol. 174, pp. 239-249.

Liebs, T.R., Herzberg, W., Ruther, W., Haasters, J., Russlies, M. & Hassenpflug, J. 2010, "Ergometer cycling after hip or knee replacement surgery: a randomized controlled trial", The Journal of bone and joint surgery.American volume, vol. 92, no. 4, pp. 814-822.

Lord, S.R., Ward, J.A., Williams, P. & Strudwick, M. 1995, "The effect of a 12-month exercise trial on balance, strength, and falls in older women: a randomized controlled trial", Journal of the American Geriatrics Society, vol. 43, no. 11, pp. 1198-1206.

Lubbeke, A., Katz, J.N., Perneger, T.V. & Hoffmeyer, P. 2007, "Primary and revision hip arthroplasty: 5-year outcomes and influence of age and comorbidity", The Journal of rheumatology, vol. 34, no. 2, pp. 394-400.

Macera, C.A., Hootman, J.M. & Sniezek, J.E. 2003, "Major public health benefits of physical activity", Arthritis and Rheumatism, vol. 49, no. 1, pp. 122-128.

Madsen, M.S., Ritter, M.A., Morris, H.H., Meding, J.B., Berend, M.E., Faris, P.M. & Vardaxis, V.G. 2004, "The effect of total hip arthroplasty surgical approach on gait", Journal of orthopaedic research : official publication of the Orthopaedic Research Society, vol. 22, no. 1, pp. 44-50.

Mahomed, N.N., Davis, A.M., Hawker, G., Badley, E., Davey, J.R., Syed, K.A., Coyte, P.C., Gandhi, R. & Wright, J.G. 2008, "Inpatient compared with home-based rehabilitation following primary unilateral total hip or knee replacement: a randomized controlled trial", The Journal of bone and joint surgery.American volume, vol. 90, no. 8, pp. 1673-1680.

Marottoli, R.A., Berkman, L.F. & Cooney, L.M.,Jr 1992, "Decline in physical function following hip fracture", Journal of the American Geriatrics Society, vol. 40, no. 9, pp. 861-866.

Meenan, R.F., Gertman, P.M. & Mason, J.H. 1980, "Measuring health status in arthritis. The arthritis impact measurement scales", *Arthritis and Rheumatism,* vol. 23, no. 2, pp. 146-152.

Montin, L., Leino-Kilpi, H., Suominen, T. & Lepisto, J. 2008, "A systematic review of empirical studies between 1966 and 2005 of patient outcomes of total hip arthroplasty and related factors", Journal of clinical nursing, vol. 17, no. 1, pp. 40-45.

Narici, M.V., Maganaris, C. & Reeves, N. 2005, "Myotendinous alterations and effects of resistive loading in old age", Scandinavian journal of medicine & science in sports, vol. 15, no. 6, pp. 392-401.

Narici, M.V., Maganaris, C.N., Reeves, N.D. & Capodaglio, P. 2003, "Effect of aging on human muscle architecture", Journal of applied physiology (Bethesda, Md.: 1985), vol. 95, no. 6, pp. 2229-2234.

National Audit Office 2003, Hip replacements: an update. HC 956.

National Joint Registry for England and Wales 2010, 7th Annual Clinical Report.

Newson, R.S. & Kemps, E.B. 2007, "Factors that promote and prevent exercise engagement in older adults", Journal of aging and health, vol. 19, no. 3, pp. 470-481.

Nilsdotter, A.K., Petersson, I.F., Roos, E.M. & Lohmander, L.S. 2003, "Predictors of patient relevant outcome after total hip replacement for osteoarthritis: a prospective study", Annals of the Rheumatic Diseases, vol. 62, no. 10, pp. 923-930.

Province, M.A., Hadley, E.C., Hornbrook, M.C., Lipsitz, L.A., Miller, J.P., Mulrow, C.D., Ory, M.G., Sattin, R.W., Tinetti, M.E. & Wolf, S.L. 1995, "The effects of exercise on falls in elderly patients. A preplanned meta-analysis of the FICSIT Trials. Frailty and Injuries: Cooperative Studies of Intervention Techniques", JAMA : the journal of the American Medical Association, vol. 273, no. 17, pp. 1341-1347.

Rasch, A., Bystrom, A.H., Dalen, N., Martinez-Carranza, N. & Berg, H.E. 2009, "Persisting muscle atrophy two years after replacement of the hip", The Journal of bone and joint surgery.British volume, vol. 91, no. 5, pp. 583-588.

Reardon, K., Galea, M., Dennett, X., Choong, P. & Byrne, E. 2001, "Quadriceps muscle wasting persists 5 months after total hip arthroplasty for osteoarthritis of the hip: a pilot study", Internal Medicine Journal, vol. 31, no. 1, pp. 7-14.

Roder, C., Parvizi, J., Eggli, S., Berry, D.J., Muller, M.E. & Busato, A. 2003, "Demographic factors affecting long-term outcome of total hip arthroplasty", Clinical orthopaedics and related research, vol. (417), no. 417, pp. 62-73.

Roder, C., Staub, L.P., Eggli, S., Dietrich, D., Busato, A. & Muller, U. 2007, "Influence of preoperative functional status on outcome after total hip arthroplasty", The Journal of bone and joint surgery.American volume, vol. 89, no. 1, pp. 11-17.

Rooks, D.S., Huang, J., Bierbaum, B.E., Bolus, S.A., Rubano, J., Connolly, C.E., Alpert, S., Iversen, M.D. & Katz, J.N. 2006, "Effect of preoperative exercise on measures of functional status in men and women undergoing total hip and knee arthroplasty", Arthritis and Rheumatism, vol. 55, no. 5, pp. 700-708.

Ryan, A.S., Treuth, M.S., Rubin, M.A., Miller, J.P., Nicklas, B.J., Landis, D.M., Pratley, R.E., Libanati, C.R., Gundberg, C.M. & Hurley, B.F. 1994, "Effects of strength training on bone mineral density: hormonal and bone turnover relationships", Journal of applied physiology (Bethesda, Md.: 1985), vol. 77, no. 4, pp. 1678-1684.

Salaffi, F., Carotti, M. & Grassi, W. 2005, "Health-related quality of life in patients with hip or knee osteoarthritis: comparison of generic and disease-specific instruments", *Clinical rheumatology,* vol. 24, no. 1, pp. 29-37.

Sashika, H., Matsuba, Y. & Watanabe, Y. 1996, "Home program of physical therapy: effect on disabilities of patients with total hip arthroplasty", Archives of Physical Medicine and Rehabilitation, vol. 77, no. 3, pp. 273-277.

Shih, C.H., Du, Y.K., Lin, Y.H. & Wu, C.C. 1994, "Muscular recovery around the hip joint after total hip arthroplasty", Clinical orthopaedics and related research, vol. (302), no. 302, pp. 115-120.

Sinaki, M. 2004, "Falls, fractures, and hip pads", Current osteoporosis reports, vol. 2, no. 4, pp. 131-137.

Skelton, D.A., Greig, C.A., Davies, J.M. & Young, A. 1994, "Strength, power and related functional ability of healthy people aged 65-89 years", Age and Ageing, vol. 23, no. 5, pp. 371-377.

Stratford, P.W., Kennedy, D., Pagura, S.M. & Gollish, J.D. 2003, "The relationship between self-report and performance-related measures: questioning the content validity of timed tests", *Arthritis and Rheumatism,* vol. 49, no. 4, pp. 535-540.

Suetta, C., Andersen, J.L., Dalgas, U., Berget, J., Koskinen, S., Aagaard, P., Magnusson, S.P. & Kjaer, M. 2008, "Resistance training induces qualitative changes in muscle morphology, muscle architecture, and muscle function in elderly postoperative patients", Journal of applied physiology (Bethesda, Md.: 1985), vol. 105, no. 1, pp. 180-186.

Suetta, C., Magnusson, S.P., Rosted, A., Aagaard, P., Jakobsen, A.K., Larsen, L.H., Duus, B. & Kjaer, M. 2004, "Resistance training in the early postoperative phase reduces hospitalization and leads to muscle hypertrophy in elderly hip surgery patients--a controlled, randomized study", Journal of the American Geriatrics Society, vol. 52, no. 12, pp. 2016-2022.

Terwee, C.B., Mokkink, L.B., Steultjens, M.P. & Dekker, J. 2006, "Performance-based methods for measuring the physical function of patients with osteoarthritis of the hip or knee: a systematic review of measurement properties", *Rheumatology (Oxford, England),* vol. 45, no. 7, pp. 890-902.

Trudelle-Jackson, E., Emerson, R. & Smith, S. 2002, "Outcomes of total hip arthroplasty: a study of patients one year postsurgery", The Journal of orthopaedic and sports physical therapy, vol. 32, no. 6, pp. 260-267.

Trudelle-Jackson, E. & Smith, S.S. 2004, "Effects of a late-phase exercise program after total hip arthroplasty: a randomized controlled trial", Archives of Physical Medicine and Rehabilitation, vol. 85, no. 7, pp. 1056-1062.

van Baar, M.E., Assendelft, W.J., Dekker, J., Oostendorp, R.A. & Bijlsma, J.W. 1999, "Effectiveness of exercise therapy in patients with osteoarthritis of the hip or knee: a systematic review of randomized clinical trials", Arthritis and Rheumatism, vol. 42, no. 7, pp. 1361-1369.

Wang, A.W., Gilbey, H.J. & Ackland, T.R. 2002, "Perioperative exercise programs improve early return of ambulatory function after total hip arthroplasty: a randomized, controlled trial", American Journal of Physical Medicine & Rehabilitation / Association of Academic Physiatrists, vol. 81, no. 11, pp. 801-806.

Wang, B.W., Ramey, D.R., Schettler, J.D., Hubert, H.B. & Fries, J.F. 2002, "Postponed development of disability in elderly runners: a 13-year longitudinal study", Archives of Internal Medicine, vol. 162, no. 20, pp. 2285-2294.

Wang, W., Morrison, T.A., Geller, J.A., Yoon, R.S. & Macaulay, W. 2009, "Predicting Short-Term Outcome of Primary Total Hip Arthroplasty A Prospective Multivariate Regression Analysis of 12 Independent Factors", The Journal of arthroplasty, .

Ware, J.E.,Jr & Sherbourne, C.D. 1992, "The MOS 36-item short-form health survey (SF-36). I. Conceptual framework and item selection", *Medical care,* vol. 30, no. 6, pp. 473-483.

Ware, J.,Jr, Kosinski, M. & Keller, S.D. 1996, "A 12-Item Short-Form Health Survey: construction of scales and preliminary tests of reliability and validity", *Medical care,* vol. 34, no. 3, pp. 220-233.

Wigerstad-Lossing, I., Grimby, G., Jonsson, T., Morelli, B., Peterson, L. & Renstrom, P. 1988, "Effects of electrical muscle stimulation combined with voluntary contractions after knee ligament surgery", Medicine and science in sports and exercise, vol. 20, no. 1, pp. 93-98.

Wijgman, A.J., Dekkers, G.H., Waltje, E., Krekels, T. & Arens, H.J. 1994, "No positive effect of preoperative exercise therapy and teaching in patients to be subjected to hip arthroplasty", Nederlands tijdschrift voor geneeskunde, vol. 138, no. 19, pp. 949-952.

Wilson, J., Charlett, A., Leong, G., McDougall, C. & Duckworth, G. 2008, "Rates of surgical site infection after hip replacement as a hospital performance indicator: analysis of data from the English mandatory surveillance system", Infection control and hospital epidemiology : the official journal of the Society of Hospital Epidemiologists of America, vol. 29, no. 3, pp. 219-226.

Wood, G.C. & McLauchlan, G.J. 2006, "Outcome assessment in the elderly after total hip arthroplasty", The Journal of arthroplasty, vol. 21, no. 3, pp. 398-404.

Young, N.L., Cheah, D., Waddell, J.P. & Wright, J.G. 1998, "Patient characteristics that affect the outcome of total hip arthroplasty: a review", Canadian journal of surgery.Journal canadien de chirurgie, vol. 41, no. 3, pp. 188-195.

Part 2

Special Topics in Hip Arthroplasty

9

Planning of Arthroplasty in Dysplastic Hips

Nevzat Selim Gokay[1], Alper Gokce[1], Bulent Alp[2] and Fahri Erdogan[2]
[1]*Namik Kemal University School of Medicine, Department of Orthopaedics and Traumatology, Tekirdag*
[2]*Istanbul University, Cerrahpasa School of Medicine, Department of Orthopaedics and Traumatology, Istanbul*
Turkey

1. Introduction

Hip dysplasia is one of the major conditions leading degenerative hip arthritis in early adulthood. Devolopmental insuffuciency of bony structures yields asymetric ball and socket formation, which usually associated with trophic changes and instability. Total hip joint replacement has successfull results in patients with hip dysplasia in adulthood. The major goal of the treatment is rebuilding of a new stable artificial joint with painless range of motion. There is a need of a meticulous preoperative planning assessing the anatomic severity of the pathology, which is consisted of involved bony and soft tissue components. Limb length discrepency, quality of bone stock, muscle atrophies, weakness and contractures should be evaluated before surgery. There are several classifications for assesment of acetabuar dysplasia. However, we are aware of a combined clasification or comprehensive allgorithym for assesment of all components of pathology in unisom.
Current devolopments in the field of radiology like Three Dimensional (3d) Computerized Tomography (CT) and Magnetic Resonance Imaging (MRI) allowed assesment of all component of hip dysplasia preoperatively. Metaphyseal and acetabular bone stock and structure, anteversion degrees and soft tissues has to be taken in consideration. The aim of this chapter is to review the present classifications and reported experiences on hip dysplasia and discuss the value of missing parts. The preoperative planning process were also reviewed regarding the role of modern radiologic examination techniques on current surgical and clinical applications.

2. Planning of arthroplasty in dysplastic hips

Patient selection is very importmant in the treatment of developmental dysplasia of the hip (DDH). In proper and young patients femoral or periacetabular osteotomy should be considered. Nevertheless total hip arthroplasty is often required for most of the patients with dysplasia. The major goal of the treatment is rebuilding of a new stable artificial joint with painless range of motion. To this end, there is a need of a meticulous preoperative planning assessing the anatomic severity of the pathology, which is consisted of involved bony and soft tissue component. The most important thing which should stick in our minds is the complexity of the anatomical abnormality complicating the reconstruction.

The orthopaedic surgeons should display a hard challenge to overcome these deformities. Serious hypoplasia of the acetabulum, femoral head deformity, short femoral neck, excessive anteversion of the neck, narrow and straight medullary canal, totally dislocation, limb leg discrepancy and highly placed trochanter are some of these deformities which makes the surgery difficult. Surgery may be further complicated by the effects of previously performed osteotomies. Therefore, an accurate guide is mandatory to solve this problem in the pre-operative planning.

2.1 An overlook to the basic science of congenital hip disease

Understanding of the embryological development of the hip, epidemiology, pathologic anatomy and the natural history of congenital hip disease (CDH) should help us to conceive the disease with accuracy and improve our skills in surgical area.

2.1.1 Embryology and normal development of the hip

The acetabulum and femoral head develope from the same mesenchymal cells in a cleft at the tenth week of the gestational period (Gardner & Gray, 1950; Strayer, 1943) Hip joint is completely formed at the 11th week of gestation. It is initially deeply set and spherical. It becomes progressively less deeply set and hemispherical until birth. The hip has maximum range of motion at birth as it is shallowest. They thought that this adaptation help the fetus pass through the birth canal. After birth these trends reverse : the acetabulum becomes deeper again and the femoral head more spherical. This process continues throughout childhood. Thus the risk of dislocation is greatest at the prenatal period.(Rális & McKibbin, 1973; Watanabe, 1974; Wedge & Wasylenko, 1978).

It is better to discuss about the normal postnatal development of the hip, before examining the pathologic anatomy of DDH. The outer two thirds of the acetabulum is formed by the acetabular cartilage. This complex is interposed between the ilium, the pubis and the ischium. It is rich from hyaline cartilage cells and contains growth plates on each side which helps the hip socket to expand during growth. (Ponseti, 1978; Watanabe, 1974; Weinstein, 1987). It is known that the concavity of the acetabulum develops in response to the presence of the spherical femoral head (Harrison, 1961; Smith et al., 1958).

2.1.2 Pathologic anatomy of DDH

The term of DDH was started to be used in the last decades, after it was understood that this disease presents in different manners;

1. Dysplasia: The articular relationship between femur and acetabulum isn't broken, consequently Shenton's line is intact. There is inadequate development of the acetabulum.
2. Subluxation: The femoral head migrates laterally and proximally, Shenton's line is broken but femoral head is still in contact with acetabulum.
3. Dislocation: The femoral head is completely out of the acetabulum. The displacement of the femoral head is usually in posterosuperior direction.

It seems that these are the different stages of a disease seen in ages. (Hartofilakidis et al, 2000; Weinstein, 1987)

Therefore the pathological anatomy of the disease differs in a wide spectrum and depends on the stage of the disease. The anatomical pathology in dysplasia is mostly at the acetabuler side of the joint. It is shallow than usual and femoroacetabular coverage is not enough.

This entity may cause osteoartrhritic changes and femoral head will become deformed in time. Secondary degerative changes may lead the dysplastic hip convert into a subluxed hip. In subluxation femoral head is proximally and laterally displaced. The major difference between dysplasia and subluxation is the intactness of Shenton's line on the graphies. In these cases bone stock of the acetabulum is less affected, and development of the femur is almost normal. In the otherhand, if a hip is dislocated, there is no relationship between the femoral head and acetabulum, acetabulum is too dysplasic and femoral head articulates to a false acetabulum on the iliac bone. The course of the abductor muscles changes to horizontally instead of lateral and vertical direction. The muscles also shorten in length due to the position of the trochanter major. Affected leg is shortened. Acetabulum is too much hypoplastic and the acetabular bone stock is remarkable diminished which is anteriorly. The bone stock is affected mostly in low dislocation cases due to the growth disruption of the acetabular lateral wall by the compression of the femoral head. Femur is also abnormal; it's hypoplastic, anteverted and femoral canal is narrow than usual. Capsule is elongated and thickened. The course of the nerve and arteries is altered. External rotators are elongated, also.

2.2 Land marks and classification methods of DDH

Various anatomical landmarks on conventional graphies were used to assess the degree of acetabular dysplasia. Center edge angle of Wiberg, acetabular angle of Sharp and femoral head extrusion index are some of these parameters measured using these landmarks (Heyman & Herndon, 1950; Sharp, 1961; Wiberg, 1939).

There are several classifications for the assesment of acetabular displasia. The classifications of Crowe and Hartofilakidis are the most used ones in the litarature. Crowe et al. described a method to determine degree of dysplasia in 1979 (Crowe et al., 1979). It was based on the degree of proximal femoral migration relative to the acetabulum on an anteroposterior radiograph of the pelvis. The authors differentiated the disease into four classes according to the distance between the teardrop and junction of the femoral neck and head. The amount of the proximal migration of the femoral head was measured as a percentage of the height of the femoral head or the pelvis (Table 1).

The classification of Hartofilakidis et al. classified dysplasia in three groups based on anatomic correlations (Hartofilakidis et al., 1988). The dislocated hip was described in two stages as low and high dislocation (Table 2). The other classification system, which was described by Eftekhar and Kerboul et al., was classified according to the shape of the acetabulum and head, and the side of dislocation respectively (Eftekhar, 1993; Kerboul et al., 1987). Along these most reliable ones are the classifications of Crowe and Hartofilakidis and their classifications have shown a better reproducibility than the systems of Eftekhar and Kerboul et al (Brunner et al., 2008; Decking et al., 2006). However, we are aware of a combined classification or comprehensive algorithym for assesment of all components of this pathology.

There isn't any classification available describing this disease with the all aspects of the deformity. Most of the classifications are focused on the shape and relation between the head of femur and acetabulum. Soft tissue disturbances were excluded during evaluation and the effects of this on the success of the treatment were overlooked. Transversely orianted and poorly developed abductor muscles, and shortened adductors are some of these conditions which complicates the treatment than expected. Also, none of these classifications in use considers the amount of femoral anteversion and metaphyseal development which results in discrepancy between the stem. These classifications should describe the deformity however they couldn't achieve any idea on the treatment method and the implant type.

Group	Description
I	Subluxation < 50% or proximal dislocation < 0.1% of the pelvic height
II	Subluxation 50% - 75% or proximal dislocation of 0.1% to 0.15 of pelvic height
III	Subluxation 75% - 100% or proximal dislocation of 0.15 to 0.20 of pelvic height
IV	Subluxation > 100% or proximal dislocation of > 0.20% of pelvic height

Table 1. The Classification of Crowe et al.

Type	Description
Dysplasia	The femoral head is not dislocated out of the acetabulum despite the degree of subluxation
Low Dislocation	The femoral head is dislocated and articulates with a false acetabulum which partially covers the true acetabulum to a varying degree
High Dislocation	The femoral head is dislocated and has migrated superiorly and posteriorly with no relation with any part of the true

Table 2. The Classification of Hartofilakidis et al.

2.3 The clinical presentation and indications in developmental hip disease

Most of the DDH patients have symptoms of other joints except the hip joint. The ipsilateral knee tends to be in valgus due to the hyper adductus of the hip. Low back pain may occur in patients with bilateral dislocations though to the hyperlordosis of the lumbar spine (Wedge & Wasylenko, 1978). As a result knee and lowback pain are mostly first symptoms of the disease. Most patients suffer from limping rather than the pain.

The indication of total hip prosthesis surgery in DDH, does not differ from the indications in primer arthrosis. The important point is that surgery in DDH patients is more complicated and the complication rate is higher than the others. So the indication of the surgery may be difficult in patients with minor symptoms. The main symptom for surgery indication should be the pain. Despite the complicity of the disease most of the patients of dislocation have no symptom rather than limping. It may be better to choose other treatment options in patients which have no or little pain. Limbing only, shouldn't be an indication for total hip arthroplasty.

2.4 Total hip arthroplasty surgery in DDH

Despite the advanced techniques and implants, the total hip arthroplasty in DDH still remains as a hardchallenge at the present time. The most difficult part of this challenge is to decide the best technique and optimum implant for each patient. Unfortunately there is no consensus of opinion on the surgical planning of these patients who present in a wide spectrum. The success of the operation mostly depends on the severity of the disease. According to the Crowe classification, the rate of survival at 20 years follow-up, was found as 72.7%, 70.7%, 36.7% and 15.6% for class 1,2,3 and 4, respectively (Chougle et al, 2005). Although total hip surgery is a succcessful operation in the treatment of dysplastic hips, it may present many problems due to the musculer contractures, abnormal location of the hip center, inadequate bone stock of acetabulum and femur, alterations in the hip anatomy, abductor insufficiency and leg length discrepancy (Charnley & Feagin, 1973; Hartofilakidis et al., 1996; Mulroy & Harris, 1990; Patterson & Brown, 1973; Symeonides et al., 1997).

2.4.1 The preoperative planning of DDH patients

Troelsen et al. drew our attention to the importance of the weight bearing pelvic radiographs and stated that it may allow us to determine the retroversion degree of the acetabulum more accurately (Troelsen et al., 2010). Although Standard Pelvis graphies and Judet graphies may tell us information about the acetabular osseous stock, the complicity of this disease induced the human being in searching new imaging modalities. The evolution in the imaging technologies, gives us the comfort of the understanding the pathology with all details before the surgery. CT has been used in preoperative planning and reported that important data about the morphology of the joint was obtained with the assistance of CT (Xenakis et al.,1996). 3d CT was also reported as an useful device in determining the acetabular anteversion and anterolateral deficiencies (Anda et al., 1991; Nakamura et al., 2000)

2.4.2 The exposure

Most methods of approache to the hip may be appropriate in DDH patients with slight deformity, for instance anterolateral and posterolateral exposures. Cameron et al. used Smith-Peterson approach to Crowe class 3 and 4 hips and they reported perfect results (Cameron et al., 1996). Despite their results they also reported a high rate of nerve complication. The surgical approach may be very dangerous due to the extraordinary anatomy in the highly dislocated patients. Trochanter major may serve as a good guide for the oriantation of the surgeon. Transtrochanteric or subtrochanteric aproachs are indicated for the highly dislocated patients who require retansion of the abductors. Kumar and Shair described an extended iliofemoral approach but found no advantage of this technique besides it results too much muscle dissection (Kumar & Shair, 1997).

2.4.3 The approach to the dysplastic asetabulum

It is without controversy that the approach to the acetabulum and acetabular component placement are the most important part of the reconstruction in DDH. It was reported that the osseous stock is much more at the true acetabuler area (Charnley & Feagin, 1973; Dunn

& Hess, 1976; Eftekar, 1978; Mendes et al., 1996). Though the ideal area of acetabuler component placement is thought to be the true acetabulum (Linde & Jensen, 1988; Yoder et al., 1988) and restoration of normal hip center of rotation provided good long-term results (Bozic et al., 2004; Yoder et al.,1988). The superior or lateral placement of the acetabuler cup was accused of being a risk factor for femoral and acetabuler loosening (Doehring et al., 1996; Yoder et al.,1988). Reaming the acetabulum deeply and using porous coated small acetabuler implants is usually enough to reconstruct the acetabulum. Although a lower rate of loosening has been reported in conjunction with medialization of the hip center, small prosthetic componenets require the use of a thin liner which are known to be responsible for polyethilen wear (Saikko, 1995). This is the reason that small cups are not appropriate to use in young and active patients with hip dysplasia (Dudkiewicz et al., 2002). The size of the acetabular component depends mostly on the severity of dislocation (Flecher et al., 2008). While the size of the acetabular cup used in Crowe 2 is the largest ones, smallest implants usually necesary in Crowe 4 patients. Moreover polyethylene wear found to be related to the cup inclination angle (Perka et al., 2004). Perka, also stated that there was no significant association between wear and the cup size or the thickness of the liner in their series.
The inadequate medialisation of the hip center seems to be an important factor modifying long term results (Kennedy et al., 1998; McQueary et al., 1988). The best position of the femoral head center is thought to be less than 35 mm vertically from the interteardrop line and 25 mm laterally from the teardrop (Hirakawa et al., 2001). Alternatively; controlled acetabuler medialisation (Hess & Umber, 1978; Paavilainen et al., 1990), acetabuler enlarging and bone greft augmentation (MacKenzie et al., 1996; McQueary & Johnston, 1988) or reinforcement cage reconstruction (Gill et al., 1998) are the other methods which can be used. But these techniques may lead to an excessive bone loss and the usage of long ofset femoral heads may be required.
High hip center concept was stated as an issue by Russotti (Russotti et al., 1991). They recommended to place the acetabular component at a more proximal but not more lateral position of the center of the hip in difficult acetabular reconstructions. It was stated that a longer stable fixation, than placement of the acetabular component at the true anatomical position, will be achieved if the latter approach necessitates reliance on large bulk allografts or autogenous grafts to provide most of the structural support. In a series of Dearborn et al., only 4 percent mechanical failure in 46 patients was reported after a mean of 10.4 years of follow-up duration (Dearborn et al., 1999). But, it was suggested that superior positioning of the acetabular component, leads to increased rates of loosening of the femoral and acetabular components (Pagnano, 1996). Also, Doehring reported that superolateral hip center relocation should be avoided and that superior-only relocation may be mechanically acceptable within the confines of the osseous anatomy of the acetabulum (Doehring et al, 1996). An attempt should be made to position the acetabular component in or near the true acetabular region. Hartofilakidis described the necessity of placement of the acetabuler component to the true acetabular level, in three entries; 1)The lever arm for body weight is much longer than the abductor lever arm at the level of false acetabulum and it results in an excessive load on the hip joint, 2)Shearing forces acting on the acetabular cup may lead to early loosening at the level of the false acetabulum, 3)The bone stock is usually better at the level of the true acetabulum than it is at more proximal levels ((Hartofilakidis & Karachalios, 2004). The hip center of rotation could be restored in only seventy eight (% 66) of 121 hips in a serie of Perka (Perka et al, 2004). Following the elongated capsule is often helpful in the location of the true acetabulum during surgery. However the localising of the normal hip

center during the operation is not always so easy. It leads the acetabuler malplacement in an inadequate coverege. To overcome this problem a method of acetabuloplasty was described (Dunn & Hess, 1976; Hartofilakidis et al., 1988; Stamos et al., 1984). They termed this technique as cotyloplasty. In this technique, they created a controlled comminuted fracture of the entire medial wall of the acetabulum with use of a reamer or a chisel after compilation of the acetabuler reaming. Perforating the internal layer of the periosteum was avoided. After obtaining a large amount of autogenous cancellous graft from femoral head, they placed the graft material over the periosteum of the fractured medial wall. They finally cemented the acetabuler component at an angle of 40-45 degrees horizontally and 10 degrees of anteversion. They adviced 3 to 4 weeks bed rest postoperatively and didn't allow full weight bearing until the graft is incorparated radiographically, considering the horizontal compressive vectors applied by the muscles of the hip. Hartofilakidis et al. used this technique in 68 total hip operation which they used Charnley implants, and Charnley technique, involves an osteotomy of the greater trochanter (Hartofilakidis et al., 1996). Forty nine of the patients were type 3, 31 were type 2 and 6 were type 1 according to their classification. They found good or excellent results in 94 % of the patients operated in a mean duration of follow-up of seven years.
Various types of implants had been attempted in the reconstruction of the acetabulum. Cemented cups were tended to be use in large series in the past. In a series of Stans et al., aseptic loosening developed in 53% of cemented acetabular components (Stans et al., 1998). They thought that this high loosening rates were related with the acetabuler component malplacement in Crowe type III patients. Insertion of the acetabuler component without cement may be preferred when the osseous cavity could provide at least 80 % osseous coverage of a cementless cup (Hartofilakidis & Karachalios, 2004).
Perka et al. used a cementless threaded cups in reconstruction of the acetabulum (Perka et al, 2004). They didn't use a bone graft material to reconstruct the superolateral margin and the cup was slightly medialized to achieve stable anchorage of at least one thread in the existing bone. Although it was found that threaded acetabuler components had high loosing results in the past (Stan et al., 1998), Perka reported a survival rate of % 97.5 at an average of 9.3 years for threaded cups. Their results were better than the those after implantation of cemented cups.
Flecher et al. reported a survival rate of 94.7% at 12 years, using a cementless pres-fit acetabuler component with an obturator hook and screws (Flecher et al., 2008). They sustained that this implant combined the principles of a reinforcement ring with those of uncemented acetabular press-fit components.

2.4.4 The usage of bone grafts in the augmentation of acetabuler component

A technique of bolting the femoral head to the wing of ilium was developed to support the acetabuler component (Harris, 1974). The acetabular cavity was reamed together with into the graft and the host bone. Screws were also used in fixing the autograft. Femoral head allografts became popular in time after the advantages of autografts Jasty & Harris, 1987). It was reported that this technique worked well for short time follow-up and gave the surgeon the possibility of overcoming with the atrophic acetabulums (Harris et al., 1977). However, a high failure rate of nearly 46% were reported at a follow-up of twenty years with the use of the femoral head as an autograft for augmenting the superolateral aspect of the acetabular rim (Harris, 1993; Mulroy & Harris, 1990). The difficulties in revascularisation and of the large grafts and the forces which the graft is exposed may be the possible reasons for the failure. Also, the high failure rates of femoral head augmentation in the reconstruction of superolateral acetabulum with cancellous bone fixation was related with mostly proximal placement of the acetabulum (Stans et al., 1998). Only cement augmentation may be an option in reconstructing the acetabulum in Crowe type III patients. It was reported that cement augmentation works well if the initial hip center is within the true acetabuler region (Stans et al., 1998).

After the cementless acetabuler components began to be used in dysplasia patients, the need to massive grafts in acetabular reconstruction, even at atrophic acetabulums, was diminished (Jasty et al., 1995). It was suggested that lack of osseous reconstruction of the lateral acetabular margin did not have any notable influence on the stability of the cup (Perka et al., 2004). In our personel experiences, if you have press-fit fixation between anterior and posterior wall or sufficient fixation with screws; it is allowed early weight bearing without any problem.

2.4.5 The approach to the deformed femur

The difficulty in reconstructing the femur of dysplastic patients mostly resulted from the alteration in the anatomy of the femur. The femur of the DDH patients were shown to have shorter necks and smaller straighter canals than the normal femurs (Noble et al., 2003). Cemented stems were used in dysplastic patients for a long time with a lesser success than the patients of primer arthrosis. Probably, the biomechanical abnormality of the hip and the persisted limbing after the surgery causes the act of abnormal forces on the cemented component. Consequently early aseptic loosening rates of cemented components increases in DDH patients. In a 20 years follow-up, 5 % aseptic loosing rate was reported with the cemented femoral components (Klapach et al., 2001). Morever evidence of aseptic loosening was observed in 40% of the femoral components of Crowe type III patients at 20 years duration (Stans et al., 1998).

Cementless femoral stems seem to be more useful in reconstruction of young patients. Furthermore usage of the cementless stems prevent the occupation of excessive thick cement in narrow medullary canals. In a series of Lai et al., 56 patients, who have Crowe type 4 DDH, were operated with cementless stems (Lai et al., 2005). They didn't report any stem revision in a follow-up period of mean 12.3 years.

Cementless Zweymüller stem was used in 121 dysplastic hips and fracture occured in the proximal part of the femur in seven cases (Perka et al., 2004). They believed that the high rate of femoral fracture was a result of incresed anteversion of the femoral neck, the tight medullary space and the the altered anatomy in the proximal femur following previous operations. However the survival rate of the stems was not influenced by this complication and it was reported as % 100 at an average follow-up duration of 9.3 years.

The porous coated S-Rom cementless moduler stem was also reported as successful in the treatment of Crowe type III and IV hips, at a 10 year follow-up (Biant et al., 2009). They used the prosthesis as an intramedullary fixation device in the patients whom were required femoral shortening, with the benefit of the straight structure of this stem.

The excessive femoral anteversion seems to be an important problem in DDH patients rather than the primer arthrosis patients (Argenson et al.,2005). Compensating for excessive anteversion of the dysplastic femur is easy with the use of cemented stems. If a cementless stem will be used, it may be better to choose a moduler or distally fixed component rather than proximally fixed femoral component. The proximally fixed components don't allow you to rotate the stem to compansate the anteversion because of the metaphyseal filling.

Moduler stems allow us the regulation of the femoral anteversion unrelated with proximal metaphsial morphology (Cameron et al., 1996). An other option in overcoming the anteversion problem is the usage of the thin conically stems. The results of Wagner conic prosthesis are also found as successful in a short term period (Ström et al, 2003). Hartofilakidis reported successfull results with CDH Charnley prosthesis, a straight thin prosthesis (Hartofilakidis & Karachalios, 2004).

2.4.6 The subtrochanteric femoral shortening osteotomy

The restoration of the acetabulum to the anatomic center of the hip is not always so easy especially in Crowe type 4 patients. Three possible alternative to solve this problem on the dislocated femur were reported; 1) Trochanteric osteotomy may be carried out with metaphysel shortening and advancement of the trochanter. Cemented stem may be the choice of use in this option, 2) A modular stem may be an option, 3) Subtrochanteric shortening and derotation, combined with an distally fixed cementless stem is the third alternative (Cabenala, 2001). Trial reduction by skeletal or skin traction was performed before the surgery, to assess the potential reduction (Symenoides et al., 1997). They also used a gradual traction technique with the use of an external fixator but pain and nerve palsy was reported in this case. According to us, subtrochanteric femoral shortening osteotomy is the best option to lower the femoral head to its original site instead of soft tissue release without damaging the nerves by streching. Non-union rates are low with the use of cementless femoral stems, especially in Crowe type 4 dysplasies. Its also useful in aligning the anteversion of the neck in such malrotated femoral metaphysises. There is more than one technique reported for the shortening of the femur (Bruce et al., 2000; Klisic & Jankovic, 1976; Sener et al., 2002; Yasgur et al.,1997). Klisic and Jankovic (Klisic & Jankovic, 1976) was first stated the usage of the femoral shortening osteotomies in the treatment of highly dislocated hips and than it was adapted into the total hip replacement operations by Sponseller and MacBeath (Sponseller & McBeath, 1988). Transvers subtrochanteric shortening osteotomy is a successful technique and none neurologic complication was reported in a series of Myung- Sik Park et al. of 24 patients operated with transvers osteotomy (Park et al., 2007). Yalcin et al. reported 79,5 % good and perfect results in 44 total hip replacements accompanied by transvers osteotomy at a meanly 62 months follow-up (Yalcin et al., 2010). In a study of Aeron et al., the patients, whom femurs were shortened, were followed up to mean 4.8 years and preoperative Harris scores found to increase from 43 to 89, postoperatively (Krych et al., 2010).

The short time requirement for bone healing, much bone contact and stability against the torsional forces are the advantages of step-cut osteotomy. Despite of these advantages, Sener et al. reported 2 non-unions after step-cut osteotomy in 28 patients (Sener et al., 2002) while one non-union was reported after transvers osteotomy in 14 hips (Onodera et al., 2006). In an other serie, Masaki Takao et al. combined cementless moduler total hip prosthesis with step-cut subtrochanteric shortening osteotomy (Takao et al., 2011). No non-union and nerve palsy were reported. Merle d'Aubigne and Postel hip score increased from 9 to 16 in this 23 cases serie. The operation found to be successfull in Crowe type IV patients. Furthermore, Grappiolo et al performed different femoral osteotomy techniques during total hip prosthesis surgery of 128 dysplastic hips (Grappiolo et al, 2007). They thought that subtrochanteric transvers osteotomy was the safest technique, after a 20 years experience.

Also, subtrochanteric transvers osteotomy is the technique which was favoured in our clinic for last 6 and 7 years. It seems to be much easy to perform, rather than the other techniques. The other advantage of this technique is that it gives you the possibility to fix the malrotation of the proximally femur.
In spite of these good results with shortening osteotomy, some authors don't favor shortening of the femoral diaphysis (Hartofilakidis & Karachalios, 2004). Osteotomy of the greater trochanter was performed in all hips except for three with dysplasia in a series of Hartofilakidis, consisted of 223 patients. They shortened the femur with progressive resection of bone from the femoral neck. Although they acquired a limb-lengthening of average 3.5 cm (1 to 7 cm) in the high dislocated patients, they only reported 2 nerve palsy which resolved within six months. They believed that nerve damage can be avoided by cautious handling of the retractors intraoperatively and by the placement of both hip and knee in flexion for three to four days after the operation. Fibrous union was seen 4%, 13% and 22% of the patients in dysplastic, low dislocated and high dislocated groups, respectively. It was stated that all of these fibrous unions were asymptomatic. Non-union and migration of the greater trochanter was observed in 2 and 1 hips in low dislocated and high dislocated groups, respectively.
Kerboull et al., also performed femoral stem mostly without shortening in 118 Crowe type IV hips (Kerboull et al., 2001). Shortening of the femur was needed only in 2 patients. Only 1 transient peroneal nevre palsy was reported although limb was lengthened more than 4 cm in 30 hips. The amount of limb lengthening causing nerve palsy, is not clear in the literature. After the operation, hip and knee flexion may help in reducing the tension in femoral and peroneal nerve, respectively. It was reported that 2.7 cm lengthening increased the risk of peroneal nerve injury, while 4.4 cm lengthening increased the risk of sciatic nerve injury (Edwards et al., 1987). They concluded that the maximal lengthening shouldn't exceed 4 cm. The 30 % of nerve palsy thought to be due to lengthening of the limb (Johanson et al., 1983). However, no correlation was observed between nerve injury and the amount of limb lengthening in a study, recently (Eggli et al, 1999). They found out the relation between nerve injury and the severity of the surgery. All cases who had nerve palsy after the operation, except one, required hard work because of different reasons like; previous operation, the severity of the disease, large acetabuler defect, serious flexion deformity of the hip. Direct or indirect mechanical trauma was thougth to be responsible in nerve palsy.

2.4.7 The resurfacing arthroplasty in DDH

Although that total hip arthroplasty is known as the golden treatment option in DDH, it was reported that resurfacing arthroplasty would be a successful alternative in Crowe type 1-2 patients (Xu et al., 2008). Amsutz et al. operated 103 hips of 90 patients whom have 94 percent Crowe type 1 displasia and reported it as a perfect method in a short and mid term period (Amstutz et al., 2008). It was interesting that the 43% of the femoral heads had a defect of more than 1 cm in their series. The vitality of the femoral head of the patients, whom were operated with Birmingham implants, was examined by fluride positron emission tomography and found that the femoral head vitality persisted after the operation (Forrest et al., 2006). However, the ALVAL reaction resulted from metal-metal implants is the drawback of this technique, because the age-group of the indicated patients are mostly young.

2.4.8 Difficulties of arthroplasty in previously operated patients

The affect of the previous operations at the childhood on arthroplasty is not clear. Highly complication and revision rates were reported after total hip arthroplasty of the patients with femoral osteotomy (Ferguson et al., 1994). Boos et al. compared the results of the total hip arthroplasty between the patients whom femoral osteomy was performed before and not performed (Boos et al., 1997). There was no difference in peri-operatif complication and revision rates but they stated that the operation time was much longer and the surgical exposure was much difficult in the previously operated group than the other.
Chiari osteotomy was thought to be as an ease in the acetabuler component placement during the arthroplasty operations (Chiari, 1974). Supporters of this opinion attract the attention on the need of long time studies to sustain their theory (Hoffman et al., 1974; Mitchell, 1974; Wedge, 1995). Despite of these supporters, more bleeding was reported in previously operated patients with Chiari technique. And it was also stated that it was time consuming and the morbidiy was higher (Minoda et al., 2006). The removal of the implants used during the osteotomy operations seems as a factor increasing the morbidity (Beaupre & Csongradi, 1996; Jago & Hindley, 1998). In our experience, it is hard to secure the primary stability of the acetabulum in patients who had periacetabular osteotomy beforehand.

3. Conclusion

There are several classification systems which may tell us the pathology very well in DDH. However none of them seems to be a candidate to guide for the surgeon in choosing the best technique and prosthesis as well. It is obvious that there is a need for a new classification method in DDH. 3D CT scans may be useful in preoperative planning. The reconstruction in DDH will remain as a challange which may be overcomed in the battle field since a new classification method is reported to help the surgeon.

4. References

Anda S., Terjesen T., Kvistad K.A. (1991). Computed tomography measurements of the acetabulum in adult dysplastic hips: which level is appropriate? *Skeletal Radiol.* Vol.20, No.4, pp.267-271, ISBN 1853218

Amstutz HC, Le Duff MJ, Harvey N, Hoberg M. (2008). Improved survivorship of hybrid metal-on-metal hip resurfacing with second-generation techniques for Crowe-I and II developmental dysplasia of the hip. *J Bone Joint Surg Am.* Vol.90, Suppl. 3, (August), pp.12-20, ISBN 18676931

Argenson JN, Ryembault E, Flecher X, Brassart N, Parratte S, Aubaniac JM. (2005). Three-dimensional anatomy of the hip in osteoarthritis after developmental dysplasia. *J Bone Joint Surg Br.* Vol.87, No.9, (September), pp.1192-1196, ISBN 16129740

Beaupre G.S., Csongradi J.J. (1996). Refracture risk after plate removal in the forearm. *J Orthop Trauma.* Vol.10, No.2, (February), pp.87-92, ISBN 8932666

Biant L.C., Bruce W.J., Assini J.B., Walker P.M., Walsh W.R. (2009). Primary total hip arthroplasty in severe developmental dysplasia of the hip. Ten-year results using a cementless modular stem. *J Arthroplasty.* Vol.24, No.1, (January), pp.27-32, ISBN 18977633

Boos N., Krushell R., Ganz R., Müller M.E. (1997). Total hip arthroplasty after previous proximal femoral osteotomy. *J Bone Joint Surg Br.* Vol.79, No.2, (March), pp.247-253, ISBN 9119851

Bozic K.J., Freiberg A.A., Harris W.H. (2004).The high hip center. *Clin Orthop Relat Res.* Vol.420, (March), pp.101-105, ISBN 15057084

Bruce W.J., Rizkallah S.M., Kwon Y.M., Goldberg J.A., Walsh W.R. (2000). A new technique of subtrochanteric shortening in total hip arthroplasty: surgical technique and results of 9 cases. *J Arthroplasty.* Vol.15, No.5, (August), pp.617-626, ISBN 10960001

Brunner A, Ulmar B, Reichel H, Decking R. (2008). The Eftekhar and Kerboul classifications in assessment of developmental dysplasia of the hip in adult patients. Measurement of inter- and intraobserver reliability. *HSS J.* Vol.4, No.1, (February), pp.25-31, ISBN 18751859

Cabanela M.E. (2001) Total hip arthroplasty for developmental dysplasia of the hip. *Orthopedics.* Vol.24, No.9, (September) pp.865-866, ISBN 11570460

Charnley J., Feagin J.A. (1973). Low-friction arthroplasty in congenital subluxation of the hip. *Clin Orthop Relat Res.* Vol.91, (March-April), pp.98-113, ISBN 4574070

Cameron H.U., Botsford D.J., Park Y.S. (1996). Influence of the Crowe rating on the outcome of total hip arthroplasty in congenital hip dysplasia. *J Arthroplasty.* Vol.11, No.5, (August), pp.582-587, ISBN 8872579

Chougle A., Hemmady M.V., Hodgkinson J.P. (2005). Severity of hip dysplasia and loosening of the socket in cemented total hip replacement. A long-term follow-up. *J Bone Joint Surg Br.* Vol.87, No.1, (January), pp.16-20, ISBN 15686231

Chiari K. (1974). Medial displacement osteotomy of the pelvis. *Clin Orthop Relat Res.* Vol.98, (January-Febuary), pp.55-71, ISBN 4817245

Crowe J.F., Mani V.J., Ranawat C.S. (1979). Total hip replacement in congenital dislocation and dysplasia of the hip. *J Bone Joint Surg Am.* Vol.61, No.1, (January), pp.15-23, ISBN 365863

Dearborn J.T., Harris W.H. (1999). High placement of an acetabular component inserted without cement in a revision total hip arthroplasty. Results after a mean of ten years. *J Bone Joint Surg Am.* Apr;81(4):469-80, ISBN 10225792

Decking R, Brunner A, Decking J, Puhl W, Günther KP. (2006). Reliability of the Crowe und Hartofilakidis classifications used in the assessment of the adult dysplastic hip. *Skeletal Radiol. Vol.35, No.5,* (May), pp.282-287, ISBN 16534641

Doehring T.C., Rubash H.E., Shelley F.J., Schwendeman L.J., Donaldson T.K., Navalgund Y.A. (1996). Effect of superior and superolateral relocations of the hip center on hip joint forces. An experimental and analytical analysis. *J Arthroplasty.* Vol.11, No.6, (September), pp.693-703, ISBN 8884445

Dudkiewicz I., Salai M., Ganel A., Blankstein A., Chechik A. (2002). Total hip arthroplasty in patients younger than 30 years of age following developmental dysplasia of hip (DDH) in infancy. *Arch Orthop Trauma Surg.* Vol.122, No.3, (April), pp.139-142, ISBN 11927994

Dunn HK, Hess WE. (1976). Total hip reconstruction in chronically dislocated hips. *J Bone Joint Surg Am.* Vol.58, No.6, (September), pp.838-845, ISBN 956229

Edwards BN, Tullos HS, Noble PC. (1987). Contributory factors and etiology of sciatic nerve palsy in total hip arthroplasty. *Clin Orthop Relat Res.* Vol.218, (May), pp.136-141, ISBN 3568473

Eftekhar N. (1978). Principles of total hip arthroplasty. C V Mosby, St. Louis, pp 437–455.

Eggli S., Hankemayer S., Müller M.E. (1999). Nerve palsy after leg lengthening in total replacement arthroplasty for developmental dysplasia of the hip. *J Bone Joint Surg Br.* Vol.81, No.5, (September), pp.843-845, ISBN 10530847

Ferguson G.M., Cabanela M.E., Ilstrup D.M. (1994). Total hip arthroplasty after failed intertrochanteric osteotomy. *J Bone Joint Surg Br.* Vol.76, No.2, pp.252-257, ISBN 8113286

Flecher X., Parratte S., Brassart N., Aubaniac J.M., Argenson J.N. (2008). Evaluation of the hip center in total hip arthroplasty for old developmental dysplasia. *J Arthroplasty.* Vol.23, No.8, (December), pp.1189-1196, ISBN 18534475

Forrest N., Welch A., Murray AD., Schweiger L., Hutchison J., Ashcroft G.P. (2006). Femoral head viability after Birmingham resurfacing hip arthroplasty: assessment with use of [18F] fluoride positron emission tomography. *J Bone Joint Surg Am.* Vol.88, Suppl.3, (November), pp.84-89, ISBN 17079372

Gardner E., Gray D.J. (1950). Prenatal development of the human hip joint. *Am J Anat.* Vol.87, No.2, (September), pp.163-211, ISBN 14771010

Gill T.J., Sledge J.B., Müller M.E. (1998). Total hip arthroplasty with use of an acetabular reinforcement ring in patients who have congenital dysplasia of the hip. Results at five to fifteen years. *J Bone Joint Surg Am.* Vol.80, No.7, (July), pp.969-979, ISBN 9698001

Grappiolo G., Spotorno L., Burastero G. (2007). Evolution of surgical techniques for the treatment of angular and torsional deviation in DDH: 20 years experience. *Hip Int.* Vol.17, Suppl.5, pp.105-110, ISBN 19197890

Harris W.H. (1974). Total hip replacement for congenital dysplasia of the hip: Technique. *In W.H. Harris (Ed). The Hip, Proceedings of the 2nd Open Scientific Session of the Hip Society.* St Louis, CV Mosby, pp.251-265

Harris W.H., Crothers O., Oh I. (1977). Total hip replacement and femoral-head bone-grafting for severe acetabular deficiency in adults. *J Bone Joint Surg Am.* Vol.59, No.6, (September), pp.752-759, ISBN 908698

Harris W.H. (1993). Management of the deficient acetabulum using cementless fixation without bone grafting. *Orthop Clin North Am.* Vol.24, No.4, (October), pp.663-665, ISBN 8414432

Harrison T.J. (1961). The influence of the femoral head on pelvic growth and acetabular form in the rat. *J Anat.* Vol.95, (January), pp.12-24, ISBN 13711848

Hartofilakidis G., Stamos K, Ioannidis T.T. (1988). Low friction arthroplasty for old untreated congenital dislocation of the hip. *J Bone Joint Surg Br.* Vol.70, No.2, (March), pp.182-186, ISBN 3346284

Hartofilakidis G., Stamos K., Karachalios T., Ioannidis T.T., Zacharakis N. (1996). Congenital hip disease in adults. Classification of acetabular deficiencies and operative treatment with acetabuloplasty combined with total hip arthroplasty. *J Bone Joint Surg Am.* Vol.78, No.5, (May), pp.683-92, ISBN 8642024

Hartofilakidis G., Karachalios T., Stamos K.G. (2000). Epidemiology, demographics, and natural history of congenital hip disease in adults. *Orthopedics*. Vol.23, No.8, (August), pp.823-7, ISBN 10952045

Hartofilakidis G., Karachalios T. (2004). Total hip arthroplasty for congenital hip disease. *J Bone Joint Surg Am.* Vol.86-A, No.2, (February), pp.242-250, ISBN 14960667

Hess W.E., Umber J.S. (1978). Total hip arthroplasty in chronically dislocated hips. Follow-up study on the protrusio socket technique. *J Bone Joint Surg Am.* Vol.60, No.7, (October), pp.948-954, ISBN 701343

Heyman C.H., Herndon C.H. (1950). Legg-Perthes disease; a method for the measurement of the roentgenographic result. *J Bone Joint Surg Am.* Vol.32, No.A4, (October), pp.767-778, ISBN 14784485

Hirakawa K., Mitsugi N., Koshino T., Saito T., Hirasawa Y., Kubo T. (2001). Effect of acetabular cup position and orientation in cemented total hip arthroplasty. *Clin Orthop Relat Res.* Vol.388, (July), pp.135-142, ISBN 11451112

Hoffman D.V., Simmons E.H., Barrington T.W. (1974). The results of the Chiari osteotomy. *Clin Orthop Relat Res.* Vol.98, (January-February), pp.162-170, ISBN 4817226

Jago E.R., Hindley C.J. (1998). The removal of metalwork in children. *Injury.* Vol.29, No.6, (July), pp.439-441, ISBN 9813700

Jasty M., Harris W.H. (1990). Salvage total hip reconstruction in patients with major acetabular bone deficiency using structural femoral head allografts. J Bone Joint Surg Br. Vol.72, No.1, (January), pp.63-67, ISBN 2298796

Jasty M., Anderson M.J., Harris W.H. (1995). Total hip replacement for developmental dysplasia of the hip. Clin Orthop Relat Res. Vol.311, (February), pp.40-45, ISBN 7634589

Johanson N.A., Pellicci P.M., Tsairis P., Salvati E.A. (1983). Nerve injury in total hip arthroplasty. *Clin Orthop Relat Res.* Vol.179, (October), pp.214-222, ISBN 6617020

Kennedy J.G., Rogers W.B., Soffe K.E., Sullivan R.J., Griffen D.G., Sheehan L.J. (1998). Effect of acetabular component orientation on recurrent dislocation, pelvic osteolysis, polyethylene wear, and component migration. *J Arthroplasty.* Vol.13, No.5, (August), pp.530-534, ISBN 9726318

Kerboul M., Mathieu M., Sauzieres P. (1987). Total hip replacement for congenital dislocation of the hip. In: Postel M., Kerboul M., Evrard J., Courpied J.P. (eds) Total hip replacement. Springer, Berlin Heidelberg New York, pp 51–66 .

Kerboull M., Hamadouche M., Kerboull L. (2001). Total hip arthroplasty for Crowe type IV developmental hip dysplasia: a long-term follow-up study. *J Arthroplasty.* Vol.16, No.8, Suppl. 1, (December), pp.170-176, ISBN 11742471

Klapach A.S., Callaghan J.J., Goetz D.D., Olejniczak J.P., Johnston R.C.(2001). Charnley total hip arthroplasty with use of improved cementing techniques: a minimum twenty-year follow-up study. *J Bone Joint Surg Am.* Vol.83-A, No.12, (December), pp.1840-1848, ISBN 11741064

Klisic P., Jankovic L. (1976). Combined procedure of open reduction and shortening of the femur in treatment of congenital dislocation of the hips in older children. *Clin Orthop Relat Res.* Vol.119, (September), pp.60-69, ISBN 954325

Krych A.J., Howard J.L., Trousdale R.T., Cabanela M.E., Berry D.J. (2010). Total hip arthroplasty with shortening subtrochanteric osteotomy in Crowe type-IV developmental dysplasia: surgical technique. *J Bone Joint Surg Am.* Suppl. 1, Pt. 2, (September), pp.176-187, ISBN 20844173

Kumar A., Shair A.B. (1997). An extended iliofemoral approach for total arthroplasty in late congenital dislocation of the hip: a case report. *Int Orthop.* Vol.21, No.4, (September), pp.265-266, ISBN 9349966

Lai K.A., Shen W.J., Huang L.W., Chen M.Y. (2005). Cementless total hip arthroplasty and limb-length equalization in patients with unilateral Crowe type-IV hip dislocation. *J Bone Joint Surg Am.* Vol.87, No.2, (February), pp.339-345, ISBN 15687157

Linde F., Jensen J. (1988). Socket loosening in arthroplasty for congenital dislocation of the hip. *Acta Orthop Scand.* Vol.59, No.3, (June), pp.254-257, ISBN 3381653

MacKenzie J.R., Kelley S.S., Johnston R.C. (1996). Total hip replacement for coxarthrosis secondary to congenital dysplasia and dislocation of the hip. Long-term results. *J Bone Joint Surg Am.* Vol.78, No.1, (January), pp.55-61, ISBN 8550680

McQueary F.G., Johnston R.C. (1988). Coxarthrosis after congenital dysplasia. Treatment by total hip arthroplasty without acetabular bone-grafting. *J Bone Joint Surg Am.* Vol.70, No.8, (September), pp.1140-1144, ISBN 3417699

Mendes D.G., Said M.S., Aslan K. (1996). Classification of adult congenital hip dysplasia for total hip arthroplasty. *Orthopedics.* Vol.19, No.10, (October), pp. 881-887, ISBN 8905863

Minoda Y., Kadowaki T., Kim M. (2006). Total hip arthroplasty of dysplastic hip after previous Chiari pelvic osteotomy. *Arch Orthop Trauma Surg.* Vol.126, No.6, (August), pp.394-400, ISBN 16628429

Mitchell G.P. (1974). Chiari medial displacement osteotomy. *Clin Orthop Relat Res.* Vol.98, (January-February), pp.146-150, ISBN 4817224

Mulroy R.D. Jr., Harris W.H. (1990). Failure of acetabular autogenous grafts in total hip arthroplasty. Increasing incidence: a follow-up note. *J Bone Joint Surg Am.* Vol.72, No.10, (December), pp.1536-1540, ISBN 2254363

Nakamura S., Yorikawa J., Otsuka K., Takeshita K., Harasawa A., Matsushita T. (2000). Evaluation of acetabular dysplasia using a top view of the hip on three-dimensional CT. *J Orthop Sci.* Vol.5, No.6, (November), pp.533-539, ISBN 11180914

Noble P.C., Kamaric E., Sugano N., Matsubara M., Harada Y., Ohzono K., Paravic V. (2003). Three-dimensional shape of the dysplastic femur: implications for THR. *Clin Orthop Relat Res.* Vol.417, (December), pp.27-40,ISBN 14646700

Onodera S., Majima T., Ito H., Matsuno T., Kishimoto T., Minami A. (2006). Cementless total hip arthroplasty using the modular S-ROM prosthesis combined with corrective proximal femoral osteotomy. *J Arthroplasty.* Vol.21, No.5, (August), pp.664-669, ISBN 16877151

Paavilainen T., Hoikka V., Solonen K.A. (1990). Cementless total replacement for severely dysplastic or dislocated hips. *J Bone Joint Surg Br.* Vol.72, No.2, (March), pp.205-211, ISBN 2312556

Pagnano W., Hanssen A.D., Lewallen D.G., Shaughnessy W.J. (1996). The effect of superior placement of the acetabular component on the rate of loosening after total hip arthroplasty. *J Bone Joint Surg Am.* Vol.78, No.7, (July), pp.1004-14, ISBN 8698717

Park M.S., Kim K.H., Jeong W.C. (2007). Transverse subtrochanteric shortening osteotomy in primary total hip arthroplasty for patients with severe hip developmental dysplasia. *J Arthroplasty.* Vol.22, No.7, (October), pp.1031-1036, ISBN 17920477

Patterson F.P., Brown C.S. (1972). The McKee-Farrar total hip replacement. Preliminary results and complications of 368 operations performed in five general hospitals. *J Bone Joint Surg Am.* Vol.54, No.2, (March), pp.257-75, ISBN 4631242

Perka C., Fischer U., Taylor W.R., Matziolis G. (2004). Developmental hip dysplasia treated with total hip arthroplasty with a straight stem and a threaded cup. *J Bone Joint Surg Am.* Vol.86-A, No.2, (February), pp.312-319, ISBN 14960676

Ponseti I.V. (1978). Growth and development of the acetabulum in the normal child. Anatomical, histological, and roentgenographic studies. *J Bone Joint Surg Am.* Vol.60, No.5, (July), pp.575-585. ISBN 681376

Rális Z., McKibbin B. (1973). Changes in shape of the human hip joint during its development and their relation to its stability. *J Bone Joint Surg Br.* Vol.55, No.4, (November), pp.780-785, ISBN 4766182

Russotti G.M., Harris W.H. (1991). Proximal placement of the acetabular component in total hip arthroplasty. A long-term follow-up study. *J Bone Joint Surg Am.* Vol.73, No.4, (April), pp. 587-592, ISBN 2013598

Sharp I. (1961). Acetabular dysplasia. *J Bone Joint Surg (Br).* Vol.43, pp.268-272.

Saikko V.O. (1995). Wear of the polyethylene acetabular cup. The effect of head material, head diameter, and cup thickness studied with a hip simulator. *Acta Orthop Scand.* Vol.66, No.6, (December), pp.501-506, ISBN 8553815

Sener N., Tozun I.R., Asik M. (2002). Femoral shortening and cementless arthroplasty in high congenital dislocation of the hip. *J Arthroplasty.* Vol.17, No.1, (January), pp.41-48, ISBN 11805923

Smith W.S., Ireton R.J, Coleman C.R. (1958). Sequelae of experimental dislocation of a weight-bearing ball- and socket joint in a young growing animal; gross alterations in bone and cartilage. *J Bone Joint Surg Am.* Vol.40-A, No.5, (October), pp.1121-1127, ISBN 13587581

Sponseller P.D., McBeath A.A. (1988). Subtrochanteric osteotomy with intramedullary fixation for arthroplasty of the dysplastic hip. A case report. *J Arthroplasty.* Vol.3, No.4, pp.351-354, ISBN 3241173

Stamos K., Hartofilakidis G., Koroneas A., Xenakis T. Mechanical strength of P.M.M.A bonding to cancellous bone graft. An experimental study in dogs. Read the combined meetings of the Hellenic Association of Orthopaedic Surgery and Traumatology and American Hip Society, Rhodes, May 4, 1984.

Stans A.A., Pagnano M.W., Shaughnessy W.J., Hanssen A.D. (1998). Results of total hip arthroplasty for Crowe Type III developmental hip dysplasia. *Clin Orthop Relat Res.* Vol.348, (March), pp.149-157, ISBN 9553547

Strayer L.M. (1943). The Embryology of the Human Hip Joint. *Yale J Biol Med.* Vol.16, No.1, (October 1943), pp. 13-26.6, ISBN 21434122

Ström H., Mallmin H., Milbrink J., Petrén-Mallmin M., Nivbrant B., Kolstad K. (2003). The cone hip stem: a prospective study of 13 patients followed for 5 years with RSA. Acta Orthop Scand. Vol.74, No.5, (October), pp.525-530, ISBN 14620971

Symeonides P.P., Pournaras J., Petsatodes G., Christoforides J., Hatzokos I., Pantazis E. (1997). Total hip arthroplasty in neglected congenital dislocation of the hip. *Clin Orthop Relat Res.* Vol.341, (August), pp.55-61, ISBN 9269155

Takao M., Ohzono K., Nishii T., Miki H., Nakamura N., Sugano N. (2011). Cementless modular total hip arthroplasty with subtrochanteric shortening osteotomy for hips with developmental dysplasia. *J Bone Joint Surg Am.* Vol.93, No.6, (March), pp.548-555, ISBN 21411705

Troelsen A, Rømer L, Jacobsen S, Ladelund S, Søballe K. (2010). Cranial acetabular retroversion is common in developmental dysplasia of the hip as assessed by the weight bearing position. *Acta Orthop.* Vol.81, No.4, (August), pp.436-441, ISBN 20809742

Watanabe RS. (1974). Embryology of the Human Hip. *Clin Orthop Relat Res.* Vol.98, (Jan-Feb), pp.8-26, ISBN 4817247

Wedge J.H. (1995). Osteotomy of the pelvis for the management of hip disease in young adults. *Can J Surg.* Vol.38, Suppl.1, (February), pp.25-32, ISBN 7874625

Wedge J.H., Wasylenko M.J. (1978). The natural history of congenital dislocation of the hip: a critical review. *Clin Orthop Relat Res.* Vol.137, (Nov-Dec), pp.154-162, ISBN 743823

Weinstein S.L. (1987). Natural history of congenital hip dislocation (CDH) and hip dysplasia. *Clin Orthop Relat Res.* Vol.225, (December), pp.62-76. ISBN 3315382

Wiberg G. (1939). Studies on dysplasiic acelabula and congenital subluxation of the hip joint. *Acta Ortbop Scand.* Vol. 58, No. Suppl, pp.1-132

Xenakis TA, Gelalis ID, Koukoubis TD, Soucacos PN, Vartziotis K, Kontoyiannis D, Tatsis C. (1996). Neglected congenital dislocation of the hip. Role of computed tomography and computer-aided design for total hip arthroplasty. *J Arthroplasty.* Vol.11, No.8, (December), pp.893-8, ISBN 8986566

Xu W.D., Li J., Zhou Z.H., Wu Y.S., Li M. (2008). Results of hip resurfacing for developmental dysplasia of the hip of Crowe type I and II. *Chin Med J (Engl).* Vol.121, No.15, (August), pp.1379-1383, ISBN 18959113

Yalcin N., Kilicarslan K., Karatas F., Mutlu T., Yildirim H. (2010). Cementless total hip arthroplasty with subtrochanteric transverse shortening osteotomy for severely dysplastic or dislocated hips. *Hip Int.* Vol.20, No.1, (January-March), pp.87-93, ISBN 20235079

Yasgur D.J., Stuchin S.A., Adler E.M., DiCesare P.E. (1997). Subtrochanteric femoral shortening osteotomy in total hip arthroplasty for high-riding developmental dislocation of the hip. *J Arthroplasty.* Vol.12, No.8, (December), pp.880-888, ISBN 9458253

Yoder S.A., Brand R.A., Pedersen D.R., O'Gorman T.W. (1988). Total hip acetabular component position affects component loosening rates. *Clin Orthop Relat Res.* Vol.228, (March), pp.79-87, ISBN 3342591

10

Hip Arthroplasty in Highly Dislocated Hips

Zoran Bascarevic[1,2], Zoran Vukasinovic[1,2],
Violeta Bascarevic[2] and Vladimir Bascarevic[1,3]
[1]*Faculty of Medicine, University of Belgrade, Belgrade*
[2]*Institute of Orthopaedic Surgery „Banjica", Belgrade*
[3]*Institute of Neurosurgery, Clinical Center of Serbia, Belgrade*
Serbia

1. Introduction

Developmental disorder of the hip (DDH) is the most frequent disease of this joint. It is manifested by dysplasia, subluxation or luxation in childhood period and arthrosis in adults. Early degenerative changes of the hip occur at the location of disordered anatomy and biomechanics already in youth, while in the childhood age they are mostly asymptomatic (Ando & Gotoh, 1990).

DDH mostly occurs in females, even 4-10 times more often than in males. Also, the disease is unevenly expanded, both ethnically and geographically, but also according to different habits in regard to the nursing care of neonates and infants. For example, the disease does not develop among the Bantu colored population, while in Canadian Indians it is very frequent rating even 12.3%, which is related to their habit of nursing babies in narrow wooden cradles. In those Indians who do not practice it the frequency is considerably lower (1.2%) (Vukasinovic et al., 1994, 2004).

In our regions data on the frequency of DDH vary between 0.5-34.8%, depending on the regional customs in nursing children, but also on the method applied in the diagnostics of the disease; clinically it is the lowest, radiographically higher, and ultrasonographically the highest (Klisic et al., 1984). Former classical term of the disease was "congenital dislocation of the hip", which, over the years became unsustainable, since it has been disclosed that the disease is not congenital, but that it often develops after birth under the influence of environmental factors. In addition, it does not always involve a total dislocation, but only disturbed interrelationship among the joint surfaces of the hip. Although the former term can be still found in the literature, today the term "developmental disorder of the hip" is accepted worldwide (Klisic, 1989).

2. Etiopathogenesis and pathoanatomy of DDH

To understand the problem faced by the arthroplastic surgeon in treating a high luxation of the hip in adults, it is necessary to be acquainted with etiopathogenesis of the disease, because it is in a direct association with its pathoanatomic substrate.

After numerous years of research, attitudes of the leading world experts on this disease have been mostly brought in accordance (Ando & Gotoh 1990; Cherney & Westin 1989; Klisic et al. 1984, 1989; Vukasinovic & Bascarevic, 2004).

There is the predominating opinion that two groups of etiological factors contribute to the development of DDH; endogenous and exogenous (mechanical). (Vukasinovic & Djoric, 1994; Vukasinovic & Bascarevic, 2004).
Endogenous factors involve acetabular dysplasia, increased anteversion of the femoral neck and head, as well as joint laxity. Beside primary acetabular dysplasia, which is one of the causes of the disease, the so called secondary acetabular dysplasia is also mentioned, which develops due to hip dislocation itself. Although a lax joint capsule can be generalized, as for example when associated with Ehlers-Danlos syndrome, in DDH it is mostly only elongated in the superior-posterior portion, thus secondary, caused by luxation instead of being its major cause. (Vukasinovic & Djoric, 1994; Vukasinovic & Bascarevic, 2004).
Exogenous (mechanical) factors involve the basis of the so called mechanical theory which has been obtaining a rising number of supporters as it can explain the frequency of luxations in first pregnancies, pelvic positions, Cesarean section, high birth weight, oligohydramnion and fetopelvic disproportion. In addition, hip luxation due to DDH is often associated with other deformities of the feet, knees, neck (torticollis) and other. (Vukasinovic & Djoric, 1994; Vukasinovic & Bascarevic, 2004).
Exogenous (mechanical) factors can affect the fetus intrauterine, during delivery and postnatally. The intrauterine factors mostly involve three luxating fetal positions, while the postnatal ones above all refer to traditional baby diapering with bent knees and extended legs. Not only can such a position induce a spontaneous reduction of unstable joint, but it can also provoke the development of luxation. The mechanical factors occurring during birth can be discarded today, because even in newborns the hips are so stable that rough manual manipulation will sooner cause femoral head epyphysiolisis or diaphyseal fracture than hip luxation. It is considered that action of two factors is necessary for DDH to develop; a specific position of the femur involving the head which is not orientated toward the base of the acetabulum and expulsion force pushing the baby's head out of the acetabulum. (Vukasinovic & Djoric, 1994; Vukasinovic & Bascarevic, 2004).
In short, DDH pathogenesis features the following: a predisposing base representing unstable genetic factors, above all acetabular dysplasia and capsular laxity, while the determinant mechanical factors exert pressure on the great trochanter in one of the luxating fetal positions. This can explain the growing incidence of bilateral luxations in pelvic births; forces act on both great trochanters, i.e. isolated left-sided luxations in normal birth (baby head down presentation with left turned back); the maternal promontorium exerting pressure on the great trochanter. (Vukasinovic & Djoric, 1994; Vukasinovic & Bascarevic, 2004).
Pathological changes involve all structures of the joint, while the pathoanatomical substrate differs depending on the degree of disorder.
The acetabulum changes in depth during physiological development becoming the shallowest in the perinatal period. Spherical formation (joint congruency) is caused by the presence and pressure of the femoral head. In DDH unfavorable intra-articular relationships lead to acetabular anterior and superior deficiency, as well as its anteversion. Consequently, the acetabulum becomes ovoid or even triangle-like insufficiently covering the femoral head. It is mostly dilated, but can be also completely undeveloped, narrowed due to the lack of

developmental stimulation caused by the absent head in the joint. (Vukasinovic & Djoric, 1994; Bascarevic & Vukasinovic, 2004).

The limbus gradually flattens and thickens first in the superoposterior portion. Gradually, a groove is formed enabling the head to slide out of the joint. It is partially grown together with the capsule and is lacking in some areas. In subluxations it is everted, while in full luxations it is inverted and interpolated between the head and the acetabulum. (Vukasinovic & Djoric, 1994; Bascarevic & Vukasinovic, 2004).

The ligamentum teres differs depending on the severity of disorder ranging from normal and occasionally hypoplastic, elongated and hypertrophic, up to fully atrophic in luxations.

The femoral head can be differently formed, from normal - spherical to flattened and deformed with limbal impression. It is most often decreased with highly expressed fovea. (Vukasinovic & Djoric, 1994; Bascarevic & Vukasinovic, 2004).

The femoral neck is usually shortened with increased anteversion. However, it can even be normal, but also retroverted. The collo-diaphyseal angle is usually normal, but can be also decreased or conversely increased.

The capsule of the joint is thickened and mostly lax, but can be also tightened. With the progression of luxation, it becomes lengthened and narrowed in the empty space between the head and the acetabulum resuming the form of a sand-clock. It grows adhering to the bones that form the acetabulum, thus impeding reduction. (Vukasinovic & Djoric, 1994; Bascarevic & Vukasinovic, 2004).

The ligamentum transversum is most frequently strong and thickened and additionally narrows the already dysplastic acetabulum. Its position is the only constant one in the pathological anatomy of the hip in high luxations and represents the major and occasionally the only orientation point in the attempt to find the true acetabulum in the total arthroplasty of the hip. (Bascarevic & Vukasinovic, 2004).

Muscular motion starters are also changed, particularly the iliopsoas; its tendon is short and thickened, while short external rotators are hypotrophic, but also shortened. However, the major hip abductors, primarily the gluteus medius, although hypotrophic, are not shortened and do not create resistance before reduction. In addition, after arthroplasty and induction of the necessary muscular length (close to physiological) they show unusual vitality in the restitution of strength and function of joints. (Vukasinovic & Djoric, 1994; Bascarevic & Vukasinovic, 2004).

Finally, when we speak of high luxations of the hip in the light of aloarthroplasty, attention should be turned to the fact that DDH is not the only condition causing high luxation of the hip in adults. Hip trauma, juvenile rheumatism, neonatal sepsis and some other similar conditions can also cause established hip luxation that can be resolved only when treated by a total hip arthroplasty (Besset et al., 2003; Betz et al., 1990; Choi et al., 1990; Learmonth et al., 1989; Maric & Haynes 1993; Ruddlesdin et al., 1986; Young-Hoo et al., 2009).

3. Classification of high hip dislocation in adults

In the literature there are several classifications that determine high hip dislocation in adults. **Crowe** classification of hip dislocation describes four stages, depending on the position of the femoral head within the joint. The first three stages define the progressive migration of the head to the level of subluxation, while the fourth stage is luxation (Crowe et al., 1979).

According to the classification by **Eftekhar** the problem of the developmental disorders of the hip is viewed through acetabular changes. Four stages are also described; A/ slightly widened and dysplastic acetabulum with milder deformation of the head, B/ intermediately positioned false acetabulum, C/ high position of the false acetabulum, and D/ high non-weight bearing dislocation with the femoral head that has never been in contact with the iliac bone (Eftekhar 1978).

The most modern and up-to-now the best classification recommending total arthroplasty in relation to joint deficiency was given by **Hartofilakidis** et al. in 1996, according to which the condition was viewed as acetabular dysplasia, low dislocation and high dislocation (Hartofilakidis et al., 1996).

4. Treatment of high hip dislocation in adults

Treatment of the developmental disorder of the hip should be initiated at the moment of the disease detection, and the best results are achieved in the earliest childhood. At that period various forms of non-operative and operative treatments by biological surgeries are possible to be applied. (Vukasinovic & Djoric, 1994; Vukasinovic & Bascarevic, 2004). However, if the treatment is initiated only after the onset of arthrosis or under the conditions of high non-weight bearing hip luxation, operative treatment modalities are only reduced to total hip arthroplasty.

The operative procedure is most challenging because of changed anatomical correlations. The topographic correlation of muscles initiators of the hip, joint capsule and neurovascular elements are changed and unstable thus making the operative approach very difficult. The identification of bone structures, primarily of the true acetabulum, is also not at all easy (Lai et al., 1996, 2005; Charnley & Feagin 1973; Crowe et al., 1979; Dunn & Hess, 1976; Eskelinen et al., 2006; Hartofilakidis et al., 1998, 2004, 2008; Holinka et al., 2010; Paavilainen et al., 1990).

The ligamentum transversum is the only reliable parameter determining, not only the height and center of the artificial hip, but also the anteversion (flexion) position of the acetabular ring.

The proximal part of the femoral bone canal is very narrow, with markedly increased anteversion. The acetabular bone mass is underdeveloped, while the bone is insufficiently firm. The joint capsule is elongated, inelastic and thickened, while the surrounding muscles are without any strength, shortened and grown to the capsule. The neurovascular structures are shortened and dislocated from their anatomic positions (Carrlson et al., 2003; Holinka et al., 2010; Paavilainen et al., 1990).

In the past there were numerous unsuccessful attempts to perform total hip arthroplasty in adults at the location of high luxation caused by developmental disorder. Exactly due to excessively changed anatomic characteristics of the acetabulum and proximal femur, the operative procedure and the entire surgical concept are most complicated. Therefore, some authors consider high hip luxation as a contraindication for total arthroplasty (Figs. 1, 2, 3).

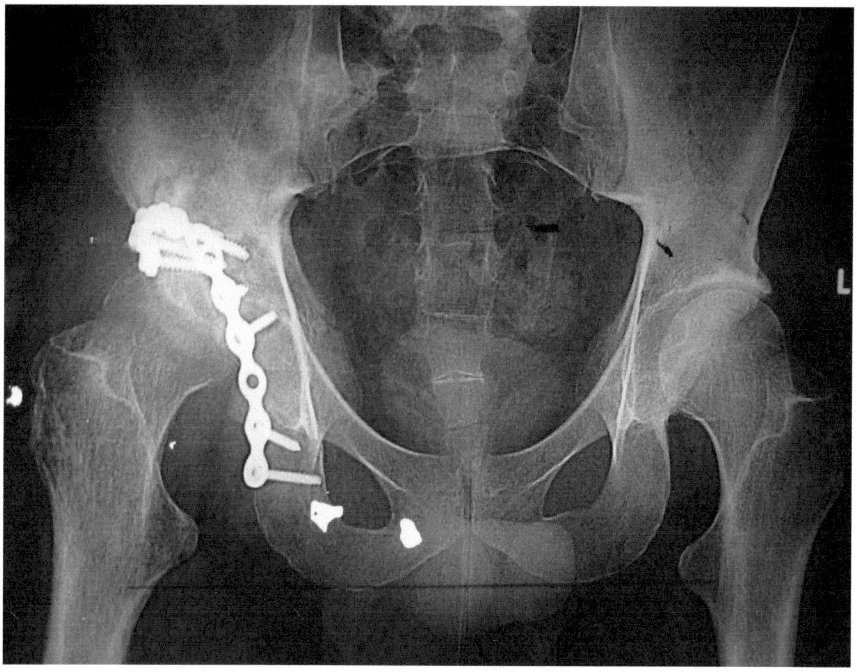

Fig. 1a. A 35-year old male after acetabular osteosynthesis performed due to traumatic dislocation of the right hip with superior and posterior acetabular wall fracture.

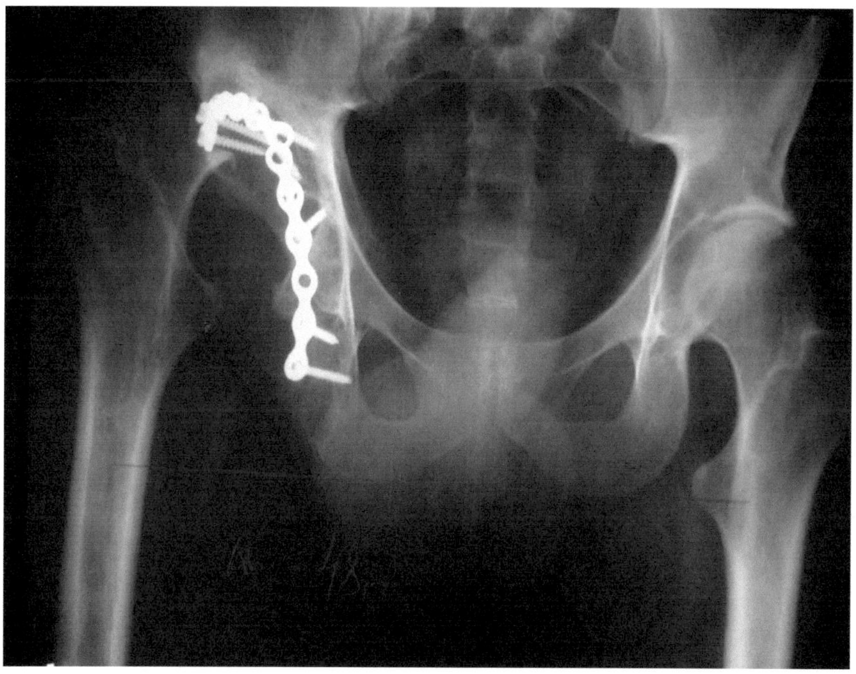

Fig. 1b.The same patient, six month later high dislocation of the hip occured due to failed osteosynthesis. Full absence of superior and posterior acetabular walls. Leg length discrepancy was 48 mm.

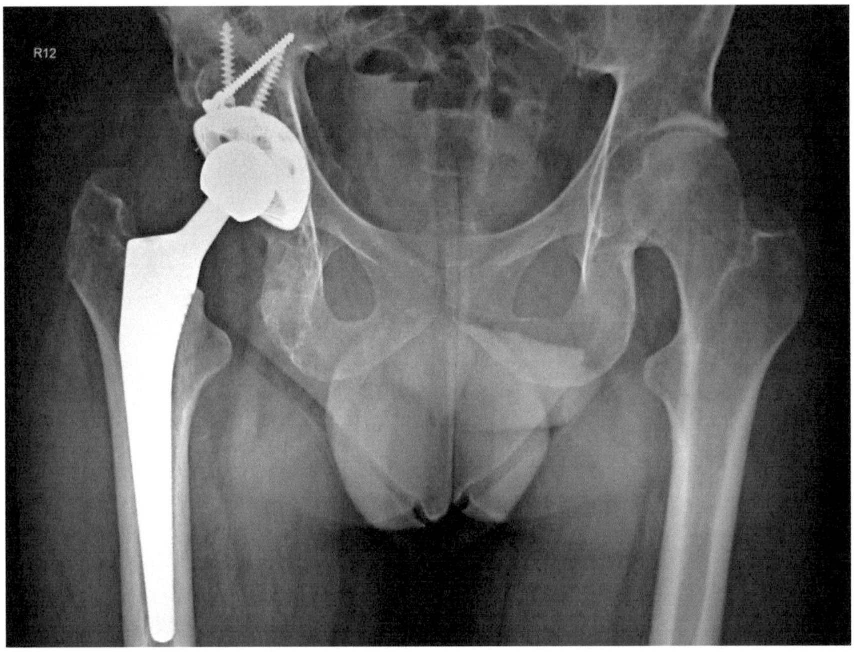

Fig. 1c. The same patient, three months after total arthroplasty of the hip, with the osteoplasty of the superior and posterior acetabular walls by solitary bone grafts from the bone bank. Restitution of leg length by positioning the acetabular component into the physiological hip rotation center.

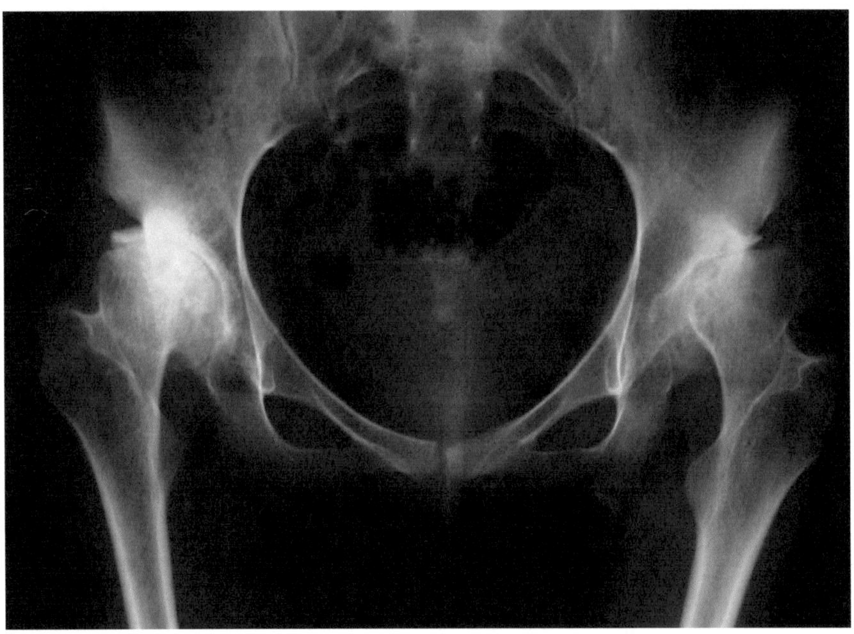

Fig. 2a. A 20-year old female with bilateral secondary arthrosis of the hips due to juvenile rheumatoid arthritis. Bilateral hip subluxation with various disorders of collo-diaphyseal femoral angle.

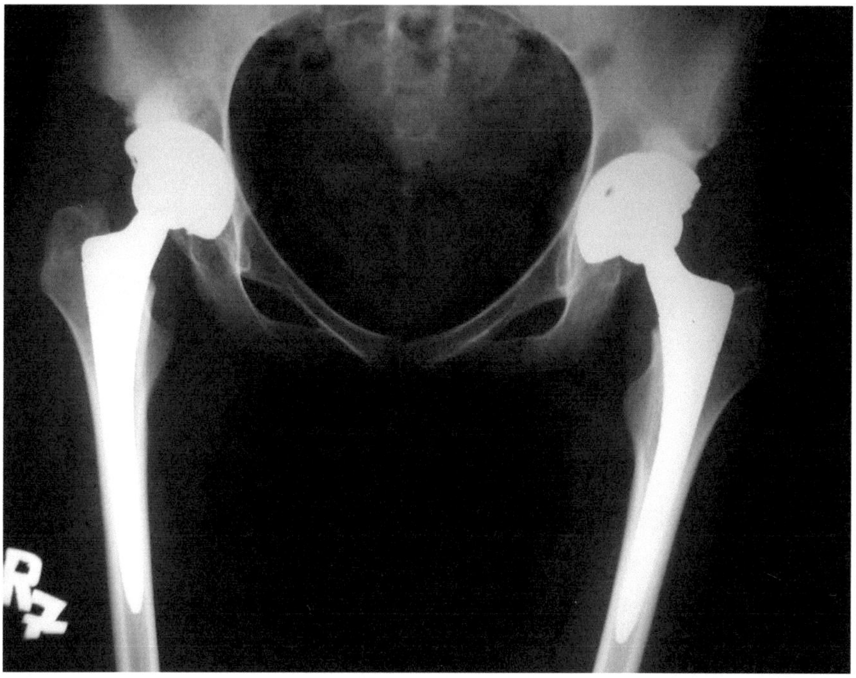

Fig. 2b. The same patient, one year after bilateral total arthroplasty of the hip with restitution of rotation centers.

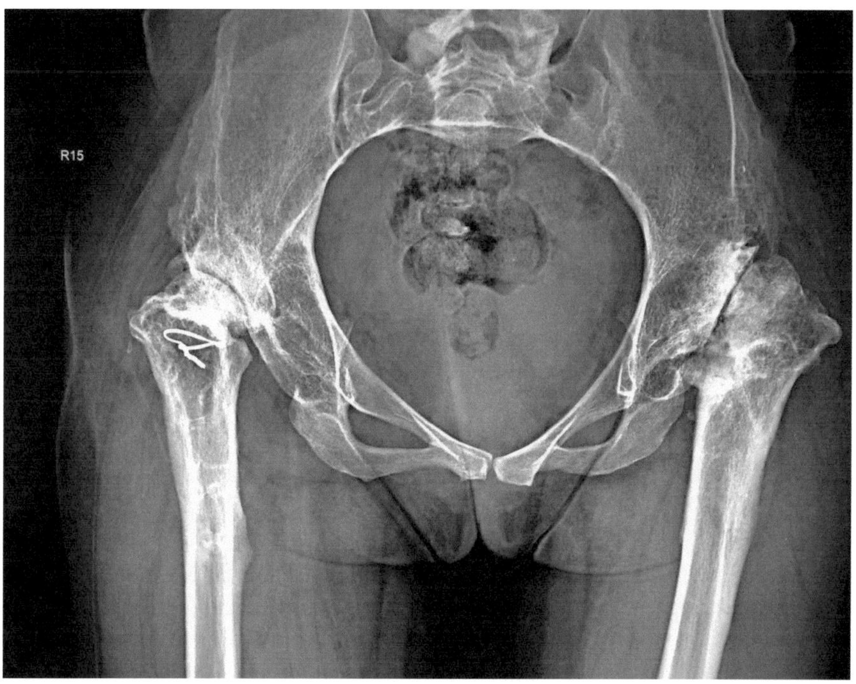

Fig. 3a. A 30-year old female with bilateral high dislocation of the hips after multiple surgeries due to neonatal sepsis.

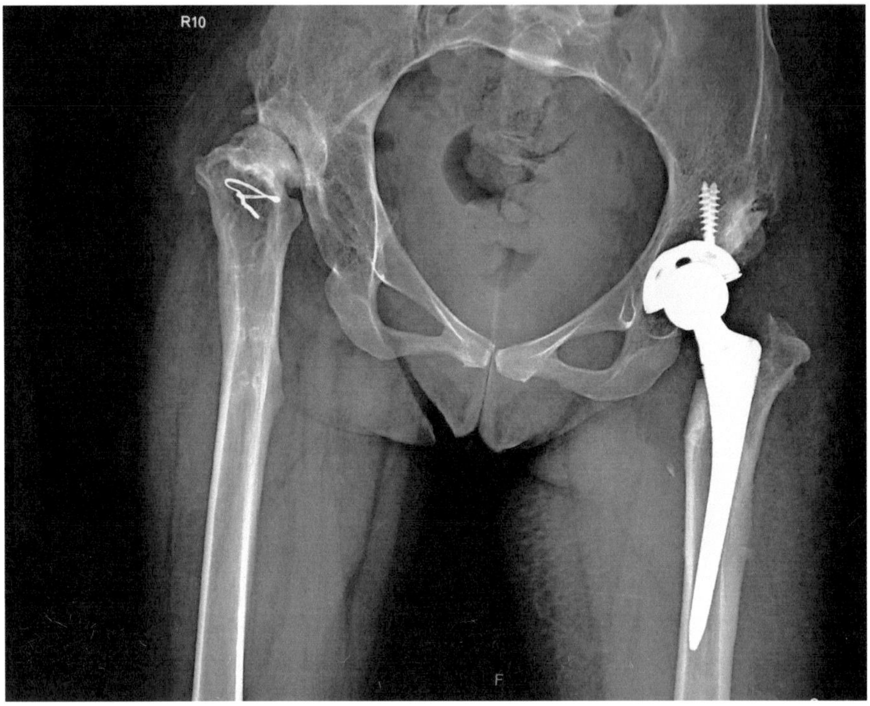

Fig. 3b. The same patient, one month after total arthroplasty of the left hip with restitution of rotation centers. The leg length equality is expected after the operation of the opposite hip.

4.1 Surgical procedures

The literature reports many operative techniques for total arthroplasty of the hip in patients with high dislocation. All agree on one point; the center of joint rotation should be restored, meaning that the acetabular component of the implant must be positioned in the primary paleo-acetabulum. This is the only way to expect good joint function, being the only mode to establish the physiological distance between the ends of the muscular initiators of hip motion, thus enabling their full strength. However, there is no full agreement as to the preparation and positioning of the proximal femur at the required level of the primary acetabulum (Carrlson et al., 2003; Crowe et al., 1979; Dunn & Hess, 1976; Eskelinen et al., 2006; Hartofilakidis et al., 1996, 1998, 2004; Holinka et al., 2010; Lai et al., 1996, 2005; Paavilainen et al., 1990).
Many surgical techniques have been described by authors discussing the type and modes of femoral abbreviation osteotomies. Some of them are performed through the very trochanteric mass (midtrochanteric), while others are done below it (subtrochanteric), with various forms of resection osteotomies with or without fixation of the proximal fragment or great trochanter. Some authors achieve the adequate position of the femur in correlation to paleo-acetabulum by extrafocal distraction after the resection of the joint. Arthroplasty is to follow as a new operative technique, where the entire operative procedure is performed in

two acts. (Carrlson et al., 2003; Eskelinen et al., 2006; Hartofilakidis et al., 1996; Holinka et al., 2010; Lai et al., 1996, 2005; Paavilainen et al., 1990).

4.1.1 Total hip arthoplasty with iliofemoral distraction in high hip dislocation

As a part of total arthroplasty, the surgical technique applied to achieve the reduction of a high luxation of the hip without using femoral osteotomy is a relatively rare operative procedure. In the literature it was described by Lai et al. in 1996 and 2005, and then by Holinka et al. in 2010 (Carrlson et al., 2003; Eskelinen et al., 2006; Holinka et al., 2010; Lai et al., 1996, 2005).

The leading idea of this surgical procedure is based on the hypothesis that operative procedures with femoral abbreviation osteotomies, regardless of the type, could generally leave a considerable leg-length discrepancy, as well as muscular weakness of hip motion starters. The authors found a back-up for this notion in the articles by Crowe et al., Charnley et al., Dunn et al., Hartofilakidis et al., Paavilainen et al.Eskelinen et al., and others (Charnley & Feagin 1973; Crowe et al., 1979; Dunn & Hess, 1976; Eskelinen et al., 2006; Hartofilakidis et al., 1998; Paavilainen et al., 1990).

The operative procedure is performed in two acts. Namely, total arthroplasty is preceded by iliofemoral distraction with the Wagner's apparatus positioned in the ilium and distal femur. Before the distraction, it is necessary to perform subcutaneous adductor tenotomy of the hip, while femoral head resection with a total soft tissue release can be done before the distraction (Holinka et al.) or in the second act, as a part of total arthroplasty (Lai et al.). The distraction is performed gradually, 2-5 mm daily with regular X-ray check-ups and follow-up of neurocircular status of extremities, until the required joint reduction is achieved, bringing the femoral small trochanter into the acetabular teardrop level. During this period the patient is kept in bed. The second surgical act is performed after a few weeks involving removal of the Wagner's distraction apparatus and total arthroplasty of the hip.

The principles of total arthroplasty with positioning of the acetabular ring into the paleo-acetabulum and the stem in the femoral channel are standard. (Carrlson et al., 2003; Holinka et al., 2010; Lai et al., 1996, 2005; Paavilainen et al., 1990).

Such a surgical procedure is very complicated and requires long-term hospitalization and inactivity of the patient. The fact itself that in achieving the goal, total arthroplasty of the hip, requires two operative acts makes it twice riskier for the patient. In addition, the positioning of an extrafocal external apparatus in the area of the hip before arthroplasty might be as such problematic, because of exposing bone tissue to external environment over a long period of time. Strong Schantz screws in the femoral diaphysis can also present areas of decreased biomechanical resistance, particularly as known that the femur is anyway dysplastic in high luxations. Problems can also arise intraoperatively if there is extensive femoral anteversion. Namely, the positioning of a stem of standard geometry under such conditions could prove impossible to perform in the correction of overextensive anteversion. A solution could found in using special stems of small dimensions and/or modular geometry; however, this does not solve the problem of the residual anterior torsion of the femoral neck.

All this is probably the reason why such operative procedure is rarely described in the literature.

4.1.2 Total hip arthoplasty with femoral abbreviation osteotomies

Today there are basically two operative techniques for total arthroplasty of the hip in high luxations with femoral abbreviation osteotomies, and both are based on osteotomies in the subtrochanteric region.

One technique involves resection of a larger part of the trochanter mass, hence the entire metaphysis and a portion of diaphysis, with preservation of the great trochanter with abductor attachments, while by other operative procedures resection osteotomy is performed only on the diaphysis below the small trochanter, with the metaphysis remaining preserved.

Femoral abbreviation osteotomies in total arthroplasty of the hip, particularly when treating high luxations due to DDH, have been described by numerous authors (Dunn et al., 1976; Crowe et al., 1979 ; Paavilainen at al., 1990, 1993; Hartofilakidis et al., 1996, 1998, 2004, 2008 ; Papagelopoulos et al., 1996; Numair et al., 1997; Carrlson et al., 2003).

The original operative technique by Paavilainen et al. has been slightly modified by Carlsson et al., but basic postulates have remained the same. After exposing the hip through the posterolateral approach, abbreviation osteotomy of the proximal femur is performed at two levels, horizontal and sagittal. The diaphysis is osteotomized transversally 7-9 cm below the top of the great trochanter, and then osteotomy of the proximal fragment at the sagittal level is performed, thus leavening abductor attachments of the hip, primarily of the gluteus medius in the lateral part, which basically represents the great trochanter. The remaining portion of the proximal fragment is removed, i.e. if necessary it can be used as a graft. The conical stem of small dimensions is implanted into the distal fragment, namely directly into the femoral diaphysis. After having positioned the acetabular component of the endoprosthesis, the remaining proximal fragment is lowered onto the proximal portion of the diaphysis and fixed with screws and/or wire serclages. Walking with partial weight-bearing is immediately allowed, while full weight-bearing can be allowed after two months (Paavilainen at al., 1990, 1993; Carrlson et al., 2003).

This operative procedure has the advantage over those described above primarily because arthroplasty of the hip is performed in one act. Hospital stay is much shorter, with more rapid rehabilitation and without any significant limitation as to weight-bearing. Although osteotomy of the proximal femur is done, the function of the gluteus medius remains preserved. Rather, its strength is reinstituted with the distalization of the trochanter attachments.

Theoretically, the problem of this operative procedure might be non-healing of the great trochanter dislocated onto the diaphysis, however, authors have reported no such incidence in any of the cases. Also, theoretically, a delayed problem of potential revisional surgery might present a full loss of the metaphyseal bone of the proximal femur. The necessity to use a slightly more specific dysplastic stems, i.e. the impossibility of standard femoral implants (due to absent metaphyseal) does not present a true problem if taken into consideration a relatively small number of patients with such a condition.

At the Institute of Orthopaedic Surgery "Banjica" in Belgrade, high dislocation of the hip in adults is treated by transverse subtrochanteric abbreviational femoral osteotomy and, of course, a mandatory implantation of the acetabular component into the primary acetabulum. The operative technique was developed in 1984, however, over the time it has undergone minor modifications. The essence has remained identical, only some details were changed regarding the extent of capsular excision and the mode of femoral osteotomy. Namely, today we do not excise the entire joint capsule, although it is cautiously prepared and freed from attached muscles, while the stability of the femoral segments is achieved by the adapted transverse osteotomy and implantation of the standard stem with distal rotational stability. Also, over the last 11 years, with the emergence of new implants, above all hemispheric press-fit acetabular rings, the need for acetabuloplasty, which was almost regularly applied at the time of screw ring usage, nowadays is almost nonexistent (Radojevic & Zlatic, 1990; Tabak et al., 2003; Zlatic et al., 1990).

The relaxation of the neuromuscular elements is achieved by the postoperative positioning of the leg with the hip and the knee in flexion which is individually adapted to each patient. Gradual stretching is done during the next days and last on average for 2-3 days. Only then the patient is allowed to stand up and to begin walking. Individually tolerant weight bearing on the operated leg is immediately allowed. Discarding the crutches is also done on individual basis, above all depending on the patient's capability to achieve a stabile weight bearing within a given time. Certainly, osteotomy bone consolidation and the incorporation of endoprosthetic components also contribute to the decision on when walking supports could be discarded. Thromboembolic profilactic therapy is applied with low molecular weight heparine from the day of surgery until elapsed 35 postsurgical days (Fig. 4).

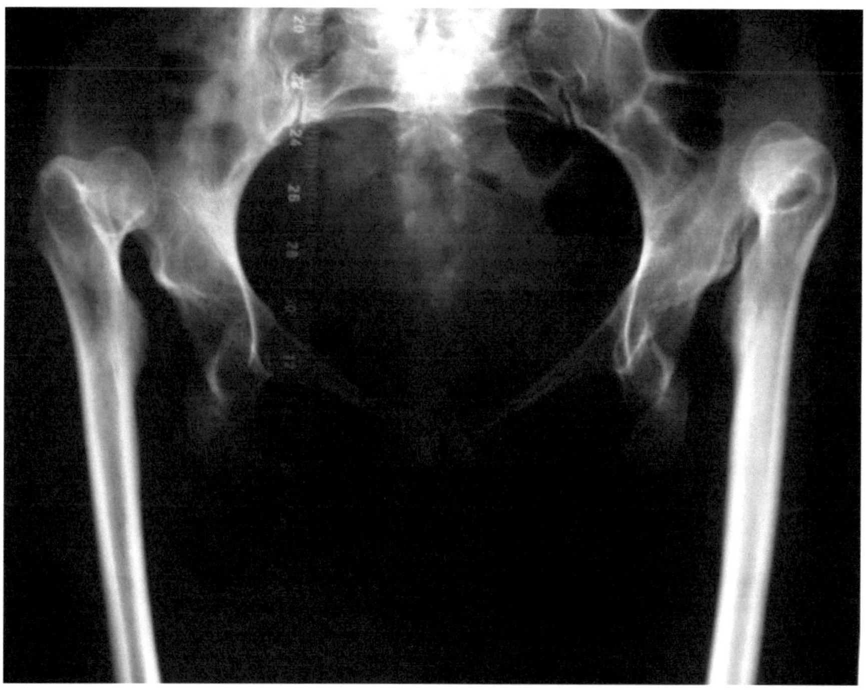

Fig. 4a. A 35-year old female with bilateral high dislocation of the hips due to DDH.

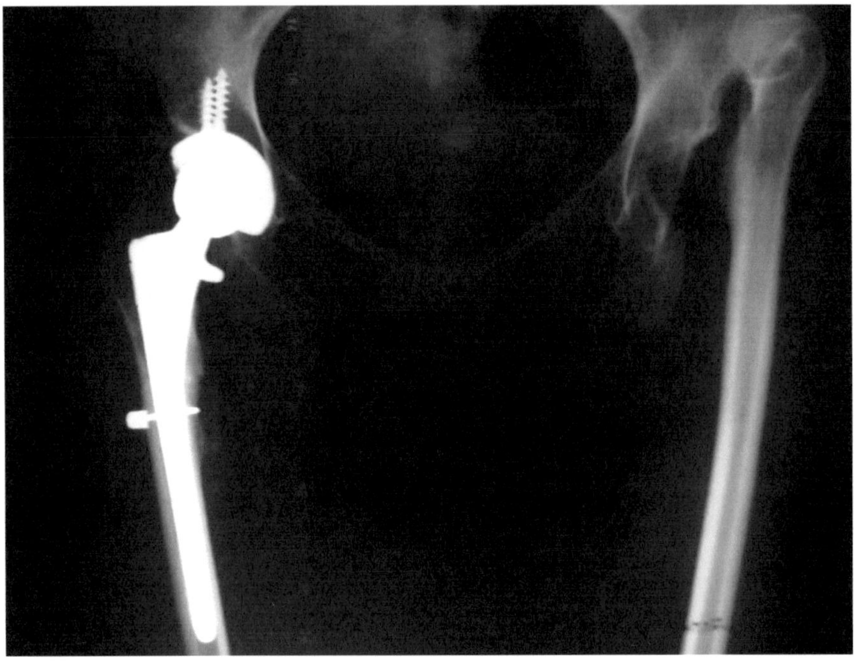

Fig. 4b. The same patient, nine months after total arthroplasty of the right hip. Good bone consolidation after four centimetres shortening subtrochanteric osteotomy.

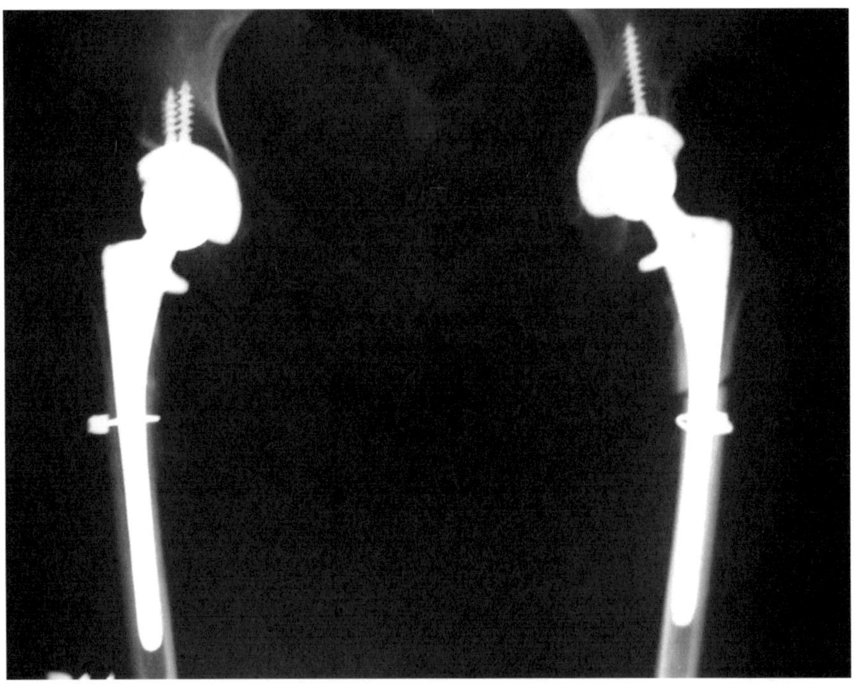

Fig. 4c. The same patient, three months after left hip arthroplasty with abreviation subtrochanteric osteotomy. Leg length equality established. Bone consolidation in progress, femoral stem stable.

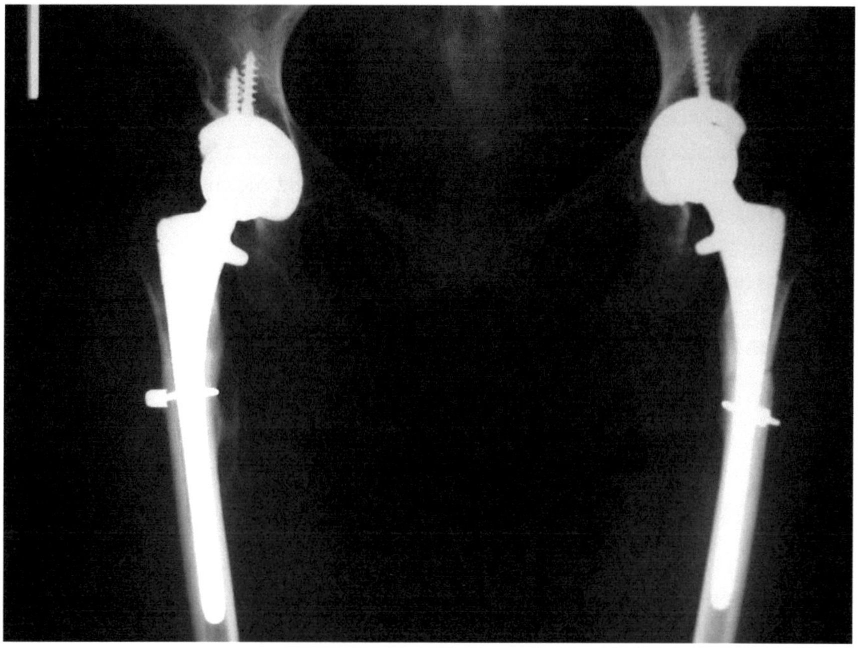

Fig. 4d. The same patient, 18 months after right total hip arthroplasty and nine month after left total hip artroplasty. Both osteotomies were fully consolidated.

5. Conclusion

As can be seen, all previously described operative techniques for high hip luxation treatment with total hip arthroplasty are reliable in hands of experienced surgeons.
According to our opinion both operative techniques with femoral abbreviation osteotomies have significant advantages over two-act operative procedures. The theoretical advantage of the latter described operative technique, with diaphyseal subtrochateric resection, over the former ones, with diaphyseal and metaphyseal resection, could be in the preservation of the bone metaphysis of the proximal femur with the possibility to use the standard midcoated implants without distal ingrowing and without additional fixation. On the other hand, the advantage of the former technique could refer to the healing of osteotomized fragments. Namely, a potentially delayed healing, and even non-healing of diaphyseal and metaphyseal bones in the subtrochanteric region is more probable than the fusion of firmly fixed great trochanter to the diaphysis.

6. Acknowledgment

This work was supported by Ministry of Education and Science, Republic of Serbia (Grant No. 41004).

7. References

Ando, M, Gotoh, E. (1990). Significance of inguinal folds for diagnosis of congenital dislocation of the hip in infants aged three to four mounts. *J Pediatr Orthop*, Vol. 10, No. 3, (May-Jun 1990) pp. (331-334), ISSN 0271-6798

Bascarevic Z, Vukasinovic Z, Slavkovic N, Dulic B, Trajkovic G, Bascarevic V, Timotijevic S. (2010). Alumina on alumina ceramic versus metal-on-highly cross-linked polyethylene bearings in total hip arthoplasty: a comparative study. *Int Orthop,* Vol. 34, No. 8, (November 2009) pp. (1129-1135), ISSN 0341-2695

Bascarevic, Z, Vukasinovic, Z. (2004). Diseases of the adult hip, In: *Special orthopaedics,* Vukasinovic, Z, pp. (275-303), Institute for orthopaedic diseases "Banjica" Belgrade, ISBN 86-82411-04-0, Belgrade

Besset, B, Fassier, F, Tanzer, M, Brooks, C. (2003). Total hip arthroplasty in patients younger than 21 years: a minimum 10 year follow up. *Can J Surg,* Vol. 46, No. 4, (August 2003), pp. (257-262), ISSN 1488-2310

Betz, R, Cooperman, D, Wopperer, J. (1990). Late sequelae of septic arthritis of the hip in infancy and childhood. *Je Pediatr Orthop,* Vol.10, No. 3, (May-Jun 1990), pp. (365-372), ISSN 0271-6798

Carrlson, A, Bjorkman, A, Ringsberg, K, Schewelov, T. (August 2003). Untreated congenital and posttraumatic high dislocation of the hip treated by replacement in adult age. *Acta Orthop Scand,* Vol. 74, No. 4, (August 2003), pp. (389-396), ISSN 0001-6470

Charnley, J, Feagin, JA. (1973). Low-friction arthroplasty in congenital subluxation of the hip. *Clin Orthop Relat Res,* Vol. 91, No. 3-4, (March-April 1973), pp. (98-113), ISSN 0009-921X

Cherney, D, Westin, G. (1989). Acetabular development in the infants dislocated hips. *Clin Orthop Relat Res,* Vol. 242, No. 5, (May 1989), pp. (98-103), ISSN 0009-921X

Choi IH, Pizzutillo PD, Bowen JR, Dragann R, Malhis T. (1990). Sequelae and reconstruction after septic arthritis of the hip in infants. *J Bone Joint Surg Am,*Vol. 72, No. 8, (September 1990), pp. (1150-1165), ISSN 0021-9355

Crowe, JF, Mani, VJ, Ranawat, CS. (1979). Total hip replacement in congenital dislocation and dysplasia of the hip. *J Bone Joint Surg Am,* Vol. 61, No. 1, (January 1979), pp. (15–23), ISSN 0021-9355

Delimar, D, Cicak, N, Klobucar, H, Pecina, M, Korzinek, K. (2002). Acetabular roof reconstruction with pedicled iliac graft. *Int Orthop,* Vol. 26, No. 6, (July 2002), pp. (344–348), ISSN 0341-2695

Dunn, HK, Hess, WE. (1976). Total hip reconstruction in chronically dislocated hips. *J Bone Joint Surg Am,* Vol. 58, No. 6, (September 1976), pp. (838–845), ISSN 0021-9355

Eftekhar, NS. (1978). *Principles of total hip arthroplasty,* CV Mosby, ISBN 0306439921, St. Louis

Eskelinen, A, Helenius, I, Remes, V, Ylinen, P, Talloroth, K, Paavilainen, T. (2006). Cementless total hip arthroplasty in patients with high congenital hip dislocation. *J Bone Joint Surg Am,* Vol. 88, No. 1, (January 2006), pp. (80-91), ISSN 0021-9355

Hartofilakidis, G, Georgiades, G, Babis, GC, Yiannakopoulos, CK. (2008). Evaluation of two surgical techniques for acetabular reconstruction in total hip replacement for congenital hip disease: results after a minimum ten-year follow-up. *J Bone Joint Surg Br,* Vol. 90, No. 6, (June 2008), pp. (724–730), ISSN 0301-620X

Hartofilakidis, G, Karachalios, T. (2004). Total hip arthroplasty for congenital hip disease. *J Bone Joint Surg Am,* Vol. 86-A, No. 2, (February 2004), pp. (242–250), ISSN 0021-9355

Hartofilakidis, G, Stamos, K, Karachalios, T. (1998). Treatment of high dislocation of the hip in adults with total hip arthroplasty. Operative technique and long-term clinical results. *J Bone Joint Surg Am,* Vol. 80, No. 4, (April 1998), pp. (510–517), ISSN 0021-9355

Hartofilakidis, G, Stamos, K, Karachalios, T, Ioannidis, TT, Zacharakis, N. (1996). Congenital hip disease in adults. Classification of acetabular deficiencies and operative treatment with acetabuloplasty combined with total hip arthroplasty. *J Bone Joint Surg Am,* Vol. 78, No. 5, (May 1996), pp. (683-92), ISSN 0021-9355

Holinka, J, Pfeiffer, M,Hofstaetter, JG, Lass, R, Kotz, RI, Giurea, A. (2010). Total hip replacement in congenital high hip dislocation following iliofemoralmonotube distraction. *Int Orthop,* Vol. 35, No. 5, (March 2010), pp. (639-645), ISSN 0341-2695

Klisic, P. (1989). Congenital dislocation of the hip: a misleading term. *J Bone Joint Surg,* Vol. 71, No. 1, (January 1989), pp. (136-139), ISSN 0301-620X

Klisic, P, Rakic, D, Pajic, D. (1984). Triple prevention of congenital dislocation of the hip. *J Pediatr Orthop,* Vol. 4, No. 6, (November 1984), pp. (759-761), ISSN 0271-6798

Lai, KA, Liu, J, Liu, TK. (1996). Use of iliofemoral distraction in reducing high congenital dislocation of the hip before total hip arthroplasty. *J Arthoplasty,* Vol.11, No. 5, (August 1996), pp. (588-593), ISSN 0883-5403

Lai, KA, Shen, WJ, Huang, LW, Chen, MY. (2005). Cementless total hip arthroplasty and limb-length equalization in patients with unilateral Crowe type-IV hip dislocation. J *Bone Joint Surg Am,* Vol. 87, No. 2, (February 2005), pp. (339-345), ISSN 0021-9355

Learmonth, ID, Heywood, AW, Kaye, J, Dall, D. (1989). Radiological loosening after cemented hip replacement for juvenile chronic arthritis. *J Bone Joint Surg Br,* Vol. 71, No. 2, (March 1989), pp. (45-55), ISSN 0301-620X

Maric, Z, Haynes, RJ. (1993). Total hip arthroplasty in juvenile rheumatoid arthritis. *Clin Orthop,* Vol. 290, No. 5, (May 1993), pp. (197-199), ISSN 0009-921X

Numair, J, Joshi, AB, Murphy, JC, Porter, ML, Hardinge, K. (1997). Total hip arthroplasty for congenital dysplasia or dislocation of the hip. Survivorship analysis and long-term results. *J Bone Joint Surg Am,* Vol. 79, No. 9, (September 1997), pp. (1352–1360), ISSN 0021-9355

Paavilainen, T, Hoikka, V, Solonen, KA. (1990). Cementless total replacement for severely dysplastic or dislocated hips. *J Bone Joint Surg Br,* Vol. 72, No. 2, (March 1990), pp. (205–211), ISSN 0301-620X

Papachristou, G, Hatzigrigoris, P, Panousis, K, Plessas, S, Sourlas, J, Levidiotis, C, Chronopoulos, E. (2006). Total hip arthroplasty for developmental hip dysplasia. *Int Orthop,* Vol. 30, No. 1, (February 2006), pp. (21–25), ISSN 0341-2695

Papagelopoulos, P, Trousdale, RT, Lewallen, DG. (1996). Cementless total hip arthroplasty with femoral osteotomy for proximal femoral deformity. *Clin Orthop,* Vol. 332, No. 11, (November 1996), pp. (151-162), ISSN 0009-921X

Pitto, RP, Schikora, N. (2004). Acetabular reconstruction in developmental hip dysplasia using reinforcement ring with a hook. *Int Orthop,* Vol. 28, No. 4, (August 2004), pp. (202–205), ISSN 0341-2695

Radojevic, B, Zlatic, M. (1990). An L-shaped bone graft for acetabular deficiency. *J Bone Joint Surg Br,* Vol. 72, No. 1, (January 1990), pp. (152-153), ISSN 0301-620X

Ruddlesdin, C, Ansell, BM, Arden, GP, Swann, M. (1986). Total hip replacement in children with juvenile chronic arthritis. *J Bone Joint Surg Br,* Vol. 68, No. 2, (March 1986), pp. (218-222), ISSN 0301-620X

Tabak, AY, Celebi, L, Muratli, H, Yagmurlu, F, Aktekin, C, Bicimoglu, A. (2003). Cementless total hip replacement in patients with high total dislocation: the results of femoral shortening by subtrochanteric segmental resection. *Acta Orthop Traumatol Turc,* Vol. 37, No.4, (April 2003), pp. (277-283), ISSN 1017-995x

Vukasinovic, Z, Bascarevic, Z. (2004). Diseases of the infant hip, In: *Special orthopaedics,* Vukasinovic Z, pp (237-273), Institute for orthopaedic diseases "Banjica" Belgrade, ISBN 86-82411-04-0, Belgrade

Vukasinovic, Z, Djoric, I. (1994). Developmental disorder of the hip, In: *Hip diseases in childhood,* Vukasinovic Z, pp. (37-78), Special orthopeadic hospital „Banjica" Belgrade, ISBN 86-82411-01-6, Belgrade

Kim YH, Seo HS, Kim JS. (2009). Outcomes after THA in patients with high hip after childhood sepsis. *Clin Orthop Relat Res,* Vol. 467, No. 9, (September 2009), pp. (2371-2378), ISSN 0009-921X

Zlatic, M, Radojevic, B, Lazovic, C. (1990). Reconstruction of the hipoplastyc acetabulum in cementless arthroplasty of the hip. *Int Orthop,*Vol. 14, No.4, (April 1990), pp. (371-375), ISSN 0341-2695

Modular Femoral Neck Fracture After Total Hip Arthroplasty

Igor Vučajnk and Samo K. Fokter
Celje General and Teaching Hospital
Slovenia

1. Introduction

In the middle of the 20th century total hip arthroplasty (THA) became the most popular and the most common reconstructive procedure of the hip. It is important as a last resort in treatment of terrible pain due to progressive hip arthritis of different etiologies. Implanting an artificial hip prosthesis, the surgeon helps the patient by releasing the pain and restoring the range of movement so that the patient can resume his normal activities.
Historically, treatment of progressive osteoarthritis evolved from arthrodesis through different osteotomies, nerve divisions, joint debridements, and interpositions of different organic or inorganic materials between the articular surfaces, towards the final introduction of total hip endoprosthesis. The first endoprostheses were made of glass. Afterwards the quality of the materials progressed from plastic, steel, to cobalt-chromium alloys and finally titanium alloys. Additionally, considerable effort was made to improve the manufacturing techniques, hip biomechanics and the usage of appropriate materials (Harkess & Crockarell, 2007). The studies of materials revealed that orthopaedic implants must be biocompatible; they have to resist all forms of corrosion (Sharan, 1999), resist degradation and withstand all forces that potentially apply. Different designs of total hip endoprostheses follow different philosophies. Two kinds of prosthesis designs are currently used in primary hip arthroplasty. Monoblock is a femoral stem prosthesis made of a single piece, while modular prostheses are made of two modules: the femoral stem and the femoral neck. The stem can be of different sizes, and the neck is of different sizes and different neck angle versions.
According to the American Academy of Orthopaedic Surgeons (AAOS), more than 193,000 total hip replacements are performed yearly in the United States alone. The prediction for the US is that the number of total hip replacements will at least double by the year 2030 (Wilson N., 2008).

2. Modular neck hip prosthesis

Modular neck hip prosthesis has been gaining popularity worldwide for the last thirty years. Modular stems are commonly used in revision hip surgery. The use of this kind of endoprosthesis was first published in 1948 by McBride, then later by Bousquet and Bornard in 1978. Several companies presently offer different versions of modular neck hip endoprostheses for primary total hip arthroplasty (Keppler, 2006). The advantage of this type of endoprosthesis is that the surgeon has an intraoperative choice of neck version and neck length independently of the stem size. The surgeon can then adjust the femoral offset, correct leg length and achieve hip stability.

Modular hip endoprostheses can be classified as proximal, mid-stem, distal and multi-modular. The proximal ones have modules for sleeve, shoulder and neck, neck, collars and proximal pads (Froehlich, 2006). In this chapter we focus on proximal modular neck endoprostheses.

Important differences exist between the two sexes in femoral neck length, femoral shaft diameter, collum-caput-diaphysis angle (CCD), neck version and offset (Traina, 2009). In order to properly restore the hip biomechanics these parameters must be kept in mind. Appropriate restoration of femoral offset and appropriate soft tissue balancing is necessary. Unsatisfactory restoration of hip biomechanics can and will lead to limping, abductor muscle imbalances, and higher rates of wearing. In order to achieve the best biomechanics of the reconstructed hip, preoperative planning is essential. However, as the femoral version cannot be appropriately and adequately assessed with standard radiographs, modular hip prosthesis offers some advantage during the operation. In addition, some benefits of modular neck hip prosthesis in developmental dysplasia of the hip (DDH) have been reported. One study showed that monoblock stems restore offset in only one out of three patients. Eight different neck shaft angle solutions are necessary to restore the anatomy in 50% of the patients (Massin, 2000).

3. Complications associated with modular neck hip prosthesis

The complications associated with modular neck hip arthroplasty are divided in medical complications and complications associated with surgery and materials. Medical complications, such as cardiovascular, thromboembolic, pulmonary, anaemic and renal complications as well as delirium can be prevented or at least minimized with careful preoperative risk assessment and proper perioperative care (Foerg, 2005). Other complications including joint infection, nerve and blood vessel injury, and bleeding during or after the surgery can be reduced by proper operative techniques. Leg length inequality, prosthesis dislocation, and prosthesis impingement can be prevented with a proper choice of offset and neck version. The highly corrosive environment of the human body demands the use of such biomaterials which will withstand degradation that could lead to another serious complication - failure of the prosthetic material.

Instability is the second most common complication after aseptic loosening (Abraham, 2005). Dislocation rates vary among reports from 0.5% to 11%. The risk of dislocation is associated with time from the operation and with traumatic events, polyethylene wear and pseudocapsule laxity.

4. Prosthesis size and materials

Modular neck hip endoprostheses are made of different numbers of modules. The prosthesis used for primary THA is made of two modules, the femoral stem and the femoral modular neck. The femoral stem comes in different sizes in order to fit different femoral dimensions. The numbers of stem sizes differ from one manufacturer to the other. The femoral neck comes in different sizes and versions as well, and the number again depends on the manufacturer. The two modules connect at the stem neck junction called the taper. The modularity gives important advantage for fine adjustments of leg length and femoral anteversion.

The materials used for modular femoral stem and modular neck are made of cobalt alloys (Co-Cr-Mo; cobalt-chromium-molybdenum) and of titanium alloys (Ti-6Al-4V; titanium-aluminium-vanadium). Cobalt alloys are among the strongest materials used for implants and can resist high-loading. The added molybdenum increases the strength even more. Chromium is added for hardness and makes the alloy more resistant to corrosion. The unique property of titanium alloys is their tissue biocompatibility. Corrosion is very limited in titanium alloys and they resist to crevice corrosion because they form a passive layer of oxide films (titanium oxide) on their surface. The biomaterials used have to resist crevice corrosion, fretting corrosion, galvanic corrosion, and pitting corrosion in order to withstand the degradation process. Also, the materials must have proper mechanical and wear properties.

5. Modular neck fracture

An increasing number of recently published case reports and studies describe catastrophic failures of modular femoral neck prostheses resulting from material fracture. The Swedish Hip Arthroplasty Register Annual Report of femoral hip stems noted overall femoral stem implant failure in 493 prostheses out of the 299,368 primary hip arthroplasties performed from 1979 to 2008 (1.4%) (Garellick et al., 2009). A report on the Metha Short Hip Stem Prosthesis (Aesculap AG, Tuttlingen, Germany) also showed a 1.4% failure rate of modular necks (68 neck failures out of 5000 THA) (Grupp, 2010). According to the Wright Company, the Profemur (Profemur Z, Wright Medical Technology, Inc., Arlington, TN, USA) modular neck fracture rate in 198,331 implanted endoprostheses has been calculated to 0.028% (Wright Medical Technology Inc., 2010). The Profemur world wide fracture rate in all necks, including long and short necks is reported to be 0.058% (6 fractures out of every 10,000 THA) (Wright Medical Technology Inc., 2010). Both in Wright and in Aesculap, the necks were made of titanium alloys. This complication is supposed to occur in almost all cases with long necks, heavier patients and male patients. Both studies concluded that titanium long necks should be replaced with cobalt chrome alloy necks because they are safer (Wright Medical Technologies Inc., 2010; Grupp, 2010). The Zimmer Company reviewed over 300,000 primary VerSys prostheses (VerSys Hip System, Zimmer Inc., Warsaw, IN, USA) implanted since the year 2000 and their fracture rate was less than 0.0018% (Hertzler et al., 2009). A center implanting Acumatch M-series cementless hip endoprostheses (Acumatch M-series, Exactech Inc., Gainesville, Florida, USA) reported on fracture rates of 1.6% (8 fractures out of 500 implanted prostheses) (Paliwal, 2010).

There are many reasons for prosthesis fracture. As mentioned in the previous section, orthopaedic implants are subject to crevice corrosion, fretting corrosion, galvanic corrosion and pitting corrosion (Sharan, 1999). The changing demographics of the patients undergoing total hip replacement surgeries could also contribute to the fracture rates. These include increased patient weight, increased physical activities, increased life expectancy, and the timing of the operation (Chrowninshield, 2006).

Fretting is a phenomenon which occurs between two contacting bodies experiencing reciprocating motion. In our case small scale reciprocating movements occur between the femoral stem and the femoral neck at the taper junction. When the main factor causing fretting is oxidation the process is called fretting corrosion. The more the neck is in varus position and the longer the neck is, the greater is the tendency for fretting because of the increased lever arm. Microscopic cracks develop in the fretting zone that can lead to femoral neck fracture. Studies in vitro show that mechanical loading accelerates the corrosion process (Goldberg and Gilbert, 2002).

Another type of process occurring at the taper connection is crevice corrosion. The crevice between two modules will be a corrosion site if there is enough space to allow the income of an aqueous solution (Colliere et al., 1992). The crevice should be sufficiently narrow to maintain a stagnant zone. As corrosion in this zone progresses, oxygen depletion will lead to an excess of positively charged ions in the surrounding aqueous environment of the crevice. The negatively charged chloride ions will migrate to balance them. As a result, hydrochloric acid will form. Hydrochloric acid can dissolve titanium or cobalt alloys which are otherwise stable. Once the crevice corrosion has begun it continues even in the absence of loading.

Concern was raised in the past that galvanic corrosion can arise from inappropriate combinations of dissimilar metal components. Galvanic corrosion is an electrochemical process in which two physically connected dissimilar metals experience metallic deterioration while being exposed to electrically conductive fluids. Different metals have different electrochemical characteristics. When two dissimilar metals are placed together, electrons will start to flow spontaneously from one metal to the other. The loss of electrons from the active metal is called oxidation and oxidation will lead to the process of corrosion (Shetty, 1989). Corrosion will start the release of metal ions and will cause among other complications damage to the prosthesis surface. This can lead to the loss of material strength and eventually to failure.

There is also a form of extremely localized, symmetric corrosion called pitting corrosion. It leads to the creation of small holes in the metal. The mechanism of pitting corrosion is probably the same as crevice corrosion.

The studies of modular neck adapters and stems showed that fretting leads to microcracks on the surface (Grupp, 2010; Wright Medical Technologies Inc., 2010). Fretting is accompanied with crevice corrosion and pitting corrosion. As mentioned above, the passive oxide film formed in titanium alloys is permanently destroyed by fretting corrosion and crevice corrosion. Fretting reduces the fatigue strength of titanium alloys. Fretting at the connection can be increased by the intraoperative contamination of taper with small particles of bone or tissue. Contamination should always be prevented by assembling the device carefully and drying the components before the assembly (Grupp, 2010). Both studies concluded that the change of femoral neck material from titanium alloys to cobalt alloys increases the safety of the connection (Grupp, 2010; Wright Medical Technologies Inc., 2010). Cobalt alloys have the same fatigue strength, they form the passive oxide layer and have excellent fretting corrosion characteristics in comparison to titanium alloys. Cobalt alloys are superior in stiffness and modules of elasticity, notch sensitivity, crack propagation, and abrasion compared to titanium alloys. However, cobalt alloys are inferior to titanium alloys in characteristics of crevice corrosion and are more allergenic. The authors recommended that heavier patients, especially those weighing more than 100 kg, and more physically active male patients require long necks made of cobalt alloys.

Froehlich et al. did a follow up of their experience with seven different modular stems implanted since 1984 (Froehlich, 2006). They implanted 2,248 stems for primary THA in cemented and uncemented way. They used S-Rom (S-Rom Modular Hip System, JMPC/DePuy, Warsaw, IN, USA), Apex Modular (Apex Modular Hip System, Global Orthopaedic Technology, Unanderra, NSW, Australia), K2 Apex (Apex K2 Modular Hip System, Omni Life Science, Inc., East Taunton, MA, USA), OTI/Encore R-120 cemented stem, OTI/Encore R-120 porous c.c. cementless stem (R-120 Modular Stem, DJO Surgical, Austin, TX, USA), UniSyn (UniSyn Total Hip System, Hayes Medical, Inc., El Dorado Hills, CA, USA) and Cremascoli Modular Neck (Wright Medical Technologies, Inc., Arlington, TN, USA). They experienced 12 femoral component failures, 2 in a c.c. proximal modular neck and 10 in proximal modular titanium shoulder neck. The authors remain enthusiastic about modularity and continue to use modular stems in their practice. The reason for failure in their cases was a single high load event and suggested quasi-static shear failure of the pin alignment. The OTI/Encore modular neck failure occurred in the distal neck engagement taper (Froehlich, 2006). The company increased the upper taper diameter, the lower taper diameter, the surface area, and the distal taper length so that the fatigue testing results improved.

Several recent case reports exist describing the failure of modular necks of the Profemur prostheses (Profemur Z, Wright Medical Technologies Inc., Arlington, TN, USA) (Atwood, 2010; Wright G., 2010; Wilson D. J., 2010). They describe a well integrated implant that could only be removed with trochanteric osteotomy. Usually the initiation site for failure was the anterior and superior part of the neck. Degradation of the polished surface was noted at the insertion point of the taper. Also, evidence of abrasion and corrosion was seen (Dangles, 2010). The Federal Drug Administration Manufacturer and User Facility Device Experience (FDA MAUDE) database describes 98 adverse effects for the Profemur modular neck prosthesis for the years 2000-2009. 37 of those include breakage of the femoral neck (FDA MAUDE, as cited in Skendzel et al., 2011). Skendzel et al. reported on two cases of fractured Profemur modular neck and concluded that the long varus necks used increased the bending moment by 32.7% when compared to short varus necks (Skendzel et al., 2011). The stress was concentrated at the modular junction. Removal of the complete femoral component was required during revision surgery because the Morse taper could not be removed. Both patients experienced a traumatic event before the failure. Atwood et al. described the fracture of a Profemur long straight neck in a man of 2 m height and 109.8 kg weight who fell on his hip (Atwood, 2010). The surgery revealed a crack of 2 mm below the stem edge. They found the initiation site near the lateral-anterior corner of the neck. They also found signs of crevice corrosion and fretting wear.

Grupp et al. studied the Metha Short Hip Stem Prosthesis (Metha Short Hip Stem Prosthesis, Aesculap AG, Tuttlingen, Germany) as a consequence of several reports of failed titanium alloy femoral necks (Grupp, 2010). Out of 5,000 THA they found 68 neck adapter failures. They found neither processing or material deviation nor incorrect dimensioning. The retrieved prostheses showed a similar fracture pattern with the fracture starting in the anterolateral area at the upper part of the cone where there is maximum biomechanical stress. The reason for failure was attributed to fretting, fretting corrosion, and crevice corrosion which lead to the loss of fatigue strength of titanium alloy. The combination of factors listed above, as well as contamination of the cone adapter with fluids or particles, increased patient weight, high activity level, male gender, and CCD angle of 135 and smaller increased the rate of failure. They concluded that the change to cobalt-based alloy modular necks increases the safety of cone connection.

However, some studies did not show any problems regarding modular femoral components. The study by Toni et al. showed no clinical complications related to modular necks (Toni et al., 2001). They studied 216 hip prostheses of AnCA Fit type (AnCA Fit, Cremascoli Ortho, Milan, Italy) which were implanted from June 1995 to December 1997. Another study by Duwelius et al. using the Zimmer M/L Taper Hip Prosthesis with Kinectiv Technology (Zimmer M/L Taper Hip Prosthesis with Kinectiv Technology, Zimmer, Warsaw, IN, USA) on 634 patients from April 2007 to November 2008 showed no complications related to modular neck failure (Duwelius et al., 2010). The stem and neck were manufactured from titanium alloy (Ti6Al4V).

6. Case report

At the Depatment of Orthopaedic Surgery and Sports Trauma, Celje General and Teaching Hospital, Celje, Slovenia, modular hip prostheses have been used since the year 1992 in selected patients. The first prosthesis used was GSP (Cremascoli Ortho, Sorem Ortho, Toulon, France) and at the time of writing the prosthesis in use is the Profemur Z (Wright Medical Technology, Inc., Arlington, TN, USA). From 1992 to 2008, 306 modular neck hip prostheses of three different types were implanted at our department. From 1992 to 2004, 88 GSP modular neck hip prostheses (Cremascoli Orthopaedics, Sorem Ortho, Toulon, France) were implanted. From 2002 to 2006 we implanted 58 Anca Dual Fit hip stems (Cremascoli Ortho, Milan, Italy). In 2006 we started implanting Profemur Z modular neck hip prostheses (Wright Medical Technology, Inc., Arlington, TN, USA) and 160 of these were implanted by the end of 2008.

In December 2010, a 69-year old male was admitted to our hospital's emergency department with acute pain in his right hip. The pain appeared after a fall on his right side from standing height. The examination revealed right inguinal tenderness and shortening of his right lower extremity with external rotation. The review of standard radiographic exams showed modular prosthesis neck fracture. This was the first such complication seen at our department (Fig. 1). The patient's height was 178 cm and he weighed 110 kg (BMI 34.7). He was treated at our institution in 1998 when he was 56 years old. At that time his BMI was 31.6 (weight 100 kg). The operation was performed because the patient suffered from rheumatoid arthritis with the involvement of his right hip. A fully modular cementless total hip endoprosthesis was implanted (fully hidroxy-apatite coated femoral stem (GSP) with modular cobalt-chromium long straight neck, 28 mm diameter ceramic head, and acetabulum of the press-fit type (ANCA-Fit) with ceramic acetabular insert, (Cremascoli Orthopaedics, Sorem Ortho, Toulon, France). None of the postoperative visits or radiographic exams showed any signs of wear or other complications. The patient was pain free before the event.

Revision surgery was scheduled as soon as we received the custom made acetabular cup inlay (ANCA-Fit, Wright Medical Technology Inc., Arlington, TN, USA). The operation was performed by the same surgeon and the previous lateral approach was used. Revision surgery confirmed the fracture of the modular prosthesis neck. It was impossible to remove only the remaining neck from the taper, so that the entire femoral stem had to be removed. The femoral stem was well integrated in the femur and femoral osteotomy was necessary in order to remove the implant. Macroscopically, the tissue showed no metal debris or granuloma. The remaining part of the fractured neck module was approximately 2 mm below the top of the taper (Fig. 2-4).

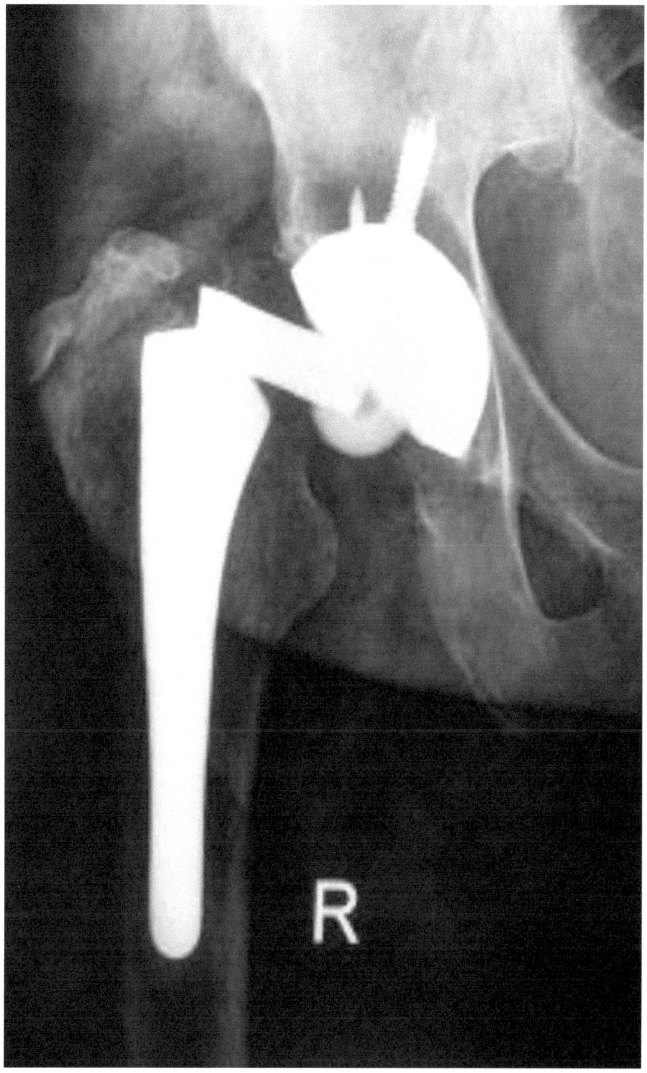

Fig. 1. Standard antero-posterior radiograph of the patient's right hip at admission. (Courtesy M. Kotnik, M. D.)

In order to properly reconstruct the biomechanics of the hip, cementless revision modular stem with ceramic head (Waldemar Link GmbH & Co, Hamburg, Germany) was used. The acetabular lining was exchanged as well and a custom made ANCA-Fit (Wright Medical Technology, Inc., Arlington, TN, USA) component implanted (Fig. 5). Standard tissue specimens were collected during the revision procedure for microbiologic cultures which showed no bacterial growth.

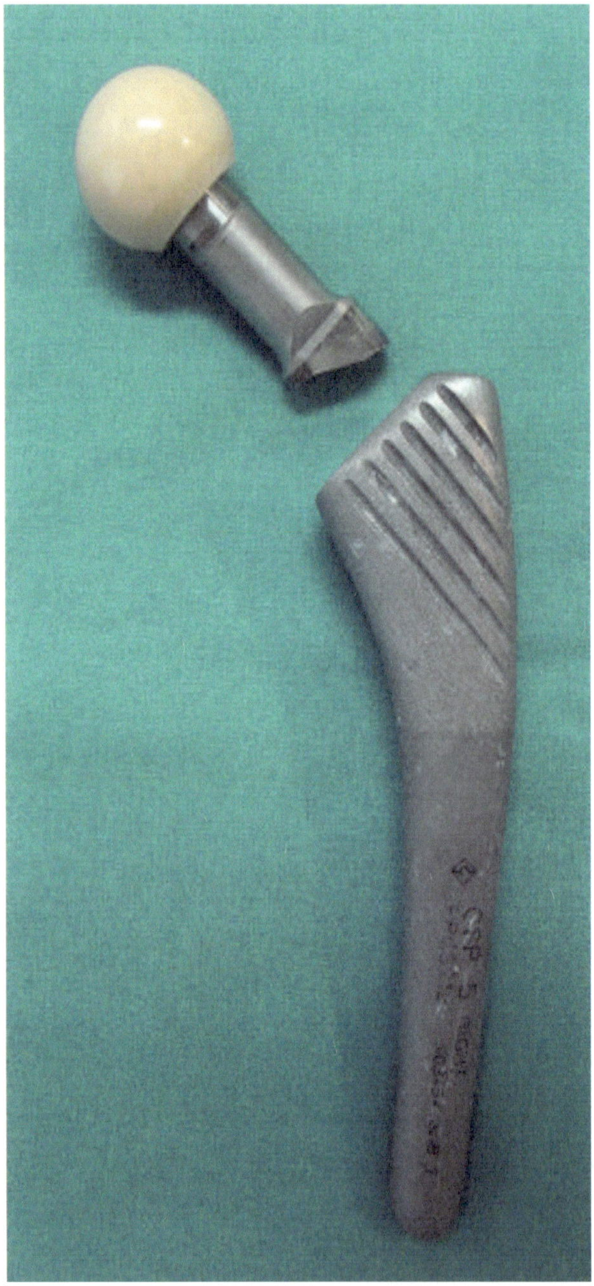

Fig. 2. Photograph of the retrieved fully-modular prosthesis showing the modular neck fracture.

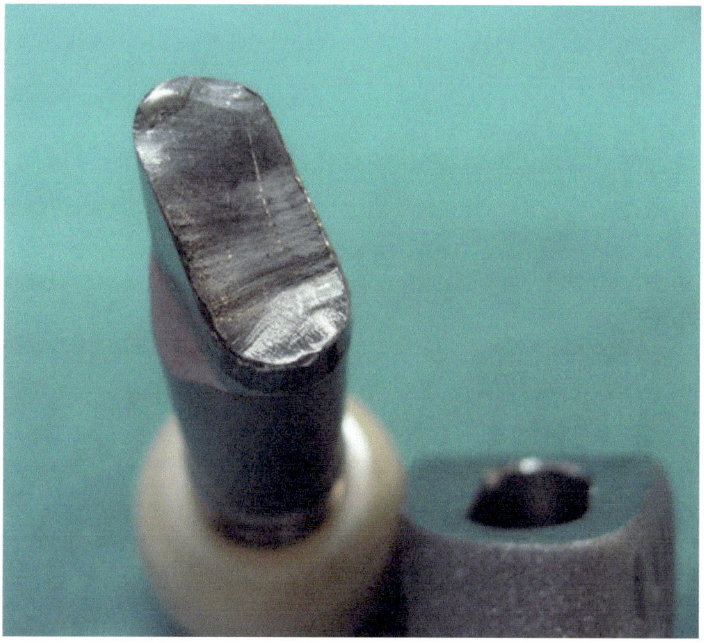

Fig. 3. A close-up photograph showing the fractured modular femoral neck.

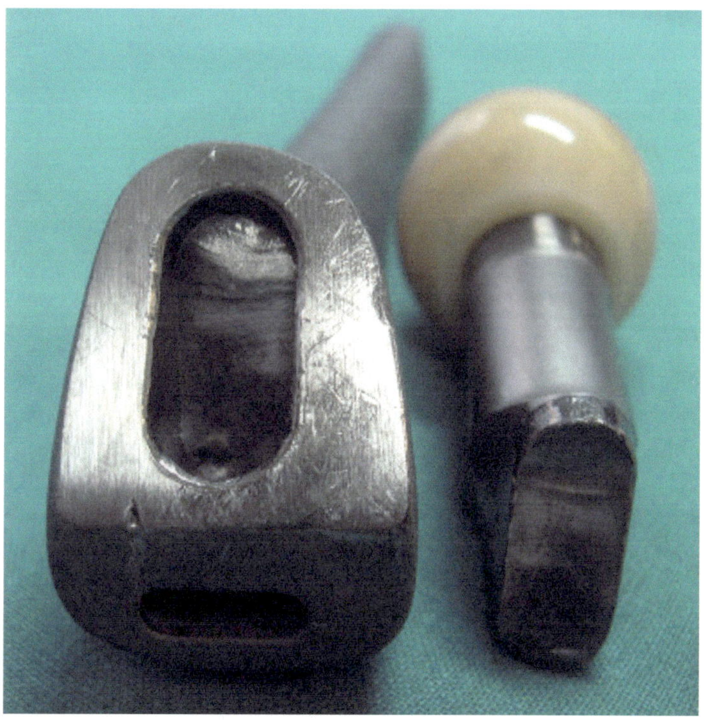

Fig. 4. Photograph showing the removed prosthesis with fractured neck and the remaining of the modular neck in the femoral stem taper.

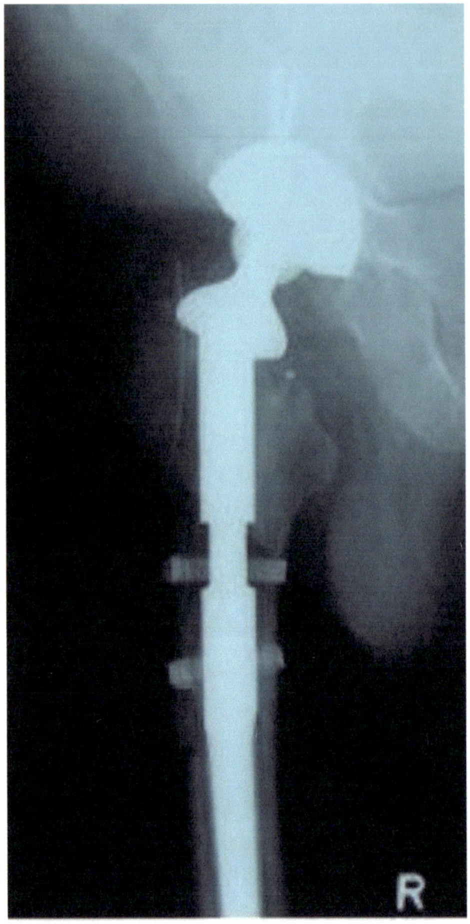

Fig. 5. Radiograph of the revised right hip with the cementless revision modular prosthesis in place. (Courtesy M. Kotnik, M. D.)

7. Conclusion

Modular neck hip prostheses are nowadays wildly used around the globe. The Profemur stem (Wright Medical Technology Inc., Arlington, TN, USA) only was sold in more than 200,000 units by the end of 2010 (Wright Medical Technologies Inc., 2010). There are many benefits in proximal modularity. The theoretical benefits of modular neck include bone and tissue conservation, restoration of joint biomechanics, reduced blood loss, easier rehabilitation, ease of revision, simple surgical technique, and different modular options (McTighe, 2008). In addition, the possibility of implanting a stem with a retroverted modular neck can prevent cup impingement and dislocation of the prosthesis. Moreover, if revision operation is necessary for the dislocated THA, only exchange of the modular neck might be required. The surgeon has an intraoperative option of choosing the appropriate neck length, neck version and CCD angle independently of the femoral stem size, taking into account the considerable differences in stem sizes between the two sexes (Traina, 2009). The proximal modular neck type of the prosthesis is useful in primary hip arthroplasty due

to the significant differences among the individuals requiring hip reconstruction. Some types of modular neck prostheses offer as much as 60 different variations with modularity compared to only about 10 options offered by monoblock stems (Duwelius, 2010).
However, added modularity brings another possibility for complication. Recent reports emphasize the need for changing the neck material from titanium alloys to the safer cobalt-chromium alloys. Constant evaluation of laboratory material should be continued, even though it does not always guarantee proper information regarding in vivo parameters. Careful preoperative planning should be performed in spite of modular neck THA allowing anatomic reconstruction of the hip. The increased variety of intraoperative surgical options with the fully-modular stems should not be an excuse for bad surgical technique and improper cup position.

8. References

Abraham R. & Arthur L. M. (2005). Instability after Total Hip Replacement. *Seminars in Arthroplasty*, Vol.16, No.2, (June 2005), pp. 132-141, ISSN 1045-4527

American Academy of Orthopaedic Surgeons, AAOS. (April 2009). Total Hip Replacement, In: *Your orthopaedic connection*, Accessed June 23 2011, Available from: <http://orthoinfo.aaos.org/topic.cfm?topic=a00377>

Atwood, S.; Patten, E.; Bozic, K.; Pruitt, L. & Ries, M. (2010). Corrosion-induced fracture of a double-modular hip prosthesis: a case report. *The Journal of Bone and Joint Surgery*, Vol.92, No.6, (June 2010), pp. 1522-1525, ISSN 0021-9355

Collier, J.; Surprenant, V.; Jensen, R.; Mayor, M. & Surprenant, H. (1992). Corrosion between the components of modular femoral hip prostheses. *The Journal of Bone and Joint Surgery, British Volume*, Vol.74, No.4, (July 1992), pp. 511-517, ISSN 0301-620X

Crowninshield, R.; Rosenberg, A. & Sporer, S. (2006). Changing demographics of patients with total joint replacement. *Clinical Orthopaedics and Related Research*, Vol.443, No.2, (February 2006), pp. 266-272, ISSN 0009-921X

Dangles, C. J. & Altstetter, C. J. (2010). Failure of the modular neck in a total hip arthroplasty. *The Journal of Arthroplasty*, Vol.25, No.7, (October 2010), pp. 5-7, ISSN 0883-5403

Duwelius, P. J.; Hartzband, M. A.; Burkhart, R.; Carnahan, C.; Blair, S.; Wu, Y. & Grunkemeier, G. L. (2010). Clinical Results of a Modular Neck Hip System: Hitting the "Bull's-Eye" More Accurately. *American Journal of Orthopedics*, Vol.39, Suppl.10, (October 2010), pp. 2-6, ISSN 1078-4519

Foerg, F. (2005). Medical Complications Associated with Total Hip Arthroplasty. *Seminars in Arthroplasty*, Vol.16, No.2, (June 2005), pp. 88-99, ISSN 1045-4527

Froehlich, J. A.; McTighe, T.; Cameron, H. U.; Kegg, K.; Keggi, J.; Kennon, R. & Woodgate, I. (2006). Defining the Role of Modular Stem Designs in THA, *ITSA 19th Annual Symposium*, New York City, October 2006

Garellick, G.; Kärrholm, J.; Rogmark, C. & Herberts, P. (October 2009). Swedish Hip Arthroplasty Register Annual Report 2008, In: *Department of Ortopaedics, Faculty of Medicine, Göteborg University*, Accessed June 24 2011, Available from: <https://www.jru.orthop.gu.se/>

Goldberg, J. & Gilbert, J. (2002). In vitro corrosion testing of modular hip tapers. *Journal of Biomedical Materials Research, Part B, Applied Biomaterials*, Vol.64, No.2, (December 2002), pp. 78-93, ISSN 1552-4973

Grupp, T.; Weik, T.; Bloemer, W. & Knaebel, H. (2010). Modular titanium alloy neck adapter failures in hip replacement - failure mode analysis and influence of implant material. *BMC Musculoskeletal Disorders*, Vol.11, No.3, (January 2010), pp. 1-12

Harkess, J. W. & Crockarell, J. R. (2007). Arthroplasty of the hip, In: *Campbell's Operative Orthopaedics*, Canale, S. T. & Beaty, J. H., (Eds.), pp. 314-351, Mosby, An Imprint of Elsevier, Retrieved from <http://www.mdconsult.com/books/page.do?eid=4-u1.0-B978-0-323-03329-9..50010-6&isbn=978-0-323-03329-9&uniqId=263852506-2#4-u1.0-B978-0-323-03329-9..50010-6>

Hertzler, J. S.; Johnson, T. S. & Meulink, S. L. (2009). *Performance evaluation of Kinectiv™ Technology*, Zimmer, Inc, Retrieved from <http://www.zimmer.com/web/enUS/pdf/Performance_Evaluation_of_Kinectiv_Technology.pdf>

Keppler, L.; Cameron, H. U. & McTighe, T. (2006). The Role of Modularity in Primary THA - Is There One?, *AAOS Scientific Exhibit*, Chicago, 2006

Massin, P.; Geais, L.; Astoin, E.; Simondi, M. & Lavaste, F. (2000). The anatomic basis for the concept of lateralized femoral stems: a frontal plane radiographic study of the proximal femur. *The Journal of Arthroplasty*, Vol.15, No.1, (January 2000), pp. 93-101, ISSN 0883-5403

McTighe, T.; Woodgate, I.; Turnbull, A.; Keggi, J.; Kennon, R.; Keppler, L.; Harrison, J.; Brazil, D.; Wu, W. & Cameron, H. U. (2008). A New Approach To Neck Sparing THA Stem. *AAOS Scientific Exhibit*, San Francisco, March 2008

Paliwal, M.; Gordon Allan, D. & Filip, P. (2010). Failure analysis of three uncemented titanium-alloy modular total hip stems. *Engineering Failure Analysis*, Vol.17, No.5, (July 2010), pp. 1230-1238, ISSN 1350-6307

Sharan, D. (1999). The problem of corrosion in orthopaedic implant materials. *Orthopaedic Update (India)*, Vol.9, No.1, (December 1999), pp. 1-5

Shetty, R. (1989). *Use of Dissimilar Metals in Orthopaedic Implants*, Zimmer, Inc., Retrieved from http://www.zimmer.co.nz/web/enUS/pdf/Use_Of_Dissimilar_Metals_in_Orthopaedic_Implants.pdf>

Skendzel, J. G.; Blaha, J. D. & Urquhart, A. G. (2011). Total hip arthroplasty modular neck failure. *The Journal of Arthroplasty*, Vol.26, No.2, (February 2011), pp. 338.e1-338.e4

Toni, A.; Paderni, S.; Sudanese, A.; Guerra, E.; Traina, F.; Antonietti, B. & Giunti, A. (2001). Anatomic cementless total hip arthroplasty with ceramic bearings and modular necks: 3 to 5 years follow-up. *Hip International*, Vol.11, No.1, (2001), pp. 1-17

Traina, F.; De Clerico, M.; Biondi, F.; Pilla, F.; Tassinari, E. & Toni, A. (2009). Sex differences in hip morphology: is stem modularity effective for total hip replacement? *The Journal of Bone and Joint Surgery*, Vol.91, Suppl.6, (November 2009), pp. 121-128

Wilson, D. J.; Dunbar, M.; Amirault, J. & Farhat, Z. (2010). Early failure of a modular femoral neck total hip arthroplasty component: a case report. *The Journal of Bone and Joint Surgery*, Vol.92, No.6, (June 2010), pp. 1514-1517

Wilson, N.; Schneller, E.; Montgomery, K. & Bozic, K. (2008). Hip and knee implants: current trends and policy considerations. *Health Affairs*, Vol.27, No.6, (2008), pp. 1587-1598

Wright, G.; Sporer, S.; Urban, R. & Jacobs, J. (2010). Fracture of a Modular Femoral Neck After Total Hip Arthroplasty. A Case Report. *The Journal of Bone and Joint Surgery*, Vol.92, No.6, (June 2010), pp. 1518–1521

Wright Medical Technology, Inc. (2010). Masters Hip Post Training Document, Amsterdam, July 2010

12

Surface Replacement of Hip Joint

Hiran Amarasekera and Damian Griffin
[1]Orthopaedic Research Fellow/PhD Student, Warwick Orthopaedics
University of Warwick Medical School
[2]Professor of Trauma and Orthopaedics, Warwick Orthopaedics
University of Warwick Medical School
United Kingdom

1. Introduction

Surface hip replacement more commonly known as hip resurfacing arthroplasty is a type of a hip replacement that is different to a total hip replacement. In a total hip replacement femoral head and neck are removed and a metal stem is inserted to the femoral shaft. In hip resurfacing articular surface is shaved and a metal cap (Fig 1) is inserted preserving most of the bone in femoral head and neck.

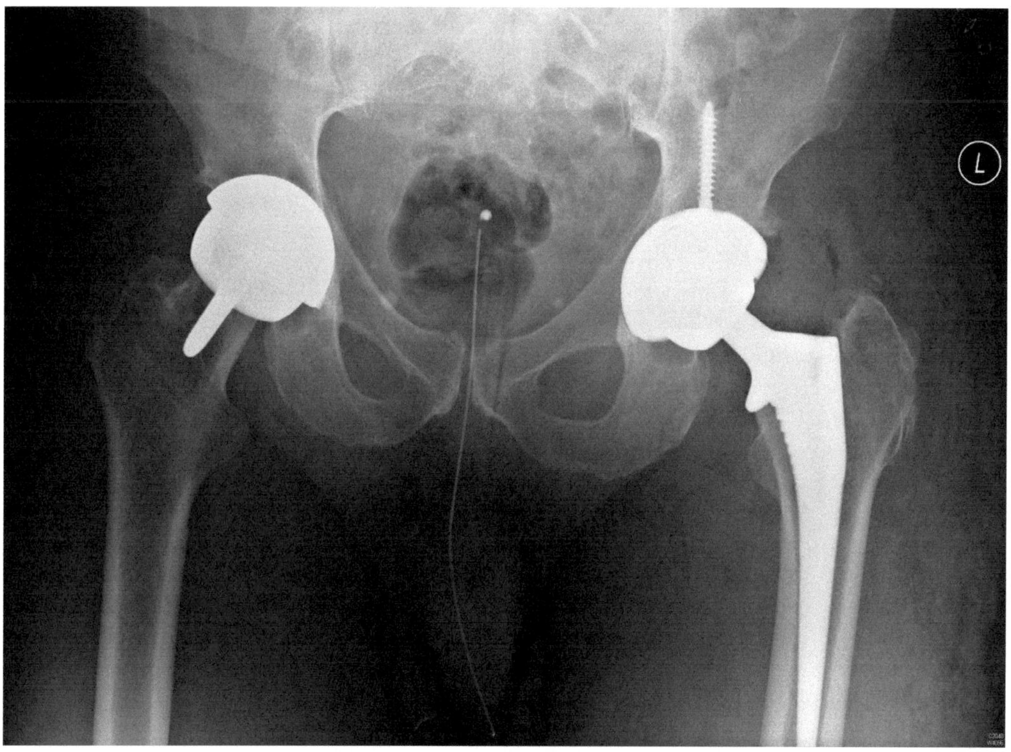

Fig. 1. X Ray shows a Hip Resurfacing arthroplasty (Right) and a Total Hip Replacement (Left)

Compared to the total hip replacement resurfacing arthroplasty preserves more bone on the femoral side (Fig.1). Acetabular replacement is similar to both procedures. Main advantages of surface replacement include preservation of femoral bone stock; increase degree of motion, and easier conversion to a total hip replacement during revision. All these make resurfacing arthroplasty an attractive alternative to a total hip replacement especially in the young active adults.

2. History

Professor Sir John in initially introduced hip resurfacing early in 1950s. (Charnley 1960; McMinn and Daniel 2006) The initial designs were uncemented PTFE (polytetrafluaroethelene) on metal. All early implants had an acetabular component made of softer material such as PFFE and femoral component made of metal. This combination of hard on soft surface caused many problems.

The previous designs failed due to two main reasons. Firstly combination of hard on soft surfaces and large diameter heads lead to increase wear, wear particle accumulation, osteolysis of the bone.

Secondly posterior approach used during the procedure damaged the blood supply to the femoral head. This lead to reduced femoral head vascularity, osteonecrosis, femoral neck fractures, and aseptic loosening of the implant.

Due to these problems hip resurfacings in the 50s through 80s were not a popular option to treat arthritis in the young adult. However in early 1990s *McMinn et al (McMinn et al. 1996)* introduced the modern hip resurfacing which used metal on metal bearings with improved instrumentation for precision placement of implants. It was believed metal on metal reduce the wear and tear of the implanted hip. Vascularity too was addressed by proposing many surgical approaches such as the trochanteric flip(Ganz et al. 2001) antero-lateral(Jacobs, Goytia, and Bhargava 2008) or direct-lateral (Hardinge 1982)as alternative approaches to the conventional posterior approach which is widely used in total hip replacement.

Hip resurfacings has been conducted in many centres since early 1990 as popular option in treating young active adults with hip problems. However with time long term results from the modern surface replacements has identified it's own set of complications(Shimmin, Bare, and Back 2005) such as femoral neck fractures aseptic loosening, avascular necrosis, osteolysis of head and increase metal ions levels.(Hing, Back, and Shimmin 2007)

Due to these factors the selection criteria for surface replacement has changed from a much broader set to a narrow and a limited set, over the last decade.(Nunley, Della Valle, and Barrack 2009)

At present even-though the selection criteria is narrowed it sill remains a key alternative to the conventional hip replacements.

3. Indications for hip resurfacing

When surface replacement was re introduced in early 1990 s the ideal candidate for the procedure was a young active adult with good hip morphology and a reasonably good bone quality, with osteoarthritis of the hip.(McMinn et al. 2011)

With a high range of motion and a low dislocation rate surface replacement seem to be the ideal option for a young adult who could have a near normal range of motion following resurfacing arthroplasty. If the patient requires a revision to total hip replacement then this could be delayed and a second revision delayed even further. As people live longer with an increasing life expectancy rate this enables the orthopaedic surgeon to delay the first total hip replacement. (Della Valle, Nunley, and Barrack 2008; Hing, Back, and Shimmin 2007)
However with the availability of the long-term complications of hip resurfacing arthroplasty the initial interest that prevailed in early 1990s has waned over the last few years and, many surgeons have narrowed selection criteria down.

3.1 Selection criteria

3.1.1 Age

55 years for women 65 years for men.(Corten et al. 2011)

3.1.2 Sex

Resurfacing is better tolerated by men than women. Pre-menopausal women have a better chance than the post menopausal women as the femoral neck fracture rate increases after menopause.(Shimmin and Back 2005) Some studies suggest that surgical technique, implant selection, and implant positioning should be modified according to the gender. If this is done there is a high possibility that gender specific bias can be eliminated, as this is a common problem in surface replacement.(Amstutz, Wisk, and Le Duff 2011; Jameson et al. 2008)

3.1.3 Pathology of the hip

Ideal candidate for a hip resurfacing is a patient with primary osteoarthritis. However most patients do not develop primary osteoarthritis at an early age. Younger patients developing osteoarthritis is mostly due to secondary causes. Surface replacement of the hip has been performed in many pathological conditions that eventually lead to secondary osteoarthritis. However conditions in which the bone may be weak such as osteoporosis, resurfacings should be avoided as this can lead to high incidence of femoral neck fractures. Avascular necrosis (AVN) is a relative contraindication for hip resurfacing. Even though some surgeons have performed hip resurfacing in AVN patients most surgeons believe that resurfacing should not be done on these patients. Partial hip resurfacing/hemi resurfacing seems to be the popular treatment option for patients with Avascular Necrosis. In partial resurfacing only the necrotic area of the articular surface is removed and replaced (Fig 2).(Siguier et al. 2001; Ushio et al. 2003) Partial resurfacing is also done for localised osteochondral defects. (Van Stralen et al. 2009)
The indications for hip resurfacing has changed during the past decade as high failure rates were observed among certain patient groups.(McMinn et al. 2011)
This has lead to a re think and development of more stringent patient selection criteria.

3.2 Surgical techniques

Surgical approach to the hip is similar to the approaches done when performing a total hip replacement. However there are many additional considerations to be kept in mind when

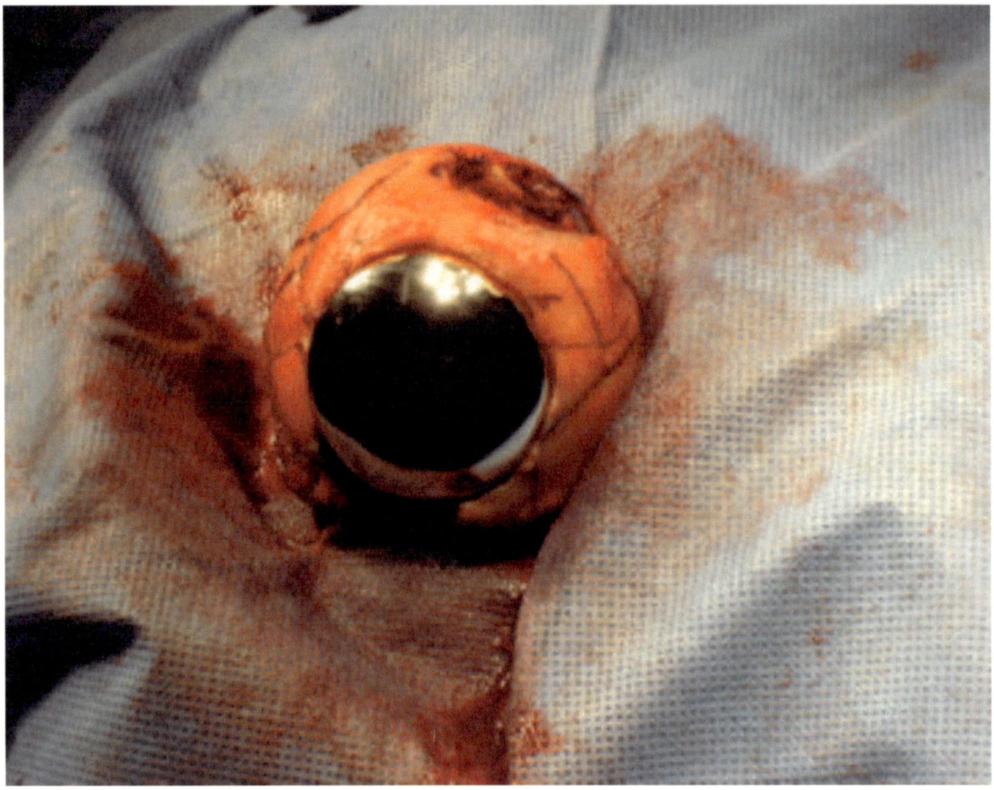

Fig. 2. Partial resurfacing done on a patient with an osteochondral defect

performing a resurfacing arthroplasty. As more bone is preserved in femoral head and the neck preserving the vascularity is a key issue. (McBryde et al. 2008) Therefore some surgeons do not use the traditional posterior approach when performing a hip resurfacing. This is because the posterior approach cuts the medial circumflex femoral artery (MCFA) main artery supplying of the femoral head and neck. This damage is believed to cause AVN of femoral head. Most studies demonstrated a fall in blood supply during posterior approach compared to other surgical approaches.(Beaule, Campbell, and Shim 2006; Bradley, Freeman, and Revell 1987; Howie, Cornish, and Vernon-Roberts 1993) However some authors including us have questioned the clinical significance of this drop as we are not clear whether the drop is transient or permanent and whether it is below the critical ischaemic level to cause the death of osteocytes in the femoral head.(Amarasekera et al. 2008)

Common alternative approach that is described to preserve blood flow was described by *Ganz et al* as the trochanteric flip approach.(Ganz et al. 2001) This is an anterior type of approach done by doing a trochanteric flip osteotomy. This approach preserves the MCFA and the main blood supply to the femoral head. Therefore it is believed in theory that the vascularity is better preserved by this approach as compared to the posterior approach. However the key disadvantage of this approach is that the patient has to be non weight bearing for four to six weeks until the trochanteric flip osteotomy heals. The other approaches describe for resurfacing include(Gerdesmeyer et al. 2008) antero lateral

approach, direct lateral approach(Hardinge 1982), and minimally invasive approaches. (McMinn et al. 2005; Mont, Ragland, and Marker 2005)
Studies have been done not only to evaluate intra-operative (Amarasekera et al. 2008) as well as post-operative blood supply (Forrest et al. 2006) following different surgical approaches in resurfacing arthroplasty patients.
Post-operative vascularity has been studied using SPECT (Single Positron Emission Computed Tomography) scanning. The attenuation factor affecting the accuracy of the results in the presence of metal implants has been addressed by performing phantom studies. (Amarasekera et al. 2011)
Once a suitable surgical approach is chosen the next steps in the surgery are fairly straightforward. The acetabular replacement is similar to a THR. However the femoral head replacement is far more a demanding task as the placement of the cup is crucial and needs accuracy. This is a technically demanding procedure compared to a placing the femoral component in a THR. Poorly positioned components will lead to high wear rates, impingement and dislocations. Due to the technically demanding nature of the procedure training surgeons is challenging and has a to slow learning curve.(Berend et al. 2011) Due to this using navigation to position implants has been tried but does not appear to have an advantage over the learning curve.(Saithna and Dekker 2009; Shields et al. 2009)
To cement or not to cement the implants is another point that has been debated over the years.
When surface replacements were re introduced most implants were cemented. Therefore cementing technique and the type of cement used, area of the component cemented, all seem to contribute to the success of surgery.(Bitsch and Schmalzried 2008; Bitsch et al. 2008) Specific cementing techniques have been described when cementing the femoral component. (Bitsch et al. 2008; Bitsch et al. 2007; Chandler et al. 2006) Achieving the correct cement mantle is a technically challenging procedure. Too much cement can cause thermal necrosis while too little cement can cause a poor penetration and femoral loosening where as an extreme thin mantle can cause mechanical failure leading to high wear particles further leading to osteolysis.(Scheerlinck, Delport, and Kiewitt 2010)
Due to these controversies some surgeons adapt partially cementing the component avoiding the pin, (Schlegel et al. 2011) and some surgeons have totally stopped using cement. This lead to development of uncemented hip resurfacings and has become the procedure of choice among some surgeons.

4. Complications of surface replacements

It is worth mentioning that all general complications associated with hip surgery such as infection, bleeding, DVT, are seen with hip resurfacings. Apart from these there is a set of complications that is unique to this procedure. These are outlined below.

4.1 Avascular necrosis of femoral head (Bradley, Freeman, and Revell 1987; Little et al. 2005)

As described earlier avascular necrosis of the femoral head and neck is a potential complication that can result in failure of the implant. The main reason for this is the damage to blood supply that occurs during posterior approach. (Amarasekera et al. 2008)Avoiding posterior approach and adapting other approaches such as antero-lateral or trochanteric flip approaches(Ganz et al. 2001, 2001) will minimise this.

4.2 Femoral neck fractures

This is a known complication that can range between 0- up to1.8% after hip resurfacing.(Steffen et al. 2009) Avascular necrosis(Steffen et al. 2010), mechanical factors such as notching, femoral neck lengthening, and varus mal alignment of the femoral component has been attributed as contributory causes for femoral neck fractures.. Some studies suggest females (3%) have a higher incidence than males (1.3%) (Jameson et al. 2008) while other studies do not find any difference between the sexes.(Steffen et al. 2009) Failure rate and revision rate too seem to be higher in females as compared to males.(Carrothers et al. 2010)

4.3 Aseptic loosening of components, osteolysis, pseudo tumours, and ALVAL (Aseptic Lymphocytic Vasculitis Associated Lesions), (Zustin et al. 2009)

Large head size in hip resurfacing causes increase wear and tear leading to high metal particles. Some escape to blood flow causing high metal ion levels in blood. Some trigger an immune response leading to metallosis, aseptic loosening, lymphocytic infiltration, and osteolysis and bone resorbtion. It is less clear whether this same reaction can be triggered by cement particles. Developing a proper cementing technique(Campbell et al. 2009) or considering uncemented implants may help to minimise these complications. However dealing with increase wear metal particles remains a challenging problem.

These complications are due to series of immune reactions that occur as the body respond to large number of wear particles or cement. In early sixties these were common when metal on plastic implants were used it was a major cause for failure but with metal on metal it was thought that these would be minimal.(Zustin et al. 2010) However long term results of modern hip resurfacings suggest that the problem still exists. Recent systematic review suggests aseptic loosening to be the most common complication reported in hip resurfacing.(van der Weegen et al. 2011) (Zustin et al. 2009)

4.4 Persistent groin pain (Bin Nasser et al. 2010; Bartelt et al. 2010; Campbell et al. 2008; Nikolaou et al. 2009) and femoroacetabular impingement(Lim et al. 2011; Yoo et al. 2011)

These are mainly caused by mechanical problems such as poor positioning of implants. (Bin Nasser et al. 2010)

Carrothers et al reported prevalence of complications following surface replacement of 5000 hips in a multi surgeon series involving 141 surgeons.(Carrothers et al. 2010)These are given below (Table 1)

Complication	Number of hips	Prevalence
Fracture Neck of femur	54	1.1%
Loosening -Acetabular	32	0.6%
Femoral head AVN	30	0.6%
Loosening-Femoral	19	0.4%
Infection	17	0.3%
ALVAL/Metallosis	15	0.3%
Loosening-Both	05	0.1%
Dislocation	05	0.1%
Revision rate	182	3.6%

Table 1. Complications reported by *Carrothers et al*

5. Conclusion

When resurface was first done initial complications were due to high wear between metal and plastic surface. This is because the surface area of the resurfacing femoral head is much larger that the surface area of a THR implant. This causes more frictional forces between the acetabular and femoral components producing increase wear particles. When the head was metal and the cup was plastic the wear rate was even higher and this lead to initially failure of the original designs. To avoid this problem the modern implants were designed as metal on metal expecting the wear to be a less significant. Recent evidence suggest collection of metal particles within the tissues causes metallosis and leaking metal to the blood stream has caused high metal ion levels, (Clarke et al. 2003; Vendittoli et al. 2010; Vendittoli, Ganapathi, and Lavigne 2007)metal allergies, and metallosis. This has been attributed to triggering immunological reactions such as ALVAL, Pseudo tumour formations, resorbtion of head finally leading to loosening and implant failure.

Due to all these complications resurfacing arthroplasty has fallen out of favour as the automatic procedure of choice to treat young active patient with hip problems.

This has re opened the debate on how best to treat young active adults with hip problems. Uncemented hip replacement, minimal invasive techniques, and arthroscopic hip procedures are a few options that should be considered as an alternative to hip resurfacing in selected patients.

Nevertheless surface replacement done on a carefully selected patient by a highly trained surgeon taking in to consideration the surgical approach, cementing technique, implant selection and implant positioning will increase the success rate of the procedure.

6. References

Amarasekera, H. W., M. L. Costa, P. Foguet, S. J. Krikler, U. Prakash, and D. R. Griffin. 2008. The blood flow to the femoral head/neck junction during resurfacing arthroplasty: A COMPARISON OF TWO APPROACHES USING LASER DOPPLER FLOWMETRY. *J Bone Joint Surg Br* 90 (4):442-5.

Amarasekera, H. W., M. L. Costa, N. Parsons, J. Achten, D. R. Griffin, S. Manktelow, and N. R. Williams. 2011. SPECT/CT bone imaging after hip resurfacing arthroplasty: is it feasible to use CT attenuation correction in the presence of metal implants? *Nucl Med Commun* 32 (4):289-97.

Amstutz, H. C., L. E. Wisk, and M. J. Le Duff. 2011. Sex as a patient selection criterion for metal-on-metal hip resurfacing arthroplasty. *J Arthroplasty* 26 (2):198-208.

Bartelt, R. B., B. J. Yuan, R. T. Trousdale, and R. J. Sierra. 2010. The prevalence of groin pain after metal-on-metal total hip arthroplasty and total hip resurfacing. *Clin Orthop Relat Res* 468 (9):2346-56.

Beaule, P. E., P. Campbell, and P. Shim. 2006. Femoral Head Blood Flow during Hip Resurfacing. *Clin Orthop Relat Res.*

Berend, K. R., A. V. Lombardi, Jr., J. B. Adams, and M. A. Sneller. 2011. Unsatisfactory surgical learning curve with hip resurfacing. *J Bone Joint Surg Am* 93 Suppl 2:89-92.

Bin Nasser, A., P. E. Beaule, M. O'Neill, P. R. Kim, and A. Fazekas. 2010. Incidence of groin pain after metal-on-metal hip resurfacing. *Clin Orthop Relat Res* 468 (2):392-9.

Bitsch, R. G., C. Heisel, M. Silva, and T. P. Schmalzried. 2007. Femoral cementing technique for hip resurfacing arthroplasty. *J Orthop Res* 25 (4):423-31.

Bitsch, R. G., T. Loidolt, C. Heisel, and T. P. Schmalzried. 2008. Cementing techniques for hip resurfacing arthroplasty: development of a laboratory model. *J Bone Joint Surg Am* 90 Suppl 3:102-10.

Bitsch, R. G., and T. P. Schmalzried. 2008. [Cementing techniques for hip resurfacing arthroplasty. What do we know?]. *Orthopade* 37 (7):667-71.

Bradley, G. W., M. A. Freeman, and P. A. Revell. 1987. Resurfacing arthroplasty. Femoral head viability. *Clin Orthop Relat Res* (220):137-41.

Campbell, P., A. Shimmin, L. Walter, and M. Solomon. 2008. Metal sensitivity as a cause of groin pain in metal-on-metal hip resurfacing. *J Arthroplasty* 23 (7):1080-5.

Campbell, P., K. Takamura, W. Lundergan, C. Esposito, and H. C. Amstutz. 2009. Cement technique changes improved hip resurfacing longevity - implant retrieval findings. *Bull NYU Hosp Jt Dis* 67 (2):146-53.

Carrothers, A. D., R. E. Gilbert, A. Jaiswal, and J. B. Richardson. 2010. Birmingham hip resurfacing: the prevalence of failure. *J Bone Joint Surg Br* 92 (10):1344-50.

Chandler, M., R. S. Kowalski, N. D. Watkins, A. Briscoe, and A. M. New. 2006. Cementing techniques in hip resurfacing. *Proc Inst Mech Eng H* 220 (2):321-31.

Charnley, J. 1960. Surgery of the hip-joint: present and future developments. *Br Med J* 1 (5176):821-6.

Clarke, M. T., P. T. Lee, A. Arora, and R. N. Villar. 2003. Levels of metal ions after small- and large-diameter metal-on-metal hip arthroplasty. *J Bone Joint Surg Br* 85 (6):913-7.

Corten, K., R. Ganz, J. P. Simon, and M. Leunig. 2011. Hip resurfacing arthroplasty: current status and future perspectives. *Eur Cell Mater* 21:243-58.

Della Valle, C. J., R. M. Nunley, and R. L. Barrack. 2008. When is the right time to resurface? *Orthopedics* 31 (12 Suppl 2).

Forrest, N., A. Welch, A. D. Murray, L. Schweiger, J. Hutchison, and G. P. Ashcroft. 2006. Femoral head viability after Birmingham resurfacing hip arthroplasty: assessment with use of [18F] fluoride positron emission tomography. *J Bone Joint Surg Am* 88 Suppl 3:84-9.

Ganz, R., T. J. Gill, E. Gautier, K. Ganz, N. Krugel, and U. Berlemann. 2001. Surgical dislocation of the adult hip a technique with full access to the femoral head and acetabulum without the risk of avascular necrosis. *J Bone Joint Surg Br* 83 (8):1119-24.

———. 2001. Surgical dislocation of the adult hip: A TECHNIQUE WITH FULL ACCESS TO THE FEMORAL HEAD AND ACETABULUM WITHOUT THE RISK OF AVASCULAR NECROSIS. *J Bone Joint Surg Br* 83-B (8):1119-1124.

Gerdesmeyer, L., H. Gollwitzer, R. Bader, and M. Rudert. 2008. [Surgical approaches in hip resurfacing]. *Orthopade* 37 (7):650-8.

Hardinge, K. 1982. The direct lateral approach to the hip. *J Bone Joint Surg Br* 64 (1):17-9.

Hing, C., D. Back, and A. Shimmin. 2007. Hip resurfacing: indications, results, and conclusions. *Instr Course Lect* 56:171-8.

Howie, D. W., B. L. Cornish, and B. Vernon-Roberts. 1993. The viability of the femoral head after resurfacing hip arthroplasty in humans. *Clin Orthop Relat Res* (291):171-84.

Jacobs, M. A., R. N. Goytia, and T. Bhargava. 2008. Hip resurfacing through an anterolateral approach. Surgical description and early review. *J Bone Joint Surg Am* 90 Suppl 3:38-44.

Jameson, S. S., D. J. Langton, S. Natu, and T. V. Nargol. 2008. The influence of age and sex on early clinical results after hip resurfacing: an independent center analysis. *J Arthroplasty* 23 (6 Suppl 1):50-5.

Lim, S. J., J. H. Kim, Y. W. Moon, and Y. S. Park. 2011. Femoroacetabular Cup Impingement After Resurfacing Arthroplasty of the Hip. *J Arthroplasty*.

Little, C. P., A. L. Ruiz, I. J. Harding, P. McLardy-Smith, R. Gundle, D. W. Murray, and N. A. Athanasou. 2005. Osteonecrosis in retrieved femoral heads after failed resurfacing arthroplasty of the hip. *J Bone Joint Surg Br* 87 (3):320-3.

McBryde, C. W., M. P. Revell, A. M. Thomas, R. B. Treacy, and P. B. Pynsent. 2008. The influence of surgical approach on outcome in Birmingham hip resurfacing. *Clin Orthop Relat Res* 466 (4):920-6.

McMinn, D., and J. Daniel. 2006. History and modern concepts in surface replacement. *Proc Inst Mech Eng H* 220 (2):239-51.

McMinn, D. J., J. Daniel, P. B. Pynsent, and C. Pradhan. 2005. Mini-incision resurfacing arthroplasty of hip through the posterior approach. *Clin Orthop Relat Res* 441:91-8.

McMinn, D. J., J. Daniel, H. Ziaee, and C. Pradhan. 2011. Indications and results of hip resurfacing. *Int Orthop* 35 (2):231-7.

McMinn, D., R. Treacy, K. Lin, and P. Pynsent. 1996. Metal on metal surface replacement of the hip. Experience of the McMinn prothesis. *Clin Orthop Relat Res* (329 Suppl):S89-98.

Mont, M. A., P. S. Ragland, and D. Marker. 2005. Resurfacing hip arthroplasty: comparison of a minimally invasive versus standard approach. *Clin Orthop Relat Res* 441:125-31.

Nikolaou, V., S. G. Bergeron, O. L. Huk, D. J. Zukor, and J. Antoniou. 2009. Evaluation of persistent pain after hip resurfacing. *Bull NYU Hosp Jt Dis* 67 (2):168-72.

Nunley, R. M., C. J. Della Valle, and R. L. Barrack. 2009. Is patient selection important for hip resurfacing? *Clin Orthop Relat Res* 467 (1):56-65.

Saithna, A., and A. P. Dekker. 2009. The influence of computer navigation on trainee learning in hip resurfacing arthroplasty. *Comput Aided Surg* 14 (4-6):117-22.

Scheerlinck, T., H. Delport, and T. Kiewitt. 2010. Influence of the cementing technique on the cement mantle in hip resurfacing: an in vitro computed tomography scan-based analysis. *J Bone Joint Surg Am* 92 (2):375-87.

Schlegel, U. J., J. Siewe, R. G. Bitsch, J. Koebke, P. Eysel, and M. M. Morlock. 2011. Influence of cementing the pin on resistance to fracture in hip resurfacing. *Clin Biomech (Bristol, Avon)* 26 (2):136-40.

Shields, J. S., T. M. Seyler, C. Maguire, and R. H. Jinnah. 2009. Computer-assisted navigation in hip resurfacing arthroplasty - a single-surgeon experience. *Bull NYU Hosp Jt Dis* 67 (2):164-7.

Shimmin, A. J., and D. Back. 2005. Femoral neck fractures following Birmingham hip resurfacing: a national review of 50 cases. *J Bone Joint Surg Br* 87 (4):463-4.

Shimmin, A. J., J. Bare, and D. L. Back. 2005. Complications associated with hip resurfacing arthroplasty. *Orthop Clin North Am* 36 (2):187-93, ix.

Siguier, T., M. Siguier, T. Judet, G. Charnley, and B. Brumpt. 2001. Partial resurfacing arthroplasty of the femoral head in avascular necrosis. Methods, indications, and results. *Clin Orthop Relat Res* (386):85-92.

Steffen, R. T., N. A. Athanasou, H. S. Gill, and D. W. Murray. 2010. Avascular necrosis associated with fracture of the femoral neck after hip resurfacing: histological assessment of femoral bone from retrieval specimens. *J Bone Joint Surg Br* 92 (6):787-93.

Steffen, R. T., P. R. Foguet, S. J. Krikler, R. Gundle, D. J. Beard, and D. W. Murray. 2009. Femoral neck fractures after hip resurfacing. *J Arthroplasty* 24 (4):614-9.

Ushio, K., M. Oka, S. H. Hyon, S. Yura, J. Toguchida, and T. Nakamura. 2003. Partial hemiarthroplasty for the treatment of osteonecrosis of the femoral head. An experimental study in the dog. *J Bone Joint Surg Br* 85 (6):922-30.

van der Weegen, W., H. J. Hoekstra, T. Sijbesma, E. Bos, E. H. Schemitsch, and R. W. Poolman. 2011. Survival of metal-on-metal hip resurfacing arthroplasty: a systematic review of the literature. *J Bone Joint Surg Br* 93 (3):298-306.

Van Stralen, R. A., D. Haverkamp, C. J. Van Bergen, and H. Eijer. 2009. Partial resurfacing with varus osteotomy for an osteochondral defect of the femoral head. *Hip Int* 19 (1):67-70.

Vendittoli, P. A., M. Ganapathi, and M. Lavigne. 2007. Blood and urine metal ion levels in young and active patients after Birmingham hip resurfacing arthroplasty. *J Bone Joint Surg Br* 89 (7):989; author reply 989-90.

Vendittoli, P. A., A. Roy, S. Mottard, J. Girard, D. Lusignan, and M. Lavigne. 2010. Metal ion release from bearing wear and corrosion with 28 mm and large-diameter metal-on-metal bearing articulations: a follow-up study. *J Bone Joint Surg Br* 92 (1):12-9.

Yoo, M. C., Y. J. Cho, Y. S. Chun, and K. H. Rhyu. 2011. Impingement between the acetabular cup and the femoral neck after hip resurfacing arthroplasty. *J Bone Joint Surg Am* 93 Suppl 2:99-106.

Zustin, J., M. Amling, M. Krause, S. Breer, M. Hahn, M. M. Morlock, W. Ruther, and G. Sauter. 2009. Intraosseous lymphocytic infiltrates after hip resurfacing arthroplasty : a histopathological study on 181 retrieved femoral remnants. *Virchows Arch* 454 (5):581-8.

Zustin, J., M. Hahn, M. M. Morlock, W. Ruther, M. Amling, and G. Sauter. 2010. Femoral component loosening after hip resurfacing arthroplasty. *Skeletal Radiol* 39 (8):747-56.

13

Retrograde Stem Removal Techniques in Revision Hip Surgery

Kálmán Tóth
Department of Orthopaedics, University of Szeged
Hungary

1. Introduction

Total hip replacement has about a 50 year old past. In recent decades the number of revision hip arthroplasties in developed countries reached 15-20% of primary replacements. The average survival for both cemented and uncemented implants is about 94-95% at ten years. At the end of that period they have to be replaced.

Removal of a well cemented femoral stem in revision total hip arthroplasty is a technically demanding procedure, which requires knowledge and proficiency in the usage of a multitude of surgical techniques and instruments. Experiences with traditional cement removing techniques have been published in numerous publications (Dennis et al., 1987; Ferguson, 1988; Laffargue et al., 2000; Lauer et al., 2002; Stühmer, 1987).

Femoral component failure and fracture is a rarely seen complication, which presents as a difficult problem for the surgical team. Because of stress shielding in the proximal femur, osteolysis is often concentrated to the proximal part of the femur, whilst the distal portion of the stem might be stable and well fixed. This eventually leads to failure of the metal and component fracture. Although removing the proximal loose fragment is relatively straightforward, removing the distal tip is difficult, and often only feasible with techniques that result in weakening of the biomechanical properties of the femur, such as distal fenestration i.e. creating a small or larger window (in the lateral cortex or an extended trochanteric osteotomy (Wagner, 1989).

The Authors use a retrograde technique in the clinical setting, in which removal of cement and stem is performed with the use of a retrograde nail passed through the knee. With this technique, removal of loose stems or broken components is both possible - when the case is appropriate for the technique. Thus further compromise can be avoided to the poor bone stock.

2. Surgical technique

The patients were positioned supine on a radio-lucent table. Using a lateral approach, the scar tissue was excised and the hip joint was exposed. After dislocating the prosthesis, the proximal broken piece of the femoral component was easily removed. The end of the distal part became visible at approximately 4 to 6 cm below the lesser trochanter (Fig. 1.).

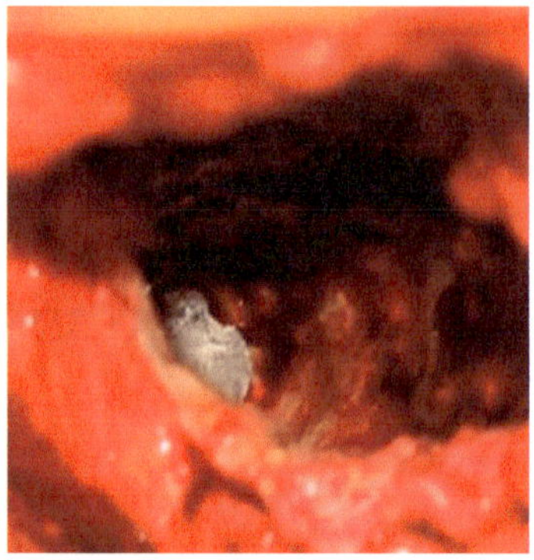

Fig. 1. The proximal end of the distal broken piece of the femoral component - there is no sufficient gap between the broken component and the femur, therefore grasping and pulling it out with a device is not feasible (intraoperative photo).

A 2-3 cm skin incision was required through the centre of the patellar ligament as described by Moed et al. (Moed & Watson, 1995) which is generally performed for osteosynthesis. The optimal entry point for retrograde femoral nailing and defined this spot 12 mm anterior to the femoral origin of the posterior cruciate ligament in sagittal plane and at the centre of the intercondylar sulcus in coronal plane. The intramedullary canal was then opened by the awl.

Under the control of a fluoroscope the 10, 12, 14 mm intramedullary nail is entered into the intramedullary canal. Reaming is not necessary, the tamp that fits best the intramedullary canal is chosen from the series. After entering the rod, it is rotated until the best alignment is obtained to the stem or the cement plug and a stable connection is achieved (Fig. 2.). To avoid deflection or perforation it is particularly important to make sure that the nail is not

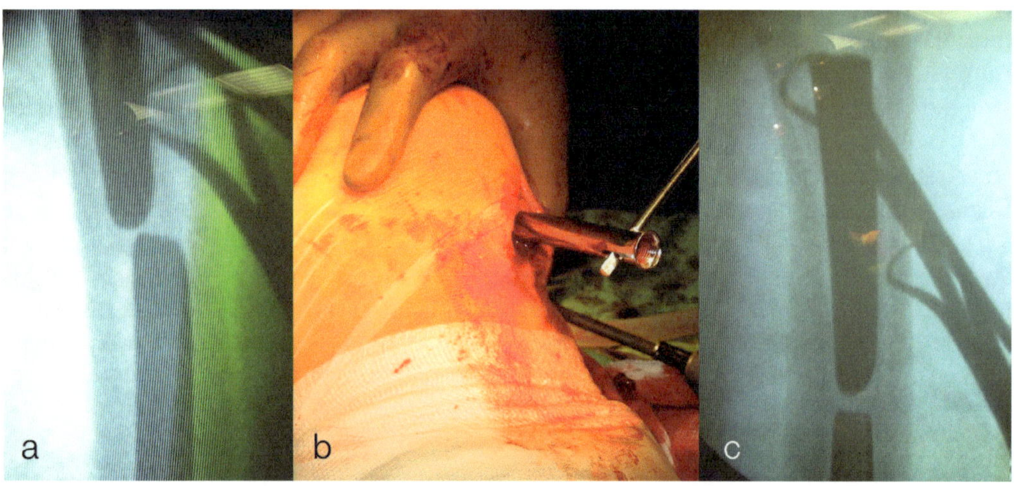

Fig. 2. a: After introducing, the alignment between the nail and the stem is poor, therefore the nail may slip from the tip of the stem causing perforation or fracture (photo taken from the image intensifier). b: Setting the rotation (intraoperative photo). c: After the nail is placed to the tip of the stem the femoral component is removed by gentle hammering (photo taken from the image intensifier).

slipped down from the stem or the distal cement plug. When the required contact between the nail and the distal part of the stem or the cement plug is visualised by the image intensifier, the femoral implant is pushed out in proximal direction by careful hammering.

Following this, the femur was reamed with a cannulated femoral reamer from the proximal end until all the granulation tissue and cement debris was removed. The intramedullary nail was pulled back during reaming without removing it from the distal femur, in order to protect the knee joint from cement particles. After thorough cleaning of the medullary canal the new femoral component was implanted. Using this method, the cortical bone is not weakened and in most cases a normal femoral stem gives sufficient stability for the revision (Fig. 3.).

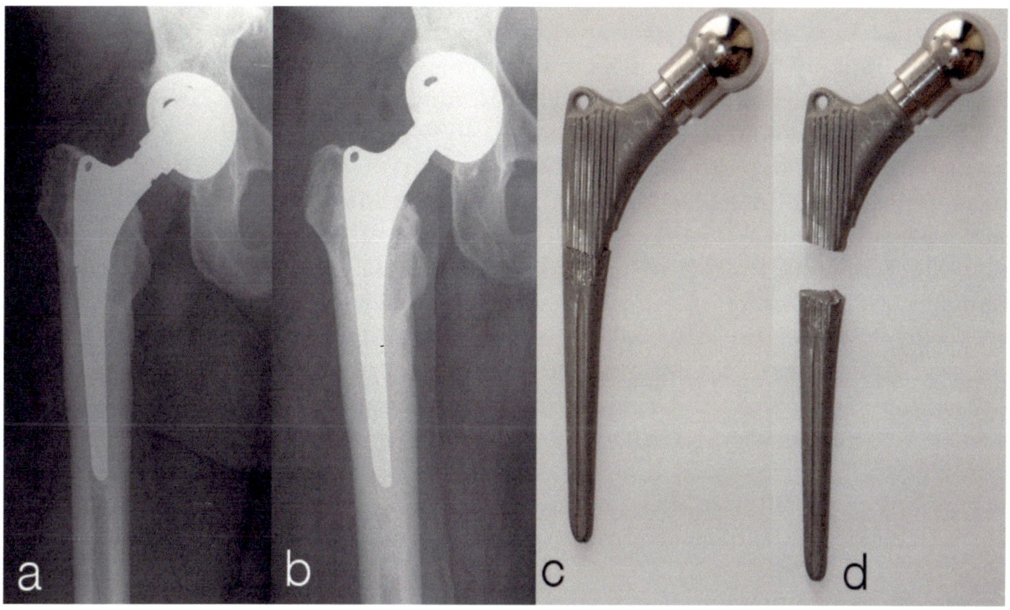

Fig. 3. a: Femoral component failure 14 years following primary surgery. b: Revision with normal femoral component following retrograde removal of broken stem. c and d: Removed, broken component.

The perioperative protocol (thrombopropylaxis, one-shot antibiotic prophylaxis, and applying antibiotic bone cement in case of cemented refixation) does not differ from the routine procedure. Occasional knee swelling occurring in the immediate postoperative period can be treated with local ice packs and applying non-steroidal anti-inflammatory drugs. Physiotherapy and mobilisation does not alter from the routine postoperative protocol.

3. Discussion

When performing revision THR, removal of the distal, often inaccessible cement or a distal fragment of a broken femoral stem is a significant concern (Engh et al., 1999). Whilst intraoperative femoral fracture remains a rare but serious complication during primary

THR, it is a significant problem during revisions (1% of 23,980 primary total hip arthroplasties compared with 7.8% of 6349 revisions in a study by Berry (Berry, 1999)). Subsequent studies have demonstrated similar results (Davis et al., 2003; Egan & Cesare, 1995; Mitchell et al., 2003; Sarvilinna et al., 2004; Taylor et al., 1978).

Farfalli (Farfalli et al., 2007) reported a series of fifty-nine intraoperative fractures that had occurred during revision total hip arthroplasty using impaction bone-grafting. The majority of the fractures (44%) occurred during cement removal.

Various new techniques have been introduced to lower the incidence of perioperative femoral fractures during cement removal, such as ultrasound (Caillouette et al., 1991; Honnart, 1996; Klapper et al., 1992; Schwaller & Elke, 2001), extra-corporal lithotripsy (Braun et al., 1992; Schmidt et al., 1998; Schreurs et al., 1991; Stranne et al., 1992; Weinstein et al., 1988), segmental cement extraction (Chin et al., 1991; Ekelund, 1992; Jingushi et al., 2000; Schurman & Maloney, 1992), application of high-energy shock waves (May et al., 1990), using a ballistically driven chiselling system (Porsch & Schmidt, 2001), or an acoustic emission-controlled milling device (Schmidt & Nordmann, 1994) or even lasers (Sherk et al., 1995). Most of these techniques had not reached widespread usage, and some authors have reported complications (Gardiner et al., 1993).

There have been three clinical studies and one experimental work published about retrograde stem removal (Piatek et al., 2007; Szendroi et al., 2010; Toth et al., 2010; Tóth et al., 2011). Tóth (Toth et al., 2010) and Szendrői (Szendroi et al., 2010) reports successful, uncomplicated application of retrograde removal technique with intact stems and distal fractured components in treatment of elective hip arthroplasty revisions, while Piatek (Piatek et al., 2007) used the technique successfully in case of periprotetic fractures.

The cadaver study compares the biomechanical effects of three different cement removing techniques, the distal fenestration (DF), the transfemoral approach (TFA) and the retrograde stem removal technique (RSR) using an experimental setup (Tóth et al., 2011). 23 paired femora were recovered from similarly aged human cadavers and were frozen. These were later subdivided into 3 groups to provide specimens of similar age and bone quality in each group (DF, TFA, RSR).

The results of the intragroup (comparison between treated and control specimens from the same cadavers from the same groups) analysis were the following: In the TFA group, the force required till fracture was significantly less than in controls ($p=0.0096$). Similar results were found in the DF group ($p=0.068$). There was no difference in the RSR group ($p=0.988$).

Intergroup analysis showed the following:

Femurs in the DF group required significantly less force to fracture than specimens in the RSR ($p=0.043$), whilst there was no difference in there respective controls ($p=0.831$).

Femurs in the TFA group required highly significantly less force to fracture than specimens in the RSR group ($p=0.0001$), whilst there was no difference in there respective controls ($p=0.178$).

That is, the cadaveric study supports the clinical experience that windowing the proximal femur, significantly decreases resistance against compression and rotational forces.

The various windowing techniques described in the literature (Arif et al., 2004; Buehler & Walker, 1998; Cameron, 1990; Hackenbroch, 1979; Kerry et al., 1999; Klein & Rubash, 1993; Moreland et al., 1986; Nelson & Barnes, 1990; Nelson & Weber, 1980; Savvidis & Löer, 1989;

Shepherd & Turnbull, 1989; Stranne et al., 1992; Tyer et al., 1987; Weber, 1981; Witt & Hackenbroch, 1976), and their modifications (Arif et al., 2004; Nelson & Barnes, 1990; Zweymüller et al., 2005) and the new instruments developed for these techniques (Brinckmann & Horst, 1985), all serve one purpose, to decrease the often inevitable weakening of the proximal femoral bone stock, preserving as much intact bone as possible. Although the more conservative windowing techniques tend to preserve more proximal bone, they still inevitably lead to decreased resistance against fracture.

The studies performed by Dennis et al. (Dennis et al., 1987) on cadaveric femora, showed that when femurs without intramedullary support are stressed to failure, fractures occur through the cortical holes 90% of the time, therefore they suggested that long revision femoral stems should be used to bypass the window by at least 2 to 2.5 times the cortical diameter measured at the fenestration level (Fig. 4/b). This has been generally accepted and is widely used in orthopaedic practice (Kerry et al., 1999; Klein & Rubash, 1993; Lotke et al., 1986; Moreland et al., 1986; Nelson & Barnes, 1990; Nelson & Weber, 1980; Savvidis & Löer, 1989; Shepherd & Turbull, 1989; Tyer et al., 1987).

The disadvantage of using a long stem with proximal opening of the femur instead of the RSR technique and a short stem (Fig. 3a, 3b.), is that long revision stems are more expensive, the necessary exposure requires a longer incision (Fig. 4c), with more soft tissue stripping, surgery is often much longer, blood loss can be extensive, and the local and general complication rate is higher.

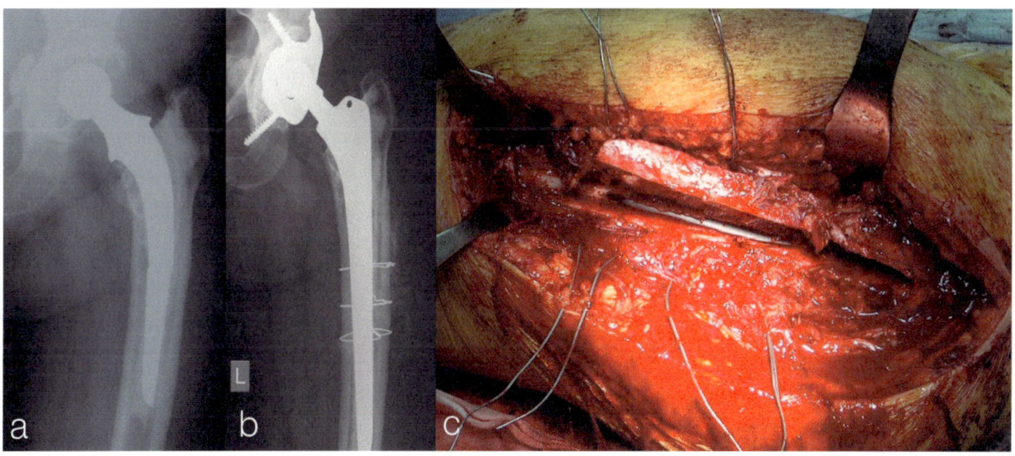

Fig. 4. a: Femoral component failure and acetabular component loosening 17 years following primary surgery. b: Distal fragment of cement and stem are removed through bone window, followed by wire refixation of the window. The long revision femoral stem distally overreaches the window by the length of 2.5 times. c: Major surgical wound with extended osteotomy (intraoperative photo).

The RSR technique cannot always be used, and is absolutely contraindicated in the case of septic loosening or if the knee or the distal femur is affected by primary or metastatic tumours. Large distal cement plugs or the presence of oblique cement at the end of the stem are relative contraindications, because these can force the nail used for removal towards the cortical bone, which can lead to unwanted perforation or even periprosthetic fracture.

In the clinical setting depending on the quality of the proximal femoral bone, both a short a long femoral stem can be used for the revision surgery after RSR. As the cortex is not violated during component removal, a short primary stem (cemented or uncemented) is a valid option and is our preference, if the cortices are not very thin, and at least some peripheral cancellous bone is present, for cement penetration. We like to reserve long stems as a final resort, to allow a possible future revision.

4. Conclusion

Our cadaver experiments clearly confirm the clinical experience, that the window technique significantly weakens resistance of femur against rotation under compression forces. In contrast, with the retrograde cement removal technique this weakening does not occur.
Our experience with retrograde cement removal in elective revisions and periprosthetic fractures shows that - taking into consideration indications and contraindications- retrograde prosthesis removal technique is a viable alternative solution in case of intact as well as failed femoral components. It is associated with less intraoperative complications and faster, safer recovery compared to traditional techniques.
However, longer follow–up time is required to confirm the durability of the observed clinical outcomes.

5. References

Arif, M., Sivananthan, S., & Choon, DS. (2004). Revision of total hip arthroplasty using an anterior cortical window, extensive strut allografts, and an impaction graft: follow-up study. *J Orthop Surg (Hong Kong),* Vol. 12, No. 1, (June, 2004), pp. 25-30, ISSN 1022-5536

Berry, DJ. (1999). Epidemiology: hip and knee. *Orthop Clin North Am,* Vol. 30, No. 2, (April, 1999), pp. 183-190, ISSN 0030-5898

Braun, W., Claes, L., Ruter, A., & Paschke, D. (1992). Effect of shock waves on the strength of connection between bone and polymethylmethacrylate. An in vitro study of human femur segments. *Z Orthop Ihre Grenzgeb,* Vol. 130, No. 3, (May-June, 1992), pp. 236–243, ISSN 0044-3220

Brinckmann, P., & Horst, M. (1985). New instruments for the removal of an artificial hip joint from the shaft. *Z Orthop Ihre Grenzgeb,* Vol. 123, No. 1, (January-February, 1985), pp. 113-114, ISSN 0044-3220

Buehler, KO., & Walker, RH. (1998). Polymethylmethacrylate removal from the femur using a crescentic window technique. *Orthopedics,* Vol. 21, No. 6, (June, 1998), pp. 697-700, ISSN 0147-7447

Caillouette, JT., Gorab, RS., Klapper, RC., & Anzel, SH. (1991). Revision arthroplasty facilitated by ultrasonic tool cement removal. Part II: histologic analysis of endosteal bone after cement removal. *Orthop Rev,* Vol. 20, No. 5, (May, 1991), pp. 435–440, ISSN 0094-6591

Cameron, HU. (1990). Tips of the trade #29. Femoral windows for easy cement removal in hip revision surgery. *Orthop Rev,* Vol. 19, No. 10, (October, 1990), pp. 909-910, 912 ISSN 0094-6591

Chin, AK., Moll, FH., McColl, MB., Hoffman, KJ., & Wuh, HC. (1991). An improved technique for cement extraction in revision total hip arthroplasty. *Contemp Orthop*, Vol. 22, No. 3, (March, 1991), pp. 255–264, ISSN 0194-8458

Davis, CM., 3rd, Berry, DJ., & Harmsen, WS. (2003). Cemented revision of failed uncemented femoral components of total hip arthroplasty. *J Bone Joint Surg Am*, Vol. 85-A, No. 7, (July, 2003), pp.1264-1269, ISSN 0021-9355

Dennis, DA., Dingman, CA., Meglan, DA., O'Leary, JF., Mallory, TH., & Berme, N. (1987). Femoral cement removal in revision total hip arthroplasty. A biomechanical analysis. *Clin Orthop Relat Res*, Vol. 220, No. 7, (July, 1987), pp. 142-147, ISSN 0009-921X

Egan, KJ., & Di Cesare, PE. (1995). Intraoperative complications of revision hip arthroplasty using a fully porous-coated straight cobalt-chrome femoral stem. *J Arthroplasty*, Vol. 10, Suppl. (November, 1995), pp. 45-51, ISSN 0883-5403

Ekelund, AL. (1992). Cement removal in revision hip arthroplasty. Experience with bone cement added to the cavity in 20 cases. *Acta Orthop Scand*, Vol. 63, No. 5, (October, 1992), pp. 549–551, ISSN 0001-6470

Engh, CA., McAuley, JP., & Engh, C. (1999). Surgical approaches for revision total hip replacement surgery: the anterior trochanteric slide and the extended conventional osteotomy. *Instr Course Lect*, Vol. 48, (1999), pp. 3-8, ISSN 0065-6895

Farfalli, GL., Buttaro, MA., & Piccaluga, F. (2007). Femoral fractures in revision hip surgeries with impacted bone allograft. *Clin Orthop Relat Res*, Vol. 462, No. 9, (September, 2007), pp. 130-136, ISSN 0009-921X

Ferguson, GM. (1988). Femoral cement removal in revision total hip arthroplasty: a biomechanical analysis. *Clin Orthop Relat Res*, Vol. 234, No. 8, (September, 1998), pp. 307-308, ISSN 0009-921X

Gardiner, R., Hozack, WJ., Nelson, C., & Keating, EM. (1993). Revision total hip arthroplasty using ultrasonically driven tools. A clinical evaluation *J Arthroplasty*, Vol. 8, No. 5, (October, 1993), pp. 517–521, ISSN 0883-5403

Hackenbroch, Jr. MH. (1979). Possibilities and limitations of exchange of hip and knee joint prostheses. *Z Orthop Ihre Grenzgeb*, Vol. 117, No. 4, (August, 1979), pp. 457-460, ISSN 0044-3220

Honnart, F. (1996). Use of ultrasound for the removal of cement in hip prosthesis reoperations. *Rev Chir Orthop Reparatrice Appar Mot*, Vol. 82, No. 2, (1996), pp. 171–174, ISSN 0035-1040

Jingushi, S., Noguchi, Y., Shuto, T., Nakashima, T., & Iwamoto Y. (2000). A device for removal of femoral distal cement plug during hip revision arthroplasty: a high-powered drill equipped with a centralizer. *J Arthroplasty*, Vol. 15, No. 2, (February, 2000), pp. 231–233, ISSN 0883-5403

Kerry, RM., Masri, BA., Garbuz, DS., & Duncan, CP. (1999). The vascularized scaphoid window for access to the femoral canal in revision total hip arthroplasty. *Instr Course Lect*, Vol. 48, (1999), pp. 9-11, ISSN 0065-6895

Klapper, RC., Caillouette, JT., Callaghan, JJ., & Hozack, WJ. (1992). Ultrasonic technology in revision joint arthroplasty. *Clin Orthop*, Vol. 285, No. 12, (December, 1992), pp. 147–154, ISSN 0009-921X

Klein, AH., & Rubash, HE. (1993). Femoral windows in revision total hip arthroplasty. *Clin Orthop Relat Res*, Vol. 291, No. 6, (June, 1993), pp. 164-170, ISSN 0009-921X

Laffargue, P., De Lestang, M., Bonnomet, F., Dupart, L., & Havet, E. (2000). Techniques of component and cement removal: osseous pitfalls and approaches. *Rev Chir Orthop Reparatrice Appar Mot,* Vol. 86, No. 9, Suppl. (September, 2000), pp. 51-54, ISSN 0035-1040

Lauer, W., Neuss, M., Wirtz, DC., & Radermacher, K. (2002). Technical principles for removal of femoral bone cements in hip prosthesis implant revision. *Biomed Tech (Berl),* Vol. 47, Suppl 1 Pt, (2002), pp. 47-48, ISSN 0013-5585

Lotke, PA., Wong, RY., & Ecker, ML. (1986). Stress fracture as a cause of chronic pain following revision total hip arthroplasty. Report of two cases. Clin Orthop Relat Res, Vol. 206, (May, 1986) pp. 147-150, ISSN 0009-921X

May, TC., Krause, WR., Preslar, AJ., Smith, MJ., Beaudoin, AJ., & Cardea, JA. (1990). Use of high-energy shock waves for bone cement removal. *J Arthroplasty,* Vol. 5, No. 1, (March, 1990), pp. 19–27, ISSN 0883-5403

Mitchell, PA., Greidanus, NV., Masri, BA., Garbuz, DS., & Duncan, CP. (2003). The prevention of periprosthetic fractures of the femur during and after total hip arthroplasty. *Instr Course Lect,* Vol. 52, (2003), pp. 301-308, ISSN 0065-6895

Moed, BR., & Watson JT. (1995). Retrograde intramedullary nailing, without reaming, of fractures of the femoral shaft in multiply injure patient. *J. Bone Joint Surg. Am,* Vol. 75, No.10, (October, 1995), pp. 1520-1527, ISSN 0021-9355

Moreland, JR., Marder, R., & Anspach, WE Jr. (1986). The window technique for the removal of broken femoral stems in total hip replacement. *Clin Orthop Relat Res,* Vol.212, (November, 1986), pp. 245-249, ISSN 0009-921X

Nelson, CL., & Weber, MJ. (1981). Technique of windowing the femoral shaft for removal of bone cement. *Clin Orthop Relat Res,* Vol. 154, (January-February, 1981), pp. 336-337 ISSN 0009-921X

Nelson, CL., & Barnes, CL. (1990). Removal of bone cement from the femoral shaft using a femoral windowing device. J Arthroplasty, Vol. 5, No. 1, (March, 1990), pp. 67-69, ISSN 0883-5403

Piatek, S., Westphal, T., Holmenschlager, F., Becker, R, & Winckler, S. (2007). Retrograde cement removal in periprosthetic fractures following hip arthroplasty. *Arch Orthop Trauma Surg,* Vol. 127, No. 7, (September, 2007), pp. 581-585, ISSN 0936-8051

Porsch, M., & Schmidt, J. (2001). Cement removal with an endoscopically controlled ballistically driven chiselling system. A new device for cement removal and preliminary clinical results. *Arch Orthop Trauma Surg,* Vol. 121, No. 5, (May, 2001), pp. 274–277, ISSN:0936-8051

Sarvilinna, R., Huhtala, HS., Sovelius, RT., Halonen, PJ., Nevalainen, JK., & Pajam¨aki, KJ. (2004). Factors predisposing to periprosthetic fracture after hip arthroplasty: a case (n = 31)-control study. Acta Orthop Scand, Vol. 75 No. 1, (February, 2004), pp. 16-20, ISSN 0001-6470

Savvidis, E., & Löer, F. (1989). Surgical technique for femur shaft fenestration in revisional surgery following total hip replacements - a comparative experimental study. *Z Orthop Ihre Grenzgeb,* Vol. 127, No. 2, (1989), pp. 228-236, ISSN 0044-3220

Schreurs, BW., Bierkens, AF., Huiskes, R., Hendrikx, AJ., & Slooff, TJ. (1991). The effect of the extracorporeal shock wave lithotriptor on bone cement. *J Biomed Mater Res,* Vol. 25, No. 2, (February, 1991), pp. 157–164, ISSN 0021-9304

Schmidt, J., & Nordmann, K. (1994). Removal of bone cement from the femoral canal using an acoustic emission-controlled milling device. *Med Biol Eng Comput*, Vol. 32, No. 3, (May, 1994), pp. 258-260, ISSN 0140-0118

Schmidt, J., Porsch, M., Hackenbroch, MH., Koebke, J., & Brimmers, P. (1998). ModiWed intracorporeal lithotripsy for cement removal in hip prosthesis exchange operations–experimental principles. *Z Orthop Ihre Grenzgeb*, Vol. 136, No. 1, (January-February, 1998), pp. 44–49, ISSN 0044-3220

Schurman, DJ., & Maloney, WJ. (1992). Segmental cement extraction at revision total hip arthroplasty. *Clin Orthop*, Vol. 285, (December, 1992), pp. 158–163, ISSN:0009-921X

Schwaller, CA., & Elke, R. (2001). Cement removal with ultrasound in revision or total hip prosthesis. *Orthopade*, Vol. 30, No. 5, (May, 2001), pp. 310–316, ISSN:0085-4530

Shepherd, BD., & Turnbull, A. (1989). The fate of femoral windows in revision joint arthroplasty. *J Bone Joint Surg Am*, Vol. 71, No. 5, (June, 1989), pp. 716-718, ISSN 0021-9355

Sherk, HH., Lane, G., Rhodes, A., & Black, J. (1995). Carbon dioxide laser removal of polymethylmethacrylate. *Clin Orthop, Vol. 310, (January, 1995), pp.* 67–71, ISSN 0009-921X

Stranne, SK., Callaghan, JJ., Fyda, TM., Fulghum, CS., Glisson, RR., Weinerth, JL., & Seaber, AV. (1992). The effect of extracorporeal shock wave lithotripsy on the prosthesis interface in cementless arthroplasty. Evaluation in a rabbit model. *J Arthroplasty*, Vol. 7, No. 2, (June, 1992), pp. 173–179, ISSN 0883-5403

Stühmer, K. (1987). Zur Technik der Zemententfernung bei Austauschoperationen von Gelenkendoprothesen. *Aktuel Probl Chir Orthop*, Vol. 31, (1987), pp. 342–346, ISSN 0378-8504

Szendrői, M., Tóth, K., Kiss, J., Antal, I., & Skaliczki G. (2010). Retrograde genocephalic removal of fractured or immovable femoral stems in revision hip surgery. *Hip Int.* Vol. 20, No. 1, (January-March, 2010), pp. 34-37, ISSN 1120-7000

Taylor, MM., Meyers, MH., & Harvey, JP Jr. (1978). Intraoperative femur fractures during total hip replacement. *Clin Orthop Relat Res*, Vol. 137, (November-December, 1978), pp. 96-103, ISSN 0009-921X

Toth, K., Sisak, K., Nagy, J., Mano, S., & Csernatony, Z. (2010). Retrograde stem removal in revision hip surgery: removing a loose or broken femoral component with a retrograde nail. *Archives of Orthopaedic and Trauma Surgery*, Vol. 130, No. 7, (July, 2010), pp. 813-818, ISSN 0936-8051

Tóth, K., Sisák, K., Wellinger, K., Manó, S., Horváth, G., Szendrői, M., & Csernátony, Z. (2011). Biomechanical comparison of three cemented stem removal techniques in revision hip surgery. *Arch Orthop Trauma Surg*. Vol. 131, No. 7, (July, 2011), pp. 1007-1012, ISSN 0936-8051

Tyer, HD., Huckstep, RL., & Stalley, PD. (1987). Intraluminal allograft restoration of the upper femur in failed total hip arthroplasty. *Clin Orthop Relat Res*, Vol. 224, (November, 1987), pp. 26-32, ISSN 0009-921X

Wagner, H. (1989). A revision prosthesis for the hip joint. *Orthopade*, Vol. 18, No. 5, (September, 1989), pp. 438–453, ISSN 0085-4530

Weber, BG. (1981). Total hip replacement revision surgery: Surgical technique and experience. In: *Hip*, E.A. Salvati, (Ed.), 3-14, Proceedings of the 9th Open Scientific Meeting of the Hip Society, ISBN 0095-7216, St. Louis, Mosby, USA

Weinstein, JN., Oster, DM., Park, JB., Park, SH., & Loening, S. (1988). The effect of the extracorporeal shock wave lithotriptor on the bone-cement interface in dogs. *Clin Orthop*, Vol. 235, (October, 1988), pp. 261-267, ISSN 0009-921X

Witt, AN., & Hackenbroch, MH. (1976). Therapeutic approaches to implant loosening in total hip arthroplasty. *Z Orthop Ihre Grenzgeb*, Vol. 114, No. 3, (June, 1976), pp. 330-341, ISSN 0044-3220

Zweymüller, KA., Steindl, M., & Melmer, T. (2005). Anterior windowing of the femur diaphysis for cement removal in revision surgery. *Clin Orthop Relat Res*, Vol. 441, (December, 2005), pp. 227-336, ISSN 0009-921X

Part 3

Knee Arthroplasty

14

History of Condylar Total Knee Arthroplasty

Luca Amendola[1], Domenico Tigani[2],
Matteo Fosco[3] and Dante Dallari[3]
[1]*Department of Orthopedic and Traumatology, Maggiore Hospital, Bologna*
[2]*Department of Orthopaedic Surgery, Santa Maria alle Scotte Hospital, Siena*
[3]*First Ward of Orthopaedic Surgery, Rizzoli Orthopaedic Institute, Bologna*
Italy

1. Introduction

The first attempt of treating patients affected by knee osteoarthritis with arthroplasty go back up to the mid-nineteenth century with the use of either a soft tissue interposed within the joint surface or resection of a different amount of bone of both distal femur and proximal tibia.

However the concept on which total joint replacement is based can be traced only after the 1880 in Berlin with Thermestocles Gluck who gave a series of lectures describing a system of joint replacement by unit made of ivory. The surgeon believed that these unit could be stabilized in bone with cement made of colophony, pumice and plaster of Paris.

The early twentieth saw the return of interposition arthroplasty with the use of autologous tissue or metallic surface and in the 1950s was developed the first surface replacement of the tibia by McKeever (McKeever, 1960). Only during the 1950s and 1960s at last the knee arthroplasty concept diverged into two theories of total joint replacement: the designer focused their effort toward constrained or hinged prosthesis or toward condylar replacement.

Condylar replacement knee prosthesis is defined as one where the femoral and tibial load-bearing surface are replaced with non connected artificial components. Work on the design of an implant that resurfaced the distal femur and proximal tibia without any direct mechanical link between the components began at the end of sixties at the Imperial College in London. The original design known as Freeman-Swanson prosthesis consisted of a metal "roller" placed on the distal femur that articulated with a polyethylene tibial tray and requires resection of both cruciate ligaments.

In other part of the world were developed different experience which carried out to Polycentric, Geomedic, Duocondylar systems (Fig.1).

Even if all of these implants were considered unsatisfactory because of a high percentage of components mobilizations, break of the components and infection the acquired experience permitted the resurfacing prosthesis planning (Insall & Scott, 2001) to occur its successive design phase followed two different ways : the anatomical approach and the functional approach. (Robinson, 2005).

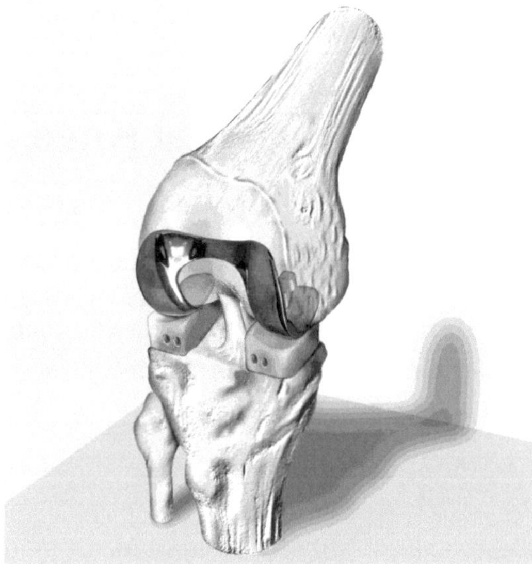

Fig. 1. Duocondylar (courtesy of Prof F. Catani).

2. Anatomical approach

Some designers studied prosthesis that preserve both cruciate ligaments, allowed the femur to roll-back on the tibia.

Yamamoto, from the Okayama University Medical School in Japan, was the first to report on implanting an anatomical femoral component with a minimally constrained single-piece polyethylene tibial component in 1970 (Yamamoto, 1979). The design called the Kodama-Yamamoto knee, consisted of an anatomical femoral mold component, including an anterior femoral flange, made of COP alloy (Co, Cr, Ni, Mo, C, and P). There was a 1-piece, mildly dished polyethylene tibial component that had a central cutout for preservation of both cruciate ligaments.

Others Authors who followed the same approach was Waugh (Waugh et al., 1973) at the University of California UCI, Townley with the cemented Anatomical knee (Townley & Hill, 1974) and Sheedom who designed the Leeds knee. All these prostheses had and horseshoe-shaped tibial component leaving a space behind and centrally for the retention of both anterior and posterior cruciate ligaments.

At the HSS, during the early seventhies, the Duocondylar knee was completely redesigned in an anatomical and symmetrical design: the Duopatellar (Fig.2).

An anterior femoral flange, patellar button, and a more dished tibial surface were added. The tibial component had a fixation peg, identical to the Total Condylar TC, the archetype of the functional approach, and, for the first time, a posterior rectangular cutout—specifically designed for the preserved posterior cruciate ligament.

Although the result of Duopatella were extremely good at the HSS the posterior cruciate-preserving approach would be developed in Boston at the Robert Breck Brigham Hospital (Scott, 1982; Sledge & Ewald, 1979). In Boston the medial tip of the femoral trochlear flange was removed, creating right and left designs based on the asymmetry of the proximal femoral flange.

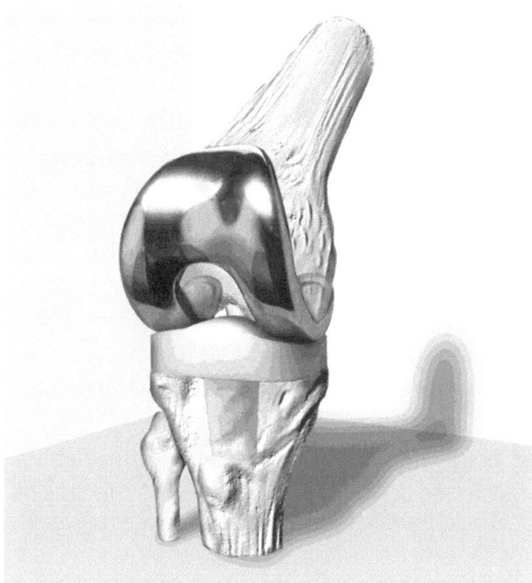

Fig. 2. Duopatellar (courtesy of Prof F. Catani).

This was done to reduce the medial overhang seen in small female rheumatoid patients. The posterior cruciate-sparing version of the Robert Brigham Hospital would later evolved in the PFC knee (Cintor Division of Codman; later, Depuy, Johnson & Johnson). At the same time Peter Walker, Clement Sledge and Fred Ewald, continued the Duopatella concept in the posteriorcruciate-retaining version of the Kinematic knee (Howmedica), which was implanted by Ewald in June 1978. This would evolve into the posteriorcruciate-sparing version of the Kinematic II, Kinemax, and Kinemax Plus systems (Howmedica).

The 80's saw the significant advances in the knee arthroplasty, particularly in the area of surgical technique and instrumentation. Kenna, Hungerford, and Krackow participated in the design of the instruments that were later called the Universal Instruments. Their tools were based on the anatomical concept of measured resection technique rather than the more functional approach of creating equal and parallel flexion and extension gaps which where used until then. The principal aspect of this new conception was that the bone and cartilage removed were to equal the thickness of the prosthetic material replacing them. Up until this time, fixation of the condylar total knee was primarily achieved with cement.

In January 1980 the first Porous-Coated Anatomical Knee (PCA) was inplanted by Hungerford at Johns Hopkins (Hungerford et al., 1982). The implant was anatomical with asymmetric medial and lateral femoral condyles similar to the Leeds and the original Townley designs. However, for the first time, it introduced porous coating in a total condylar knee for a cementless fixation. Each of the 3 components was backed with metal and a 1.5-mm-thick sintered porous coating of cobalt chrome beads.

The Miller-Galante total knee, one of the first knee replacement designed for use with cement or cementless fixation, was first implanted in 1986. The principal innovation of this implant was the choice of a titanium fiber composite for the bony ingrowth surface, because of its well-recognized biocompatibility, and the use of a Titanium Aluminums and Vanadium alloy (Ti6Al4V). The implant is fixed to the tibia with titanium screws and pegs. The uncemented version for patellar resurfacing consists of a metal-backed patella which is

fixed with fiber-mesh pegs. Modularity of tibial polyethylene inserts was incorporate in order to allow better ligamentous tension and possibility of future isolated polyethylene replacement.
"Cruciate retaining" prosthesis developed from the anatomical concept were different: some consisted of a relatively flat surface on the sagittal and transversal plane (Kinemax e PCA) while others maintained a more congruent surface on the sagittal plane. Genesis II (Smith&Nephew), Duracon (Howmedica), Nexgen CR (Zimmer), PFC CR (Depuy) represent some actual examples of this conception.

3. Functional approach

Designers of the functional approach tried to simplify the knee biomechanics by removing both cruciate ligaments.
The first system derived from the functional concept is represented by the Total Condylar prosthesis (TC; Fig.3) developed in 1973 at the Hospital for Special Surgery of New York (Insall et al., 1976).

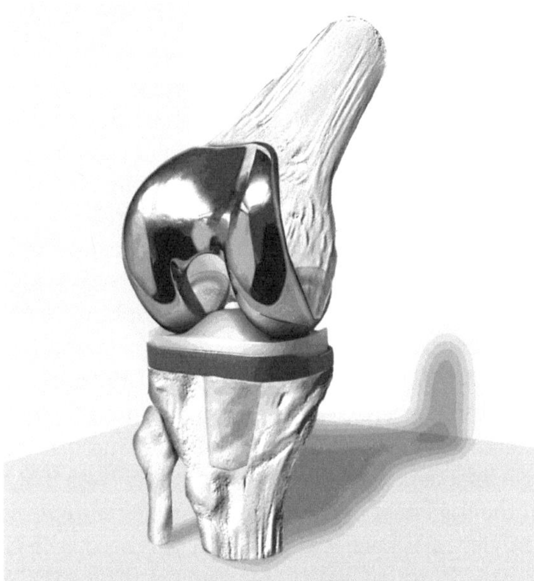

Fig. 3. Total condylar (courtesy of Prof F. Catani).

TC prosthesis consisted of two symmetric condylar surfaces with a posterior decreasing radius of curvature and an articular surface made of polyethylene, perfectly congruent in extension and partially congruent in flexion.
The TC knee would prove to be highly successful, widely used, and would later demonstrate long survival (Vince et al., 1989). Two concerns, however, pointed out the early fases of its clinical use. The femoral component would shift forward, particularly in flexion. In rare cases, this would even result in tibial loosening or anterior dislocation. The second concern was the limited flexion achieved. Average knee flexion with the TC knee was in fact 90° degrees (Robinson, 2005).

In 1978 prosthesis Insall-Burstein was designed to correct these problems by replacing the posterior cruciate ligament with a mechanical lock to reduce posterior translation of the femoral component by using a mechanism of a cam articulated with a post on the tibial component (Fig.4).

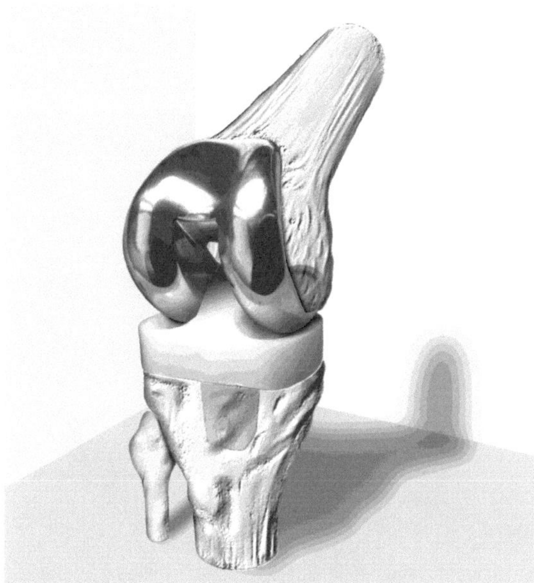

Fig. 4. IB-I allpoly (courtesy of Prof F. Catani).

The cam of the femoral component connected with the tibial central spine at about 70 degrees of flexion and then the femur could roll-back so to increase flexion.
The first IBPS knee was implanted in 1978 by Insall at the HSS.
The IBPS knee become one of the most successful total condylar knee design (Abdeen et al., 2010). Anterior femoral subluxation was eliminated and average flexion would be 115°. A metal-backed monoblock IBPS tibial component with direct-molded polyethylene was introduced in November 1980: the Insall-Burstein Modular (IBPS II) knee (Stern & Insall, 1992).
The HSS posterior-stabilized knee design would evolve into the Insall-Burstein Modular (IBPS II) knee (Zimmer; Fig.5) in 1988, the Optetrak Posterior-Stabilized knee (Exactech; Fig.6) in 1994, and the Advance Posterior- Stabilized knee (Wright Medical) in 1994.
In the 1980s and 1990s, many variations of these functional designs were introduced by different manufacturers. All of them had the characteristic to produce their motion through a so called guided motion, which mean that some characteristics of the motion, such as rollback, are produced by mechanical interaction between the femoral and tibial components.
In the Kyocera Bi-Surface knee (Kyocera Corp, Kyoto, Japan; Fig.7) (Akagi et al., 2000), for the major part of the flexion range, the knee behaves as a standard condylar replacement with moderately conforming bearing surfaces. Beyond that, the load is transferred to a spherical surface protruding behind from the femoral intercondylar region, contacting within a spherical depression at the posterior of the plastic tibial component.

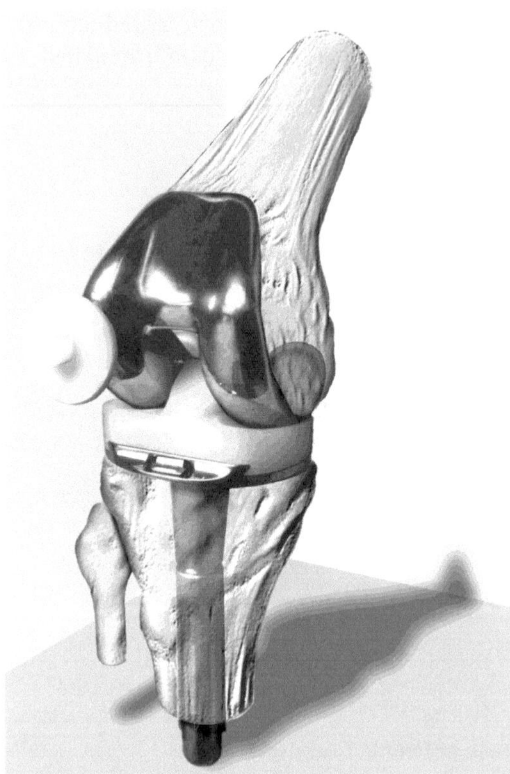

Fig. 5. IB-II PS (courtesy of Prof F. Catani).

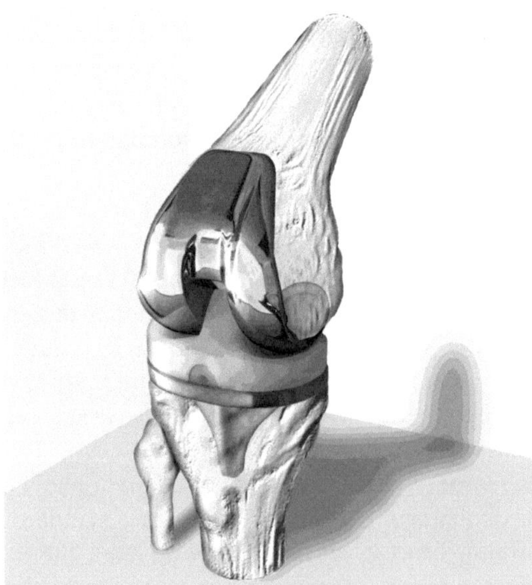

Fig. 6. Optetrak (courtesy of Prof F. Catani).

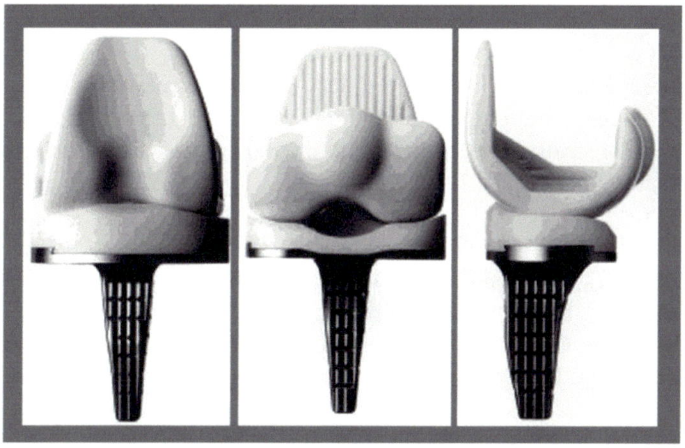

Fig. 7. The Bisurface knee prosthesis (courtesy of Kyocera Corp).

Another example of guided motion knee is represented by The Medial Pivot knee (Wright Mfg Co, Memphis, TN; Fig.8). In that prosthesis the femoral component owns a single radius of femoral curvature and a high level of conformity in the medial compartment where a ball and socket configuration is present. In reason of that configuration the medial side remains in the same position during flexion, but the lateral femoral condyle can displace behind with flexion. The porpoise of the medial pivot design is to reproduce a more physiological kinematics.

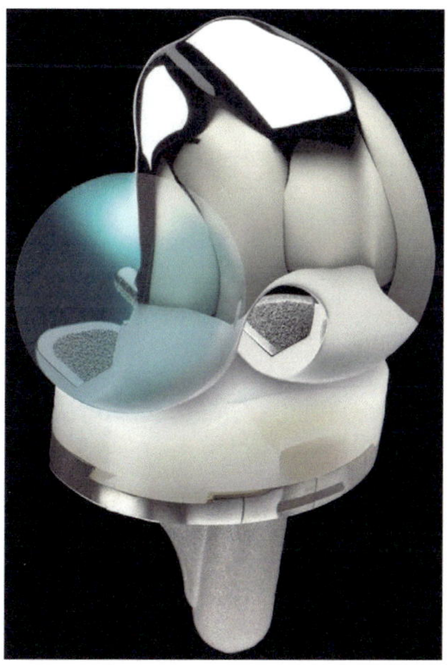

Fig. 8. Spherical condylar surface contacting within a spherical depression at the posterior of the polyethylene (courtesy of Wright Medical).

In contrast with this type of solution more recently has been introduce on the market a new design, the 3D Knee, which provides A/P stability similar to ACL deficient valgus knees

through a concave lateral compartment. The lateral compartment is fully congruent in extension and allows 15o of axial rotation. As the knee flexes, a greater range of femoral motion is possible, but is controlled by the concave lateral compartment.
The aim of the 3D Knee is then to accommodate and controls the cruciate deficient patterns of motions without constrain in stripe to reproduce the normal kinematic of the knee.
One of the most innovative functional approaches to condylar total knee design evolved from a collaboration between an orthopedic Surgeon at the New Jersey Medical School Frederic Buechel and a professor of mechanical engineering Michael Pappas. Their project to achieve a low polyethylene contact stresses while maintaining knee flexion and avoiding overload of the implant bone interfaces started in 1977 (Buechel & Pappas, 1986) with the introduction of the Low Contact Stress (LCS) knee system (fig.9). It was the first complete systems approach to total knee replacement using meniscal bearing surfaces.

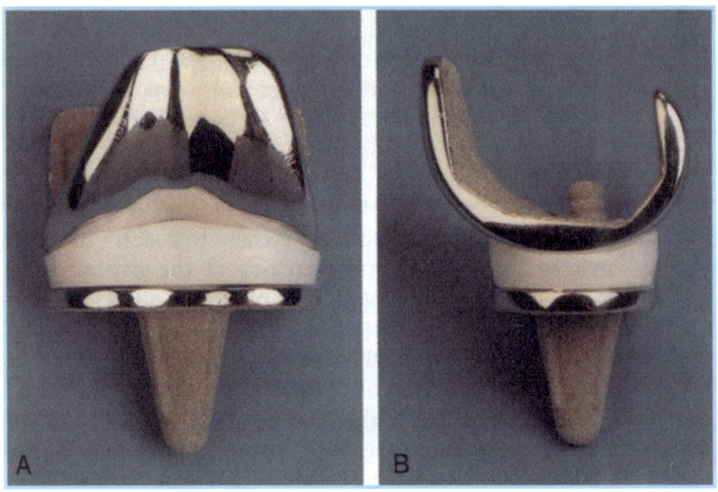

Fig. 9. LCS (courtesy of Depuy J& J).

3.1 Mobile bearing (MB) knee

The principal characteristic of the femoral component was based on the same spherical surface on the mediolateral plane while a decreasing radius of curvature from extension to flexion was present on the lateral side. This shape maintained full area contact on the upper meniscal bearing from the 0 to 45° at which walking loads are encountered, and maintaining at least spherical line at deeper flexion angles. In its origin, the LCS, was proposed as a system inclusive of both cruciate-sparing meniscal bearing and PCL-sacrificing rotating platform variant, with the latter gaining the majority of popular usage over the time.
Afterward the introduction of the LCS system, several types of Mobile bearing knees were produced. They are categorized in according of their conformity: either partially or fully conforming, then a third group is represented by the posterior stabilized MB.

3.2 Partially conforming MB

The LCS other to be the ancestor of all the MB prostheses is also, with its second version featured by a single plastic bearing that freely rotates about its post setaed whitin a hole in the tibial tray, the prototype of the partially conforming one.

Belongs to partially conforming knees the Self Aligning MB (Sulzer) designed by Bourne and Rorabeck in 1987. This prosthesis is characterized by an oval recess in posterior aspect of the polyethylene which allows unlimited rotation and limited AP translation about a tibial tray peg.
The mobile bearing knee produced by the Waldemar Link in Hamburg in 1990, called TACK, is characterized by the presence in the tibial tray of two semicircular guide that engage circular tracks on both sides of the polyethylene platform, permitting wide rotational movement.
The Interax Integrated Secure Asymmetric (Howmedica) prosthesis has nearly fully conformity between femoral condyle and tibial surface in extension and whereas the conformity gradually decrease in flexion. The tibial baseplate has two central posts that engages a curved, t-shaped guide track whitin the meniscal bearing.
In Italy Prof Ghisellini designed the Total Rotating Knee (TRK) (Cremascoli) characterized by a central tibia post projecting from the center of the tibial tray. Two type of plastic bearing were available the R type to allow freedom of rotation was intend to be use incase of PCL excision, whereas the RS allowing 10 mm of AP sliding and freedom of rotation, was indicated when the PCL was retained.

3.3 Fully conforming MB

The progenitor of fully conforming MB knees is certainly the Rotaglide Total knee System (Corin, Cirencester, UK) designed in 1986 by Polyzoides and Tsakonas: the rotaglide femoral component has a constant flexion radius of curvature in the femoro-meniscal articulation, each condyle being part of a sphere of 24 mm radius. This design ensures that congruency is retained throughout the range of flexion. The mobile meniscal bearing has two undercuts which permit up to 5mm of antero-posterior translation and 25° of rotation, 12,5° for each side. The tibial plateau has an anterior bollard that prevents anterior dislocation while restricting the rotation of the platform and another bollard in the middle of the tray that resists posterior dislocation.

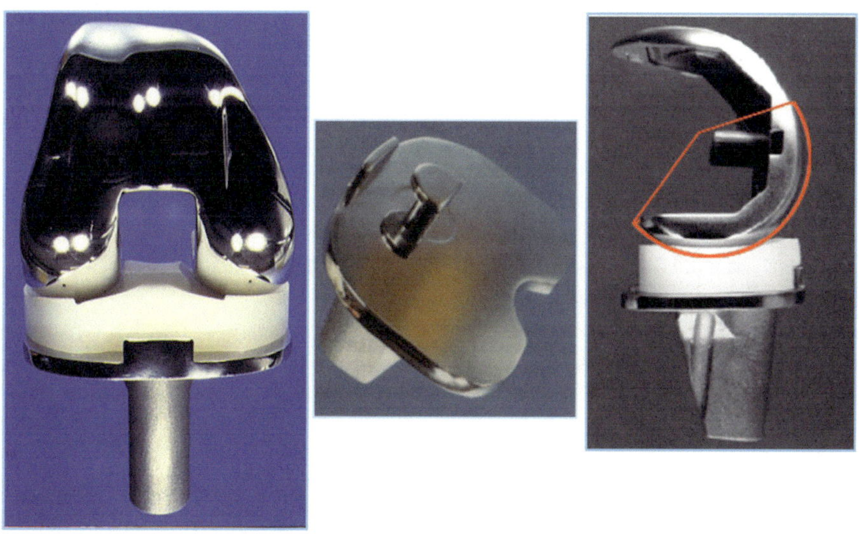

Fig. 10. a) MBK designs (courtesy of Zimmer).

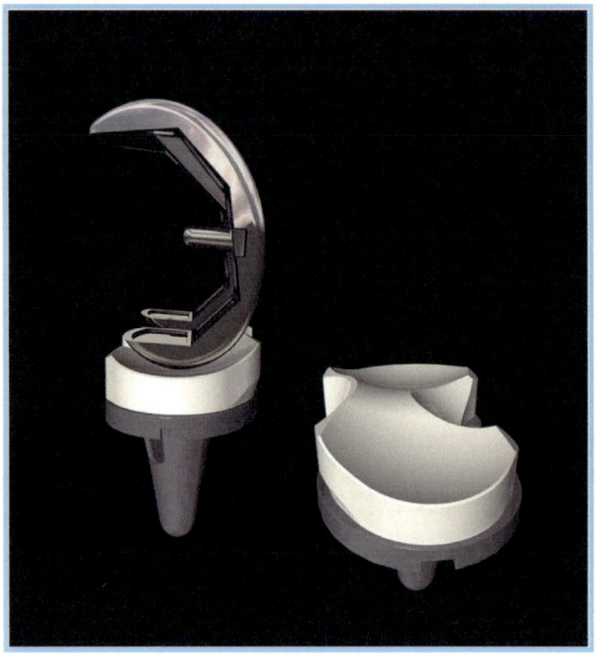

Fig. 10. b) MBK schematic.

The Medially Biased Kinematics Knee (MBK) was developed by J Insall, P Aglietti e P Walker in 1992 (Fig.10a-b). The design concept of this prosthesis is complete conformity between the femoral component and the polyethylene insert at any degree of flexion and during rotation and AP translation of the tibial insert on the tibial tray. The prosthesis design allow a medially biased kinematics guided by the natural knee's stronger medial structures and greater lateral mobility. The polyethylene has approximately 20 degrees of both internal and external rotation on the tibial baseplate about a D-shaped "mushroom" post. The tibial baseplate translates 4,5 mm in an AP direction. An anterior stop prevents the plastic bearing from sliding off the tibial tray.

3.4 Posterior stabilized MB

These design are based on the "cam and post" mechanism on a rotating polyethylene platform. The common feature is the presence of a cam situated between the posterior femoral condyles that engages a post projecting from the mobile polyethylene platform. The "cam and post" mechanism acts as a third weight-bearing condyle to help improve, load transfer and minimize polyethylene stress.
Belongs to this category the Two Radii Area Contact (TRAC, Biomet) which was indroduced in 1997. More recent designs are the P.F.C. Sigma RPF (DePuy) and the LPS mobile Flex (Zimmer).

4. Patellofemoral joint

Symptoms related to the patello-femoral joint have been reported to be a frequent cause of failure following total knee arthroplasty.

During 1980s, up to 30% of patients suffered of complication associated with the patella-femoral joint (Rhoads et al., 1990).
This disappointing feature of what was otherwise a successful procedure led between surgeons to a debate as to whether the articular surface of the patella should be replaced and, in event of the replacement , exactly how this should be performed.
At the some time various authors (Grace & Rand, 1988; Yoshii et al., 1992) pointed out the importance of prosthetic femoral and patella components.
As this problem started off with the improvement of flexion allowed by the second generation of resurfacing condylar knee, so that minimal patellofemoral problems were associate with the TC which permitted at least 90° of flexion, the principal concern of designers was to perform a deeper trochlea which floor could extend behind so as to roof of the intercondylar notch, thereby providing a surface against which the patella can articulate in full extension.
In effort to obtain a suitable designed trochlea Kulkarni and Freeman (Kulkarni et al., 2000) stressed out the importance that the trochlear surface would extended proximally sufficiently to enable even the highest patella to articulate with the femur in full extension. In their philosophy this part of the femoral prosthesis should be provided with a lateral wall and floor to ensure that the patella remains in contact with the floor of the trochlea from 0° to 20° of flexion. Lastly, the Kulkarni and Freeman trochlea surface should have a lateral wall of the trochlear groove sufficiently steep to provide a distinct resistance to lateral subluxation.
According to these criteria most of the design introduced during the nineties have incorporated multiple changes in the geometry of the trochlear groove, which have been shown to have a positive impact on the patellar complication rate (Bindelglass & Dorr, 1998; Kavolus et al., 2008; Mont et al., 1999).
An important contribution to lowering the rate of patello-femoral complication was correlate with greater attention that since that time was given to the rotational alignment of the femoral component (Anouchi et al., 1993; Scuderi et al., 1994).

5. Polyethylene

In spite of the success of designer in solving some the mentioned problems the 90's marked a period of concern regarding the catastrophic failure of the polyethylene.
Polyethylene (UHMW) has been chosen to create articular insert used for knee prosthesis. It's a low friction polymer, very resistant while articulating with metallic and extremely smooth surfaces of prosthesis.
Knee Prosthesis survival curve after 15 years arrives over 94% using this material (Insall & Scott, 2001).
Despite of these characteristics material usury it's a problem especially considering young active patients.
Damage mechanism of polyethylene are: delamination, usury caused by adhesive and abrasive wear mechanism.
Many factors can affect negatively the mechanical properties of polyethylene; some of them are due to type of prosthesis and material, others depend by clinical conditions (post-operatory alignment, weight, age of patient, ecc).
Polyethylene properties can be modified by sterilization by radiation and by exposition to oxidative environment; the effects are increase in density and elasticity of the materials itself.

Since 1995 all the industries virtually modified polyethylene sterilization procedures, by getting rid of gamma ray sterilization.
Sterilization in inert environment, gas plasma, ethylene oxide, represent at the moment the most common sterilization methods. On the same time , packaging and conserving systems has been modified.
Radiation damage on polyethylene underlined cross-link techniques advantages on usury effects.
Cross-linked polyethylene is widely used in hip prosthesis but it didn't reach the same application in knee prosthesis.
In fact a recent study performed on untimely mobilized components of prosthesis do not underlined significant differences concerning usury between conventional polyethylene and cross-linked polyethylene (Muratoglu et al., 2003).

6. High flexion knee and new materials

Some important issues have characterized the beginning of the new millennium as the effort to improve movement and the research for new materials. Both these issues are direct for better-performing prostheses for younger more active patients who wish to run, play tennis, and downhill ski.
Range of motion (ROM) after total knee arthroplasty is an important issue in determining clinical outcome and a better satisfaction from the patient. In association to expanding the indication of total knee arthroplasty to more young and active patients, their demands and expectations have increased including secondary goals other than pain relief, such as restoration of "normal-like" joint function, especially weight bearing range of motion, to suit their desired lifestyle (Noble et al., 2006).
Apart from being influenced by the condition of the patient and surgical technique, the final outcome, at least in part, depends on the implant design. Therefore, more recently, implant manufacturers have attempted to design TKAs that better accommodate knee mechanics in high flexion up to 155°.
Since it has been shown that in general posterior cruciate ligament retaining designs have erratic motion with potential for paradoxical roll forward, most of them belong to the posterior cruciate substituting prostheses (Dennis et al., 1998).
These new high-flexion designs are not radically different from their traditional (non high-flexion designs) counterparts but incorporate subtle changes in the geometry of the components to allow improved contact mechanics in the high-flexion ranges compared to traditional designs.
Regarding the sagittal geometry of the femoral component a reduction of the femoral condyles radii in the mid- and high-flexion ranges has been showed some advantage when compared with the traditional implants. In order to eliminate edge loading on the femoral component, on the posterior tibial articular surface, was necessary to extend the posterior femoral condyles. In addition an extended posterior femoral condyle help to restore the posterior condylar offset which has been previously emphasized (Bellemans et al., 2002) as an important factor in achieving high flexion. In that study the Authors observed that for every 2 mm decrease in posterior condylar offset, the maximal obtainable flexion was reduced by a mean of 12.2°.
Some designers prefer mobile bearings for the assumption that for achieving deep knee flexion is the need for large internal rotation of the tibia, which occurs with extreme

posterior shift of the lateral femoral condyle over the posterior tibial plateau increased tibial rotation with deep flexion and the theoretical advantage of improved contact area (Kurosaka et al., 2002; Nakagawa et al., 2000).
These changes are associated to a modified cam/post mechanism which allow a more jump distance and avoids dislocation at deep flexion angles (Fig. 11a-b).

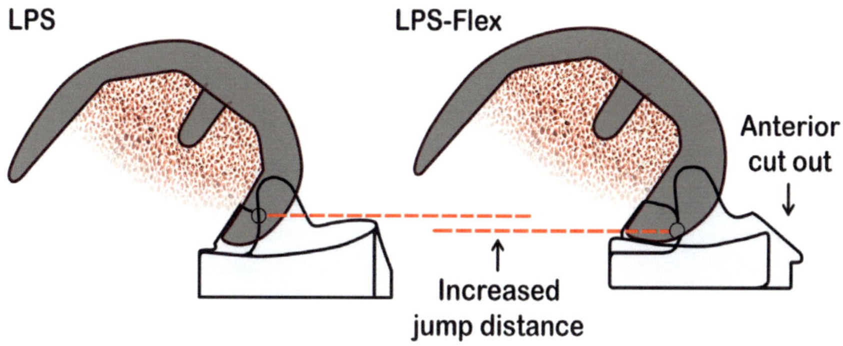

Fig. 11. a) Difference in height distance of the post/cam mechanism between LPS and LPS-Flex designs.

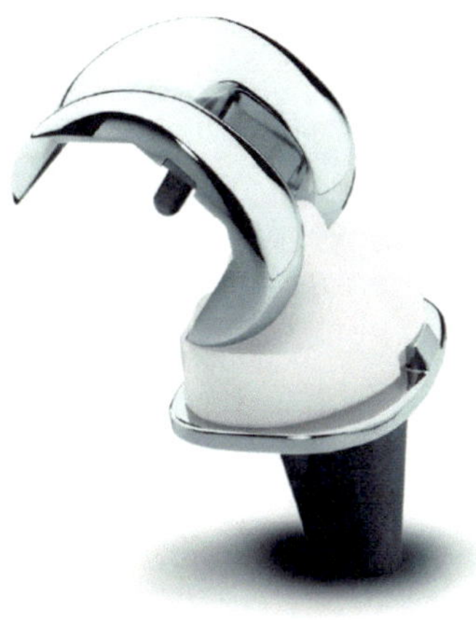

Fig. 11. b) LPS-Flex designs (courtesy of Zimmer).

Other characteristics of high flex design include the patellofemoral joint which should be designed to accommodate high angles of knee flexion. The femoral trochlear articulation should be deep enough to reduce the contact stresses on the patella and the patella should glide smoothly through a full range of motion. These kinds of prostheses in fact, in order to reduce extensor mechanism impingement during deep flexion, the anterior margin of the tibial articular component has been recessed.
In Japan with the aim to accommodate the oriental lifestyle where people sit more often on the floor than on a chair in 1989 was developed a new design originally called KU knee

(Kyoto University knee). The most outstanding feature of this model is that it has an auxiliary joint of a ball and socket at the center of the posterior part not only to facilitate a rollback movement but also to add a rotational function. During a gait under the load, the femorotibial articulation surface in a conventional design works as for standard design, but when the flexion becomes more, the auxiliary joint takes a part as a rotation center in the flexion motion. This auxiliary joint represents a certain type of posterior-stabilized knee and works to achieve a rollback, and when in flexion, rotation of tibia can be also achieved. Because this knee was unique in its biphasic surface structure for the different purposes, weight bearing, and flexion movement, it was later called bisurface knee (BS knee). Another characteristic of this prosthesis is the presence of zirconia ceramics (ZrO2) for femoral component.

Others companies modified design incorporating a lateral compartment which is fully congruent in extension, but relatively lax in flexion (Fig.12) (Mikashima et al., 2010).

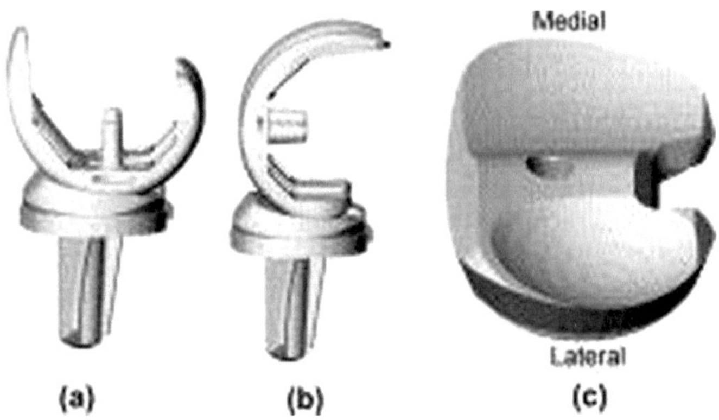

Fig. 12. From Mikashima: the lateral tibiofemoral joint is completely conforming in extension (a), but less conforming at 90 degrees of flexion (b); the tibial insert has an AP curved medial surface and a spherically recessed lateral surface (c).

This lateral congruency constrains the lateral condyle to a central antero-posterior (AP) position in extension, but allows posterior translation in flexion. This articular geometry provides antero-posterior stability and acts through the lateral femoral condyle, thus there is rough analogy with the location and stabilizing role of the anterior cruciate ligament (ACL). In addition, the modified design has a more posterior tibial sulcus (Banks & Hodge, 2004) and the maximum femoral posterior condylar offset occurs later in the flexion arc (Bellemans et al., 2002).

TKA is an effective, well-established treatment for severe arthrythis of the knee. However, further improvement in the longevity in the longevity of the arthroplasty can be achieved with more durable bearing materials.

Due to the non-conforming shape of the bearing surface, hard-on-hard bearing are unlikely to have a role in TKA and polyethylene (PE) still remain an important bearing surface material.

Despite the improvement in manufacturing and elimination of gamma-irradiation in air have already resulted in fewer wear-related problems, concerns remain about adhesive and abrasive wear caused by the hard counterface of the femoral component.

Previous studies have shown that roughening of the cobalt-chromiun (CoCr) alloy can potentiate wear of the PE (Fisher et al., 2004; White et al., 1994).
This wear can then lead to osteolysis, instability, and loosening of the implants from the underlying bone.
Designers are now concentrated on the research of different alloys for femoral components, alternative to the classic CoCrMo one (Stellite), both for complete ceramic or for ceramic surfaces.
A longer lasting of prosthesis with ceramic femoral components should be useful for younger patients with higher functional demands.
Moreover ceramic is useful when dealing with patients affected by allergies to metallic iones (Stellite) (Spector et al., 2001).
The advantages of ceramic bearing surfaces in terms of superior lubrication, friction, and wear properties compared to cobalt-chrome alloy (CoCr) surfaces in total joint arthroplasty are well recognized (Greenwald et al., 2001; Jacobs et al., 1994).
Laboratory and clinical data have demonstrated that ceramic bearings are associated with fewer wear particles that incite a less intense inflammatory host immune response than the metal-on-polyethylene articulations that are the accepted standard in total hip arthroplasty and total knee arthroplasty (Mont et al., 2003; Spector et al., 2001). The brittle nature of ceramics and the inability of ceramic materials to withstand high-impact tensile forces is of concern in clinical applications.
However, more than 10 years' long-term follow-up of cemented different ceramic knees, were performed in Japan and showed satisfactory results with low rate fractures of ceramic component (Akagi et al., 2000; Koshino et al., 2002).
An important improvement has been recently introduced in Europe by CeramTec (AG, Polchingen, Germany) with the BIOLOX Delta a composite matrix material containing 82% vol. alumina (Al_2O_3) and 17% vol. zirconia (ZrO_2) providing good mechanical characteristics in terms of strength and resistance (Dalla Pria, 2007).
Using this material it was possible to develop a femoral component with a tensile strength that meets the demands for application in TKR (Kluess et al., 2009).

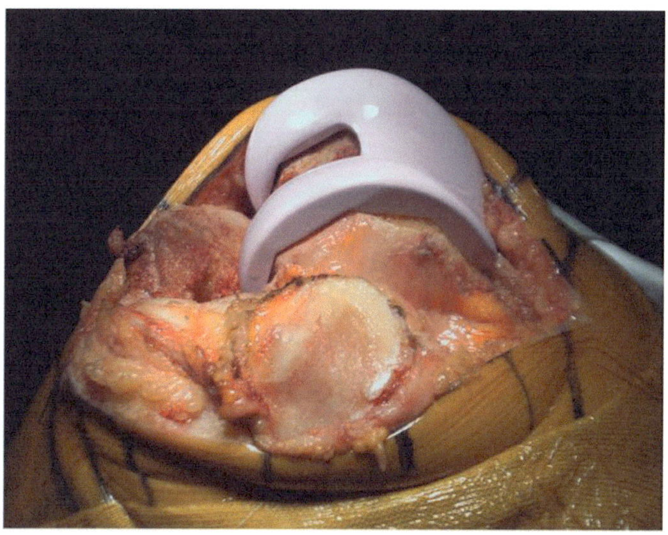

Fig. 13. a) Intraoperative photo of Biolox Delta ceramic femoral component.

A prospective international multicentre study started in 2008 with the aim to evaluate the clinical and radiological outcomes of the unconstrained Multigen Plus total knee system (Lima-Lto) with the new BIOLOX Delta ceramic femoral component (Fig.12a-b).

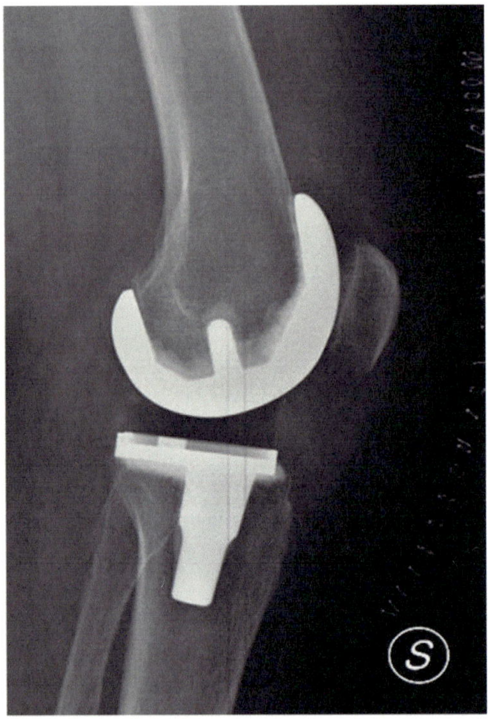

Fig. 13. b) Post-operative x-Ray of Multigen Plus total knee system (sagittal view).

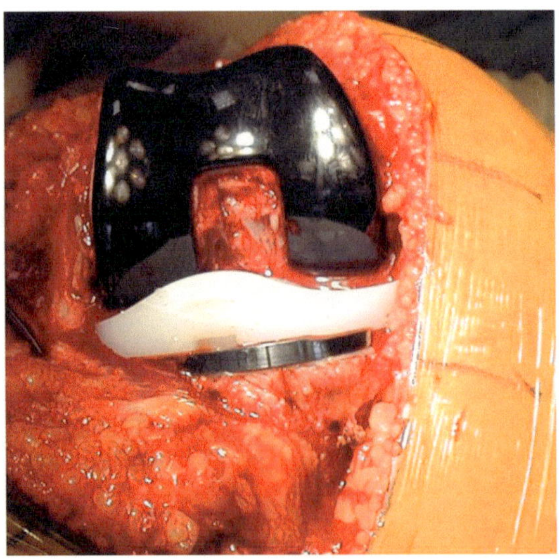

Fig. 14. Intraoperative photo of Genesis II: Oxinium femoral component.

In USA an alternative strategy has been followed to decrease PE wear in THA and TKA, which consists in the surface transformation of metal to oxidized zirconium. A wrought zirconium alloy (Zr-2.5% Niobium) is oxidized by thermal diffusion to create a 5-mm oxidized zirconium layer (Oxinium, Smith & Nephew, Memphis, TN; Fig.14) (Laskin, 2003).

Although existing data are encouraging, with both strategies (Innocenti et al., 2010), further studies are needed to define the precise indications and outcomes of ceramic surfaces in TKA.

7. Conclusions and future perspective

Technological developments in the field of knee replacement continues to increase the range of solutions for the recovery of joint mobility of the painful knee arthritis.

Particularly research and development efforts are focusing on designing effective prosthesis, allowing the movement ever closer to physiological ones, which are well tolerated and long lasting, and are implanted with less invasive interventions.

Explains the considerable attention, first, the morphological aspects of prosthetic components, and second, the quality of materials, with the aim of ensuring greater wear resistance and improved biocompatibility. This is a necessary condition for stability of the prosthetic implant and for the success of the intervention.

8. References

Abdeen, AR., Collen, SB., & Vince, KG. (2010). Fifteen-year to 19-year follow-up of the Insall-Burstein-1 total knee arthroplasty. *J Arthroplasty,* Vol.25, No.2, pp. 173-178.

Akagi, M., Nakamura, T., Matsusue Y., Ueo, T., Nishijyo, K., & Ohnishi, E. (2000). The Bisurface total knee replacement: a unique design for flexion. Four-to-nine-year follow-up study. *J Bone Joint Surg Am,* Vol.82, No.11, pp. 1626-1633.

Anouchi, YS., Whiteside, LA., Kaiser, AD., & Milliano, MT. (1993). The effects of axial rotational alignment of the femoral component on knee stability and patellar tracking in total knee arthroplasty demonstrated on autopsy specimens. *Clin Orthop Relat Res,* Vol.287, pp. 170-177.

Banks, SA., & Hodge, WA. (2004). Implant design affects knee arthroplasty kinematics during stair-stepping. *Clin Orthop Relat Res,* Vol.426, pp. 187-193.

Bellemans, J., Banks, S., Victor, J., Vandenneucker, H., & Moemans, A. (2002). Fluoroscopic analysis of the kinematics of deep flexion in total knee arthroplasty. Influence of posterior condylar offset. *J Bone Joint Surg Br,* Vol.84, No.1, pp. 50-53.

Bindelglass, DF., & Dorr, LD. (1998). Current concepts review: symmetry versus asymmetry in the design of total knee femoral components - an unresolved controversy. *J Arthroplasty,* Vol.13, No.8, pp. 939-944.

Buechel, FF., & Pappas, MJ. (1986). The New Jersey Low-Contact-Stress Knee Replacement System: biomechanical rationale and review of the first 123 cemented cases. *Arch. Orthop Trauma Surg,* Vol.105, No.4, pp. 197-204.

Dalla Pria, P. (2007). Evolution and new application of the alumina ceramics in joint replacement. *Eur J Orthop Surg Traumatol,* 17:253-256 Vol.17, pp. 253-256.

Dennis, DA., Komistek, RD., Stiehl, JB., Walker, SA., & Dennis, KN. (1998). Range of motion after total knee arthroplasty: the effect of implant design and weight-bearing conditions. *J Arthroplasty,* Vol.13, No.7, pp. 748-752.

Fisher, J., McEwen, HM., Tipper, JL., Galvin, AL., Ingram, J., Kamali, A., Stone, MH., & Ingham E. (2004). Wear, debris, and biologic activity of cross-linked polyethylene in the knee: benefits and potential concerns. *Clin Orthop Relat Res,* Vol.428, pp. 114-119.

Grace, JN., & Rand, JA. (1988). Patellar instability after total knee arthroplasty. *Clin Orthop Relat Res,* Vol.237, pp. 184-189.

Greenwald, AS., & Garino, JP. (2001). Alternative bearing surfaces: the good, the bad, and the Ugly. *J Bone Joint Surg Am,* Vol.83, No.2, pp. 68-72.

Hungerford, DS., Kenna, RV., & Krackow, KA. (1982). The porous-coated anatomic total knee. *Orthop Clin North Am,* Vol.13, No.1, pp. 103-122.

Innocenti, M., Civinini, R., Carulli, C., Matassi, F., & Villano, M. (2010). The 5-year Results of an Oxidized Zirconium Femoral Component for TKA. *Clin Orthop Relat Res,* Vol.468, pp. 1258-1263.

Insall, J., Ranawat, CS., Scott, WN., & Walker, P. (1976). Total condylar knee replacement: preliminary report. *Clin Orthop Relat Res,* Vol.120, pp. 149-154.

Insall, J., & Scott WN. (2001). *Surgery of the Knee* (third edition), Churchill-Livingstone, New York.

Jacobs, JJ., Shanbhag, A., Glant, TT., Black, J., & Galante, JO. (1994). Wear debris in total joint replacements. *J Am Acad Orthop Surg,* Vol.2, No.4, pp. 212-220.

Kavolus, CH., Hummel, MT., Barnett, KP., & Jennings, JE Jr. (2008). Comparison of the Insall-Burstein II and NexGen legacy total knee arthroplasty systems with respect to patella complications. *J Arthroplasty,* Vol.23, No.6, pp. 822-825.

Kluess, D., Souffrant, R., Fritsche, A., Mittelmeier, W., & Bader, R. (2009). Explicit Finite-Element-Analysis of the Impaction Behavior of a Ceramic Femoral Component in Total Knee Replacement. *Proceedings 55th Annual Meeting of the Orthopaedic Research Society,* Las Vegas.

Koshino, T., Okamoto, R., Takagi, T., Yamamoto, K., & Saito, T. (2002). Cemented ceramic YMCK total knee arthroplasty in patients with severe rheumatoid arthritis. *J Arthroplasty,* Vol.17, No.8, pp. 1009-1015.

Kulkarni, SK., Freeman, MA., Poal-Manresa, JC., Asencio, JI., & Rodriguez, JJ. (2000). The patellofemoral joint in total knee arthroplasty: is the design of the trochlea the critical factor? *J Arthroplasty,* Vol.15, No.4, pp. 424-429.

Kurosaka, M., Yoshiya, S., Mizuno, K., & Yamamoto, T. (2002). Maximizing flexion after total knee arthroplasty: the need and the pitfalls. *J Arthroplasty,* Vol.17, No.4, pp. 59-62.

Laskin, RS. (2003). An oxidized Zr ceramic surfaced femoral component for total knee arthroplasty. *Clin Orthop Relat Res,* Vol.416, pp. 191-196.

McKeever, DC. (1960). Tibial plateau prosthesis. *Clin Orthop Rel Res,* Vol.192, pp. 3-12.

Mikashima, Y., Tomatsu, T., Horikoshi, M., Nakatani, T., Saito, S., Momohara S., & Banks, SA. (2010). In vivo deep-flexion kinematics in patients with posterior-cruciate retaining and anterior-cruciate substituting total knee arthroplasty. *Clin Biomech (Bristol, Avon),* Vol.25, No.1, pp. 83-87.

Mont, MA., Yoon, TR., Krackow, KA., & Hungerford, DS. (1999). Eliminating patellofemoral complications in total knee arthroplasty: clinical and radiographic results of 121 consecutive cases using the Duracon system. *J Arthroplasty,* Vol.14, No.4, pp. 446-455.

Mont, MA., Booth, RE. Jr, Laskin, RS., Stiehl, JB., Ritter, MA., Stuchin, SA., & Rajadhyaksha, AD. (2003). The spectrum of prosthesis design for primary total knee arthroplasty. *Instr Course Lect.* Vol.52, pp. 397-407.

Muratoglu, OK., Mark, A., Vittetoe, DA., Harris, WH., & Rubash, HE. (2003). Polyethylene damage in total knees and use of highly crosslinked polyethylene. *J Bone Joint Surg Am,* Vol.85, No.1, pp. 7-13.

Nakagawa, S., Kadoya, Y., Todo, S., Kobayashi, A., Sakamoto, H., Freeman, MA., & Yamano, Y. (2000). Tibiofemoral movement 3: full flexion in the living knee studied by MRI. *J Bone Joint Surg Br,* Vol.82, No.8, pp. 1199-1200.

Noble, PC., Conditt, MA., Cook, KF., & Mathis KB. (2006). The John Insall Award: Patient expectations affect satisfaction with total knee arthroplasty. *Clin Orthop Relat Res,* Vol.452, pp. 35-43.

Rhoads, DD., Noble, PC., Reuben, JD., Mahoney, OM., & Tullos, HS. (1990). The effect of femoral component position on patellar tracking after total knee arthroplasty. *Clin Orthop Relat Res,* Vol.260, pp. 43-51.

Robinson, RP. (2005). The early innovators of today's resurfacing condylar knees. *J Arthroplasty,* Vol.20, No.1, pp. 2-26.

Scott, RD. (1982). Duopatellar total knee replacement: The Brigham experience. *Orth Clinic North Am,* Vol.13, No.1, pp. 89-102.

Scuderi, GR., Insall, JN., & Scott, NW. (1994). Patellofemoral pain after total knee arthroplasty. *J Am Acad Orthop Surg,* Vol.2, No.5, pp. 239-246.

Sledge, CB., & Ewald, FC. (1979). Total knee arthroplasty experience at the Robert Breck Brigham Hospital. *Clin Orthop Relat Res,* Vol.145, pp. 78-84.

Spector, BM., Ries, MD., Bourne, RB., Sauer, WS., Long, M., & Hunter, G. (2001) Wear performance of ultra-high molecular weight polyethylene on oxidized zirconium total knee femoral components. *J Bone Joint Surg Am,* Vol.83, No.2, pp. 80-86.

Stern, SH., & Insall, JN. (1992). Posterior stabilized prosthesis. Results after follow-up of nine to twelve years. *J Bone Joint Surg Am,* Vol.74, No.7, pp. 980-986.

Townley, C., & Hill, L. (1974). Total knee replacement. *Am J Nurs,* Vol.74, No.9, pp. 1612-1617.

Vince, KG., Insall, JN., & Kelly, MA. (1989). The total condylar prosthesis. 10- to 12-year results of a cemented knee replacement. *J Bone Joint Surg Br,* Vol.71, No.5, pp. 793-797.

Waugh, TR., Smith, RC., Orofino, CF., & Anzel, SM. (1973). Total knee replacement: operative technic and preliminary results. *Clin Orthop Relat Res,* 94:196-201 Vol.94, pp. 196-201.

White, SE., Whiteside, LA., McCarthy, DS., Anthony, M., & Poggie, RA. (1994). Simulated knee wear with cobalt chromium and oxidized zirconium knee femoral components. *Clin Orthop Relat Res,* Vol.309, pp. 176-184.

Yamamoto, S. (1979). Total knee replacement with the Kodama-Yamamoto knee prosthesis. *Clin Orthop Relat Res,* Vol.145, pp. 60-67.

Yoshii, I., Whiteside, LA., & Anouchi, YS. (1992). The effect of patellar button placement and femoral component design on patellar tracking in total knee arthroplasty. *Clin Orthop Relat Res,* Vol.275, pp. 211-219.

15

The UniSpacer™: Correcting Varus Malalignment in Medial Gonarthrosis

Joern Bengt Seeger[1] and Michael Clarius[2]
[1]*Center for Musculoskeletal Surgery, Charité - Universitätsmedizin Berlin, Campus Charité Mitte (CCM), Berlin*
[2]*Department of Orthopaedic and Trauma Surgery, Vulpius Klinik GmbH, Bad Rappenau*
Germany

1. Introduction

The most commonly used operative treatments of osteoarthritis of the medial compartment of the knee joint, especially in younger patients, are arthroscopy, high tibial osteotomy (HTO) and unicompartmental knee arthroplasty (UKA). The last two procedures require resection of bone stock (Iorio & Healy, 2003).

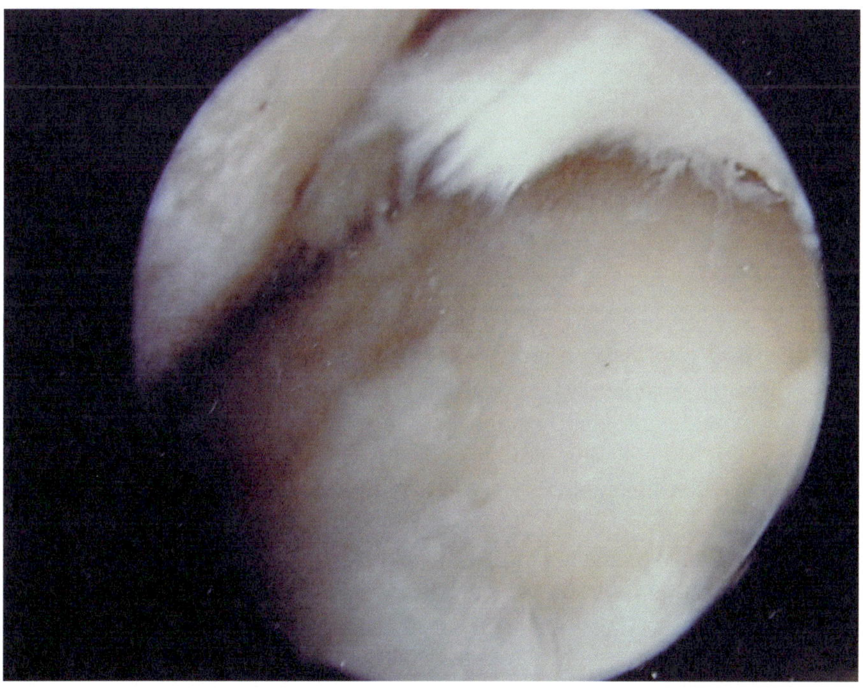

Fig. 1. Typical arthroscopic view of a patient with anteromedial osteoarthritis of the knee and degenerative lesion of the medial meniscus

A less invasive alternative to these procedures has been introduced in 2000 by Rick Hallock and Barry Fell: the UniSpacer™ implant (Zimmer, Inc., Warsaw, IN, USA), which is essentially a modern version of early metallic hemiarthroplasty as described by McKeever (McKeever, 1960) or MacIntosh (MacIntosh, 1958). However, due to a high failure rate between 16 and 44% as described by Bailie and Sisto, the implant is not available any more (Bailie et al., 2008; Sisto & Mitchel 2005).

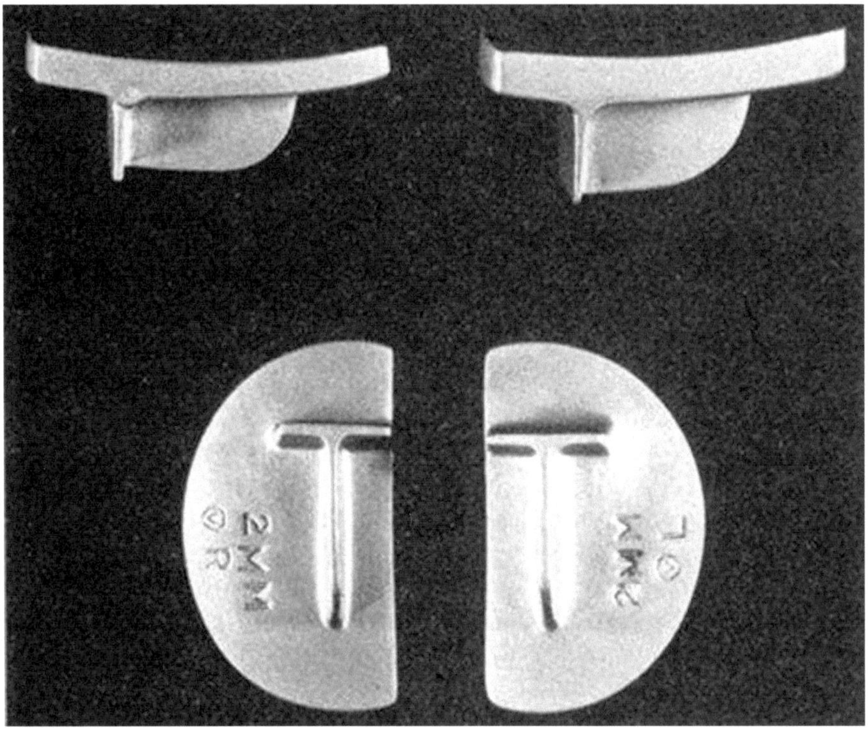

Fig. 2. Early interpositional hemiarthroplasty (Springer et al., 2006)

Implantation of this self-centering, one-piece interpositional device into the knee joint does not require any resection of bone stock and is performed via minimally-invasive surgery (Scott, 2003). Initially, a cementless metal or polyethylene interpositional device has been implanted into the medial or lateral compartment.
The Unispacer is available in several thicknesses (between 2 and 5 mm) and sizes (38 - 58 mm) and adapts to knee kinematics (Marx et al., 2009). There are special models for the left and ride side.
The UniSpacer™ is a device that is not fixed to any structures and therefore self-centering; it is used to relieve pain and to correct or minimize varus malalignment in unicompartmental osteoarthritis of the knee. The upper surface of the implant postoperatively adapts to the femoral condylus (Scott, 2003).
The UniSpacer™ is indicated in patients with isolated moderate degeneration of the medial compartment with minimal degeneration, and no significant loss of joint space in the patellofemoral compartment.

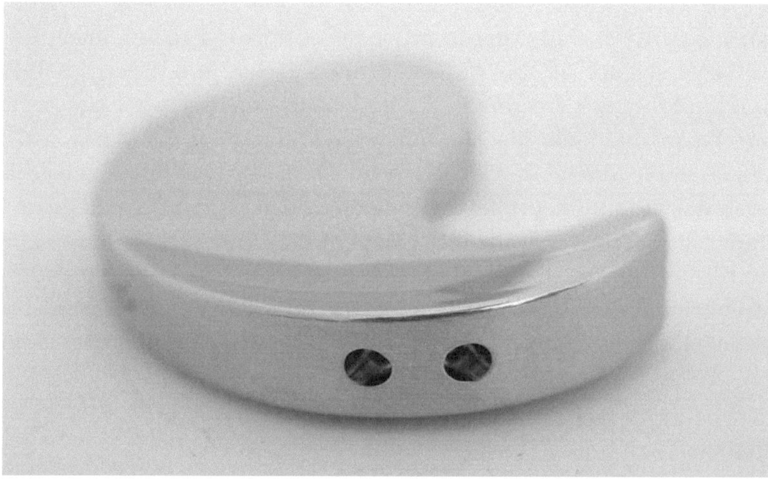

Fig. 3. UniSpacer™ metallic interpositional device

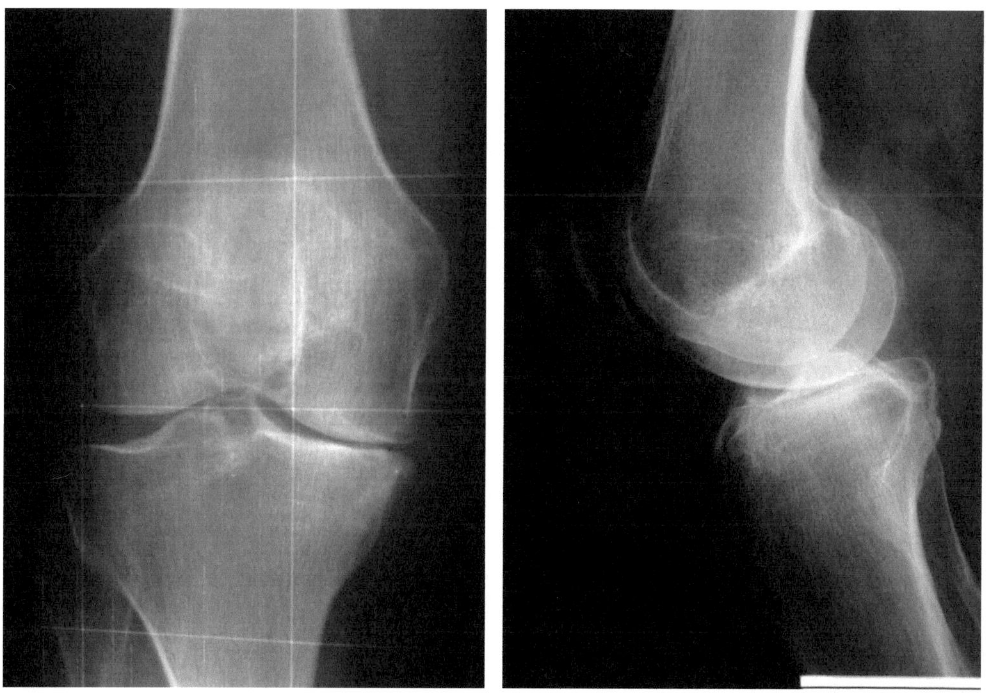

Fig. 4. and 5. Patient with medial osteoarthritis of the knee: a.p. stance and lateral view of the knee

Contraindications are inflammatory arthritis, severe instability due to advanced loss of osteochondral structure or the absence of collateral cruciate ligament integrity, as well as flexion/contracture greater than 15 degrees.

2. Operation technique (Hallock & Fell, 2003)

An arthroscopy is performed in order to prove the correct indication, intact ACL and PCL and medial meniscectomy of the posterior horn. After arthroscopy a 6-7cm medial parapatellar arthrotomy is performed. The rest of the medial meniscus is resected and osteophytes of the medial tibial plateau, the notch and around the patella are removed in order to avoid an impingement of the Unispacer. The size of the tibial plateau is measured with a special device and a probe is implanted. The correct size of the implant is controlled under fluoroscopy and the movement of the Unispacer in flexion and extension is documented. The whole medial tibial plateau should be covered in a.p. radiographs and a ventral impingement of the Unispacer with the femoral condyle should be ruled out. After implanting the original Unispacer, the wound closure is performed under usual conditions.

2.1 Rehabilitation

Weight bearing as tolerated can be performed with the use of crutches. A thrombosis prophylaxis is obligatory.

3. Results

The first results have been published by the designers group on 71 Unispacer knee system implants implanted in 67 patients. (Hallock & Fell, 2003).
The mean Knee Society knee score improved 169% in the 1-year group and 193% in the 2-year group. The mean Knee Society function score improved 31% and 65%, respectively. The mean Lysholm score improved 88% and 140%, respectively. Five implants (7%) were revised to total knee arthroplasty (TKA) and 10 implants (14%) were revised to another Unispacer Knee System implant.
Marx et al. implanted 14 Unispacer in 13 patients (4 women and 9 men). In 8 cases the left and in 6 cases the right knee joint was operated. There were no intra- or postoperative complications. There was no mobilization under anesthesia necessary. A dislocation of the spacer was not observed.
The notion of a self-centering mobile component correcting the varus knee internally without any need for bone resection has been, and still is, appealing. Clarius et al. evaluated clinical and radiological results and whether appropriate alignment change can be achieved by UniSpacer™ implantation (Clarius et al., 2003). In addition they examined the alignment change in the first 5 years after surgery.
In a retrospective study, 18 patients (19 legs) presenting with moderate stage isolated medial gonarthrosis, who had received UniSpacer™ hemiarthroplasty between 2002 and 2004, were assessed (implant thickness: 2, 3 or 4 mm); one patient received bilateral implantation; 12 right and 7 left knees had been treated. The average age of the patients (7 women and 11 men) at the time of surgery was 60.8 (48 to 72) years.
The clinical scores (Lysholm, AKS knee and function) preoperatively and at 1-, 2- and 5 year follow-up are shown in tab. 1.
Only 15 legs could be evaluated, as 4 patients had undergone revision UKA or TKA due to persistent pain. Average time to revision for the knees revised to TKA or UKA was 23.8 (±18.0) months. So far, no dislocations have been observed in this study.

Clinical Scores	preoperative	1 year postop.	2 years postop.	5 years postop
Lysholm	59.1	85.4	90.2	97.2
AKS knee	60.1	87.4	88.7	96.6
AKS function	70.0	93.8	98.5	96.4

Table 1. Clinical scores preoperative, at 1 year-, 2 year- and 5 year follow-up

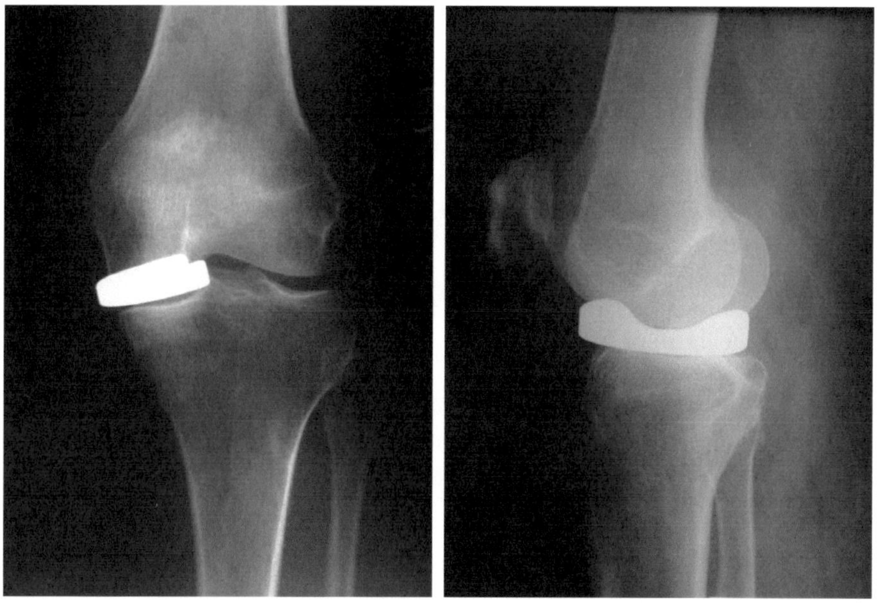

Fig. 6. and 7. Postoperative implant position

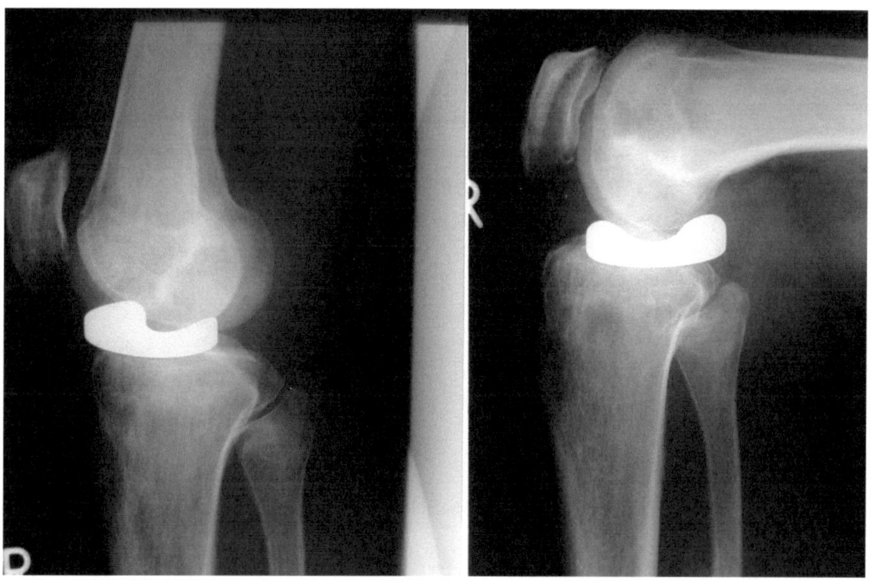

Fig. 8. and 9. Movement of the device during flexion due to the self-centering effect of the Unispacer

4. Conclusion

The use of HTO in the treatment of symptomatic varus malaligned knees has been propagated and thoroughly documented for several decades: it is a well-established therapeutic option (Nelissen et al., 2009). UKA has recently experienced a renewal of interest, with improved prostheses and techniques used. There have been reports of good long-term results for these methods. However, both can lead to distinct issues patients may be troubled with over the course of time. UKA comes with loss of bone matter in the medial compartment and, if conversion to TKA becomes necessary, bone grafts or metal wedge augmentation might be required in some cases (Springer et al., 2006).

Hemiarthroplasty with metallic interpositional devices, while first described over half a century ago, is also currently experiencing a renaissance as a treatment option of varus unicompartmental OA, the idea being to provide a means of treatment that minimizes the disadvantages of other procedures. It is used in cases where HTO is contraindicated or patients are too young for TKA. The ConforMIS iForma™ device, following the MacIntosh and McKeever rationale in being functionally fixed to the tibial surface, has had one favorable review; altogether, there are still few reports examining the use of the self-centering UniSpacer™ device in medial gonarthrosis.

Use of the UniSpacer™ in unicompartmental OA was initially recommended for young and active patients (Hallock & Fell, 2003). The role of this procedure still is not certain as it has been considered suitable for only few patients (1%) (Scott & Deshmukh, 2005) and there have been reports of poor postoperative results due to implant dislocation (up to 44%) (Bailie et al., 2005; Sisto & Mitchell, 2005).

Clarius et al. showed in their study a significant, slightly over-adjusting, correction of moderate varus alignment by UniSpacer™ arthroplasty, which does not correlate with the thickness of the implant used (Clarius et al., 2003). In the first postoperative year, a varus shift into a more neutral position could be observed, which is most likely due to adaptation of the implant to the joint. This effect is partly reversed in the following years by another slight valgus change, resulting, 5 years after surgery, in an average leg axis close to the one first achieved by UniSpacer™ implantation.

A high revision rate of 4 out of 19 UniSpacer™ implants in the first 5 postoperative years has been shown, which is unacceptably high compared to other treatment options. The reason for revision was persistent pain. There were no cases of dislocations. All revisions were technically easy to operate and uncomplicated. In all cases either UKA (2) or TKA (2) was performed and the patients were satisfied with the clinical results achieved after revision.

Looking at the high revision rates of the UniSpacer implant reported in the literature and in our study this metallic interposition arthroplasty does not seem to be a treatment option for patients with medial osteoarthritis of the knee. As there are reproducible good and excellent clinical and functional results reported with UKA after 10-15 years this operation should be preferred. However the clinical results of our remaining 14 patients with 15 operated knees were good and comparable to patients after UKA. Similar to the results of the metallic interpositional device of Mc Keever good results can be possible however the results are not predictable.

As a minimally invasive procedure, UniSpacer™ arthroplasty was seen as an alternative for treatment of varus malaligned knees in isolated medial gonarthrosis, due to good revision and conversion options.

5. References

Bailie AG, Lewis PL, Brumby SA et al (2008) The Unispacer knee implant: early clinical results. *J Bone Joint Surg Br* 90(4), pp. 446-450

Cooke TD, Li J, Scudamore RA (1994) Radiographic assessment of bony contributions to knee deformity. *Orthop Clin North Am* 25(3), pp. 387-393

Cooke TD, Scudamore RA, Bryant JT et al (1991) A quantitative approach to radiography of the lower limb. Principles and applications. *J Bone Joint Surg Br* 73-B(5), pp. 715-720

Cooke TD, Scudamore RA, Li J et al (1997) Axial lower-limb alignment: comparison of knee geometry in normal volunteers and osteoarthritis patients. *Osteoarthritis Cartilage* 5(1), pp. 39-47

Coventry MB, Ilstrup DM, Wallrichs SL (1993) Proximal tibial osteotomy. A critical long-term study of eighty-seven cases. *J Bone Joint Surg Am* 75(2), pp. 196-201

Deshmukh RV, Scott RD (2001) Unicompartmental Knee Arthroplasty: Long-Term Results. *Clin Orthop Relat Res* 392, pp. 272-278

Hallock RH, Fell BM (2003) Unicompartmental Tibial Hemiarthroplasty. Early Results of the UniSpacer(TM) Knee. *Clin Orthop Relat Res* 416, pp. 154-163

Hernigou P, Medevielle D, Debeyre J et al (1987) Proximal tibial osteotomy for osteoarthritis with varus deformity. A ten to thirteen-year follow-up study. *J Bone Joint Surg Am* 69(3), pp. 332-354

Insall JN, Joseph DM, Msika C (1984) High tibial osteotomy for varus gonarthrosis. A long-term follow-up study. *J Bone Joint Surg Am* 66(7), pp. 1040-1048

Iorio R, Healy WL (2003) Unicompartmental Arthritis of the Knee. *J Bone Joint Surg Am* 85(7), pp. 1351-1364

Kennedy WRMD, White RPMD (1987) Unicompartmental Arthroplasty of the Knee Postoperative Alignment and its Influence on Overall Results. *Clin Orthop Relat Res* 221, pp. 278-285

Koeck F, Perlick L, Luring C et al (2009) Leg axis correction with ConforMIS iForma™ (interpositional device) in unicompartmental arthritis of the knee. *Int Orthop* 33(4), pp. 955-960

MacIntosh DL (1958) Hemiarthroplasty of the knee using a space occupying prosthesis for painful varus and valgus deformities. In: of the Joint Meeting of the Orthopaedic Associations of the English-Speaking World. *J Bone Joint Surg Am* 40(6), pp. 1428-1441

McKeever DC (1960) Tibial plateau prosthesis. *Clin Orthop Relat Res* 18, pp. 86-95

Moreland JR, Bassett LW, Hanker GJ (1987) Radiographic analysis of the axial alignment of the lower extremity. *J Bone Joint Surg Am* 69(5), pp. 745-749

Scott RD (2003) UniSpacer: insufficient data to support its widespread use. *Clin Orthop Relat Res* 416, pp. 164-166

Scott RD (2003) UniSpacer(TM): Insufficient Data to Support its Widespread Use. *Clin Orthop Relat Res* 416, pp.164-166

Scott RD, Deshmukh RV (2005) Metallic hemiarthroplasty of the knee. *Curr Opin Orthop* 16(1), pp. 35-37

Sisto DJ, Mitchell IL (2005) UniSpacer Arthroplasty of the Knee. *J Bone Joint Surg Am* 87(8), pp. 1706-1711

Springer BD, Scott RD, Thornhill TS (2006) Conversion of Failed Unicompartmental Knee Arthroplasty to TKA. *Clin Orthop Relat Res* 446, pp. 214-220

Tunggal JA, Higgins GA, Waddell JP (2009) Complications of closing wedge high tibial osteotomy. *Int Orthop* 10.1007/s00264-009-0819-9

Whiteside LA (2005) Making Your Next Unicompartmental Knee Arthroplasty Last: Three Keys to Success. *The Journal of Arthroplasty* 20 (Supplement 2), pp. 2-3

16

Posterior Stabilized Total Knee Arthroplasty

Fabio Orozco and Alvin Ong
Atlanticare Care Regional Medical Center, Pomona, New Jersey
Joint Replacement, Rothman Institute, Thomas Jefferson University, Philadelphia, Pennsylvani
USA

1. Introduction

The posterior cruciate ligament (PCL) in total knee arthroplasty (TKA) functions to prevent posterior translation of the tibia and aids in femoral roll-back[1]. Roll-back allows for increased quadriceps lever arm and more efficient use of extensor musculature, permitting more normal stair climbing. Because of this, PCL retaining knees have the advantage of maintenance of ligamentous proprioception, load transfer by the native PCL and anterior-posterior stability. However, retaining the PCL also has several disadvantages. Surgical exposure of the tibia, gap balancing and reliance on diseased ligament morphology make consistent TKA results difficult. The posterior stabilized design in TKA was introduced in the mid-1970s. Surgeons who use this system believed that the results obtained are more consistent because they do not have to rely on abnormal PCL morphology. Consequently, exposure, joint line restoration and appropriate balancing of the knee are easier with PCL stabilized designs. These components are a popular treatment for patients requiring primary TKA. Improvements in implant design, a technically easier procedure in the face of deformity, restoration of knee kinematics and reported very good long-term outcomes may all be reasons for the increased use of this design.

2. History and design rationale

Most of the current total knee implants were derived from the Total Condylar Prosthesis (TCP; Zimmer, Warsaw, Indiana, USA), which was introduced in 1974. This prosthesis was a cruciate sacrificing cemented design. Technique of implantation of the TCP requires excision of the PCL but without substitution. Stability in this implant design was achieved by soft tissue balance in flexion and extension and articular conformity in the coronal and sagittal plane[2]. Consequently, the success of this implant was highly dependent of surgical technique. In 1978, the TCP was modified to the Insall Burstein Posterior Stabilized Prosthesis (IB I) to address posterior subluxation of the tibia and instability. The IB I is the

---

[1] Dorr LD Ochsner JL, Gronley J, Perry J. Functional comparison of posterior curciate-retained versus cruciate-sacrificedot al knee arthroplasty. CORR 1988; 236:36-43.

[2] Scuderi GR, Pagnano MR: Review Article: The rationale for posterior cruciate substituting total knee arthroplasty. J Orthopedic Surgery 2001, 9(2):81-88

first posterior stabilized/substituting TKA design. It incorporated a femoral cam that articulates with a polyethylene tibial post to act as a substitute for the excised native PCL. Most posterior stabilized knee designs evolved from the IB I - incorporating a cam-post mechanism to aid in roll back, increase the amount of distraction tolerated before subluxation occurs, and increase varus-valgus constraint. The cam-post mechanism improves both anterior-posterior and translational stability. Multiply studies have shown that function of the TKA is improved with PCL substitution. PCL substitution allowed for better stability, increased ROM, reduced quadriceps force in extension, improved stair-climbing ability, and improved patellofemoral function.[3] [4] [5]

3. Advantages of posterior stabilized TKA

There are several advantages with use of posterior stabilized TKA designs. These include: I) easier surgical exposure and ligament balancing, II) predictable restoration of knee kinematics, III) improved range of motion, IV) less polyethylene wear, and V) avoiding the possibility of PCL rupture.

3.1 Easier surgical exposure and ligament balancing

Adequate exposure of the tibia may not be possible with PCL retention. Excision of the PCL aids in exposing the tibia for adequate visualization by releasing the tethering effect of a tight contracted PCL. Moreover, the PCL can be excised from the femoral and tibial attachment in a reproducible way, making the ligamentous balancing and correction of the deformity easier since it is not complicated by the tethering effect of the PCL. Abnormal PCL morphology is often encountered in the diseased knee making predictable gap balancing difficult in PCL retaining designs. If the patient has a "tight", contracted PCL, the knee may be relatively tight in flexion with excessive femoral roll-back. On the other hand, if the PCL is lax or incompetent, the knee may experience posterior sag with no roll-back with knee flexion. Thus, use of posterior stabilized TKA makes balancing more predictable eliminating the reliance on abnormal PCL morphology and function.

3.2 Predictable restoration of knee kinematics

In posterior stabilized TKA, the tibial post articulates with the transverse femoral cam predictably with knee flexion, preventing posterior subluxation of the tibia while maintaining femoral roll back. Many studies report more normal kinematics with the use of posterior stabilized designs.[6] [7] [8] Fluoroscopic kinematics showed that the posterior

---

[3] Insall JN, Lachiewicz PF, Burstein AH. The posterior stabilized condylar prosthesis: a modification of the total condylar design. J Bone Joint Surg Am. 1982;64:1317

[4] Scott WN, Rubinstein M, Scuderi G. Results after knee replacement with a posterior cruciate-substituting prosthesis. J Bone Joint Surg Am. 1998;70:1163

[5] Scuderi GR, Insall JN. The posterior stabilized knee prosthesis. Orthop Clin North Am. 1989;20:71

[6] Stiehl JB, Komistek RD, Dennis DA, et al. Fluoroscopic analysis of kinematics after posterior cruciate retaining knee arthroplasty. J Bone Joint Surg Br 1995; 77B:884-889.

[7] Dennis DA, Komistek RD, Hoff WA. In vivo knee kinematics derived using an inverse perspective technique. Clin Orthop 1996; 331:107-117.

[8] Ranawat CS, Komistek RD, Rodriguez JA, et al. In vivo kinematics for fixed and mobile-bearing posterior stabilized knee prostheses. Clin Orthop Relat Res 2004; 418:184-190.

stabilized TKA experienced AP femoro-tibial translation more similar to the normal knee during normal gait and deep knee bend.[9] Moreover, studies have shown no significant difference between posterior stabilized TKA and normal knees with regard to spatio-temporal gait parameters, knee range of motion during stair climbing or in isokinetic muscle strength.[10]
A study comparing cruciate retaining, cruciate sacrificing and posterior stabilized TKA found that posterior stabilized designs produced more roll back and better quadriceps efficiency than cruciate retaining knee designs[11]. Posterior stabilized TKA predictably restores more normal knee kinematics when compared to either PCL substituting or PCL sacrificing designs.

3.3 Improved range of motion

Both cruciate retaining and posterior stabilized TKA designs can provide excellent range of motion. However, range of motion may be better when a posterior stabilized TKA is used to maintain femoral roll back. It appears, according to most comparative studies, that posterior stabilized designs may provide more predictable motion, with greater flexion under fluoroscopic visualization.[12] [13] In a very well done meta-analysis Jacobs *et al.* analyzed eight randomized controlled trials comparing posterior stabilized with cruciate retaining TKA and found that the range of motion was 8° higher (105 versus 113°) in the posterior stabilized group than the cruciate retaining group (P = 0.01, 95% confidence interval 1.7-15).[14]

3.4 Less polyethylene wear

Retention of the PCL requires that the prosthetic kinematics closely match that of the normal knee. This obligates the implant to have a "flat" polyethylene component relative to the radius of curvature of the femur. This "round on flat" design allows for minimal constraint on tibial component enabling roll back of the femur on tibia with knee flexion. This less forming design can lead to excessive point contact pressure and increase polyethylene wear. In contrast, in posterior-stabilized design, it is possible to use more conforming polyethylene articulation with minimal point contact stress. Increasing the conformity of the implant, increases the contact area, and decreases the stress to which the polyethylene is subjected. This can potentially minimize polyethylene wear and increase the long-term survival of the TKA. Cases of severe polyethylene wear in cruciate retaining implants with less conforming

---

[9] Udomkiat P, Meng BJ, Dorr LD, Wan Z. Clin Orthop 2000 Sep;(378):192-201

[10] Wilson SA, McCann PD, Gotlin RS, Ramakrishnan HK, Wootten ME and Insall JN. Comprehensive gait analysis in posterior stabilized knee arthroplasty. J Arthroplasty 1996, 11:359–67.

[11] Mahoney OM, Noble PC, Rhoads DD, Alexander JW, Tullos HS. Posterior cruciate function following total knee arthroplasty: A biomechanical study. J Arthroplasty 1994, 9:569-78.

[12] Jacobs WC, Clement DJ, Wymenga AB. Retention versus removal of the posterior cruciate ligament in total knee replacement: a systematic literature review within the Cochrane framework. Acta Orthop 2005; 76:757-768.

[13] Maruyama S, Yoshiya S, Matsui N, Kuroda R, Kurosaka M. Functional comparison of posterior cruciate retaining versus posterior stabilized total knee arthroplasty. J Arthroplasty 2004; 19:349-353.

[14] Jacobs WC, Clement DJ, Wymenga AB. Retention versus removal of the posterior cruciate ligament in total knee replacement: a systematic literature review within the Cochrane framework. Acta Orthop 2005; 76:757-768.

tibial inserts have been reported.[15] [16] Additionally, technical issues may contribute to wear in cruciate retaining TKA if the PCL is left too tight in flexion. This can lead to asymmetric posterior polyethylene wear from posterior femoral subluxation and may predispose to osteolysis.

3.5 Avoiding the possibility of posterior cruciate ligament rupture

The PCL can rupture postoperatively with the use of cruciate retaining TKA. This can occur by trauma or inflammatory disease process. Late flexion instability can occur if the PCL fails over time. This complication can also occur iatrogenically when the PCL it is overzealously recessed intraoperatively or excessive proximal tibial resection is perfomed. When too much proximal tibia is resected, the PCL insertion site can be jeopardized. The PCL can also be is damaged by synovitis from inflammatory arthropathy, resulting in failure.[17] Thus, avoiding the use PCL retaining implants can eliminate failure and instability by avoiding reliance on the integrity of the native PCL.

4. Disadvantages of posterior stabilized TKA

There are several disadvantages with use of posterior stabilized TKA designs. These include: I) tibial post wear and breakage, II) excessive bone resection, III) patellar clunk syndrome, and IV) tibio-femoral dislocations.

4.1 Tibial post wear and breakage

A potential problem with posterior stabilized design is tibial post polyethylene wear from the cam-post articulation. Excessive wear particulate debris can lead to osteolysis. In a wear analysis of retrieved posterior stabilized TKA components, evidence of wear or damage was observed on all specimens of stabilizing posts, including those revised because of infection.[18] Wear caused premature failure and early revision. Moreover, wear can lead to catastrophic failure of the tibial post through fracture. The authors concluded that the cam-post articulation in posterior stabilized implants can be an additional source of polyethylene wear debris. The variability in wear patterns observed among designs may be due to differences in cam-post mechanics, post location, and post geometry. [19]

4.2 Excessive bone resection

It is necessary to remove bone from the intercondylar notch inorder to accommodate the tibial post in most posterior stabilized TKA designs. This obligatory "box" cut can be significant in smaller sized femurs especially is TKA systems where the post remains a

[15] Collier JP, Mayor MB, McNamara JL, et al. Analysis of the failure of 122 polyethylene inserts from uncemented tibial knee components. Clin Orthop Relat Res 1991; 273:232-242.

[16] Kilgus DJ, Moreland JR, Finerman GA, et al. Catastrophic wear of tibial polyethylene inserts. Clin Orthop Relat Res 1991; 273:223-231.

[17] Waslewski GL, Marson BM, Benjamin JB. Early, incapacitating instability of posterior cruciate ligament-retaining total knee arthroplasty. J Arthroplasty 1998; 13:763-767.

[18] Puloski SK, McCalden RW, MacDonald SJ, et al. Tibial post wear in posterior stabilized total knee arthroplasty. An unrecognized source of polyethylene debris. J Bone Joint Surg Am 2001; 83A:390-397.

[19] Dolan MM, Kelly NH, Nguyen JT, Wright TM, Haas SB. Implant design influences tibial post wear damage in posterior-stabilized knees. Clin Orthop Relat Res. 2011 Jan;469(1):160-7.

constant size for each femoral component size.[20] The consequence is that there will be a relatively large notch cut for a small femoral component greatly weakening the condyle and increasing the risk of femoral condyle bone loss and periprosthetic fracture. Surgeons who chose to use posterior stabilized TKA should familiarize themselves with relative "box" cut volume to avoid intra-operative and post-operative periprosthetic fractures, especially in small, osteoporotic femurs.

4.3 Patellar clunk

Patella clunk is a complication that is more prevalent in posterior stabilized TKA designs. A prominent fibrous nodule can form at the junction of the proximal patellar pole and the quadriceps tendon. During deep flexion, this fibrous nodule can "catch" in the intercondylar notch of the femoral component causing a catching sensation on the end of the groove as the patella moves back with knee extension. It is this catching and then forceful release with extension that results in the "clunk" and pain characteristic of this condition.[21] Recommended treatment consists of physical therapy and arthroscopic debridement. Arthrotomy and possible revision surgery is reserved for recurrent clunks, malposition or loose components.[22]

4.4 Tibio-femoral dislocations

One of the disadvantages of posterior stabilized TKA is the potential for dislocation in flexion as the tibial post rides underneath the femoral cam. This occurs when there is significant extension-flexion gap mismatch. More specifically, dislocations occur when the flexion gap is larger than the corresponding extension gap, allowing the post to "jump" over the cam. The incidence of dislocation with posterior stabilized TKA is very rare with modern designs (0.2%).[23] To prevent knee dislocation it is mandatory that the surgeon balance the knee both in flexion and extension. When dislocation occurs, closed and sometimes open reduction is required. If recurrent dislocation occurs, revision surgery to correct flexion extension mismatch is imperative.

5. Alternative to cam post design

The "deep-dish" tibial insert, introduced by Hoffman et al in 2000, is an alternative to the cam post posterior stabilized TKA design. This type of design eliminated the need for resection of the intercondylar notch bone stock and use of a tibial post. AP stability is achieved by using highly conforming tibial inserts with anterior build-up[24]. Some advantages of this ultra-congruent design include: bone preservation by eliminating the

---

[20] Haas S, Nelson C, Laskin R. Posterior stabilized TKA: an assessment of bone resection. The Knee 2000; 7: 25-29.

[21] Hozack WJ, Rothman RH, Booth RE Jr, Balderston RA. The patellar clunk syndrome. A complication of posterior stabilized total knee arthroplasty. Clin Orthop Relat Res 1989; 241:203-208.

[22] Beight JL, Yao B, Hozack WJ, et al. The patellar 'clunk' syndrome after posterior stabilized total knee arthroplasty. Clin Orthop Relat Res 1994; 299:139-142.

[23] Lombardi AV Jr, Mallory TH, Vaughn BK, et al. Dislocation following primary posterior-stabilized total knee arthroplasty. J Arthroplasty 1993; 8:633-639.

[24] Hofmann AA, Tkach TK, Evanich CJ, Camargo MP: Posterior stabilization in total knee arthroplasty with use of an ultracongruent polyethylene insert. J Arthroplasty 2000;15:576-583

need for box cut, elimination of post breakage and wear, elimination of tibio-femoral dislocation and patella clunk syndrome. In addition, the ultracongruent tibial component has the advantage of distributing the loads over a larger surface area of the polyethylene insert, hypothetically limiting and distributing more evenly the loads at the bone—implant interface. Moreover, because femoral box preparation is eliminated, femoral bone stock is preserved, decreasing the potential for fracture and operative time.[25] Several studies comparing the stability, range of motion and stair climbing ability found no significant difference with ultracongruent design TKA when compared to traditional cam post design TKA.

6. Outcomes

Despite the dissimilarities between cruciate retaining and posterior stabilized TKA designs, most comparative studies have found no significant differences in function, patient satisfaction, or survivorship of the two designs in unselected patient cohorts.[26] We have divided the reported results after posterior stabilized TKA into specific outcomes to facilitate the review. Specific outcomes include the performance of posterior stabilized TKA designs in terms of proprioception, wear, loosening, and stability. Also the results with the use of posterior stabilized TKA in two particular subgroups of patients: varus-flexion deformity and postpatellectomy are included in this section.

7. Proprioception

Proprioception after TKA may be improved with the preservation of the native PCL. Mechanoreceptors have been identified in the native posterior cruciate ligament may aid in feedback mechanism improving proprioception.[27] Hystological analysis, however, suggests that marked neurologic degeneration occurs within the posterior cruciate ligament as part of the arthritic process [13]. Clinical studies are not conclusive as to which implant design has better proprioception. Warren *et al.* [14] observed that proprioception improved after TKA with either a posterior stabilized or cruciate retaining design, but suggested that greater improvement occurred in the cruciate retaining group. In contrast, Simmons *et al.* [15] noted that in patients with severe arthritis better postoperative proprioception was obtained with a posterior stabilized TKA. Becker *et al.* [16] compared patients with bilateral paired cruciate retaining and posterior stabilized TKA. Fifty percent of the patients were unable to express a preference for one knee or the other. The other 50% were equally divided between those who preferred the cruciate retaining and those who preferred the posterior stabilized knee. Most recently Swanik *et al.* [17] performed a prospective, randomized study on 20 patients to assess proprioception, kinesthesia, and balance following TKA comparing posterior stabilized

---

[25] Laskin RS, Maruyama Y, Villaneuva M, Bourne R. Deep-dish congruent tibial component use in total knee arthroplasty: a randomized prospective study. Clin Orthop Relat Res. 200 Nov;(380):36-44.

[26] Jacobs WC, Clement DJ, Wymenga AB. Retention versus removal of the posterior cruciate ligament in total knee replacement: a systematic literature review within the Cochrane framework. Acta Orthop 2005; 76:757-768.

[27] Warren PJ, Olanlokun TK, Cobb AG, Bentley G. Proprioception after knee arthroplasty: the influence of prosthetic design. Clin Orthop Relat Res. 1993;297:182-187.

versus cruciate retaining designs Joint position sense, the threshold to detect joint motion, and the patient's ability to balance on an unstable platform were assessed prior to and at least 6 months after the operation. They found that after TKA all patients detected motion significantly faster, reproduced joint position with less error and had balance improvement. The group treated with the posterior stabilized TKA more accurately reproduced joint position when the knee was extended from a flexed position. The authors conclude that retention of the PCL does not appear to improve proprioception and balance.

7.1 Loosening

At long-term follow-up there appears to be no significant difference in the aseptic loosening rates of posterior stabilized and cruciate retaining TKA designs. The cemented posterior stabilized TKA has a reported 98.1% survival rate at 14 years [19]. In the most recent study Rasquinha *et al.* [20••] reported the long-term results of a series of 150 consecutive posterior stabilized TKA that were performed in 118 patients They found a good to excellent result in 90% of patients at mean follow-up of 12 years. At 12 years, the survival rate was 94.6 ± 4.0% with failure for any reason as the end point and 98.3 ± 2.4% with mechanical failure as the end point. Revision surgery was necessary in five cases: two because of infection, one for dislocation and two for polyethylene wear and osteolysis.

7.2 Stability

As mentioned above with posterior stabilized TKA if the knee is not properly balanced dislocation in flexion can occur. This a very rare event, and can be avoided with careful balancing of the flexion and extension gaps. In terms of instability, posterior or flexion instability may in fact be a greater, although less recognized, problem with cruciate retaining TKA designs. Rupture of the PCL after surgery can cause pain and disability. Flexion instability can also result when the flexion space is left too loose, resulting in marked anterior-posterior translation of the tibia on the femur in flexion. Pagnano *et al.* [21] reported on 25 cruciate retaining TKAs treated for flexion instability. These patients presented with a typical constellation of symptoms that included a sense of knee instability without true give-way, recurrent knee joint effusions, and anterior knee pain. On exam, these knees had obvious anteroposterior instability when tested at 90° of flexion, and even demonstrated a marked posterior sag sign. They all underwent revision surgery to a posterior stabilized design and 22 of the 25 had significant symptomatic improvement after revision surgery.

7.3 Correction of deformity

Most series of patients with varus deformities have shown excellent results after 10-15 years, with either cruciate retaining or posterior stabilized TKA. There is, however, only one comparative study [22] that evaluated the results of cruciate retaining and posterior stabilized implants in the context of severe varus or varus-flexion deformities. In this series, survivorship, range of motion, and pain-related outcomes were worse in patients with fixed varus (or varus-flexion) deformities over 15° who were treated with cruciate retaining devices, compared with patients treated with posterior stabilized implants or with those who did not have such varus deformities and were treated with cruciate retaining devices.

7.4 Postpatellectomy patients

Most authors suggest that a posterior stabilized design is most appropriate in patients with previous patellectomy. The tibial post and femoral cam mechanism limits the posterior translation of the tibia that can occur without the patella. Patellectomy leads to the disruption of the normal kinematics of the knee. In the context of knee replacement, it has been hypothesized that loads on the PCL in the years following surgery may be increased, potentially resulting in late attenuation and instability [23,24]. Patellectomy also can cause decreased extensor mechanism power because of the loss of the fulcrum provided by the intact patella. A retrospective study showed that patellectomized patients treated with posterior stabilized implants had better functional and pain scores than did those treated with cruciate retaining implants [23]. In comparison to cruciate retaining designs, posterior stabilized devices lead to better results when TKA is performed in patients with prior patellectomies [25].

8. Rheumatoid arthritis

Total knee arthroplasty is a proven technique for the management of deformity and unremitting pain in the rheumatoid arthritic knee. Many important considerations must be taken into account in order to maximize the results of total knee replacement in this challenging patient population. In a retrospective study, Laskin et al[28] reported that cruciate retaining implants in patients with rheumatoid arthritis were associated with inferior results compared with posterior stabilized implants, principally because of late instability and progressive recurvatum deformity. The tendency for generalized ligamentous laxity and attenuation and joint deformity in these patients make successful TKA difficult with PCL retaining designs. These patients may present with severe or fixed valgus deformities. Most patients with rheumatoid arthritis typically have poor quality of the soft tissues and the potential for synovitis to cause late attenuation and rupture of the PCL.

9. Conclusion

The use of posterior stabilized TKA has several advantages. Potential benefits of a posterior stabilized TKA over a cruciate retaining TKA include easier surgical exposure and ligament balancing, predictable restoration of knee kinematics, improved range of motion, less wear, and avoiding the possibility of PCL rupture. In addition, the use of posterior stabilized TKA appears to be advantageous in correction of severe varus – valgus deformity. A potential problem with posterior stabilized TKA is tibial post polyethylene wear from the cam-post mechanism. Excessive wear can lead not only to osteolysis but also post fracture. Other disadvantage of posterior stabilized TKA is patellar 'clunk' syndrome, risk of dislocation or flexion instability and bone loss and peri-prosthetic condylar fracture. Despite the dissimilarities between cruciate retaining and posterior stabilized TKA designs, most studies have found no significant differences in function, patient satisfaction, or survivorship of the two designs in unselected patient cohorts. Posterior stabilized TKA outcomes appear to be better in a particular subgroup of patients including patients with patellectomy, large varus or varus-flexion deformity, and rheumatoid arthritis.

---

[28] Laskin RS, O'Flynn HM. The Insall Award. Total knee replacement with posterior cruciate ligament retention in rheumatoid arthritis: Problems and complications. Clin Orthop 1997; 345:24-28.

10. References

[1] Stiehl JB, Komistek RD, Dennis DA, *et al.* Fluoroscopic analysis of kinematics after posterior cruciate retaining knee arthroplasty. J Bone Joint Surg Br 1995; 77B:884-889.

[2] Dennis DA, Komistek RD, Hoff WA. In vivo knee kinematics derived using an inverse perspective technique. Clin Orthop 1996; 331:107-117.

[3] Ranawat CS, Komistek RD, Rodriguez JA, *et al.* *In vivo* kinematics for fixed and mobile-bearing posterior stabilized knee prostheses. Clin Orthop Relat Res 2004; 418:184-190.

[4] Jacobs WC, Clement DJ, Wymenga AB. Retention versus removal of the posterior cruciate ligament in total knee replacement: a systematic literature review within the Cochrane framework. Acta Orthop 2005; 76:757-768.

[5] Collier JP, Mayor MB, McNamara JL, *et al.* Analysis of the failure of 122 polyethylene inserts from uncemented tibial knee components. Clin Orthop Relat Res 1991; 273:232-242.

[6] Kilgus DJ, Moreland JR, Finerman GA, *et al.* Catastrophic wear of tibial polyethylene inserts. Clin Orthop Relat Res 1991; 273:223-231.

[7] Waslewski GL, Marson BM, Benjamin JB. Early, incapacitating instability of posterior cruciate ligament-retaining total knee arthroplasty. J Arthroplasty 1998; 13:763-767.

[8] Puloski SK, McCalden RW, MacDonald SJ, *et al.* Tibial post wear in posterior stabilized total knee arthroplasty. An unrecognized source of polyethylene debris. J Bone Joint Surg Am 2001; 83A:390-397.

[9] Hozack WJ, Rothman RH, Booth RE Jr, Balderston RA. The patellar clunk syndrome. A complication of posterior stabilized total knee arthroplasty. Clin Orthop Relat Res 1989; 241:203-208.

[10] Beight JL, Yao B, Hozack WJ, *et al.* The patellar 'clunk' syndrome after posterior stabilized total knee arthroplasty. Clin Orthop Relat Res 1994; 299:139-142.

[11] Lombardi AV Jr, Mallory TH, Vaughn BK, *et al.* Dislocation following primary posterior-stabilized total knee arthroplasty. J Arthroplasty 1993; 8:633-639.

[12] Fantozzi S, Catani F, Ensini A, *et al.* Femoral rollback of cruciate-retaining and posterior-stabilized total knee replacements: *in vivo* fluoroscopic analysis during activities of daily living. J Orthop Res 2006; 24:2222-2229.

[13] Kleinbart FA, Bryk E, Evangelista J, *et al.* Histologic comparison of posterior cruciate ligaments from arthritic and age matched knee specimens. J Arthroplasty 1996; 6:726-731.

[14] Warren PI, Olanlokun TK, Cobb AG, Bentley G. Proprioception after knee arthroplasty: The influence of prosthetic design. Clin Orthop 1993; 297:182-187.

[15] Simmons S, Lephart S, Rubash H, *et al.* Proprioception after unicondylar knee arthroplasty versus total knee arthroplasty. Clin Orthop 1996; 331:179-184.

[16] Becker MW, Insall JN, Faris PM. Bilateral total knee arthroplasty: one cruciate retaining and one cruciate substituting. Clin Orthop 1990; 271:122-124.

[17] Swanik CB, Lephart SM, Rubash HE. Proprioception, kinesthesia, and balance after total knee arthroplasty with cruciate-retaining and posterior stabilized prostheses. J Bone Joint Surg Am 2004; 86A:328-334.

[18] Scott RD, Thornhill TS. Posterior cruciate supplementing total knee replacements using conforming inserts and cruciate recession: effect on range of motion and radiolucent lines. Clin Orthop 1994; 309:146-149.
[19] Colizza WA, Insall JN, Scuderi GR. The posterior stabilized total knee prosthesis: Assessment of polyethylene damage and osteolysis after a 10-year minimum follow-up. J Bone Joint Surg Am 1995; 77A:1713-1720.
[20] Rasquinha VJ, Ranawat CS, Cervieri CL, Rodriguez JA. The press-fit condylar modular total knee system with a posterior cruciate-substituting design. A concise follow-up of a previous report. J Bone Joint Surg Am 2006; 88A:1006-1010. This was a long-term follow-up study with 118 patients that had a posterior stabilized TKA.
[21] Pagnano MW, Hanssen AD, Stuart MJ, Lewallen DG. Flexion instability after primary posterior cruciate retaining total knee arthroplasty. Clin Orthop 1998; 356:39-46.
[22] Laskin RS. The Insall Award. Total knee replacement with posterior cruciate ligament retention in patients with a fixed varus deformity. Clin Orthop 1996; 331:29-34.
[23] Paletta GA Jr, Laskin RS. Total knee arthroplasty after a previous patellectomy. J Bone Joint Surg Am 1995; 77A:1708-1712.
[24] Cameron HU, Hu C, Vyamont D. Posterior stabilized knee prosthesis for total knee replacement in patients with prior patellectomy. Can J Surg 1996; 39:469-473.
[25] Bayne O, Cameron HU. Total knee arthroplasty following patellectomy. Clin Orthop 1984; 186:112-114.
[26] Laskin RS, O'Flynn HM. The Insall Award. Total knee replacement with posterior cruciate ligament retention in rheumatoid arthritis: Problems and complications. Clin Orthop 1997; 345:24-28.

17

Mobile Bearing Concept in Knee Arthroplasty

Nahum Rosenberg[1,2],
Arnan Greental[1] and Michael Soudry[1,2]
[1]*Orthopaedic Surgery "A" Dept., Rambam - Health Care Campus, Haifa*
[2]*Ruth and Bruce Rappaport Faculty of Medicine, Technion - Israel Institute of Technology, Haifa*
Israel

1. Introduction

The rationale for mobile bearing design of knee replacement prosthesis is to increase its survival by reducing the rate of aseptic loosening and to improve the range of movement of the treated knee. The theoretical basis for the achievement of the first goal is the expected lower rates of the polyethylene insert wear in the mobile design in comparison to a fixed design, due to lower contact and constraint forces. A better range of movements following mobile bearing arthroplasty is expected as the result of additional moving surface between to fixed planes at the ends of the articulating bones, allowing mobility with congruency.These expected advantages of the mobile bearing design should be judged cautiously since the initial mobile bearing implants caused higher rates of breakage and disarrangement of the polyethylene inserts, when the implantation method wasn't strictly followed. In order to resolve these technical problems the rotating platform mobile prosthesis was developed.

Mobile bearing concept was implemented in a three compartment replacement prostheses and also in unicompartamental designs, especially for the medial compartment of the knee. Currently, following the more than two decades of the rising experience with implantation of a large number of mobile bearing prostheses, there is a significant amount of data for evaluation of the survival of these prosthetic designs. In order to declare on their higher expected efficiency these implants should show higher than 96-97% of ten year clinical survival, which should remain relatively stable up to 20 years of follow up, as reported in the several of fixed bearing designs. Unfortunately this data is not readily available, because only few well designed survivorship reports on mobile knee implants have been published yet. Furthermore the published data failed to provide a clear evidence of the superiority of mobile bearing design.

The endoprosthetic arthroplasty is the most popular surgical modality for treatment of advanced knee joint disease, either degenerative or inflammatory. The reason for this clinical trend is the ability to reduce pain and to restore the patient's ability to walk.

Although it has been shown that the improvement in ambulation, following knee arthroplasty, is mostly subjective, because other restrictions of a capacity to walk might be revealed following elimination of the pain in the knee (1), the reduction of the pain level while walking is considered by the patients as a significant improvement in the quality of life. For this reason a major effort is exerted by the clinicians and the industry to develop the most effective surgical techniques and prosthetic designs aiming to improve immediate postsurgical outcome of knee prosthetic arthroplasty and the longevity of the implanted prostheses. Several of the currently used prosthetic designs have already reached long term, above 10 years, survivorship of above 95%, therefore the "straggle" for the improvement in the prostheses longevity is aimed to the marginal 5% improvement of long term survivorship following the implantation by reducing the prostheses failure rate in long time scale. The success of this multidisciplinary effort of clinicians and engineers can't be overemphasized because the success will not only eliminate the need for revision surgery in patients, who are mostly in the age above sixty years, because of the expected prostheses' longevity consideration, but also will provide a prosthetic solutions for the younger patients with degenerative knees, who seek for a better treatment modality for their disability.

Therefore logically the widely used generic design of unconstrained knee prosthesis, with metal femoral component and polyethylene insert fixed on metal back-plate on tibia, with cemented or cementless fixation into articulating surfaces, should be improved in one or in several of its components in order to improve its long term clinical performance . Clearly these considerations do not related to the short term prosthetic failures, which are mostly attributed to a basically fault prosthetic design, as observed in the early constrained prostheses (2), to deficient surgical technique or to a complicated general medical condition of the patient that might lead to the prosthesis disarrangement, peri-prosthetic fracture or local infection.

Long standing clinical success of prosthetic knee replacement is dependent on the ability to provide stability with good range of movement, to resist the loosening processes and to provide material longevity of all prosthetic components. Near satisfactory range of movement and stability have been successfully achieved with widely used fixed bearing designs, however, component loosening remains their main long term problem (3,4). Although the early loosening processes, common in the original constrained designs, have been eliminated in the second generation unconstrained prostheses, late loosening, due to osteolysis caused by polyethylene wear of the fixed tibial bearings, remains unresolved (5). Therefore it is logical that the main target that should be addresses in order to reduce the late aseptic loosening of the knee prostheses would be the polyethylene insert and its susceptibility for wear following long standing and continuous exposure to compressing forces from the adjacent metal components. One of the steps for reducing the polyethylene wear was directed to improve the material characteristics of the polyethylene in order to avoid the free radicals release during the gamma sterilization by using a manufacturer process with high temperature towards the melting point with crosslinking induction and generation of ultrahigh molecular weight polyethylene that reduces the plastic insert susceptibility to mechanical wear (6). A high level of crosslinking had been used in several acetabular polyethylene designs in the last decade and showed less surface wear but, on the other hand, presented alteration in the mechanical properties of the bearing insert. For this reason this method is of limited role in the knee prostheses.

Therefore other tribulogical factors should be addressed in order to reduce the cross shear and surface pressure of the polyethylene insert. High conformation between the femoral and tibial surfaces in the prosthesis can reduce the surface pressure and polyethylene wear. But in fixed bearing design the elevation of conformation causes restriction in the range of movement of the knee. Therefore in the fixed bearing prostheses some unconformity is deliberately allowed in order to provide a reasonable range of knee movement.

Another mechanical concept to reduce the bearing component wear, which is mainly induced by the high point and line contact forces between moving metal femoral component and static polyethylene tibial insert, has been developed . By this concept an "area" contact pattern has been introduced (7). The rationale of the "area" contact pattern is based on the assumption that the forces between the prostheses components may be distributed more efficiently by using a mobile bearing polyethylene insert (8). Subsequently the hypothetical advantage is in reduction of material wear and elimination of aseptic loosening (Figure 1).

According to this concept Pappas MJ and Buechel FF developed a total knee prosthesis with mobile bearing (7), and Goodfellow JW and O'Connor J developed the unicompartamental mobile bearing "Oxford Knee" design (9).

The expectation from the later unicompartamental design was to develop a prosthetic method that will replace the technically demanding osteotomies in younger patients with unicompartamental degenerative disease. This goal was achieved only partially, since the unicompartamental design could be successful only in patients who answer to the very strict clinical and radiographic criteria.

The former, LCS® mobile meniscal bearing total knee replacement system, has been designed to lower contact stress with preservation of the crucial low constraint properties. Initially after the introduction of this system for the widespread clinical use in 1977-80 one large multicenter (10) and three independent (11,12,13) middle term follow up studies have been published showing favorable subjective outcome results in 90-97.5% of patients with 94.6 - 95.3% of six to eight years survivorship of cementless LCS® mobile bearing posterior cruciate retaining prostheses. These outcome results are close to the survivorship data reported by the system designers, that showed 97.9% and 95.1% of five and twelve years survivorship rates respectively (14).

Conversely there have been a number of reports of high rate mechanical failures of the LCS® system (8,15). These short term follow up studies showed a tendency for mobile bearing dislocation and breakage. These findings can also be supported by cadaveric biomechanical testing (16). Thus the potential susceptibility of LCS® posterior cruciate retaining design for early mechanical failure may overcome the benefits of long term low loosening rates. In an additional later report on a medium term experience with 35 cementless LCS® mobile meniscal bearing total knee replacements in patients with osteoarthritis there was an evidence of 97.1% five year survivorship (17). This high survival rate, with a satisfactory functional outcome, at middle term follow up, has been achieved by following an optimal technique of implantation, according to the designers recommendations, i.e. the tibial component should be situated perpendicularly to

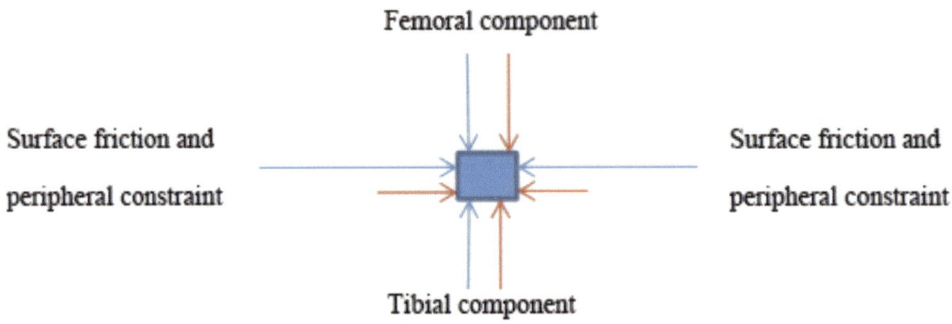

A

A: A schematic representation of vectors of forces on a unit of polyethylene tibial insert in a sagittal plane during knee loading. Blue arrows are the vectors of forces in fixed bearing design and red arrows in a mobile bearing insert, where less magnitude of force from the peripheral constrain should reduce the overall magnitude of force and to reduce the development of the polyethylene insert wear, as represented in B.

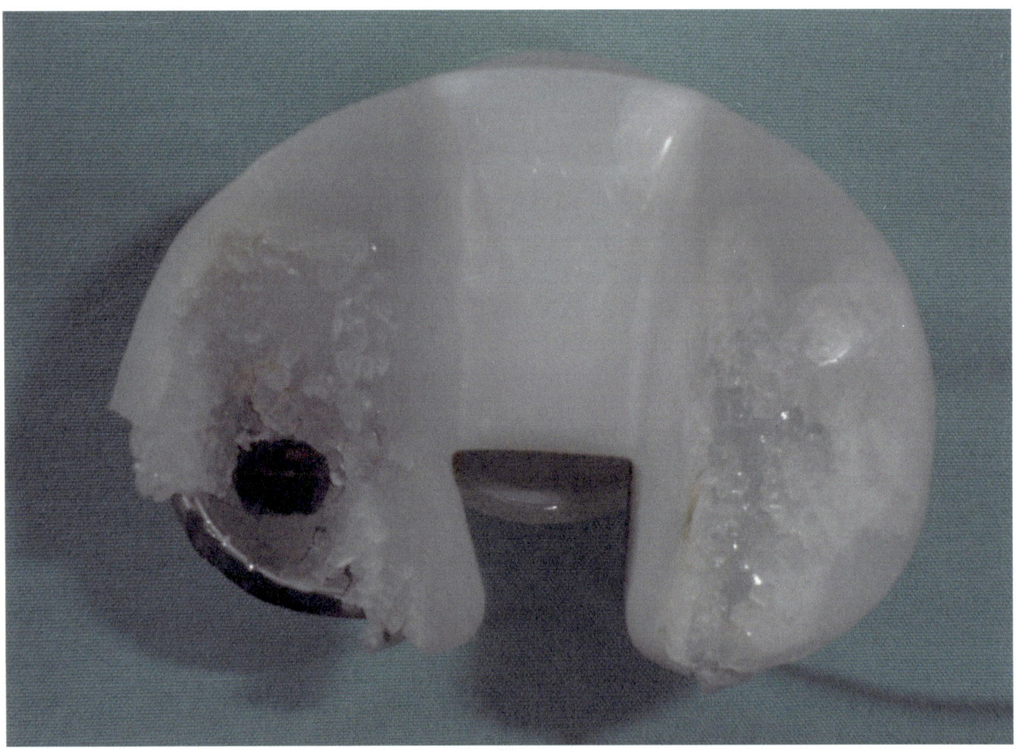

B

B: Reprehensive example of an advanced wear of a polyethylene insert of a fixed bearing design.

Fig. 1. Rationale for mobile bearing concept in knee arthroplasty prosthesis:

longitudinal axis of tibial metaphysis with 5 ^{o} - 10 ^{o} of posterior inclination relatively to the anatomical axis of tibia in the sagittal plane, the sagittal flexion angle of the femoral component should be close to 5 ^{o} relatively to the anatomical axis of femur and overall coronal alignment of the components should be around 5 ^{o} of valgus (18). The average three dimensional component alignment in this study group has not deviated more than 3 ^{o} from the recommended by the designers' optimal orientation. Therefore it might be suggested that the high survival rates of the prosthesis and good functional outcome in the majority of evaluated patients in this study should be attributed to the effective surgical technique. This was reflected by the satisfactory functional knee scores in 77% and complete pain elimination in 89% of the evaluated knees. Therefore there is evidence that in the middle term the mobile bearing design of total knee replacement can be as effective as the conventional fixed bearing designs. Additional reports on short and middle term outcome of knee replacement with LCS® mobile meniscal bearing cementless design revealed rates of aseptic loosening in the range of 0.4 - 1.8% (8,14), which are compatible with most of the effective fixed bearing designs (19). However, the real advantage of mobile bearing system in reducing the rate of osteolysis should be established in the long term survivorship studies.

The emerged susceptibility of mobile bearing meniscal surfaces to early failure due to dislocation or breakage (8) may provoke a reasonable hesitation to its widespread use. Although the designers of the LCS® mobile meniscal bearing prosthesis claimed that strict operative technique and precise prosthetic placement should avoid its mechanical failure (18), there are only few independent studies that support this claim by showing 0.6% rate of meniscal bearing failure in 2 - 10 years of follow up (13, 17). And on the other hand there is some evidence that greater deviation from the desired three dimensional placement of the mobile bearing prosthesis does not significantly reduce its 10 years survivorship and preferable functional outcome (20). Therefore there is no clear evidence of the precise precise factors contributing to the mobile inserts disarrangement.

In order to reduce the revealed possibility of mechanical failure of meniscal type mobile bearings, a more stable "rotating platform" mobile polyethylene bearing was designed. In this design a single polyethylene insert, without rotational constraint, was used. The rotating platform knee is assumed to follow the normal femoral rotation upon the tibial axis during knee flexion, which is normally between 16^{0}-23^{0} degrees (21). But it was found that the measured rotation of the bearing surface in the implanted prostheses is significantly less than expected, e.g. only in 12% of the knees there was more than 10 degrees of rotation.

Additional theoretical advantage of a mobile bearing prosthesis is the expected better patellar tracking due to the self-alignment of the mobile bearing. But this assumption has not been proven in patients, because there was no clinical evidence of a diminished post-operative anterior knee pain even in the first year after surgery (22).

The cautious approach for the efficiency of mobile bearing prostheses is even supported by the results of their biomechanical testing. It has been shown by a simulator based experiment, utilizing six million cycles of repetitive testing of prosthesis movement of mobile bearing designs with rotating platform and one fixed bearing implant, that there was no difference in the amount of in vitro wear (23).

Therefore, according to the published data it is still unclear if the theoretical advantage of the mobile bearing design is reflected in the improved clinical outcome (24,25).
Furthermore a meta-analyses of 33 studies assessing 3532 operated knees failed to present an evidence of a better clinical outcome, including the complication rate, functional and radiological results, of the mobile bearing design for knee arthroplasty in a comparison to standard fixed bearing devices (26).
This disappointing fact is probably related to the original intention to improve the current fixed bearing design survival at its marginal failure occurrence part by addressing mostly the mechanics of the polyethylene bearing insert. It seems that the differences in the bearings' fixation shouldn't be addressed for this purpose, in spite of the theoretical mechanical advantage of the mobile bearing. This suggests that different innovative methods for improvement of the prosthetic longevity should be investigated. These methods will probably be related to the other mechanical or material components of the knee prosthesis design. On this stage there is no clear evidence that the mobile bearing concept of knee prosthesis has justified the advantageous theoretical expectation for its superiority over the fixed bearing implants.

2. References

[1] Rosenberg N, Nierenberg G, Lenger R, Soudry M. Walking ability following knee arthroplasty. A prospective pilot study of factors affecting the maximal walking distance in 18 patients before and six months after total knee arthroplasty. Knee, 2007; 14(6):489-92.

[2] Riley D, Woodyard JE. Long-term results of Geomedic total knee replacement. J Bone Joint Surg, 1985; 67B: 548-50.

[3] Wright TM, Bartel DL. The problem of surface damage in polyethylene total knee components. Clin Orthop, 1986;205: 67-74.

[4] Peters PC, Engh GA, Dwyer KA, Vinh TN. Osteolysis after total knee arthroplasty without cement. J Bone Joint Surg, 1992; 74A: 864-876.

[5] Ayers DC. Polyethylene wear and osteolysis following total knee replacement. Instr Course Lect 1997;46: 205-213

[6] Fisher JD, Jennings LM, Galvin AL, Jin ZM, Stone MH, Ingham E . 2009 Knee Society Presidential Guest Lecture: Polyethylene wear in total knees. Clin Orthop Relat Res, 2010; 468:12–18.

[7] Buechel FF, Pappas MJ. New Jersey low contact stress knee replacement system. Ten year evaluation of meniscal bearings. Orth Clin N Am, 1989;20(2): 147-177.

[8] Weaver JK, Derkash RS, Greenwald AS. Difficulties with bearing dislocation and breakage using a movable bearing total knee replacement system. Clin Orthop Relat Res , 1993; 290: 244-252.

[9] Goodfellow JW, O'Connor J. The mechanics of the knee and prosthesis design. J Bone Joint Surg, 1978; 60B: 864-876.

[10] Sorrells RB, Fenning JB, Davenport JM. Comparison of the clinical results and survivorship of noncemented cruciate sacrificing versus cruciate sparing total knee

replacements. Presented at The American Academy of Orthopaedic Surgeons, San Francisco, California, February 1993.
[11] Huang CH, Lee YM, Su RY, Lai JH. Clinical results of the New Jersey low contact stress knee arthroplasty with two to five years follow-up. J Orth Surg ROC, 1991;8: 295-299.
[12] Jordan LR, Olivo JL, Voorhorst PE. Survivorship analysis of cementless meniscal bearing total knee arthroplasty. Clin Orthop Relat Res, 1997; 338: 119-123.
[13] Keblish PA, Schrei C, Ward M. Evaluation of 275 low contact stress (LCS) total knee replacements with 2- to 8- year follow up. Orthopaedics, 1993;1(2): 168- 173.
[14] Buechel FF, Pappas MJ: Long-term survivorship analysis of cruciate-sparing versus cruciate sacrificing knee prostheses using meniscal bearings. Clin Orthop Relat Res, 1990; 260: 162-169.
[15] Bert JM. Dislocation/subluxation of meniscal bearing elements after New Jersey low-contact stress total knee arthroplasty. Clin Orthop Relat Res ,1990;254: 211-215.
[16] Matsuda S, Whiteside LA, White SE, McCarthy DS: Knee stability in meniscal bearing total knee arthroplasty. J Arthroplasty 1999;14: 82-90.
[17] Rosenberg N, Henderson I. Medium term outcome of the LCS cementless posterior cruciate retaining total knee replacements. Follow up and survivorship study of 35 operated knees. The Knee, 2001; 8(2): 123-128.
[18] Buechel FF. Letters to the editor. Clin Orthop Relat Res ,1991; 264: 309-311.
[19] Lemaire R. Will bearing mobility result in a decreased incidence of TKR loosening? J Bone Joint Surg , 1999; 81B(suppl 2): 127.
[20] Vogt JC, Saarbach C. LCS mobile-bearing total knee replacement. A 10-year's follow-up study. Orthop Traum: Surg Res, 2009;95:177-82.
[21] Wasielewski RC, Komistek RD, Zingde SM, Sheridan KC, Mahfouz MR. Lack of axial rotation in mobile-bearing knee designs. Clin Orthop Relat Res, 2008; 466:2662–8.
[22] Breugem SJM, Sierevelt IN, Schafroth MU, Blankevoort L, Schaap GR, van Dijk CN. Less anterior knee pain with a mobile-bearing prosthesis compared with a fixed-bearing prosthesis. Clin Orthop Relat Res ,2008; 466:1959–65.
[23] Haider H, Garvin K. Rotating Platform versus Fixed-bearing Total Knees. An In Vitro Study of Wear. Clin Orthop Relat Res. 2008; 466:2677–85.
[24] Smith H, Jan M, Mahomed NN, Davey JR,Gandhi R. Meta-analysis and systematic review of clinical outcomes comparing mobile bearing and fixed bearing total knee arthroplasty. J Arthroplasty, 2011 – *in press*
[25] Jacobs W, Anderson PG, van Limbeek J, Wymega AAB. Mobile bearing vs fixed bearing prostheses for total knee arthroplasty for post- operative functional status in patients with osteoarthritis and rheumatoid arthritis (Review). The Cochrane collaboration, 2008;(3):1-15.

[26] Smith TO, Ejtehadi F, Nichols R, Davies L, Donell ST, Hing CB. Clinical and radiological outcomes of fixed- versus mobile-bearing total knee replacement: a meta-analysis. Knee Surg Sports Traumatol Arthrosc, 2010;18(3):325-40.

18

Soft Tissue Balance in Total Knee Arthroplasty

Tomoyuki Matsumoto[1], Hirotsugu Muratsu[2], Seiji Kubo[1],
Masahiro Kurosaka[1] and Ryosuke Kuroda[1]
[1]*Department of Orthopaedic Surgery, Kobe University Graduate School of Medicine, Kobe*
[2]*Department of Orthopaedic Surgery, Nippon Steel Hirohata Hospital, Himeji*
Japan

1. Introduction

The primary goal of total knee arthroplasties (TKAs) is the achievement of stable tibiofemoral and patellofemoral (PF) joints, which relies on accurately aligning these joint components and balancing the soft tissues. In order to achieve these criteria, it is important to utilize appropriate surgical techniques and well-designed implants [1-3]. To this end, using the more traditional intra- and extra-medullary alignment devices, the proper alignment of each joint component further relies on performing accurate femoral and tibial osteotomies along ideal levels and angles. Recently, computer-assisted and robot-assisted surgeries have been developed and reported to improve the accuracy of osteotomies in TKA [4-7]. We similarly reported on a CT-free navigation system which significantly improved the accuracy of implantations in relation to the mechanical axis, and achieved an early and mid-term clinical outcome equivalent to that of a manual group [8-10].

In contrast, the management of soft tissue balance during surgery remains difficult, leaving much to the surgeon's subjective feel. TKA is a well-established procedure, which generally results in relief of pain, improved physical function, and a high level of patient satisfaction. However, knee instability after primary TKA is considered an important factor for early TKA failure. Fehring et al. studied 279 revision surgeries within 5 years of their index arthroplasty and reported 74 revision cases (27%) caused by instability [11]. In a retrospective study of revision surgery, Sharkey et al. reported instability in 21.2% of their early revision knee arthroplasty failures [12]. They concluded that the instability might be due to inadequate correction of soft tissue imbalances in both the sagittal and coronal planes. As a result, soft tissue balancing has been recognized as an essential surgical intervention for improving the outcomes of TKA.

2. Traditional soft tissue balance assessment

Although several methods and devices for assessing soft tissue balance such as manual distraction [13], traditional tensor [13], space block [14], and lamina spreaders [15] have been described in previous papers, assessment has not been quantitative and has mainly depended on the subjective feeling of the surgeons. The second generation of tensor devices which were quantitatively applied and objective with the measurement under fixed torque or load were commercially available [16-20] or individually developed or modified [21-24].

Asano et al. [25] used a commercially available tensor combined with their original measured torque-driver was and were able to measure the load at every 1 mm interval of gap distance. However, their method could only be used for measurement with an everted, and thereby unphysiological, patellar orientation, without the prosthesis, and only at extension or 90° of flexion.

D'Lima DD et al. developed a knee arthroplasty tibial tray with force transducers and a telemetry system to directly measure tibiofemoral compressive forces in vivo [26, 27]. From 1996, the study group spent time refining manufacturing techniques, improving durability, and safety testing and then reported the first electronic knee prosthesis implant in 2004. Recently, they summarized the design, development, and in vivo use of two generations of electronic knee prosthesis with activities of daily living, rehabilitation, exercise, and athletic activities from their many studies [28]. Although this device provides a lot of useful information on kinematics after TKA, it is too specialized and expensive for routine clinical use. The implantable tibial tray with force transducers and telemetry system is useful for research, but needs a bulky implant with an extension stem-like structure, and cannot be used with other TKA systems, limiting to the population used.

3. New soft tissue balance assessment with offset type tensor

3.1 Design and parameters

In order to permit soft tissue balancing under more physiological conditions, in a surgeon friendly manner, we developed a new third-generation tensor to obtain soft tissue balancing throughout the range of motion with reduced patella-femoral (PF) and aligned tibiofemoral joints [29]. The offset type tensor consists of three parts: an upper seesaw plate, a lower platform plate with a spike and an extra-articular main body (Fig 1). Both plates are placed at the center of the knee, and we apply one of two tensioning devices that are catered to appropriately fit either a cruciate-retaining (CR) or a posterior-stabilized (PS) TKA. The PS TKA tensor consists of a seesaw plate with a proximal post along the center that fits the inter-condylar space, as well as a cam for the femoral trial prosthesis. This post and cam mechanism controls the tibiofemoral position in both the coronal and sagittal planes. The CR TKA tensor consists of a seesaw plate with a proximal convex shaped centralizer that fits the inter-condylar space and controls coronal joint alignment. These mechanisms permit us to reproduce the joint constraint and alignment after implanting the prostheses. This device is ultimately designed to permit surgeons to measure the ligament balance in varus and joint center/joint component gap, while applying a constant joint distraction force. Joint distraction forces ranging from 30lb (13.6 kg) to 80lb (36.3 kg) can be exerted between the seesaw and platform plates through a specially made torque driver which can change the applied torque value. After sterilization, this torque driver is placed on a rack that contains a pinion mechanism along the extra-articular main body, and the appropriate torque is applied to generate the designated distraction force; in preliminary *in-vitro* experiments, we obtained an error for joint distraction within ± 3 %. Once appropriately distracted, attention is focused on two scales that correspond to the tensor: the angle (°, positive value in varus ligament balance) between the seesaw and platform plates, and the distance (mm) between the center midpoints of upper surface of the seesaw plate and the proximal tibial cut (mm, joint center/joint component gap). By measuring these angular deviations and distances under a constant joint distraction force, we are able to measure the ligament balance and joint center/joint component gaps, respectively.

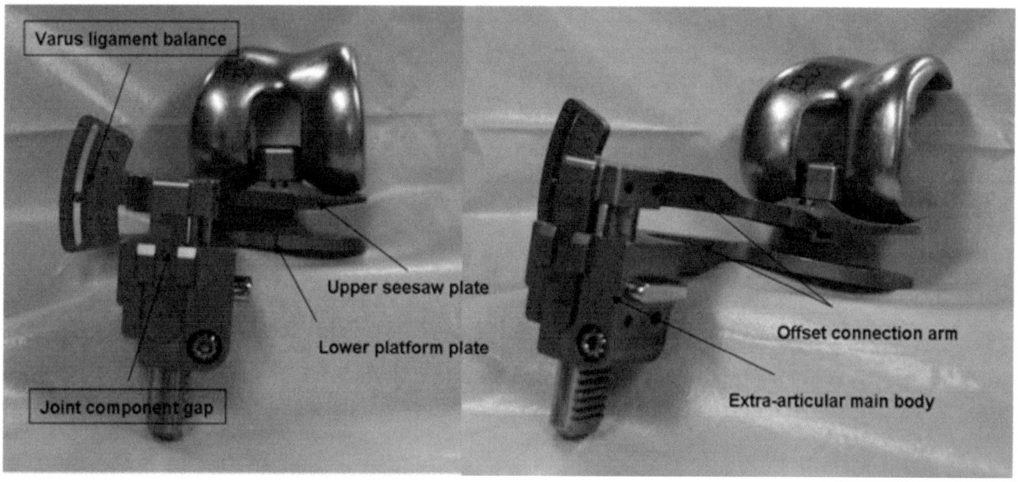

Fig. 1. Offset type tensor
The tensor consists of three parts: upper seesaw plate, lower platform plate and extra-articular main body. Two plates are connected to the extra-articular main body by the offset connection arm.

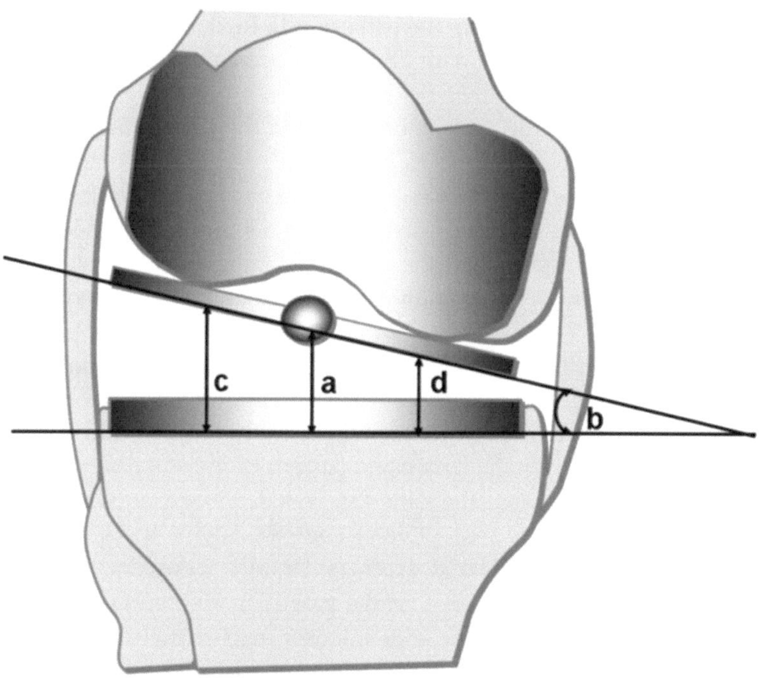

Fig. 2. Illustration showing parameters obtained and calculated.
a. Joint center gap/ joint component gap.
b. Varus ligament balance/ varus angle.
c. Lateral compartment gap
d. Medial compartment gap

Using the tensor, the following parameters can be calculated from the values: *joint component gap (joint center gap)* and *varus ligament balance (varus angle)* (Fig 2).

Joint looseness = "Component gap" - "Insert thickness"

Medial compartment gap = "Component gap" - 0.5× "Width between medial and lateral apex of femoral component representing the contact points to polyethylene insert" ×sin(varus angle)

Lateral compartment gap = "Component gap" + 0.5× "Width between medial and lateral apex of femoral component representing the contact points to polyethylene insert" ×sin(varus angle)

3.2 Soft tissue balance with reduced PF joint

We reported our experience using this device for intra-operative measurement with the PS TKA and further discussed the clinical relevance of this tensor [30-32]. First, we reported joint component gap kinematics in PS TKA with and without patellar eversion. The component gap showed an accelerated decrease during full knee extension. With the PF joint everted, the component gap increased throughout knee flexion. In contrast, the component gap with the PF joint reduced increased with knee flexion but decreased after 60° of flexion [30]. Secondly, we reported that intra-operative joint component gap kinematic assessment with reduced PF joint has the possibility to predict the post-operative flexion angle and thus allows evaluation of the surgical technique throughout the range of knee motion. Both an increased value during the extension to flexion gap and a decreased value during the flexion to deep flexion gap with PF joint reduced, not everted, showed an inverse correlation with the post-operative knee flexion angle, not pre-operative flexion angle [31]. Thirdly, we demonstrated that the correlations between the soft tissue balance assessed by the tensor and the navigation system were higher with reduced PF joint than everted PF joint, suggesting that surgeons should assess soft tissue balance during PS TKA with the PF joint reduced when using a navigation system [32]. In a series of intraoperative soft tissue balance assessments, we emphasized the importance of maintaining a reduced and anatomically oriented PF joint in order to obtain accurate and more physiologically-relevant soft tissue balancing.

Recent studies have emphasized the importance of the physiological post-operative knee condition in assessing soft tissue balance with PF joint reduction and femoral trial replacement in place [33-35]. Using our tensor with a 5-mm-long minute uniaxial foil strain gauge, Gejyo et al. reported a similar kinematic pattern of intra-operative joint component gap; when the patella was reduced, the joint gap was decreased at 90 and 135 degrees of flexion (by 1.9 mm and 5.5 mm, respectively) compared with the gap with the patella everted. Patellar tendon strain at 90 degrees of flexion, increasing with knee flexion, correlated with the joint gap difference with the patella in everted and reduced positions. Based on their study, they concluded the knee extensor mechanism might have an influence on the joint gap and be important in achieving the optimal joint gap balance during TKA [33]. With the use of an original tensor device which can measure the load of the spread joint gap, Yoshino et al. reported a significant difference between the loads in the patella everted position and thr reset position in flexion, not in extension, in PS TKA. However, in CR-TKA, they reported no significant difference between the loads in patella everted position and in patella reset position at either extension or flexion. Therefore, they concluded that the load in the flexion gap will increase in PS TKA or, in other words, the flexion gap distance will decrease by resetting [34]. With the use of an offset type tensor which has been developed based on our tensor, Kamei et al. reported a joint gap size and inclination measured intraoperatively on a knee in 90° flexion, with and without patellar eversion [35]. In the condition after tibial and distal femoral cut, they showed that the joint gap with patella in situ (17.0±3.4 mm) was significantly greater than with patellar eversion (15.4±3.0 mm), as was gap inclination at 90° flexion with the patella in situ (4.9±3.1°) compared to with patellar eversion (4.0±2.9°). Based on the results, they speculated that the steeper flexion gap inclination obtained without patellar eversion than with patellar eversion induced more externally rotated femoral positioning in the absence of patellar eversion. They emphasized that these results ought to be taken into account by surgeons considering switching from conventional to MIS-TKA.

3.3 Soft tissue balance with femoral component in place

The main concepts of measurement using the new tensor are, different from the conventional tensioning devise, with femoral trial component in place as well as a reduced PF joint. As the next step, accordingly, we focused on the difference in soft tissue balancing between the femoral trial component in place and the conventional osteotomized condition. In the intraoperative assessment of soft tissue balance, the joint gap showed significant decrease at extension, not flexion, after femoral trial prosthesis placement, and varus ligament balances were significantly reduced at extension and increased at flexion after femoral trial placement [36]. These changes at extension might be caused by the tensed posterior structures of the knee with the posterior condyle of the externally rotated aligned femoral trial. At knee flexion, a medial tension in the extensor mechanisms might be increased after femoral trial placement with PF joint repaired, and increased ligament balance in varus. We measured the "joint component gap", which is remarkably different from more conventional gap measurement. The joint component gap is measured with the femoral component in place, whereas the conventional gap measurement is made between the cutting surfaces of the femur and tibia. By keeping the femoral component in place, the knee is afforded a greater degree of extension because of its curving arc. In this arrangement, the posterior condyles of the component tighten the posterior capsule, resulting in a smaller joint gap at full extension. In addition, due to the 7 degree posterior slope of the tibia and a slight femoral anterior bowing, we can consider the "conventional extension gap" to be at about 10 degrees of the knee flexion angle. Mihalko et al. stated that the release of more posterior structures had a greater effect on the extension gap than on the flexion gap in explaining the importance of the relationship between posterior structures and the extension gap in a cadaver study [37]. Sugama et al. reported in their operative study that a bone cut from the posterior femoral condyles could change the tension of the posterior soft tissue structures and so alter the width and shape of the extension gap [38]. These previous reports support our hypothetical mechanism.

4. Soft tissue balance in CR and PS TKA

The Our above mentioned series of studies were only implemented with PS TKA. The long term results of CR and PS TKAs have shown an ability to relieve pain and improve function.

Nevertheless, the superiority of the CR or PS TKA remains a source of great controversy in the field of TKA. Proponents of the CR TKA advocate maintaining the PCL in order to increase stability, promote femoral rollback, and thereby enhance the patient's ability to climb stairs [39-43], while proponents of the PS TKA highlight studies in which patients with a resected PCL display a greater post-operative range of motion [43-45]. It is important to note in this debate, however, that investigators have been unable to show a difference in clinical outcome between both types of knees [41, 42, 46]. We have previously shown that among patients undergoing bilateral TKAs performed by the same surgeon, including a CR and PS TKA in alternate knees of the same patient, there was no difference in the post-operative knee score, yet the post-operative range of motion was significantly superior after resecting the PCL [47]. Accordingly, we extended our previous study and report on our experience with this device for the intra-operative soft tissue balance measurements of CR and PS TKAs, performed with both a reduced and everted patella.

While the joint component gap measurements with a reduced patella of PS TKA increased from extension to flexion, these values remained constant for CR TKA throughout the full range of motion. Additionally, the joint component gaps at deep knee flexion were significantly smaller for both types of prosthetic knees when the PF joint was reduced [48]. From our data, the CR TKA had stable joint kinematics from extension into deep flexion, while the joint kinematics for the PS TKA were more dynamic. Our data thereby supports prior studies indicating that the CR TKA affords patients greater stability. Our data further indicate that, compared to a CR TKA, a PS TKA with a reduced patella results in significantly larger gaps when the arc of motion ranges from mid- to deep-flexion.

In the assessment of varus/vagus balance, while the measurements of varus ligament balance with a reduced patella in PS TKA slightly increased from extension to flexion, these values slightly decreased for CR TKA from extension to flexion [49]. The data showed that CR TKA produced constant soft-tissue tension from extension into deep flexion, whereas PS TKA produced soft-tissue tension that tended to be more in varus during flexion. The PCL in knees with osteoarthritis is considered relatively rigid and shortened, despite being relatively macroscopically intact. Our findings indicate that compared with CR TKA, PS TKA with the patella reduced results in a significantly larger varus angle when the arc of motion is between midrange and deep flexion. After performing the independent cut procedure, we applied 3 or 5° of external rotation in the series of studies when setting the femoral component, which may have caused a decreasing varus balance in flexion for those patients who underwent CR TKA. Some studies indicated that the flexion gap in healthy knees is not rectangular and that the lateral joint gap is significantly lax [50-53]. The use of both a traditional soft-tissue release and the measured resection technique for knees with osteoarthritis in varus produces a pattern of soft-tissue tension that may at least partly explain why PS TKA produces a better postoperative range of motion.

Taken together, the kinematic patterns of soft tissue balance differ between the patellae everted and reduced, as well as between PS and CR TKA (Fig. 3). In light of these findings, we should carefully select patients according to the condition of their PCL, set an appropriate angle of external rotation, or do both if we wish to obtain good outcomes in CR TKA.

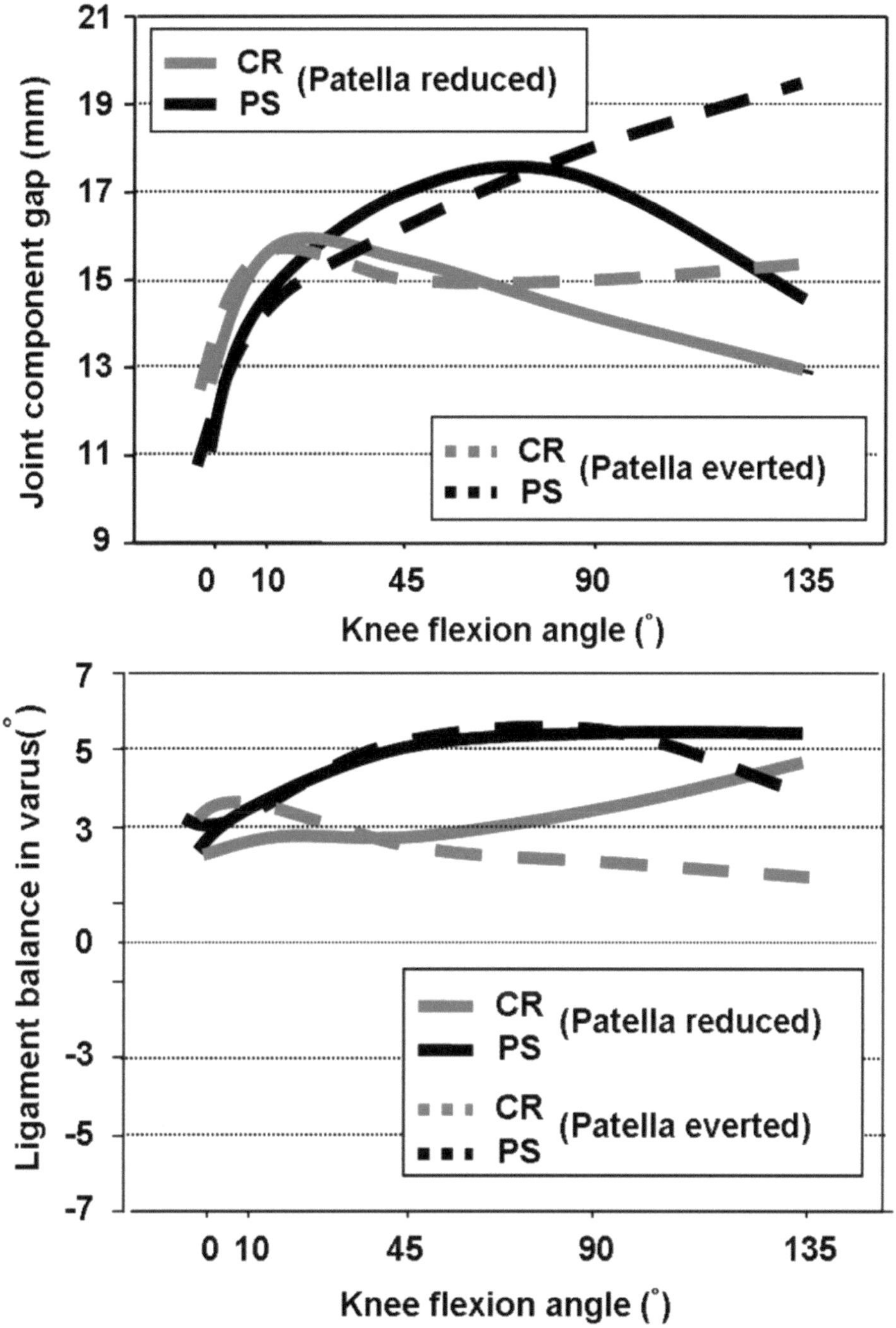

Fig. 3. Soft tissue balance in CR and PS TKA
a. Joint component gap pattern throughout the range of motion differs between CR and PS TKA as well as between the everted and reduced PF joint condition.
b. Varus ligament balance throughout the range of motion differs between CR and PS TKA as well as between the everted and reduced PF joint condition.

5. Soft tissue balance in MIS TKA

Recently, minimal incision surgery (MIS) TKA is widely promoted as a possible improvement over conventional TKA. The major advantages of MIS TKA over conventional TKA is the smaller skin incision required, and the avoidance of patellar eversion and quadriceps muscle splitting, leading to reduced blood loss, less perioperative pain, shorter length of hospital stay, and earlier return of knee function [54-61]. Although traditional TKA allow for excellent visualization, component orientation, and fixation, and have been associated with remarkable long-term implant survival, MIS TKA is attractive because of the small incision, and minimal or no pain and discomfort associated with surgery. However, while there is some evidence that these short-term benefits occur with MIS TKA [49-56], there is concern because of an increase in complications using the MIS technique, including vascular injury [62], patellar tendon injury [63, 64], condylar fracture [65], wound dehiscence and necrosis [65, 66], and component malalignment [54, 67-69]. In particular, the quadriceps-sparing (QS) approach has been developed as the least-invasive approach to the extensor mechanism by limiting medial parapatellar arthrotomy to the superior pole of the patella [70]. Although new surgical instrument designs enable surgeons to use this approach, this technique remains challenging to perform without causing damage to the vastus medialis obliquus (VMO) due to the limited working space [71, 72].

Accordingly, we compared intraoperative soft tissue balance measurements of MIS QS and conventional TKA, performed with the patella and femoral component in place. Whereas the joint component gap in MIS QS-TKA was significantly larger through the entire arc of flexion compared with conventional TKA, the pattern of joint looseness (joint component gap-polyethylene insert thickness) showed no difference between the two procedures. The varus ligament balance in MIS QS-TKA was significantly larger than that in conventional TKA at 0, 90, and 135 degrees of knee flexion [73]. The study suggested that MIS-TKA may lead to ligament imbalance due to the difficulties induced by a limited working space.

6. Influence of intra-operative soft tissue balance on post-operative flexion angle

Factors influencing the range of flexion after TKA can mainly be classified as intra-capsular or extra-capsular factors. Among extra-capsular factors the importance of pre-operative motion for post-operative results has been previously recognized [74-78]. Similarly, the pre-operative tightness of the extensor mechanism is an important factor influencing the post-operative knee flexion angle [79]. In contrast, intra-capsular factors, including implant design, ligament balancing, flexion-extension gap balance, height of the joint line, and patella resurfacing, have also been discussed by many authors [80-85]. Among such factors, although soft tissue balancing has been recognized as the essential surgical intervention for improving the outcome of TKA, the direct relationship between soft tissue balance and postoperative outcomes has never been clarified. As another concept of the joint condition, posterior condylar offset has recently been described as a determinant for flexion [86-88]. A mean reduction in flexion of 12° was reported to be found with every 2 mm decrease in offset [86]. Although posterior condylar offset is thought to be related to flexion gap, this relationship has not been discussed.

In the series of studies in PS TKA, joint gap change value ($90\text{-}0^{o}$) with PF joint reduced, not everted, showed inverse correlation with post-operative knee flexion angle ($R=-0.484$, p=0.019) and posterior condylar offset (R=-0.62, p=0.002) [31]. However, in another series of studies in CR TKA, the post-operative flexion angle was positively correlated with the joint gap change value (90-0°). In either case, multivariate regression analysis among various values including various joint gap change values, ligament balance, and pre-operative knee flexion angle demonstrated the pre-operative knee flexion angle and the joint gap change value (90-0°) had a significant independent result on post-operative knee flexion angle [89]. One of the reasons for this discrepancy may be the different patterns of soft tissue balance between PS and CR TKA [48, 49]. In that report, CR TKA showed significantly smaller gaps when the arc of movement ranged from mid- to deep flexion, compared to PS TKA [48]. The posterior cruciate ligament in osteoarthritic knee is considered relatively rigid and shortened despite being relatively macroscopically intact. When we consider flexion gap tightness, Ritter et al. reported that 30% of CR TKA required ligament balancing to obtain a smooth flexion arc [90]. If the PCL was too tight, excessive femoral rollback resulted in anterior lift-off of the tibial trial in flexion, leading to a limitation of flexion [91]. To make a better post-operative flexion angle, balancing the flexion gap can result in a satisfactory range of motion [92, 93]. In our series of studies in CR TKA, it was identified that 16% more flexion gap tightness (smaller flexion gap than extension gap) resulted in a smaller flexion angle. Similarly, using a commercially available knee balancer with the measurement under 80 N distraction force, Higuchi et al reported flexion medial/lateral gap tightness led to restriction of the flexion angle [94]. Therefore, in these cases, surgeons are advised to avoid flexion gap tightness by soft tissue release such as PCL [90, 91, 95].

7. Influence of preoperative deformity on intra-operative soft tissue balance

Pre-operative deformity of the knee differs from patient to patient. In the varus knee especially, many surgeons recognize that progressive shortening or contraction of soft tissue structures on the medial side may occur, whereas the lateral structures may become stretched [96-99]. Although severe intra-operative varus deformity needs substantial soft tissue release on the medial side during TKA, the ideal amount of medial release is still controversial; two strategies exist for soft tissue balancing in the varus knee. Some surgeons believe it is best to create equal medial and lateral gaps even in severely deformed knees [2, 100, 101]. Others accept some degree of lateral laxity is permissible, as long as proper alignment is maintained, based on evidence showing post-operative diminishment with time of lateral laxity after TKA [102, 103].

Accordingly, we compared intra-operative soft tissue balance measurements in various grades of preoperative varus deformity (10° < varus deformity, 10° < varus deformity < 20°, varus deformity >20°) during PS TKA, performed with a reduced patella. In the comparison of the changing pattern of joint component gap among the three different pre-operative deformity groups, we observed similar kinematic patterns showing an increase until 90° of knee flexion and a decrease towards deep knee flexion, and no difference among the groups throughout the flexion angle of the knee. In the comparison of medial-lateral ligamentous balance, on the other hand, the varus angle showed significant larger values in the varus alignment > 20° group compared to that of the other two groups throughout knee flexion in spite of similar patterns showing slight increases in the varus angle to 90° of knee flexion and constant balance after that. These results indicate that appropriate medial-lateral balancing is difficult in knees with severe pre-operative varus deformity, especially with varus alignment > 20° [104].

Even in normal knees, lateral ligamentous laxity and medial ligamentous laxity are not balanced and more lateral ligamentous laxity than medial ligamentous laxity has been observed [105-107]. To restore the joint line, we believe lateral laxity of less than 5 degrees is permissible in the varus alignment < 20° groups as long as proper alignment is maintained [102, 103, 108]. In such severely deformed varus knees, some surgeons may recommend the complete release of medial-sided structures including an MCL cut for achievement of a well-balanced knee [109]. However, we avoided this procedure due to the potential widening of the joint gap with elongation of the lower extremity, and subsequent patella baja as a result of joint line elevation due to a thicker polyethylene insert. Therefore, results in this series may be based on these operative procedures.

8. Soft tissue balance in gap technique

In the above mentioned study, soft tissue balance measurements were only performed in posterior-stabilized (PS) or cruciate-retaining (CR) TKAs using the measured resection technique. However, the best method of obtaining rotational alignment of the femoral component in flexion remains controversial. Some investigators favor a measured resection technique in which bony landmarks (femoral epicondyles, posterior femoral condyles, or the anteroposterior axis) are the primary determinants of femoral component rotation [110-115]. Others recommend a gap-balancing methodology in which the femoral component is positioned parallel to the resected proximal tibia with each collateral ligament equally tensioned [116-118]. Under such debate, several surgeons recently reported more consistent equalization of extension and flexion gaps with the use of computer-assisted gap balancing technique, compared with conventional measured resection technique [119, 120]. In contrast, in the comparison between the navigation-assisted measured resection and navigation-assisted gap balancing technique, some surgeons reported a better restoration of the joint line position in the navigation-assisted measured resection technique despite no differences in short-term clinical outcomes [120, 121].

Using the offset type tensor, which can be used in the gap technique [123], we performed soft tissue balance assessment during CR TKA using the tibia first gap technique with navigation system. With the tibia first gap technique, the kinematics of the component gap showed a similar pattern to the measured resection technique during CR TKA; following a significant increase during the initial 30° of knee flexion, the joint component gap showed a gradual decrease toward 120° of flexion [48, 89]. After that, soft tissue balance was assessed at extension and flexion between the basic value after tibial cut and the final value following femoral cut and with femoral component in place. The basic value of the joint gap before femoral osteotomy reflected the final value following femoral cut and with femoral component in place (unpublished data). Accordingly, the tibia first gap technique may have the advantage that surgeons can predict the final soft tissue balance from that before femoral osteotomies.

9. Summary

In the series of study using offset type tensor with PF joint reduced and femoral component in place, the kinematic pattern of intraoperative joint gap and ligament balance can be observed in TKA when they are performed while preserving a more physiological condition of the knee. Additionally, various factors influencing soft tissue balance such as patellar orientation, PS/CR type of prosthesis design, MIS/conventional technique, grade of preoperative deformity, and operation procedures, measured resection or gap technique can be examined. We believe the information provided by the use of the offset type tensor is useful and essential for providing insight into true post-operative kinematics, and thus by maintaining a reduced patella for each intra-operative measurement, the surgeon will be able to adjust the soft tissue balance more accurately and thereby expect a better post-operative outcome.

10. References

[1] Insall JN, Tria AJ, Scott WN. The total condylar knee prosthesis: the first 5 years. *Clin Orthop Relat Res.* 1979; 145: 68

[2] Insall JN, Binazzi R, Soudry M, Mestriner LA. Total knee arthroplasty. *Clin Orthop Relat Res.* 1985; 192: 13

[3] Dorr LD, Boiardo RA. Technical consideration in total knee arthroplasty. *Clin Orthop Relat Res.* 1986; 205: 5

[4] Stulberg SD, Loan P, Sarin V. Computer-assisted navigation in total knee replacement: results of an initial experience in thirty-five patients. J Bone Joint Surg Am 2002;84-A Suppl 2:90-8.

[5] Sparmann M, Wolke B, Czupalla H, Banzer D, Zink A. Positioning of total knee arthroplasty with and without navigation support. A prospective, randomised study. J Bone Joint Surg Br 2003;85:830-5.

[6] Laskin RS, Beksac B. Computer-assisted navigation in TKA: where we are and where we are going. Clin Orthop Relat Res 2006;452:127-31.

[7] Lutzner J, Krummenauer F, Wolf C, Gunther KP, Kirschner S. Computer-assisted and conventional total knee replacement: a comparative, prospective, randomised study with radiological and CT evaluation. J Bone Joint Surg Br 2008;90:1039-44.

[8] Matsumoto T, Tsumura N, Kurosaka M, Muratsu H, Kuroda R, Ishimoto K, Tsujimoto K, Shiba R, Yoshiya S. Prosthetic Alignment and Sizing in Computer-Assisted Total Knee Arthroplasty. *Int Orthop.* 28: 282-285, 2004

[9] Matsumoto T, Tsumura N, Kurosaka M, Muratsu H, Yoshiya S, Kuroda R. Clinical Values in Computer-Assisted Total Knee Arthroplasty. *Orthopedics.* 29(12): 1115-1120, 2006

[10] Ishida K, Matsumoto T, Tsumura N, Kubo S, Kitagawa A, Iguchi T, Kurosaka M, Kuroda R. Clinical Outcomes of Computer-assisted Total Knee Arthroplasty: Mid-term Results of Minimum 5 Years. *Knee Surg Sports Traumatol Arthrosc.* [Epub ahead of print]

[11] Fehring TK, Odum S, Griffin WL, Mason JB, Nadaud M. Early failures in total knee arthroplasty. *Clin Orthop Relat Res* 392: 315-318, 2001

[12] Sharkey PF, Hozack WJ, Rothman RH, Shastri S, Jacoby SM. Insall award paper. Why are total knee arthroplasties failing today? *Clin Orthop Relat Res* 404: 7–13, 2002

[13] Griffin FM, Insall JN, Scuderi GR. Accuracy of soft tissue balancing in total knee arthroplasty. *J Arthroplasty.* 15: 970-973, 2000

[14] Insall JN (1984) Total knee replacement. In: Insall JN (ed) Surgery of the knee. Churchill-Livingstone, New York

[15] Freeman MAR, Todd RC, Bamert P, Day WH (1978) ICLH arthroplasty of the knee: 1968–1977. J Bone Joint Surg 60-B:339–344

[16] Attfield SF, Warren-Forward M, Wilton T, Sambatakakis A (1994) Measurement of soft tissue imbalance in total knee arthroplasty using electronic instrumentation. Med Eng Phys 16:501–505
[17] Booth RE (2003) Tensioners: essential for accurate performance of TKA. Orthopedics 26:962–964
[18] Winemakaer MJ (2002) Perfect balance in total knee arthroplasty. J Arthroplasty 17:2–10
[19] Sambatakakis A, Attfield SF, Newton G. Quantification of soft-tissue imbalance in condylar knee arthroplasty. *J Biomed Eng.* 15: 339-343, 1993
[20] Unitt L, Sambatakakis A, Johnstone D, Briggs TW; Balancer Study Group. Short-term outcome in total knee replacement after soft-tissue release and balancing. *J Bone Joint Surg Br.* 90:159-65, 2008
[21] Viskontas DG, Skrinskas TV, Johnson JA, King GJ, Winemaker MJ, Chess DG (2007) Computer-assisted gap equalization in total knee arthroplasty. J Arthroplasty 22:334–342
[22] Wasielewski RC, Galat DD, Komistek RD (2005) Correlation of compartment pressure data from an intraoperative sensing device with postoperative fluoroscopic kinematic results in TKA patients. J Biomech 38:333–339
[23] Yagishita K, Muneta T, Ikeda H (2003) Step-by-step measurement of soft tissue balancing during total knee arthroplasty for patients with varus knees. J Arthroplasty 18:313–320
[24] Zalzal P, Papini M, Petruccelli D, de Beer J, Winemaker MJ (2004) An in vivo biomechanical analysis of the soft-tissue envelope of osteoarthritis knees. J Arthroplasty 19:217–223
[25] Asano H, Hoshino A, Wilton T (2004) Soft-tissue tension total knee arthroplasty. J Arthroplasty 19:558–561
[26] D'Lima DD, Patil S, Steklov N, Slamin JE, Colwell CW Jr (2006) Tibial force measured in vivo after total knee arthroplasty. J Arthroplasty 21:255–262
[27] Morris BA, D'Lima DD, Slamin J, Kovacevic N, Arms SW, Townsend CP, Colwell Jr CW (2001) e-Knee: evolution of the electronic knee prosthesis. J Bone Joint Surg 83-A(supplement 2, Part 1):62–66
[28] D'Lima DD, Patil S, Steklov N, Colwell CW Jr. The 2011 ABJS Nicolas Andry Award: 'Lab'-in-a-Knee: In Vivo Knee Forces, Kinematics, and Contact Analysis. Clin Orthop Relat Res. 2011 May 20. [Epub ahead of print]
[29] Muratsu H, Tsumura N, Yamaguchi M, Mizuno K, Kuroda R, Harada T, Yoshiya S, Kurosaka M. Patellar eversion affects soft tissue balance in total knee arthroplasty. *Trans Orthop Res Soc.* 28: 242, 2003
[30] Matsumoto T, Muratsu H, Tsumura N, Mizuno K, Kuroda R, Yoshiya S, Kurosaka M. Joint gap kinematics in posterior-stabilized total knee arthroplasty measured by a new tensor with the navigation system. *J Biomech Eng.* 128 (6): 867-871, 2006
[31] Matsumoto T, Mizuno K, Muratsu H, Tsumura N, Fukase N, Seiji K, Yoshiya S, Kurosaka M, Kuroda R. Influence of Intra-operative Joint Gap on Post-operative Flexion Angle in Osteoarthritis Patients Undergoing Posterior-Stabilized Total Knee Arthroplasty. *Knee Surg Sports Traumatol Arthrosc.* 15(8): 1013-1008, 2007
[32] Matsumoto T, Muratsu H, Tsumura N, Mizuno K, Kurosaka M, Kuroda R. Soft tissue balance measurement in posterior-stabilized total knee arthroplasty with a navigation system. *J Althroplasty.* 24(3): 358-64, 2009

[33] Gejo, R., Y. Morita, I. Matsushita, K. Sugimori, and T. Kimura. Joint gap changes with patellar tendon strain and patellar position during TKA. *Clin Orthop Relat Res.* 466:946-51, 2008

[34] Yoshino, N., N. Watanabe, Y. Watanabe, Y. Fukuda, and S. Takai. Measurement of joint gap load in patella everted and reset position during total knee arthroplasty. *Knee Surg Sports Traumatol Arthrosc.* 17:484-90, 2010

[35] Kamei G, Kamei G, Murakami Y, Kazusa H, Hachisuka S, Inoue H, Nobutou H, Nishida K, Mochizuki Y, Ochi M. Is patella eversion during total knee arthroplasty crucial for gap adjustment and soft-tissue balancing? *Orthop Traumatol Surg Res.* 97(3):287-91, 2011.

[36] Muratsu H, Matsumoto T, Maruo A, Miya H, Kurosaka M, Kuroda R. Femoral component placement chnges soft tissue balance in posterior-stabilized total knee arthroplasty. *Clin Biomech.* 25(9): 926-30, 2010

[37] Mihalko, W.M., L.A. Whiteside, and K.A. Krackow. 2003. Comparison of ligament-balancing techniques during total knee arthroplasty. *J Bone Joint Surg Am.* 85-A Suppl 4:132-5.

[38] Sugama, R., Y. Kadoya, A. Kobayashi, and K. Takaoka. 2005. Preparation of the flexion gap affects the extension gap in total knee arthroplasty. *J Arthroplasty.* 20:602-7.

[39] Andriacchi TP, Andersson GB, Fermier RW, Stern D, Galante JO. A study of lower-limb mechanics during stair-climbing. *J Bone Joint Surg Am.* 1980; 62(5); 749-757.

[40] Andriacchi TP, Galante JO, Fermier RW. The influence of total knee-replacement design on walking and stair-climbing. *J Bone Joint Surg Am.* 1982; 64(9): 1328-1335.

[41] Becker MW, Insall JN, Faris PM. Bilateral total knee arthroplasty. One cruciate retaining and one cruciate substituting. *Clin Orthop Relat Res.* 1991; 271: 122-124.

[42] Dorr LD, Ochsner JL, Gronley J, Perry J. Functional comparison of posterior cruciate-retained versus cruciate-sacrificed total knee arthroplasty. *Clin Orthop Relat Res.* 1988; 236: 36-43.

[43] Maloney WJ, Schurman DJ. The effects of implant design on range of motion after total knee arthroplasty. Total condylar versus posterior stabilized total condylar designs. *Clin Orthop Relat Res.* 1992; 278: 147-152.

[44] Hirsch HS, Lotke PA, Morrison LD. The posterior cruciate ligament in total knee surgery. Save, sacrifice, or substitute? *Clin Orthop Relat Res.* 1994; 309: 64-68.

[45] Insall JN, Hood RW, Flawn LB, Sullivan DJ. The total condylar knee prosthesis in gonarthrosis. A five to nine-year follow-up of the first one hundred consecutive replacements. *J Bone Joint Surg Am.* 1983; 65(5): 619-628.

[46] Udomkiat P, Meng BJ, Dorr LD, Wan Z. Functional comparison of posterior cruciate retention and substitution knee replacement. *Clin Orthop Relat Res.* 2000; 378:192-201.

[47] Maruyama S, Yoshiya S, Matsui N, Kuroda R, Kurosaka M. Functional comparison of posterior cruciate-retaining versus posterior stabilized total knee arthroplasty. *J Arthroplasty.* 2004; 19(3): 349-53.

[48] Matsumoto T, Kuroda R , Kubo S, Muratsu H, Mizuno K, Kurosaka M. The intra-operative joint gap in cruciate-retaining compared with posterior-stabilizsed total knee replacement. *J Bone Joint Surg Br.* 91(4): 475-80, 2009

[49] Matsumoto T, Muratsu H, Kubo S, Matsushita T, Kurosaka M, Kuroda R. Soft-tissue tension in cruciate-retaining and posterior-stabilized total knee arthroplasty. *J Arthroplasty*. [Epub ahead of print]
[50] Malkolf KL, Mensch JS, Amstutz HC. Stiffness and laxity of the knee—the contributions of the supporting structures. A quantitative in vitro study. J Bone Joint Surg Am 1976;58:583
[51] Seering WP, Piziali RL, Nagel DA, Schurman DJ. The function of the primary ligaments of the knee in varus-valgus and axial rotation. J Biomech 1980;13:785
[52] Moore TM, Meyers MH, Harvey JP Jr. Collateral ligament laxity of the knee. Long-term comparison between plateau fractures and normal. J Bone Joint Surg Am 1976;58:594
[53] Tokuhara Y, Kadoya Y, Nakagawa S, Kobayashi A, Takaoka K. The flexion gap in normal knees. An MRI study. J Bone Joint Surg Br 2004;86:1133
[54] Chen AF, Alan RK, Redziniak DE, Tria AJ Jr (2006) Quadriceps sparing total knee replacement. The initial experience with results at two to four years. J Bone Joint Surg Br 88: 1448-1453
[55] Hass SB, Cook S, Beksac B (2004) Minimally invasive total knee replacement through a mini midvastus approach: A comparative study. Clin Orthop Relat Res 428: 68-73
[56] Kashyap SN, Van Ommeren JW (2008) Clinical experience with less invasive surgery techniques in total knee arthroplasty: a comparative study. Knee Surg Sports Traumatol Arthrosc 16: 544–548
[57] Laskin RS, Beksac B, Phongjunakom A, Pittors K, Shim JC, Pavlov H, Petersen M (2004) Minimally invasive total knee replacement through a mini-midvastus incision; an outcome study. Clin Orthop Relat Res 428: 74-81
[58] Lombardi AV Jr, Viacava AJ, Berend KR (2006) Rapid recovery protocols and minimally invasive surgery help achieve high knee flexion. Clin Orthop Relat Res 452:117–122
[59] Luring C, Beckmann J, Haibo¨ck P, Perlick L, Grifka J, Tingart M (2008) Minimal invasive and computer assisted total knee replacement compared with the conventional technique: a prospective, randomized trial. Knee Surg Sports Traumatol Arthrosc 16: 928–934
[60] Schroer WC, Diesfeld PJ, Reedy ME, Lemarr AR (2010) Isokinetic strength testing of minimally invasive total knee arthroplasty recovery. J Arthroplasty 25: 274–279
[61] Tria Jr AJ, Coon TM (2003) Minimal incision total knee arthroplasty: early experience. Clin Orthop Relat Res 416: 185-190
[62] Tria Jr AJ. Advancements in minimally invasive total knee arthroplasty (2003) Orthopedics 26: s859
[63] Aglietti P, Baldini A, Sensi L (2006) Quadriceps-sparing versus mini-subvastus approach in total knee arthroplasty. Clin Orthop Relat Res 452: 106-111
[64] Boerger TO, Aglietti P, Mondanelli N, Sensi L (2005) Mini-subvastus versus medial parapatellar approach in total knee arthroplasty. Clin Orthop Relat Res 440: 82-87
[65] Kolisek FR, Bonutti PM, Hazack WJ, Purtill J, Sharkey PF, Zelicof SB, Ragland PS, Kester M, Mont MA, Rothman RH (2007) Clinical experience using a minimally invasive approach for total knee arthroplasty: early results of a prospective randomized study compared to a standard approach. J Arthroplasty 22: 8-13
[66] Pagnano MW, Meneghini RM (2006) Minimally invasive total knee arthroplasty with an optimized subvastus approach. J Arthroplasty 21: 22-26

[67] Dalury DF, Dennis DA (2005) Mini-incision total knee arthroplasty can increase risk of component malalignment. Clin Orthop Relat Res 440: 77-81

[68] Lin WP, Lin J, Horng LC, Chang SM, Jiang CC (2009) Quadriceps-sparing, minimal-incision total knee arthroplasty. A comparative study. J Arthroplasty 24: 1024-1032

[69] Yau WP, Leung A, Liu KG, Yan CH, Wong LS, Chiu KY (2008) Errors in the identification of the transepicondylar and anteroposterior axes of the distal femur in total knee replacement using minimally-invasive and conventional approaches. J Bone Joint Surg Br 90: 520-526

[70] Tria Jr AJ, Coon TM (2003) Minimal incision total knee arthroplasty: early experience. Clin Orthop Relat Res 416: 185-190

[71] Pagnano MW, Meneghini RM, Trousdale RT (2006) Anatomy of the extensor mechanism in reference to quadriceps-sparing TKA. Clin Orthop Relat Res 452: 102-105

[72] Robert VI, Mereddy PKR, Donnachie NJ, Hakkalamani S (2007) Anatomical variations in vastus medialis obliquus and its implications in minimally invasive total knee replacement. J Bone Joint Surg Br 89: 1462-1465

[73] Matsumoto T, Muratsu H, Kubo S, Mizuno K, Kinoshita K, Ishida K, Matsushita T, Sasaki K, Tei K, Takayama K, Sasaki H, Oka S, Kurosaka M, Kuroda R. Influence of minimum invasive approach of total knee arthroplasty on the soft tissue balance. *Knee Surg Sports Traumatol Arthrosc.* 19(6): 880-6, 2011

[74] Anouchi YS, McShane M, Kelly F Jr, Elting J, Stiehl, J. Range of motion in total knee replacement. *Clin Orthop Relat Res* 1996; 331: 87-91.

[75] Lizaur A, Marco L, Cebrian R. Preoperative factors influencing the range of movement after total knee arthroplasty for severe osteoarthritis. *J Bone Joint Surg [Br]* 1997; 79-B: 626-9.

[76] Harvey IA, Barry K, Kirby SP, Johnson R, Elloy MA. Factors affecting the range of movement of total knee arthroplasty. *J Bone Joint Surg [Br]* 1993; 75-B: 950-5.

[77] Parsley BS, Engh GA, Dwyer KA. Preoperative flexion. Dose it influence postoperative flexion after posterior-cruciate-retaining total knee arthroplasty? *Clin Orthop Relat Res* 1992; 275: 204-10.

[78] Ritter MA, Stringer EA. Predictive range of motion after total knee replacement. *Clin Orthop Relat Res* 1999; 143: 115-9.

[79] Matsumoto T, Tsumura N, Kubo S, Shiba R, Kurosaka M, Yoshiya S (2005) Influence of hip position on knee flexion angle in patients undergoing total knee arthroplasty. J Arthroplasty 20:669-673

[80] Dennis DA: *Problems After Knee Arthroplasty*. The Stiff Total Knee Arthroplasty: Causes and Cures. *Orthopedics* 2001; 24: 901-2.

[81] Harvey IA, Barry K, Kirby SPJ, Johnson R, Elloy MA: Factors affecting the range of movement of total knee arthroplasty. *J Bone Joint Surg [Br]* 1993; 75-B: 950-5.

[82] Kawamura H, Bourne RB. Factors affecting range of flexion after total knee arthroplasty. *J Orthop Sci* 2001; 6: 248-52.

[83] Schurman DJ, Matityahu A, Goodman SB, Maloney W, Woolson S, Shi, H, Bloch DA: Prediction of postoperative knee flexion in Insall-Burstein II total knee arthroplasty. *Clin Orthop Relat Re* 1998; 353: 175-84.

[84] Schurman DJ, Parker JN, Orstein D: Total condylar knee replacement. A study of factors influencing range of motion as late as two years after arthroplasty. *J Bone Joint Surg [Am]* 1985; 67-A: 1006-14.
[85] Joshi AB, Lee CM, Markovic L, Murphy JCM, Hardinge K: Total knee arthroplasty after patellectomy. *J Bone Joint Surg [Br]* 1994; 76-B: 926-9.
[86] Bellemans J, Banks S, Victor J, Vandenneucker H, Moemans A. Fluoroscopic analysis of the kinematics of deep flexion in total knee arthroplasty. Influence of posterior condylar offset. *J Bone Joint Surg [Br]* 2002; 84-B:50-3.
[87] Victor J, Bellemans J. Physiologic Kinematics as a Concept for Better Flexion in TKA. *Clin Orthop Relat Res* 2006 Aug 17; [Epub ahead of print]
[88] Kim YH, Sohn KS, Kim JS. Range of motion of standard and high-flexion posterior stabilized total knee prostheses. A prospective, randomized study. *J Bone Joint Surg [Am]* 2005; 87-A: 1470-5.
[89] Takayama K, Matsumoto T, Kubo S, Muratsu H, Ishida K, Matsushita T, Kurosaka M, Kuroda R. The Influence of Intra-operative Joint Gap on Post-operative Flexion Angle in Cruciate-retaining Total Knee Arthroplasty. Knee Surg Sports Traumatol Arthrosc [Epub ahead of print]
[90] Ritter MA, Faris PM, Keating EM (1988) Posterior cruciate ligament balancing during total knee arthroplasty. J Arthroplasty 3:323-326
[91] Kim H, Pelker RR, Gibson DH, Irving JF, Lynch JK (1997) Rollback in posterior cruciate ligament-retaining total knee arthroplasty. A radiographic analysis. J Arthroplasty 12:553-561
[92] Arima J, Whiteside LA, Martin JW, Miura H, White SE, McCarthy DS (1998) Effect of partial release of the posterior cruciate ligament in total knee arthroplasty. Clin Orthop Relat Res 353:194-202
[93] Lombardi AV, Jr., Berend KR, Aziz-Jacobo J, Davis MB (2008) Balancing the flexion gap: relationship between tibial slope and posterior cruciate ligament release and correlation with range of motion. J Bone Joint Surg Am 90 Suppl4. 121-132
[94] Higuchi H, Hatayama K, Shimizu M, Kobayashi A, Kobayashi T, Takagishi K. Relationship between joint gap difference and range of motion in total knee arthroplasty: a prospective randomised study between different platforms. Int Orthop. 2009;33(4):997-1000.
[95] Yamakado K, Kitaoka K, Yamada H, Hashiba K, Nakamura R, Tomita K (2003) Influence of stability on range of motion after cruciate-retaining TKA. Arch Orthop Trauma Surg 123:1-4
[96] Krackow KA, Mihalko WM. The effect of medial release on flexion and extension gaps in cadaveric knees: implications for soft-tissue balancing in total knee arthroplasty. *Am J Knee Surg*. 1999; 12(4) : 222
[97] Mihalko WM, Miller C, Krackow KA. Total knee arthroplasty ligament balancing and gap kinematics with posterior cruciate ligament retention and sacrifice. *Am J Orthop*. 2000; 29(8): 610
[98] Siston RA, Goodman SB, Delp SL, Giori NJ. Coronal plane stability before and after total knee arthroplasty. *Clin Orthop Relat Res*. 2007; 463: 43
[99] Mihalko WM, Saleh KJ, Krackow KA, Whiteside LA. Soft-tissue Balancing During Total Knee Arthroplasty in the Varus Knee. *J Am Acad Orthop Surg*. 2009; 17(12): 766

[100] Teeny SM, Krackow KA, Hungerford DS, Jones M. Primary total knee arthroplasty in patients with severe varus deformity. A comparative study. *Clin Orthop Relat Res.* 1991; 273: 19
[101] Winemaker MJ. Perfect balance in total knee arthroplasty: the elusive compromise. *J Arthroplasty.* 2002; 17(1): 2
[102] Lotke PA. Primary total knees: standard principles and techniques. In: Lotke PA, Lonner JH, eds. *Knee Arthroplasty.* Philadelphia, PA: Lippincott Williams & Wilkins; 2003: 49
[103] Sculco TP. Soft tissue balancing in total knee arthroplasty. In: Goldberg VM, ed. *Controversies of Total Knee Replacement.* New York, NY: Raven Press; 1991: 167
[104] Matsumoto T, Muratsu H, Kubo S, Matsushita T, Kurosaka M, Kuroda R. The Influence of Pre-operative Deformity on Intra-operative Soft Tissue Balance in Posterior-Stabilized Total Knee Arthroplasty. *J Arthroplasty.* [Epub ahead of print]
[105] Okazaki K, Miura H, Matsuda S, Takeuchi N, Mawatari T, Hashizume M, Iwamoto Y. Asymmetry of mediolateral laxity of the normal knee. *J Orthop Sci.* 2006; 11(3): 264
[106] Tokuhara Y, Kadoya Y, Nakagawa S, Kobayashi A, Takaoka K. The flexion gap in normal knees. An MRI study. *J Bone Joint Surg Br.* 2004; 86(8): 1133
[107] Nagamine R, Kondo K, Nomura H, Kanekasu K, Sonohata M, Sugioka Y. Shape of the joint gap for 90 degrees and 120 degrees knee flexion after total knee arthroplasty. *J Orthop Sci.* 2008; 13(4): 354
[108] Sekiya H, Takatoku K, Takada H, Sasanuma H, Sugimoto N. Postoperative lateral ligamentous laxity diminishes with time after TKA in the varus knee. *Clin Orthop Relat Res.* 2009; 467(6): 1582
[109] Mihalko WM, Saleh KJ, Krackow KA, Whiteside LA. Soft-tissue Balancing During Total Knee Arthroplasty in the Varus Knee. *J Am Acad Orthop Surg.* 2009; 17(12): 766
[110] Berger RA, Rubash HE, Seel MJ, Thompson WH, Crossett LS.Determining the rotational alignment of the femoral component in total knee arthroplasty using theepicondylar axis. Clin OrthopRelat Res. 1993;286:40–47.
[111] Griffin FM, Math K, Scuderi GR, Insall JN, Poilvache PL. Anatomy of the epicondyles of the distal femur: MRI analysis of normal knees. J Arthroplasty. 2000;15:354-359.
[112] Mantas JP, Bloebaum RD, Skedros JG, Hofmann AA. Implications of reference axes used for rotational alignment of the femoral component in primary and revision knee arthroplasty. J Arthroplasty. 1992;7:531–535.
[113] Poilvache PL, Insall JN, Scuderi GR, Font-Rodriguez DE. Rotational landmarks and sizing of the distal femur in total knee arthroplasty. Clin Orthop Relat Res. 1996;331:35–46.
[114] Schnurr C, Nessler J, Ko¨nig DP. Is referencing the posterior condyles sufficient to achieve a rectangular flexion gap in total knee arthroplasty? Int Orthop. 2008 Oct 28. [Epub ahead of print].
[115] Whiteside LA, Arima J. The anteroposterior axis for femoral rotational alignment in valgus total knee arthroplasty. Clin Orthop Relat Res. 1995;321:168–172.
[116] Dennis, DA. Measured resection: An outdated technique in total knee arthroplasty. Orthopedics. 2008;31:940, 943–944.
[117] Fehring TK. Rotational malalignment of the femoral component in total knee arthroplasty. Clin Orthop Relat Res. 2000;380: 72–79.

[118] Katz MA, Beck TD, Silber JS, Seldes RM, Lotke PA. Determining femoral rotational alignment in total knee arthroplasty: reliability of techniques. J Arthroplasty. 2001;16:301–305.
[119] Pang HN, Yeo SJ, Chong HC, Chin PL, Ong J, Lo NN. Computer-assisted gap balancing technique improves outcome in total knee arthroplasty, compared with conventional measured resection technique. Knee Surg Sports Traumatol Arthrosc. 2011 Mar 30. [Epub ahead of print]
[120] Seon JK, Song EK, Park SJ, Lee DS. The use of navigation to obtain rectangular flexion and extension gaps during primary total knee arthroplasty and midterm clinical results. J Arthroplasty. 2011 Jun;26(4):582-90. Epub 2010 Jun 26.
[121] Tigani D, Sabbioni G, Ben Ayad R, Filanti M, Rani N, Del Piccolo N. Comparison between two computer-assisted total knee arthroplasty: gap-balancing versus measured resection technique. Knee Surg Sports Traumatol Arthrosc. 2010 Oct;18(10):1304-10.
[122] Lee HJ, Lee JS, Jung HJ, Song KS, Yang JJ, Park CW. Comparison of joint line position changes after primary bilateral total knee arthroplasty performed using the navigation-assisted measured gap resection or gap balancing techniques. Knee Surg Sports Traumatol Arthrosc. 2011 Mar 23. [Epub ahead of print]
[123] Tanaka K, Muratsu H, Mizuno K, Kuroda R, Yoshiya S, Kurosaka M. Soft tissue balance measurement in anterior cruciate ligament-resected knee joint: cadaveric study as a model for cruciate-retaining total knee arthroplasty. J Orthop Sci. 2007 Mar;12(2):149-53. Epub 2007 Mar 30.

19

The Role of Drainage After Total Knee Arthroplasty

Ta-Wei Tai, Chyun-Yu Yang and Chih-Wei Chang
Department of Orthopedics,
National Cheng Kung University Hospital,
Tainan
Taiwan

1. Introduction

Total knee arthroplasty (TKA) is associated with significant postoperative blood loss for which blood transfusion might be necessary. The role of wound drainage is controversial. The use of drainage was believed to be effective in decreasing hematoma formation (Drinkwater and Neil 1995; Holt et al. 1997; Martin et al. 2004), which has been theoretically thought to decrease postoperative pain, swelling, and incidence of infection(Kim et al. 1998). However, a closed suction drainage system inevitably increases bleeding because the tamponade effect of a closed and undrained wound is eliminated. Though some studies have shown that drainage after TKA is not necessary(Adalberth et al. 1998; Niskanen et al. 2000; Esler et al. 2003; Parker et al. 2004; Jones et al. 2007), it is still widely used by orthopedic surgeons(Canty et al. 2003).

Surgeons who routinely drain total knee replacements may also use adjunctive measures such as autologous blood transfusion, use of fibrin tissue adhesive, compression bandaging and local ice packing(Gibbons et al. 2001; Kullenberg et al. 2006; Radkowski et al. 2007) to reduce the excessive blood loss from the drain. Recently, drain clamping has received increasing attention. Since most of the blood loss in TKA occurs during the first few postoperative hours (37% in 2 hours and 55% in 4 hours)(Jou IM 1993; Senthil Kumar et al. 2005), it seems reasonable to clamp the drain tube in the first few hours after TKA to temporarily create a tamponade effect for bleeding control. Various methods of clamping drain have been reported in the literature. However, no consensus has been achieved to date.

To clarify the role of drainage system after total knee arthroplasty, we conduct a review process in the present project. A comprehensive search was carried out and the articles regarding the drainage after surgery were reviewed. This review article focused on:

1. Effectiveness of postoperative drainage in TKA.
2. Safety and complications of postoperative drainage in TKA.
3. Effect of temporary drain clamping.

The purpose of this article is to analyze the pros and cons in using the drainage system after total knee arthroplasty and to provide practical information for orthopedic surgeons and medical care givers.

2. Search of literature

Our review team completed the search of electronic databases, including the Cochrane Central Register of Controlled Trials (2010), PubMed Medline (1966 to May 2011), and Embase (1980 to May 2011). We used the following search terms and Boolean operators: (drain OR drainage) AND (knee OR arthroplasty OR joint replacement). We also searched the reference lists of the relevant articles for any further associated studies. The criteria for inclusion in our study were: 1) reports dealing with patients undergoing primary TKA, 2) studies about postoperative drainage. After reviewing the titles and abstracts of the studies, we then determined if the study was appropriate for retrieval. These retrieved articles were reviewed by our review team. A consensus about the content of this review article was reached through out series of discussion.

3. Postoperative drainage

The effectiveness of wound drainage following TKA is still controversial. Some authors believed drains would reduce postoperative hematoma formation.(Drinkwater and Neil 1995; Holt et al. 1997; Martin et al. 2004) Postoperative drainage have been shown to provide a better wound outcome in orthopedic surgery.(Berman et al. 1990) Serous discharge from the wounds in TKA without drainage was a major concern of postoperative care.(Ovadia et al. 1997) Using a drain theoretically decreased postoperative pain, swelling, and incidence of infection(Kim et al. 1998).

Using a drain would facilitate the postoperative wound management. It is probably the most established benefit of the drainage in TKA. The number of dressing reinforcement was reported to be less in the drainage group.(Holt et al. 1997; Ovadia et al. 1997; Kim et al. 1998) Some other articles assessed the volume of blood in the dressing by measuring the weight of the dressing and found less weight in the drainage group.(Esler et al. 2003; Tao et al. 2006) In addition, Holt et al and Kim et al found that the area of ecchymosis is significant less in the drainage group.(Holt et al. 1997; Kim et al. 1998) Omonbude et al applied musculoskeletal ultrasound to measure the formation of hematoma and effusion on the fourth post-operative day and reported that the range of hematoma was less in the drainage group than the non-drainage group.(Omonbude et al. 2010) The above results of reinforcement of dressings and degree of ecchymosis and hematoma indicated the using a drain may reduce the leakage of blood from the joints and wounds.

According to a previous survey, most surgeons used closed suction drainage and believed that it would prevent from infection.(Canty et al. 2003) Many articles addressed this issue but failed to prove its effectiveness in the prevention of infection.(Holt et al. 1997; Ovadia et al. 1997; Kim et al. 1998; Esler et al. 2003; Tao et al. 2006; Cao et al. 2009; Lin et al. 2009; Tai et al. 2010a) A recent meta-analysis showed that the incidence of infection was 0.5% in the drainage group and 1.2% in the non-drainage group, but pooled data demonstrated no significant difference.(Zhang et al. 2011)

Thromboembolism is one of the most common complications after TKA, and is of great concern because of the associated increases in morbidity and mortality reported in the literature. To date, no approach to venous thromboembolic prophylaxis has been universally accepted by orthopedic surgeons. The methods of prophylaxis varied among the included studies. Using a drain in TKA theoretically reduces postoperative knee swelling

and may reduce the risk of thromboembolism. However, the evidence provided in the literature seems not to support this claim. Several studies compared the incidence of deep vein thrombosis between the drainage and non-drainage groups and all of them found no significant difference.(Holt et al. 1997; Adalberth et al. 1998; Mengal et al. 2001)
Dose using a drain increase the postoperative range of motion through reducing swelling? Several studies mentioned this issue but the results were disappointed.(Ovadia et al. 1997; Adalberth et al. 1998; Tao et al. 2006; Lin et al. 2009) All reports stated no significantly better range of motion after application of drainage. We believe that postoperative range of motion is influenced by many perioperative factors. Using a drain cannot alter the long-term range of motion.
Recently, more and more articles against the use of the drain in TKA have been published. (Adalberth et al. 1998; Crevoisier et al. 1998; Niskanen et al. 2000; Esler et al. 2003; Parker et al. 2004; Jones et al. 2007) These articles compared the outcomes of the conventional continuing drainage and non-drainage and showed that the drain system not only had no major benefits but also increased blood loss.
The number of patients requiring homologous blood transfusion was provided in several studies. Compared to the non-drainage group, the patients of the drainage group showed higher risk for excessive blood loss which required blood transfusion.(Ovadia et al. 1997; Esler et al. 2003; Cao et al. 2009) The postoperative drop of hemoglobin was also more severe in the drainage group.(Tai et al. 2010a) Longer hospital stay of the drainage group has also been reported in the same article. One possible reason was that the patients were unwilling to do physical activities with a drain inserted in their knees. Delayed rehabilitational programs kept them in the hospital for a longer time. However, this is still a controversial issue because hospital stay is affected by many confounding factors.

4. Make balance between pros and cons of drainage

According to the current evidence, we could not make a conclusion to either support using drainage or non-drainage strategies. The literature indicated that drainage after TKA reduced soft tissue ecchymosis and requirement for dressing reinforcement, but caused more blood loss and increased the blood transfusion rate. The literature also failed to support that drainage could reduce incidence of infection, deep venous thrombosis, or increase postoperative range of motion. Whether using drainage or not depends on each patient's clinical condition, surgeon's preference and consideration.

5. Effect of temporary drain clamping

Several reports regarding the delayed release of the drain have been published in the last decade. After surgery, reactive blood flow increases, with the peak flow appearing within five minutes once the tourniquet is deflated(Larsson et al. 1977). Most of the blood loss in TKA occurs during the first few postoperative hours.(Jou IM 1993; Senthil Kumar et al. 2005) Control of the bleeding is very important during this period. This may be the reason that temporary clamping of the drain tube can significantly reduce the volume of the drained blood.
The ideal drainage system would decrease hematoma formation and not cause excess blood loss. Some blood-saving strategies such as the autologous blood reinfusion, fibrin

sealant, pharmacological intervention, or other additional management have been reported to achieve this goal. The drain clamping method, if it is effective, is a much easier way to reduce blood loss compared to these interventions. The initial clamping provides a temporary tamponade effect, as well as the delayed release prevents hematoma formation.

An earlier study(Kiely et al. 2001) about the clamping drainage was reported in 2001 and it claimed that there was no significant difference between the clamping and non-clamping drainage groups in volume of drained blood, transfusion requirements, knee motion or wound status. However, several following studies(Shen et al. 2005; Tsumara et al. 2006; Raleigh et al. 2007; Stucinskas et al. 2008) showed that the drained volume was decreased by temporarily clamping the drain tubes. The other one(Eum et al. 2006) involving the 1-hour clamping method demonstrated a significant decrease in the drained volume in the clamping group during the postoperative 24 hours, but not 48 hours. The total drained blood volume ranged from 297 to 807 ml in the clamping group and 586 to 970 ml in the non-clamping group in the literature.

No matter clamping or not, most of the patients showed similar postoperative hemoglobin levels.(Kiely et al. 2001; Shen et al. 2005; Eum et al. 2006; Tsumara et al. 2006; Stucinskas et al. 2008) Only one study revealed higher postoperative hemoglobin level in the clamping group.(Raleigh et al. 2007) The number of patients requiring transfusion was provided in four studies(Shen et al. 2005; Eum et al. 2006; Tsumara et al. 2006; Stucinskas et al. 2008). One study(Eum et al. 2006) claimed that no transfusions were administered in either group. Shen et al.(Shen et al. 2005) reported similar transfusion rates in the both group. The other two articles(Tsumara et al. 2006; Stucinskas et al. 2008) showed slightly lower transfusion rates with clamped drains. Recently, administration of tranexamic acid and carbazochrome sodium sulfonate hydrate in the drain-clamping method was reported to reduce bleeding after TKA without increasing the risk of deep venous thrombosis.(Onodera et al. 2011)

It seemed that the results about blood loss were heterogeneous. One of the main reason might be the various clamping time in these trials. The debate on the length of time for which the drain should be clamped is still going on. Periods of between 1 and 24 hours have been reported.(Ryu et al. 1997; Kiely et al. 2001; Yamada et al. 2001; Prasad et al. 2005; Shen et al. 2005; Roy et al. 2006; Tsumara et al. 2006; Raleigh et al. 2007; Stucinskas et al. 2008) Some intermittent clamping methods have also showed their effectiveness in bleeding control(Prasad et al. 2005; Tsumara et al. 2006). A meta-analysis of the randomized controlled trials showed that the clamping methods could reduce the true blood loss only when the drain was clamped for four hours or more.(Tai et al. 2010b) We found three trials dealing with the two-hour, one-hour, and half-hour clamping methods and then showing no reduction in true blood loss.(Kiely et al. 2001; Eum et al. 2006; Tsumara et al. 2006) These findings suggest that when using the clamping methods to manage the drainage system after TKA, the ideal clamping period should be four hours or more. However, the patients managed with the longer duration of drain-clamping may have less blood loss but may also eliminate the potential advantages of the drainage. In addition, the situation of long clamping is similar to that of non-drainage; therefore, it is not logical for clinical practice.

Some studies(Kiely et al. 2001; Shen et al. 2005; Tsumara et al. 2006; Stucinskas et al. 2008) mentioned the effect of clamping drainage on postoperative range of motion of the knee. In these studies, the timing of measuring the range of motion varied from 6 to 83 days postoperatively. However, no significant difference was found in this issue. This finding suggested that although clamping the drain might potentially keep the knee swollen and reduce the range of motion shortly after operation, the influence did not persist.

For incidence of thromboembolic events, the previous trials demonstrated no difference in the between of the clamping and non-clamping groups. The pooled results of a recent meta-analysis also suggested that the temporary clamping methods did not significantly increase the risk of thromboembolic events. The symptomatic events occurred in 2.9% (7/244) of patients in the clamping group and 1.2% (3/259) in the non-clamping group (relative risk: 2.25, $p = 0.17$). The reported wound problems of these trials included severe oozing, bruising, blistering, partial breakdown, wound infection, and cellulitis. Another study reported an episode of transient hypotension upon release of the drain that resolved spontaneously.(Kiely et al. 2001) Again, no significant difference was found between the clamping and non-clamping groups regarding these complications.

In summary, the available evidence indicated that temporarily clamping the drains after TKA decreased the volume of drainage, but only clamping for not less than four hours decreased the reduction in hemoglobin levels. Although clamping does not increase the complication rate, its effectiveness and necessity is still questionable.

6. Authors' preference

For the past decade, we have focused on the studies about the role of the drainage system after total knee arthroplasty. In the first observational study, we found then most of the blood loss in TKA occurs during the first four postoperative hours.(Jou IM 1993; Senthil Kumar et al. 2005) Then we conducted a randomized controlled trial to check the effectiveness of four-hour temporary clamping drainage and found it is an effective method to reduce postoperative blood loss after total knee arthroplasty.(Shen et al. 2005) We also published a meta-analysis of the randomized controlled trials comparing outcomes between the various drain-clamping methods and immediately open drainage after TKA.(Tai et al. 2010b) We focused on blood loss and complications to evaluate the pros and cons of drain clamping. A trial comparing four-clamping drainage and non-drainage was conducted and revealed the role of drainage is still questionable after total knee arthroplasty.(Tai et al. 2010a) Despite clamping the drain for the first four hours after TKA, we found that the patients with drainage showed more blood loss and gained no other benefit compared with those without a drain. Although the clamping drainage was superior to the conventional drainage according to previous literature, we found no advantage of using this method compared with non-drainage. Thus, we did not routinely use the drainage system in primary total knee arthroplasty in our daily practice.

7. References

Adalberth G, Bystrom S, Kolstad K, Mallmin H, Milbrink J. Postoperative drainage of knee arthroplasty is not necessary: a randomized study of 90 patients. Acta Orthop Scand 1998;69:475-8.

Berman AT, Fabiano D, Bosacco SJ, Weiss AA. Comparison between intermittent (spring-loaded) and continuous closed suction drainage of orthopedic wounds: a controlled clinical trial. Orthopedics 1990;13:309-14.

Canty SJ, Shepard GJ, Ryan WG, Banks AJ. Do we practice evidence based medicine with regard to drain usage in knee arthroplasty? Results of a questionnaire of BASK members. Knee 2003;10:385-7.

Cao L, Ablimit N, Mamtimin A, Zhang KY, Li GQ, Li G, Peng LB. [Comparison of no drain or with a drain after unilateral total knee arthroplasty: a prospective randomized controlled trial]. Zhonghua Wai Ke Za Zhi 2009;47:1390-3.

Crevoisier XM, Reber P, Noesberger B. Is suction drainage necessary after total joint arthroplasty? A prospective study. Arch Orthop Trauma Surg 1998;117:121-4.

Drinkwater CJ, Neil MJ. Optimal timing of wound drain removal following total joint arthroplasty. J Arthroplasty 1995;10:185-9.

Esler CN, Blakeway C, Fiddian NJ. The use of a closed-suction drain in total knee arthroplasty. A prospective, randomised study. J Bone Joint Surg Br 2003;85:215-7.

Eum DS, Lee HK, Hwang SY, Park JU. Blood loss after navigation-assisted minimally invasive total knee arthroplasty. Orthopedics 2006;29:S152-4.

Gibbons CE, Solan MC, Ricketts DM, Patterson M. Cryotherapy compared with Robert Jones bandage after total knee replacement: a prospective randomized trial. Int Orthop 2001;25:250-2.

Holt BT, Parks NL, Engh GA, Lawrence JM. Comparison of closed-suction drainage and no drainage after primary total knee arthroplasty. Orthopedics 1997;20:1121-4; discussion 4-5.

Jones AP, Harrison M, Hui A. Comparison of autologous transfusion drains versus no drain in total knee arthroplasty. Acta Orthop Belg 2007;73:377-85.

Jou IM LK, Yang CY. Blood loss associated with total knee arthroplasty. J Orthop Surg (ROC) 1993;10:213.

Kiely N, Hockings M, Gambhir A. Does temporary clamping of drains following knee arthroplasty reduce blood loss? A randomised controlled trial. Knee 2001;8:325-7.

Kim YH, Cho SH, Kim RS. Drainage versus nondrainage in simultaneous bilateral total knee arthroplasties. Clin Orthop Relat Res 1998;188-93.

Kullenberg B, Ylipaa S, Soderlund K, Resch S. Postoperative cryotherapy after total knee arthroplasty: a prospective study of 86 patients. J Arthroplasty 2006;21:1175-9.

Larsson J, Lewis DH, Liljedahl SO, Lofstrom JB. Early biochemical and hemodynamic changes after operation in a bloodless field. Eur Surg Res 1977;9:311-20.

Lin J, Fan Y, Chang X, Wang W, Weng XS, Qiu GX. [Comparative study of one stage bilateral total knee arthroplasty with or without drainage]. Zhonghua Yi Xue Za Zhi 2009;89:1480-3.

Martin A, Prenn M, Spiegel T, Sukopp C, von Strempel A. [Relevance of wound drainage in total knee arthroplasty--a prospective comparative study]. Z Orthop Ihre Grenzgeb 2004;142:46-50.

Mengal B, Aebi J, Rodriguez A, Lemaire R. [A prospective randomized study of wound drainage versus non-drainage in primary total hip or knee arthroplasty]. Rev Chir Orthop Reparatrice Appar Mot 2001;87:29-39.

Niskanen RO, Korkala OL, Haapala J, Kuokkanen HO, Kaukonen JP, Salo SA. Drainage is of no use in primary uncomplicated cemented hip and knee arthroplasty for osteoarthritis: a prospective randomized study. J Arthroplasty 2000;15:567-9.

Omonbude D, El Masry MA, O'Connor PJ, Grainger AJ, Allgar VL, Calder SJ. Measurement of joint effusion and haematoma formation by ultrasound in assessing the effectiveness of drains after total knee replacement: A prospective randomised study. J Bone Joint Surg Br 2010;92:51-5.

Onodera T, Majima T, Sawaguchi N, Kasahara Y, Ishigaki T, Minami A. Risk of Deep Venous Thrombosis in Drain Clamping With Tranexamic Acid and Carbazochrome Sodium Sulfonate Hydrate in Total Knee Arthroplasty. J Arthroplasty 2011;

Ovadia D, Luger E, Bickels J, Menachem A, Dekel S. Efficacy of closed wound drainage after total joint arthroplasty. A prospective randomized study. J Arthroplasty 1997;12:317-21.

Parker MJ, Roberts CP, Hay D. Closed suction drainage for hip and knee arthroplasty. A meta-analysis. J Bone Joint Surg Am 2004;86-A:1146-52.

Prasad N, Padmanabhan V, Mullaji A. Comparison between two methods of drain clamping after total knee arthroplasty. Arch Orthop Trauma Surg 2005;125:381-4.

Radkowski CA, Pietrobon R, Vail TP, Nunley JA, 2nd, Jain NB, Easley ME. Cryotherapy temperature differences after total knee arthroplasty: a prospective randomized trial. J Surg Orthop Adv 2007;16:67-72.

Raleigh E, Hing CB, Hanusiewicz AS, Fletcher SA, Price R. Drain clamping in knee arthroplasty, a randomized controlled trial. ANZ J Surg 2007;77:333-5.

Roy N, Smith M, Anwar M, Elsworth C. Delayed release of drain in total knee replacement reduces blood loss. A prospective randomised study. Acta Orthop Belg 2006;72:34-8.

Ryu J, Sakamoto A, Honda T, Saito S. The postoperative drain-clamping method for hemostasis in total knee arthroplasty. Reducing postoperative bleeding in total knee arthroplasty. Bull Hosp Jt Dis 1997;56:251-4.

Senthil Kumar G, Von Arx OA, Pozo JL. Rate of blood loss over 48 hours following total knee replacement. Knee 2005;12:307-9.

Shen PC, Jou IM, Lin YT, Lai KA, Yang CY, Chern TC. Comparison between 4-hour clamping drainage and nonclamping drainage after total knee arthroplasty. J Arthroplasty 2005;20:909-13.

Stucinskas J, Tarasevicius S, Cebatorius A, Robertsson O, Smailys A, Wingstrand H. Conventional drainage versus four hour clamping drainage after total knee arthroplasty in severe osteoarthritis: a prospective, randomised trial. Int Orthop 2008;

Tai TW, Jou IM, Chang CW, Lai KA, Lin CJ, Yang CY. Non-Drainage Is Better Than 4-Hour Clamping Drainage in Total Knee Arthroplasty. Orthopedics 2010a;156-60.

Tai TW, Yang CY, Jou IM, Lai KA, Chen CH. Temporary drainage clamping after total knee arthroplasty: a meta-analysis of randomized controlled trials. J Arthroplasty 2010b;25:1240-5.

Tao K, Wu HS, Li XH, Qian QR, Wu YL, Zhu YL, Chu XB, Xu CM. [The use of a closed-suction drain in total knee arthroplasty: a prospective, randomized study]. Zhonghua Wai Ke Za Zhi 2006;44:1111-4.

Tsumara N, Yoshiya S, Chin T, Shiba R, Kohso K, Doita M. A prospective comparison of clamping the drain or post-operative salvage of blood in reducing blood loss after total knee arthroplasty. J Bone Joint Surg Br 2006;88:49-53.
Yamada K, Imaizumi T, Uemura M, Takada N, Kim Y. Comparison between 1-hour and 24-hour drain clamping using diluted epinephrine solution after total knee arthroplasty. J Arthroplasty 2001;16:458-62.
Zhang QD, Guo WS, Zhang Q, Liu ZH, Cheng LM, Li ZR. Comparison Between Closed Suction Drainage and Nondrainage in Total Knee Arthroplasty A Meta-Analysis. J Arthroplasty 2011;

20

Proximal Tibiofibular Joint in Knees with Arthroplasty

Hakan Boya
*Başkent University, Faculty of Medicine,
Department of Orthopaedics and Traumatology,
Zübeyde Hanım Hospital, İzmir
Turkey*

1. Introduction

Because proximal tibiofibular joint (PTFJ) is a diarthrodial joint encased in a synovial-lined articular capsule, it is possible to observe disorders at synovial joints, such as traumatic dislocation, osteoarthritis, inflammatory arthritis, ganglion cysts, pigmented villonodular synovitis, and infection.

Because of its close proximity to the knee joint, PTFJ may be the cause of lateral knee pain. This issue is important, especially in knees with arthroplasty. However, knee arthroplasty may exacerbate PTFJ. Consequently, the joint should be examined in detail before and after knee arthroplasty operations.

2. Embryology and postnatal development

Before 12 weeks of fetal age, PTFJ does not create a cavity (Bozkurt et al., 2003; Resnick et al., 1978). Subsequently, narrow cavities, which may be separated from the lateral femorotibial joint by a small amount of loose fibrous or areolar tissue, are apparent (Resnick et al., 1978). Subsequent development of the PTFJ includes the formation of articular cartilage, synovial tissue, synovial recesses, and a fibrous capsule (Resnick et al., 1978). Ossification usually begins in the proximal tibia within the first three months following birth. The tibiofibular joint morphology has considerable morphologic variation, and the joint may communicate with the knee joint (Ogden, 1984).

3. Anatomy

PTFJ is a diarthrodial joint between the lateral tibial condyle and fibular head; it is located posterolaterally on proximal tibia (Bozkurt et al., 2003). PTFJ has certain characteristics of synovial joints, such as synovial membrane, hyaline cartilage, and a fibrous capsule (Bozkurt et al., 2003; Resnick et al., 1978). The stability of the joint is provided by anterosuperior and posterosuperior capsular ligaments (Ogden, 1974; Resnick et al., 1978; Gray, 1977). The tendon of the biceps femoris muscle inserts into the anterior part of the fibular head and enforces the anterosuperior ligament of the joint (Bozkurt et al., 2003; Marshall et al., 1972).

Communication between the knee joint and PTFJ is reported to be 10-63% (Bozkurt et al., 2003; De Franca, 1992; Eichenblat et al., 1983, Veth et al., 1984). Communication between the

proximal tibiofibular and the knee joint occurs via the subpopliteal recess-associated defect in the posterior ligament of the fibular head (Dirim et al., 2008). The relation of the defect to trauma or developmental deficiency is unclear (Dirim et al., 2008).
Two types of PTFJ were defined according to joint line inclination; oblique (inclination > 20^0) and horizontal (inclination < 20^0) (Ogden, 1974). Moreover, planar, trochoid and double trochoid types of PTFJ have been reported (Espregueira-Mendes & Vieira, 2006).

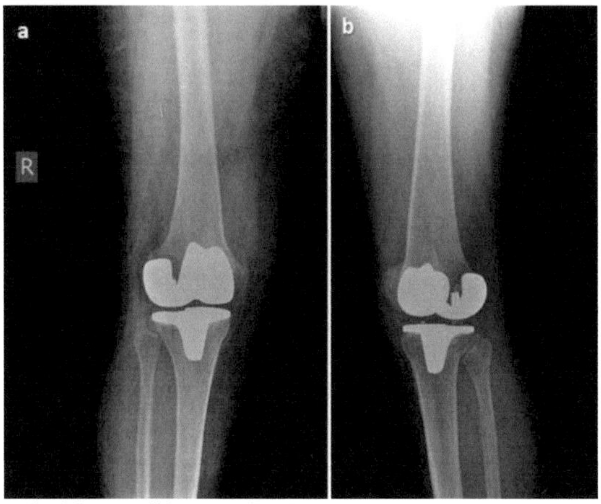

Fig. 1. Horizontal (a) and oblique (b) type PTFJ

3.1 Functional anatomy

Primary functions of PTFJ include the following:
1. Dissipation of torsional stresses applied at the ankle. With external rotation of the fibula about its longitudinal axis during dorsiflexion of the ankle joint, the proximal fibula rotates a few degrees externally (Barnett & Napier, 1952). The amount of external rotation is much greater in horizontal-type PTFJs (Barnett & Napier, 1952).
2. Dissipation of lateral tibial bending movements. Tensile and torsional forces influence the proximal-middle fibula in contrast to the distal fibula, which is affected by compressive forces (Ogden, 1974).
3. Transmitting axial loads in weight-bearing. Approximately one-sixth of the static load is applied at the ankle being transmitted to the PTFJ (Lambert, 1971).

4. Pathologies of PTFJ

It is possible to observe all disease at the PTFJ, similar to other synovial joints. Pathologies of this joint include primary osteoarthritis (Bozkurt et al., 2004; Öztuna et al., 2003; Özcan et al., 2009), trauma (Ogden, 1974; Resnick et al., 1978), infection, and inflammatory arthritis (Resnick & Niwayama,1995), synovial osteochondromatosis (Bozkurt et al., 2007; Heybeli et al., 2009; Weiss et al., 1975), neoplasms (Forster et al., 2007), ganglion cysts (Miskovsky et al., 2004; Mortazavi et al., 2006; Ward & Echardt, 1994), and pigmented villonodular synovitis (Ryan et al., 2004).

4.1 PTFJ in knees with severe primary osteoarthritis

PTFJ can be affected by primary osteoarthritis (Öztuna et al., 2003). The degree of osteoarthritis of the proximal tibiofibular joint strongly correlates with the degree of arthritis in tibiofemoral joints (TFJ) that have severe degenerative joint disease (Boya et al., 2008). Inflammatory enzymes passing between the joint spaces through possible anatomical communication between the TFJ and PTFJ may contribute to the advancement of arthritis in the respective compartments (Boya et al., 2008; Bozkurt et al., 2003). As with other joints, osteophytes, subchondral cysts, subchondral sclerosis, and joint-space narrowing are typical imaging findings (Forster et al., 2007).

Although primary degenerative disease of the PTFJ is commonly associated with primary degenerative disease of the knee joint, radiographic findings of the PTFJ in patients with severe degenerative knee osteoarthritis and varus misalignment do not correlate with clinical findings (Özcan et al., 2009).

4.2 PTFJ in other pathologies

Various neoplasms can affect the proximal tibiofibular joint, including osteochondroma, osteoblastoma, osteosarcoma, and nerve sheath tumors (Schwannomas and neurofibromas) (Forster et al., 2007).

Tuberculosis lesions at the fibular head can destroy PTFJ and mimic tumoral lesions (Abdelwahab et al., 2003-2004).

Synovial chondromatosis is a chronic, progressive disease of the synovial tissue in which free chondral loose bodies are formed after metaplasia (Bozkurt et al., 2007; Heybeli et al., 2009; Weiss et al., 1975).

A ganglion is a tumorlike, cystic lesion that arises from the joint, tendon sheath, or muscle (Miskovsky et al., 2004). It is a rare pathology at the PTFJ but can cause three different pathologies: asymptomatic mass, symptomatic fluctuant mass, and mass with peroneal nerve dysfunction (Forster et al., 2007).

PTFJ is affected similarly to other synovial joints in rheumatoid arthritis. Peroneal nerve dysfunction due to subluxation, dislocation of dextruted PTFJ is a pathologic entity of the joint with RA (Ishikawa & Hirohata, 1984). Moreover, it is possible to observe radiological deterioration of the PTFJ in patients with ankylosing spondylitis (Hong et al., 2009).

Pigmented villonodular synovitis (PVNS) is an uncommon proliferative disease of the synovium, which is usually monoarticular, presenting as chronic monoarthritis of the knee (Forster et al., 2007). PVNS is characterized by synovial hypertrophy with diffuse or focal hemosiderin deposition in the joint (Ryan et al., 2004). The disease can affect the PTFJ similarly to other synovial joints.

5. Importance of PTFJ in knees with arthroplasty

The PTFJ can be considered the fourth compartment of the knee joint because of its communication with the knee joint cavity (Bozkurt et al., 2003). PTFJ can be a source of lateral knee pain because of its pathologies. However, frequently it is overlooked because of its lack of emphasis in the literature (Forster et al., 2007). For this reason, the PTFJ should be carefully evaluated for osteoarthritis in patients being considered for a total knee arthroplasty operation. If it is overlooked as an etiology of a patient's lateral knee pain, pain from the diseased PTFJ may continue post-operatively. Furthermore, pathologies of the PTFJ may cause peroneal nerve dysfunction in patients with knee arthroplasty (Gibbon et al., 1999). PTFJ stability is important in cases with knee arthroplasty, especially in patients with rheumatoid arthritis. In those patients, the PTFJ may became unstable. Because of proximal movement of the fibular head, it may impinge to extruded bone cement under the tibial base

plate posterolaterally (Otani et al., 1998). This possibility should be considered during cementing of the tibial base plate; posterolateral cement excursion should be avoided in patients with inflammatory arthritis.
PTFJ pathologies can affect the arthroplasty results. Conversely, knee arthroplasty can produce PTFJ pathologies. It is possible to inadvertently destroy the PTFJ during an erroneous lower-level tibial cut; this may produce joint-related symptoms after a knee arthroplasty operation. Knees with aseptic loosening of the prosthesis produce inflammatory mediators and polyethylene particles can migrate to the PTFJ via communication between the knee and proximal tibiofibular joints. This can result in deterioration of the PTFJ and subsequent symptoms (Crawford et al., 1998).

6. Conclusion

The degree of osteoarthritis of the proximal tibiofibular joint strongly correlates with the degree of arthritis in tibiofemoral joints that have severe degenerative joint disease. Although primary degenerative disease of the PTFJ is commonly associated with primary degenerative disease of the knee joint, radiographic findings of the PTFJ in patients with severe degenerative knee osteoarthritis and varus misalignment do not correlate with clinical findings. It is possible to observe all disease at the PTFJ, similar to other synovial joints. Because of its close proximity to the knee joint, PTFJ may be the cause of lateral knee pain. This issue is important, especially in knees with arthroplasty. However, knee arthroplasty may exacerbate PTFJ. Consequently, the joint should be examined in detail before and after knee arthroplasty operations.

7. References

Abdelwahab, IF., Poplaw, S., Abdul-Quader, M. & Naran, D. (2003). Tuberculous pseudotumor of the proximal end of the fibula. A case report. *Bull Hosp Jt Dis*, Vol.61, No.3-4, pp. 145-147, ISSN 0883-9344

Barnett, CH. & Napier, JR. (1952) The axis of rotation of the ankle joint in man. Its influance upon the form of the talus and mobility of the fibula. *J Anat*, Vol.86, No.1, (January1952), pp. 1-9, ISSN 1136-4890

Boya, H., Ozcan, O. & Oztekin, HH. (2008). Radiological evaluation of the proximal tibiofibular joint in knees with severe primary osteoarthritis. *Knee Surg Sports Traumatol Arthrosc*, Vol.16, No.2, (February 2008), pp. 157-159, ISSN 0942-2056

Bozkurt, M., Yılmaz, E., Atlihan, D., Tekdemir, I., Havitçioğlu, H. & Günal, I. (2003). The proximal tibiofibuar joint: An anatomic study. *Clin Orthop Relate Res*, Vol.406, No.1 (January 2003), pp. 136-140, ISSN 0009-921X

Bozkurt, M., Yılmaz, E., Akseki, D., Havıtcıoğlu, H. & Günal, I. (2004). The evaluation of the proximal tibiofibular joint for patients with lateral knee pain. *The Knee*, Vol.11, No.4, (August 2004), pp. 307-312, ISSN 0968-0160

Bozkurt, M., Uğurlu, M., Doğan, M. & Tosun, N. (2007) Synovial chondromatosis of four compartments of the knee: medial and lateral tibiofemoral spaces, patellofemoral joint and proximal tibiofibular joint. *Knee Surg Sports Traumatol Arthrosc*, Vol.15, No.6, (June 2007), pp. 753-755, ISSN 0942-2056

Crawford, R., Sabokbar, A., Wulke, A., Murray, DW. & Athanasou, NA. (1998). Expansion of an osteoarthritic cyst associated with wear debris: a case report. *J Bone Joint Surg Br*,Vol.80, No.6, (November 1998), pp. 990-993, ISSN 0301-620X

De Franca, GG. (1992). Proximal tibiofibular joint dysfunction and chronic knee and low back pain. *J ManipPhysiol Ther*, Vol.15, No.6, (July-August 1992), pp. 382-387, ISSN 0161-4754

Dirim, B., Wangwinyuvirat, M., Frank, A., Cink, V., Pretterklieber, ML., Pastore, D. & Resnick, D.(2008). Communication between the proximal tibiofibular joint and knee via the subpopliteal recess: MR arthrography with histologic correlation and stratigraphic dissection. *AJR Am J Roentgenol*, Vol.191, No.2, (August 2008), pp. W44-51, ISSN 1546-3141

Eichenblat, M. & Nathan, H. (1983). The proximal tibiofibular joint. An anatomical study with clinical and pathological considerations. *Int Orthop*, Vol.7, No.1, pp. 31–39, ISSN 0341-2695

Espregueira-Mendes, JD. & da Silva, MV. (2006). Anatomy of the proximal tibiofibular joint. *Knee Surg SportsTraumatol Arthrosc*, Vol.14, No.3, (March 2006), pp. 241-249, ISSN 0942-2056

Forster, BB., Lee, JS., Kelly, S., O'Dowd, M., Munk, PL., Andrews, G. & Marchinkow, L. (2007) Proximal tibiofibular joint: an often-forgotten cause of lateral knee pain. *AJR Am J Roentgenol*, Vol.188, No.4, (April 2007) pp. W359-366, ISSN ISSN 1546-3141

Gibbon, AJ., Wardell, SR. & Scott, RD. (1999). Synovial cyst of the proximal tibiofibular joint with peroneal nerve compression after total knee arthroplasty. *J Arthroplasty*, Vol.14, No.6, (September 1999), pp. 766-768, ISSN 0883- 5403

Gray, H. (1977). *The classic Collector's Edition. Gray's Anatomy*, Churchill Livinstone Inc, ISBN 978-051-7223-65-9, New York, USA

Heybeli, N., Ozcan, M., Copuroğlu, C. & Yalniz, E. (2009). Isolated synovial chondromatosis of the proximal tibiofibular joint. *Acta Orthop Traumatol Turc*, Vol.43, No. 5, (November-December 2009), pp. 448-452, ISSN 1017-995X

Hong, HP., Chung, HW., Choi, BK., Yoon, YC. & Choi, SH. (2009) Involvement of the proximal tibiofibular joint in ankylosing spondylitis. Acta Radiol, Vol.50, No.4, (May 2009), pp. 418-422, ISSN 0284-1851

Ishikawa, H. & Hirohata K. (1984). Bilateral peroneal nerve palsy secondary to posterior dislocation of the proximaltibiofibular joint in rheumatoid arthritis. *Rheumatol Int*, Vol.5, No.1, pp. 45-47, ISSN 0172-8172

Lambert KL. (1971). The weight-bearing function of the fibula. A strain gauge study. *J Bone Joint Surg Am*, Vol.53, No.3, (April 1971), pp. 507-513, ISSN 0021-9355

Marshall, JG., Girgis, FG. & Zelko, RR. (1972). The Biseps Femoris tendon and its functional significance. *J Bone Joint Surg Am*, Vol.54, No.7, (October 1972), pp. 1444-1450, ISSN 0021-9355

Miskovsky, S., Kaeding, C. & Weis, L. (2004) Proximal tibiofibular joint ganglion cysts: excision, recurrence, and joint arthrodesis. *Am J Sports Med*, Vol.32, No.4, (June 2004), pp.1022-1028, ISSN 0363-5465

Mortazavi, SM., Farzan, M. & Asadollahi, S. (2006). Proximal tibiofibular joint synovial cyst--one pathology with three different presentations. *Knee Surg Sports Traumatol Arthrosc*, Vol.14, No.9, (September 2006), pp. 875-879, ISSN 0942-2056

Ogden, JA. (1974). The anatomy and function of the proximal tibiofibular joint. *Clin Orthop,* Vol.101, No.6, (June 1974), pp. 186-191, ISSN 0009-921X

Ogden, JA. (1984). Radiology of postnatal skeletal development. IX. Proximal tibia and fibula. *Skeletal Radiol,* Vol.11, No.3, pp. 169-177, ISSN 0364-2348

Otani, T., Fujii, K., Ozawa, M., Kaechi, K., Funaki, K., Matsuba, T. & Ueno, H. (1998). Impingement after total knee arthroplasty caused by cement extrusion and proximal tibiofibular instability. *J Arthroplasty,* Vol.13, No.5, (August 1998), pp. 589-591, ISSN 0883-5403

Özcan, O., Boya, H. & Oztekin, HH. (2009) Clinical evaluation of the proximal tibiofibular joint in knees with severe tibiofemoral primary osteoarthritis. *The Knee,* Vol.16, No.4, (August 2009), pp. 248-250, ISSN 0968- 0160

Öztuna, V., Yıldız, A., Özer, C., Milcan, A., Kuyurtar, F. & Turgut, F. (2003). Involvement of the proximal tibiofibular joint in osteoarthritis of the knee. *The Knee,* Vol.10, No.4, (December 2003), pp. 347-349, ISSN 0968-0160

Resnick, D., Newell, JD., Guerra, J Jr., Danzing, LA., Niwayama, G. & Goergen, TG. (1978) Proximal tibiofibular joint: Anatomic-pathologic-radiographic correlation. *Am J Roentgenol,* Vol.131, No.1, (July 1978), pp. 133-138, ISSN 0361-803

Resnick, D. & Niwayama, G. (1995). Anatomy of individual joints, In: *Diagnosis of bone and joint disorders,* Resnick, D. & Niwayama, G. pp. 741-750, WB Saunders, ISBN 072165066X, 9780721650661, Philadelphia

Ryan, RS., Louis ,L., O'Connell, JX. & Munk, PL. (2004). Pigmented villonodular synovitis of the proximal tibiofibular joint. *Australas Radiol,* Vol.48, No.4, (December 2004), pp. 520-522, ISSN 0004-8461

Ward, WG. & Eckardt, JJ. (1994) Ganglion cyst of the proximal tibiofibular joint causing anterior compartment syndrome. A case report and anatomical study. *J Bone Joint Surg Am,* Vol.76, No.10, (October 1994), pp. 1561- 1564, ISSN 0021-9355

Weiss, C., Averbuch, PF., Steiner, GC. & Rusoff, JH. (1975). Synovial chondromatosis and instability of the proximal tibiofibular joint. *Clin Orthop Relat Res,* Vol.108, No.5, (May 1975), pp. 187-190, ISSN 0009-921X

Veth, RP., Kingma. LM. & Nielsen, HK. (1984). The abnormal proximal tibiofibular joint. Arch Orthop Trauma Surg, Vol.102, No.3, pp. 167-171, ISSN 0936-8051

Part 4

Special Topics in Knee Arthroplasty

21

Special Situations in Total Knee Arthroplasty

Orlando M. de Cárdenas Centeno and Felix A. Croas Fernández
"Frank País" International Scientific Orthopedic Complex
Medical Sciences University, Havana
Cuba

1. Introduction

Total Knee Arthroplasty TKA has become a highly successful joint reconstruction procedure.
Surgical outcomes, patients satisfaction and implant survival have improved, and the operation has become widely accepted to afford relief pain, restoration of range motion and function. TKA has been shown to have durable and predictable results in elderly patients.
The principals indications for TKA are severe pain and functional disability. Others indications include deformity, instability and loss of motion.
The diagnosis associated with this features for which TKA has been successfully performed include osteoarthritis, rheumatoid arthritis, inflammatory arthritis, osteonecrosis, and others disability disorders, including tumors and fractures.
The indications and contraindications to perform a TKA have been well established and documented.
Nevertheless there are situations well-known as special or complex, where sometimes could be considered controversial or relative contraindications, and require a deep analysis and take difficult decision.
Up today, specials situations are not presented in elderly patient only. These situations occur in young patient less than 55 or 40 years old too. (De Cárdenas et al 2009) at present, on the basis of obtained results and different reported, the indications for TKA have been expanded eventually to younger people.
Total Joint Arthroplasty continues to confer immense benefits upon patients with joint disease, and it is considered as one of the most cost-effective surgical procedures (Dunbar et al 2009).
In special situations, TKA may be performed in patients in any age to salvage a knee or even to restore motion and relief pain where other procedures are not possible. This indication, however, remains controversial and could be considered relatives contraindications.
The aim of this study is present our modest experience and valuate a group of patients with different situations to whom were performed a complex TKA in specials situations using a Kalisté Knee System.

1.1 Special situations

Complex TKA in specials situations have been presented and development by differents Orthopaedics Surgeons and although controversial criterions have been collected, the concept and the outcomes has been well accepted by orthopedic community.

While the literature does not resolve all the controversies in TKA, sometimes we will encounter apparently disparate advice in some areas; some of which is due to honest differences in opinion and personal experiences and some related to the type of implants.
Based in the evidence of scientific papers, literature, experts opinion and by consensus, we would like to present our modest experience and results.
Different representative patients with specials situations: Fig. 1

- Stiff and ankylosed Knee
- Knee angular deformity: Varus / Valgus (figure 1.a / figure 1.b)
- High Tibial Osteotomy HTO (after) (figure 1.c)
- Patellar problems (after Maquet osteotomy or patellectomy)
- Rheumatoid Arthritis (Total Joint Collapsed) (figure 1.d)
- Post-traumatic Osteoarthritis
- Arthrodesed Knee
- Achondroplasic

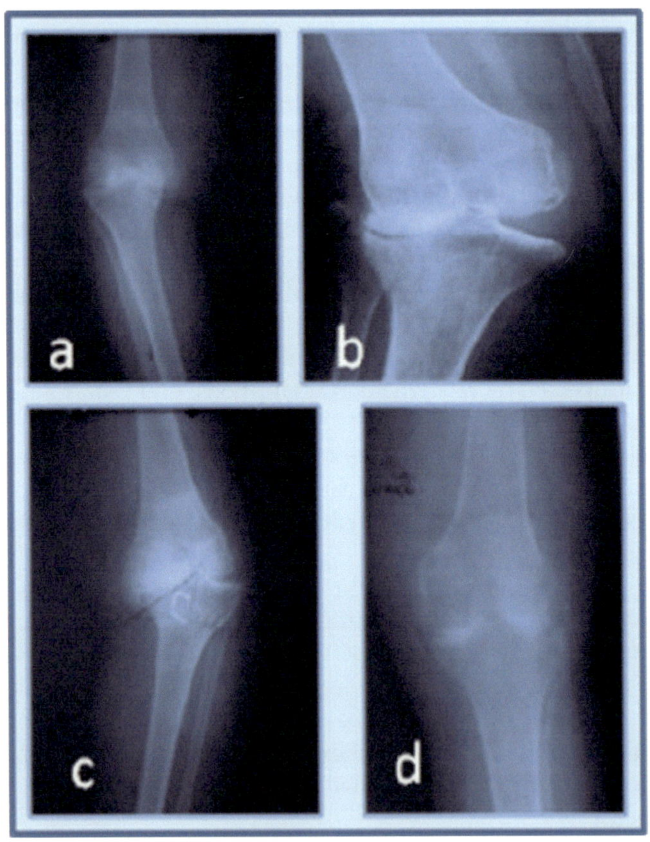

Fig. 1. Different special situations of the knee.

Many of these conditions are associated or combined with:
Instability, flexed or extended painful rigid knee and/or bone defect.
In summary all this patients have diagnosis of Severe Osteoarthritis of the Knee. (figure 2.)

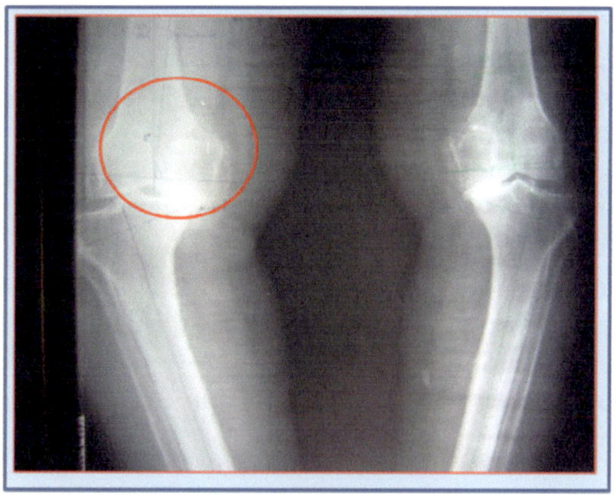

Fig. 2. Severe Bilateral Osteoarthritis of the Knee

2. Material and method

This is a longitudinal, prospectively and follow-up study. Between January 2004 and January 2010 the authors did 636 consecutive Total Knee Arthroplasty in 582 patients with moderate to severe Osteoarthritis of the Knee. They were treated using Kalisté Knee System (FHorthopedic. France).

From this group were selected 132 patients (146 TKA) to be included in this study. They were 14 Bilateral in two stage and 118 Unilateral, 69 left Knee and 49 right Knee. 81patients (61,4 %) were female and 51 (38,6 %) male, with a mean age of 62.5 years old (range 25 to 82 years old).

2.1 Patient selection

The patient selected to be included in this study has been patients with specials situations as was descripted.

All of them has severe primary knee osteoarthritis IV-V Alback's radiographic classification or secondary to others conditions like post-traumatic, rheumatic arthritis with total joint collapse, angular deformity: varus / valgus.

Stiff or ankylosed knee, patellar problems as after Maquet osteotomy or patellectomy, history or failured high tibial osteotomy, arthrodesed knee and achondroplasic.

Gender, race or age not were criteria to exclude. The authors excluded patients with ligth or moderate primary knee osteoarthritis and varus / valgus/ flexed deformity less than 10 degrees, additional exclusion criteria included history of septic arthritis of the knee, neuropathic knee, and hemophilic arthritis not was criteria to be included.

2.2 Ethical considerations

The study was approved by the institutional review board.

All the patients were well informed and documented about the methodology, purpose and procedure of this study, and have given their consent in writing.

2.3 Clinical assessment

Pre-operative clinical evaluation include detailed medical history, full name, identification card number, gender, race, age and all dates according to the standard file to all patients

admitted in this hospital, and thorough clinical-functional and radiographic examination using the Knee Society Scoring KSS, because it is one of the more acceptable and standardized instruments to evaluation of results, and it is a powerful tool for comparing specific dynamics of the knee arthroplasty.
The Knee Society Clinical Rating System available since 1989 (Insall et al.1989), have been the preferred method of outcome assessment after knee replacement for many surgeons.
The new KSS is being validated and updated to reflect current trend in Knee Arthroplasty and contemporary expectation and activities levels that were not well addressed in earlier assessment models. It includes visual analog and pain assessment, as well as objective measures of knee motion and stability.
The functional component of the KSS is relevant to contemporary patients of any demographic background (Lonner JH, 2009).

2.4 Radiographic evaluation

Pre-operative image evaluation includes standard differents Knee radiographs:
Comparative anterior-posterior AP standing view (if the patient could be stand) or in supine position, lateral view in 25-30 flexion degree (each one) and patella axial view (all of this, if it was possible according to the knee joint condition).
Additionally radiographic studies of the both hip and both ankle were taken to know the conditions of these joints.
Pangonogramme not was possible, and anterior-posterior radiographic views were done standing or supine position with 14" x 17" cassettes.
Radiographic analysis permitted the determination of the preoperative knee osteoarthritis classification (Alback S, 1968) and included measurement of the mechanical axis, measurement of the femorotibial axis and assessment of the degree of correction.
On standing AP radiographic view, were measured the varus or valgus deformity.
On lateral radiographic view, were measurement the posterior slope of the tibia and observed the posterior knee aspect and the patella localization.
On axial radiographic view were observed patellofemoral alignment, joint space and joint surface.
All this measurements were done using a goniometer.
To the determination of the preoperative osteoarthritis classification an co-author (RJTR) who did not do surgeries reviewed all available radiograph taken before surgery, and at the most recent follow-up for evidence of component loosening, radiolucencies, and overall alignment, using the Knee Society total knee roentgenographic evaluation and Scoring System (Ewald FC, 1989).
Using the X-Ray template (transparences) of the Kalisté components systems were calculated the size of the each component during pre-operative plannification.

2.5 Surgical technique

2.5.1 Kalisté Total Knee System

Kalisté Total Knee System (FHorthopedic.France) is a tricompartmental resurfacing prosthesis.
The femoral and tibial resections are independent.
This design allows the surgeons to begin with either the tibial stage or the femoral stage.
It is mainly based on intramedullary femoralalignment. Pre-operative control of the femoral guide alignment is performed with the help of extramedullary rods.

The pre-operative plannification (radiographic studies) allow the surgeon to calculate the anatomical axis of the leg, in order to calculate the angle o femoral valgus.
The resections (distal femoral and proximal tibial) are perpendicular to the mechanical axis of the leg. Tibial viewing in intramedullary, if the entry point used is located at the level of the insertion of the anterior cruciate ligament or external (tibia varus). Definition of the axes and estimation of the size of the implants are determined thanks to X-Rays template at a 1.15 scale.
The Kalisté Total Knee System was designed to admit posterior cruciate ligaments PCL-retaining or posterior stabilized PS Knee prosthesis. (Fig. 3.a, 3.b)

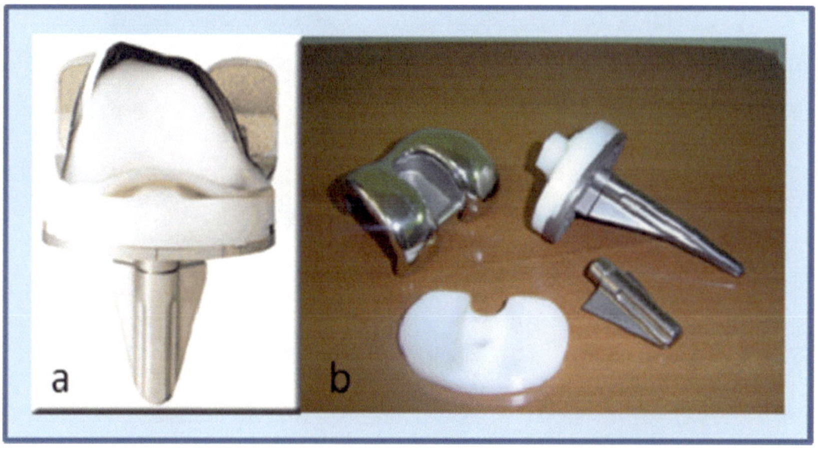

Fig. 3. a. Kaliste Total Knee System (PCL retaining), b. Kaliste Total Knee System (Posterior Stabilized) (with permission FHorthopedic. France)

The accessories, augmentation devices, and short or long stem for the operative technique are available in the instrumentation sets.
The surgeon decides if use or not use the patellar prosthesis component and it is available too.

2.5.2 Surgical protocol

All surgeries were done by one surgeon (OMCC), the same surgical team and at one institution (CCOI Frank Pais, La Habana, Cuba) all procedures followed a standard operative protocol. Surgeries were done with the patient in supine position.
All surgical procedures were performed in a standard operation theatre with standard air conditions (not ultra-clean air, not laminar flow). Standard clothing was used by the surgical team. 87% of the surgeries were with spinal, epidural anesthesia using intravenous sedation too, and only in selective patients with specific clinical conditions were under general anesthesia as anesthesiologist advised. Pneumatic tourniquet not were used in nobody case. Hemostasis achieved with use of cauterization and diathermy.
The limb washed and draping technique for TKA was done as usually. Ancilliary leg-holding device was placed on the limb and operating table to provide stable and gradual positioning of the Knee during surgery.
In all cases of this study were used posterior-stabilized Kalisté Knee System cemented with Polymethylmethacrylat.

The procedure to implant the components was according to the standards total knee arthroplasty, using the instrumentation designed to it. Variants were used as advisable in each special situation (Lotke PA, 1999, 2002, Nelson CL 2002, Scuderi GR 2002, Padgell D. 2002, Griffin FM 2002, Lombardi AV et al. 2009).
In general, a straight anterior longitudinal (midline) skin incision was the most appropriate performed when skin condition was possible, followed by a medial parapatellar capsular arthrotomy (Fig. 4).

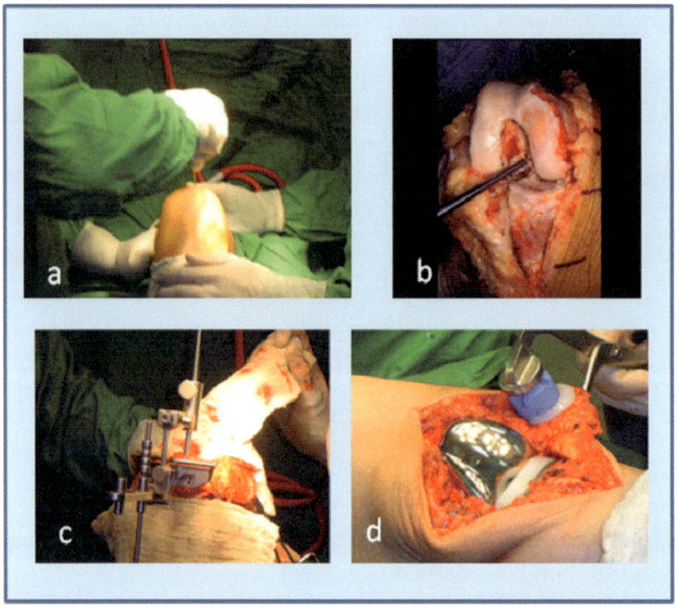

Fig. 4. a. b. c. d. Different phases of the surgical procedure to implant the knee prosthesis.

It provides adequate access to medial or lateral aspect of the limb. In some cases was necessary a variant, selected of classical approach options according the need.
All patients had placement of drain 24-48 hours post-operation according to standard practice peri-operative prophylaxis consisted of intravenous cephalosporin (Cephazoline 1 gr) starting one hour prior to surgery and continue for 24 to 72 hours. Patients also received subcutaneous low molecular weight heparin LMWH for prophylaxis again deep vein thrombosis DVT started in the evening of the operation day till 10 days according to the conditions of the patients.

2.6 Rehabilitation protocol

All the patients were assigned to regimen for post-operative early mobilization.
Day of the operation: Following skin closure and wound dressing, the knee was placed straight on the bed until early next morning, in an extension splint, with a pillow under the foot, in order to increase the venous backflow and decrease edema. An ice bag over the knee is allowed for the reduction of the hyperemia, the edema and the inflammation.
Post-operative day 1: The regime of rehabilitation program consists in “to leave make” or “allow make” by him/her self (patient) under physiotherapist guide.
We never used continues passive motion CPM machine.

The physiotherapist passively and actively moved the Knee and taught the patient to repeat different exercises during the day alone (5 times daily, at least 3 times), and after each, ice bag over Knee. (figure 5 a, b, c, d)

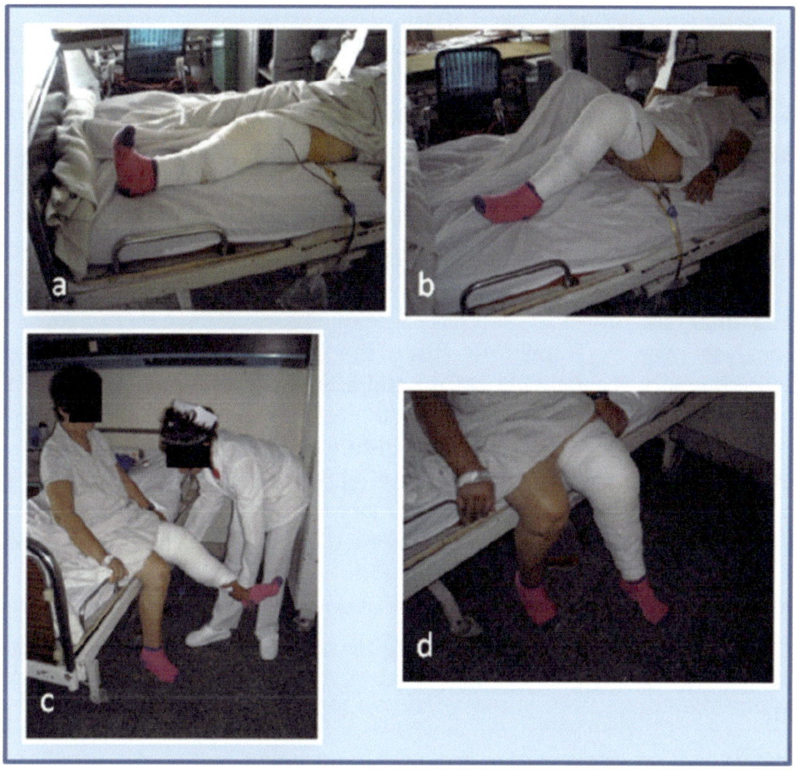

Fig. 5. a. b. c. d. The patient in the postoperative first day, doing exercises intensive rehabilitation program under the guidance of the physiotherapist.

The patient is allowed to sit on the bed or on a seat, bending the knee as tolerated, isometric strengthening of the quadriceps and concentric dynamic exercises of periarticular hip and ankle muscles were encouraged. The knee was placed in the extension splint again overnight.

Post-operative day 2: Continue the same as day 1, increasing the range of motion ROM. The patient started to walk with walker and muscular strengthening recovery was intensified.

Post-operative day 3: The same as day 2, but increasing the ROM, bending the knee to 90° and started to walk with two crutches.

Between the post-operative days 3 to day 5, the patient can go at home with Doctor's orderly and exercises program written and follow-up by outpatient department OPD.

2.7 Evaluation and follow-up

To evaluate the patients, they were checked and recorded according to the KSS all categories were collected in data base and processed in the Med Cal program.

Clinical and functional assessment was performed pre-operatively and post-operative at 3, 6, 12 months and yearly. Patients were evaluated prospectively by means of the Knee

Society Scoring System KSSS and by Analogical Visual Scale AVS to the Health Perception Criteria.
A locally-designed patient satisfaction questionnaire was also given to all patients before operation and yearly after operation, asking them to rate their replacement on a scale from 0 to 10, with 0 being very dissatisfied and 10 being very satisfied.
A deep infection was any infection that concurred inside the knee joint, requiring prosthesis removal.
A superficial infection was any infection of the skin that responded well to antibiotic with not residual problems.
Aseptic loosening was considered to be the presence of a radiolucent line larger than 2 mm around the entire prosthesis which was not related to infection.
Fatal deep venous thrombosis was an acute thromboembolism episode that ended in death.

2.8 Statistical analysis

Statistical analysis was performed to study the possible differences between clinical-functional conditions of the patients before and after operation and radiographic changes for evidence of component loosening, radiolucencies and overall alignment. Before operation each patient was valuated clinical-functionally according KSS. Postoperative were repeated the valuation with the same Scoring System (KSS) at 3, 6 months and yearly. The obtained results were compared. The primary information was recorded in data base elaborated for this study. The results were presented in tables and graphics performed using Microsoft Office Excel and Word program, Window seven operative systems.
Statistical technique of absolute and relative frequency were applied, odds ratio and p-value.

3. Results

All the patients in this study had substantial pain and functional limitation before the surgery. Some of them used wheelchair and many used walker, crutches or cane (support dependence).
This study is one of the largest series of specials situations in TKA. Several authors has reported on the results of total knee arthroplasty in patients with specials situations and reported significant improvement in KSS and ROM.
The study population of this series composed by 132 patients (100%) are summarized in the table 1, and were according gender 81 (61,4%) female and 51 (38.6) male and the age distribution were 38 (28.8%) less than 50 years old and 94 (71,2%) more than 50 years old.

	AGE (Years Old)					
	< 50		> 50		TOTAL	
GENDER	N	%	N	%	N	%
Female	29	22.0	52	39.4	81	61.4
Male	9	6.8	42	31.8	51	38.6
TOTAL	38	28.8	94	71.2	132	100

Table 1. Study population between age and gender distribution (Sources: Data Base)

The primary diagnosis distributions have been summarized in table 2.

"Special Situations" Diagnosis	PATIENTS	
	N	%
After High Tibial Osteotomy	42	31.8
Rheumatoid Arthritis (Joint Collapsed)	14	10.6
Post-traumatic Osteoarthritis	19	14.4
After Patellectomy	5	3.8
Severe Knee deformity Varus/Valgus	31	23.5
Stiff and Ankylosed Knee	18	13.6
After Maquet Osteotomy	3	2.3
TOTAL	132	100

Table 2. "Special Situations". Diagnosis Distribution

In our series study, the side distribution of the knees operated was as showed the Table 3 and Graphic 1.

Number operated knee							
Bilateral		Unilateral					
		Left		Right		Total	
N	%	N	%	N	%	N.	%
14	10,6	67	56,8	51	42,2	118	89,4
Odds ratio	1,0742	Odds ratio	2,4219	Odds ratio	2,3355		
p value	0,0593	p value	0,0374	p value	0,0453		

Table 3. Number of Knee operated with "Special Situations" CCOI Frank País. January 2004 - January 2010. (Source: Data Base)

In the sample, 118 patients were operated unilaterally on one knee to 56.8% and 42.2% distributed left knee and right knee respectively. As the number of patients who underwent bilateral knee represent 10.6% of the total. Patients undergoing unilateral knee had both left and right odds ratio of 2.4219 and 2.3355 respectively, indicating that there are two times more likely a patient could be operated on one knee than both, particularly, the left knee.

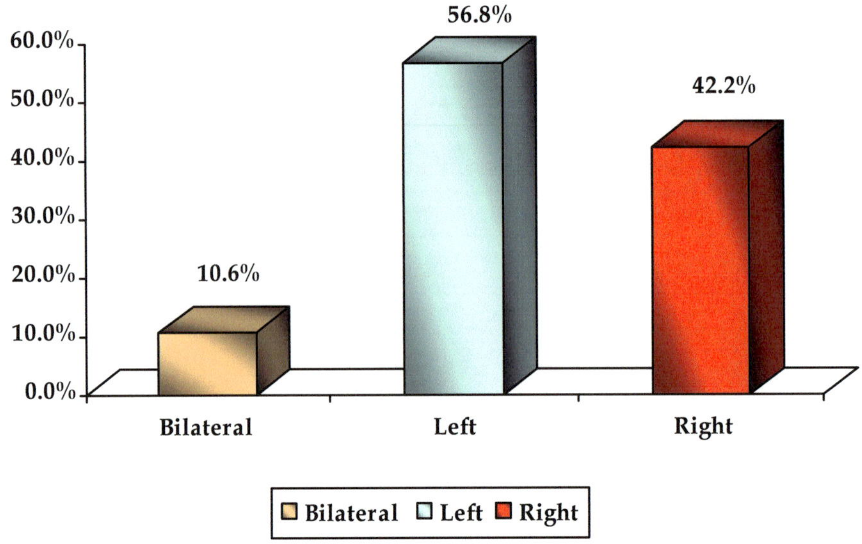

Graphic 1. Number of knees operated according to location

The clinical and functional pre-operative (1 year to follow-up) results according KSS were summarized in the Table 4 and Graphic 2.

Indicator	Clinical				Functional			
	Pre operative	Post operative	Odds ratio	P - value	Pre operative	Post operative	Odds ratio	P - value
Mean	29	89	3,4673	0,0321	23	88	4,0284	0,0382
Range	14 - 49	64 - 100	3,1632	0,0493	0 - 58	62 – 100	4,4570	0,0302

Table 4. Clinical and Functional pre-operative and post-operative (1 year follow-up) Results according KSS. CCOI "Frank País" January 2004 – January 2010 **(Source: Data Base).**

The mean preoperative scale application in clinical phase KSS was 29, indicating that there is a limited deterioration in the knee as a result of joint degeneration, a year is a significant improvement of this parameter as it close to 100 which is the optimum value (89), indicating a favourable clinical evolution of these patients after total knee arthroplasty. According to the level in the preoperative stage, it is appreciated that there was a path of the mean values in the clinical assessment between 14 and 49 points, and in the postoperative phase was reached 64 to 100 points, which is evidence of clinical improvement of patients after surgery. For the value that represents the odds ratio 3.1632 of the clinical phase is to infer that a patient operated year total knee arthroplasty has 3 times more likely to improve in the KSS scale score that if does not apply this surgical procedure.

As for the functional parameter the patients were on average 23 points which shows result in loss of function after knee surgery, and in the postoperative phase is reached near 88 to 100, showing a significant recovery in the functional state of the knees operated patients. The functional range of this phase before the operation is relatively moderate to low once the replacement will elevate this range from 62 to 100 which show functional improvement in knee patients after surgery. For the value 4.4570 represents the odds ratio in this functional setting. We must infer that a patient per year to operate for total knee arthroplasty has 4 times more probabilities to improve his-her functionality according to the KSS scale score that if does not apply this surgical procedure.

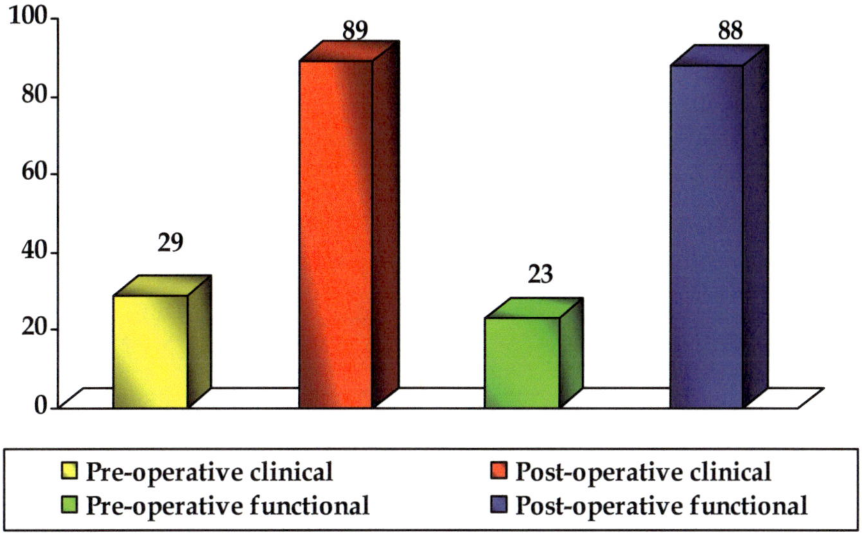

Graphic 2. Graphic behaviour and the year according to preoperative level in patients with knee osteoarthritis KSS operated by ATR.

And finally clinical-functional pre-operative and post-operative, evolution according KSS during 6 years follow up study were showed as a total mean punctuation in the Table 5 and Graphic 3.

Indicator	Pre-operative total mean punctuation	Post-operative total mean punctuation	Follow-up (months)	Odds ratio	P - value
	51	166	3	4,0932	0,0352
		176	6		
		177	12		
		174	24		
		176	36		
		180	48		
		182	60		
		180	72		
Reference Value	200	200	.		
Mean	51	177			

Table 5. Clinical – functional pre-operative and post-operative. Evolution according KSS during 6 years follow-up study. **(Source: Data base).**

It is observed in the preoperative average score achieved on average in the six years was 51 points, and in the postoperative period shows that every year the score is close to 200, the average score is 177, significantly favourable outcome once the total knee arthroplasty. For the odds ratio value reached 4.0932 as can be inferred that a patient operated for total knee arthroplasty from 3 months of surgery is four times more likely to improve their clinical and functional rating scale that a patient KSS not yet been operated with this procedure.

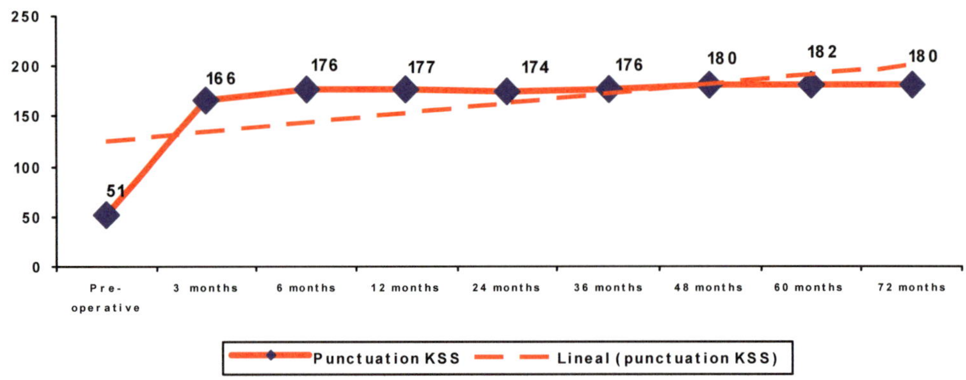

Graphic 3. Graphic trends in overall behavior and functional clinical phases, of the knee as punctuation in the KSS scale.

The graph shows trends as there is a significant evolution (P <0.05) clinical and functional satisfactory phases in the recovery of patients undergoing knee for knee replacement as early as three months after surgery, where this evolution remains a tendency to increase average scale score as KSS.

The final radiographic evaluation showed that 138 (94,5%) of the 146 (100%) operated knee were in neutral alignment, 4 were in valgus and 4 flexed less than 10 degrees each one.

About complications, were 2 deep infection that required revision, prosthesis removed and arthodesis. 3 were superficial infection, 3 mechanical problems: 1 patellar tendon rupture (revision and reconstruction) and 2 patella dislocation (1 arthroscopy to release and 1 revision and realignment).About death (before 90 days post-operative): 1 multiple organic failure in a 78 years old man with high risk and 1 fatal deep venous thrombosis DVT (suddenly).

Our results showed not significant differences in complications between others reported in the medical literature in terms of death, infections, dislocations or revision.

None of the knees had evidence of aseptic loosening, radiolucent or implant migration at the time of the lasted follow up. It may be that a longer follow-up will be required to reveal any difference in outcome.

An efficient surgery, with an aggressive post-operative rehabilitation program and a proper patient selection should maximize favorable results and limit perioperative morbidity.

Every surgeon must evaluate the risk-to-benefit ratio for each individual patient; by the way, the management of these specials conditions has changed over the last years.

Up-today TKA is considered "high tech" procedures.

All patients in our study had functional improvement at the time of latest follow-up. There was a substantial improvement in pain relief and in the range of motion of the knees after TKA in specials situations and the degree of satisfaction of patients significantly improved according to criteria autopersección as shown in Table 6 according to the visual analog scale and of course, improved the quality of life.

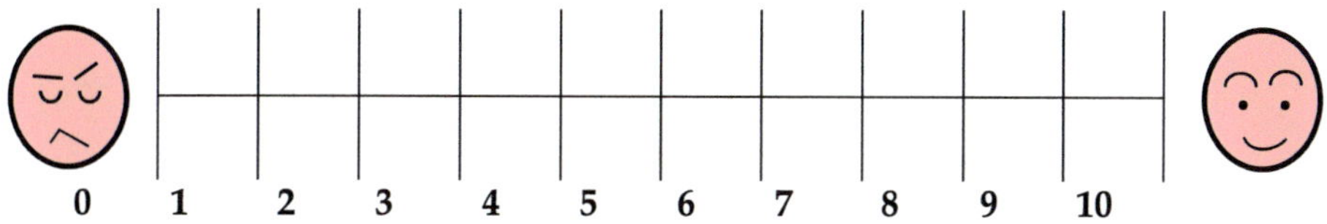

PRE-OP	VS	POST-OP
MEAN: 1.5	VS	MEAN: 8.7
RANGE: 0 - 3	VS	RANGE: 7 - 10

Table 6. Analogical visual scale avs. (Source: Data Base)

3.1 Evolutive cases presentation.

Finally, as evidence of the results were showed some evolutive cases off this study.
The first case, was 64 years old, female, with that diagnosis severe bilateral osteoarthritis of the knee, combined with genus varus and flexion contracture, she has history of high tibial osteotomy in her left knee eight years ago. A sequence evolutive was showed in the figure 6. a, b, c, d, e, f, g, h.

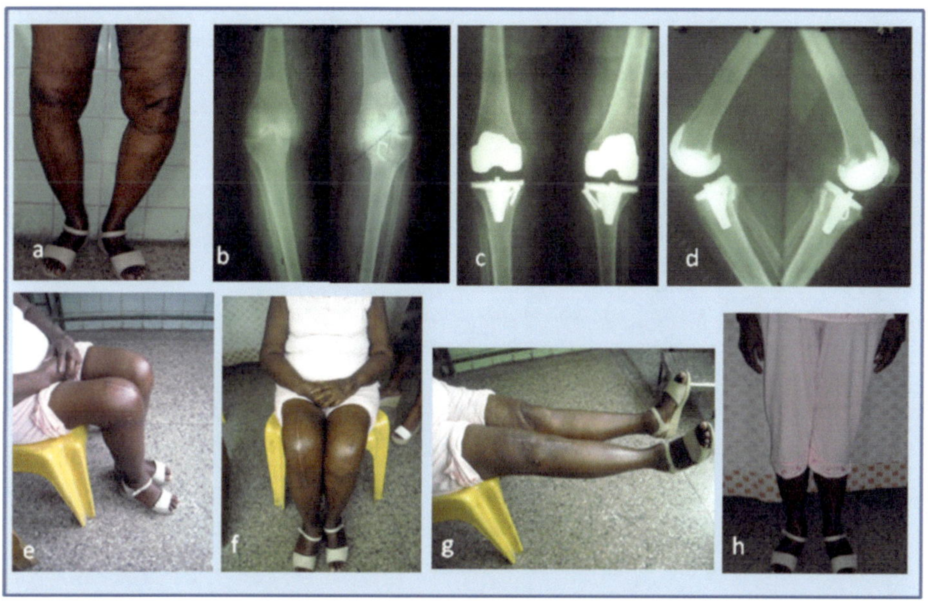

Fig. 6. a. Genus varus deformity, b. X-ray AP view showed severed OA in both knee with HTO in the left, c. X-ray AP view showed bilateral TKA implanted in both knee with two screw reinforced the medial side of the tibial to solve the bone loose and corrected deformity, d. Lateral view of both knee whit TKA implanted, e. f. g. h. the patient rehabilitated with range of motion and full stability.

The second case showed was a 34 years old, female with diagnosis of Rheumatoid arthritis and total joint collapse of both knee in wheelchair the last 3 years, and of course both knee were in fixed flexion the figure 7 a, b, c, d, e, f, g, h showed the sequence of follow - up.

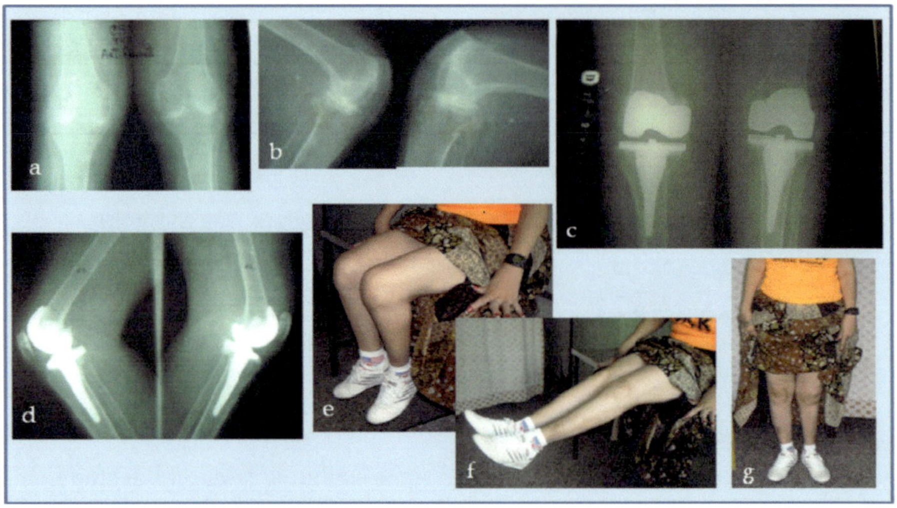

Fig. 7. a. b. Pre-operative AP and Lateral view X-ray of both knee showed the total joint collapse and fixed flexion deformity, c. d. Post-operative bilateral TKA implanted, and e. f. g restored the patient, showing full extension.

The last case presented was a 32 years old, male, with history of multiple injured patient involved in route traffic accident RTA 2 years ago, that actually has diagnosis of post traumatic severe ostearthritis , with stiff and posterior subluxated left knee. The figure 8 a. b. c. d. e. f. g. h. showed the sequence of pre and post operative results to recovery assessed at one year of evolution.

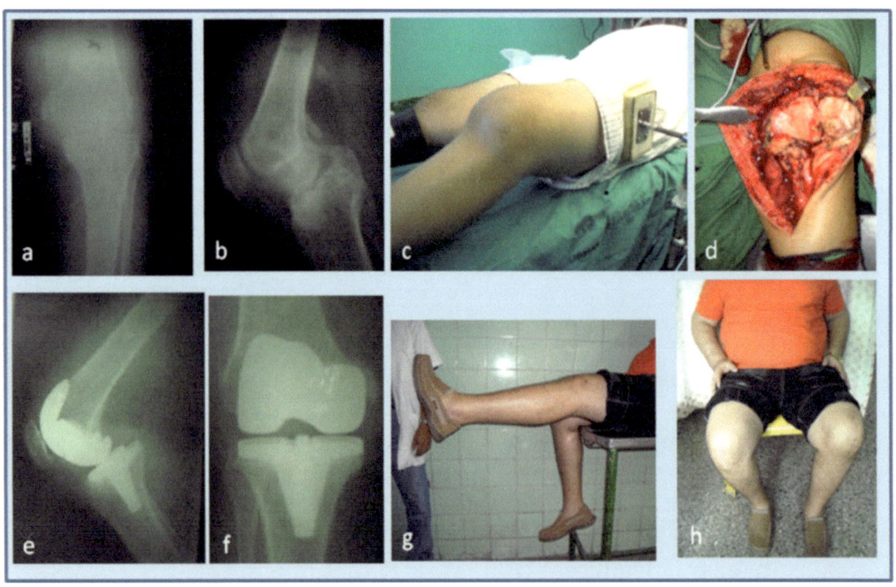

Fig. 8. a. b. c. Evident deformity of the left knee sequel of trauma that required extensive soft tissue release (d.) and TKA implanted (e. f.) and final recovery of the patient with excellent range of motion.

4. Conclusion

In this study about complex Total Knee Arthroplasty in special situation according to our results an outcome, till now the evidence permitted arrive to the following conclusions: patients with specials situations in the knee may look complex or difficult, but the Total Knee Arthroplasty using Kalisté System has been a very successful operation with a high level of patient satisfaction and functional improvement like others reports.

Best results were achieved when the surgeon has carefully evaluated all the factors influencing in each individual special situation and did a preoperative plannification according to it.

The selections of patient and prosthesis design were very important, but we believe that efficient surgery and overall the experience and skill of the surgeon could be more important.

At one to six years follow-up postoperative, the functional outcome between before and after operation appears to be significant different, nevertheless we considered the weakness of this study is the short-mid time's follow-up and need further investigation and follow-up at least ten to fifteen years after implantation.

We believe that the use of Kalisté Knee System improved our results and we can advice this design as an excellent system of TKA.

Finally, our study showed the aim of the evaluation and the evidence: improved the Quality of Life of the Patient in Relation with Health QLPRH.

5. Acknowledgment

The first acknowledgment and gratitude is to Professor Sc. Dr. Rodrigo J.Alvarez Cambras, my mentor, and to Dr. Ricardo J. Tarragona too,for their participation in this study.

I gratefully acknowledge Margarita Garcia, Mayra Leon, Emma Sanchez, Isabel Vega and Gonzalez Liuba for your time, patience and support during the writing, language, as well as making the graphs, tables and photos. And special thanks to Ms Adriana Pecar for her invitation to submit this chapter.

6. References

Agencia de Evaluación Tecnologías Sanitarias (AETS) (2002). Índice y escalas utilizadas en ciertas tecnologías de la prestación ortoprotésica. (Protetización del Sistema Osteoarticular). AETS Instituto de Salud Carlos III. Ministerio de Sanidad y Consumo. Madrid. Noviembre. pp. 5.8, 55-64, 120-28 ISBN 84-95463-14-8

Aglietti P.; Windsov RE.; Buzzi R. and Insall JN (1989). Arthroplasty for stiff or ankylosed Knee. J. Arthroplasty. 41(1):1-5

Aglietti P.; Buzzi R.; Segoni F., et al (1995). Insall-Burstein posterior-stabilized Knee prosthesis in rheumatoid arthritis. J. Arthroplasty; 10:217-25

Alhback S (1968). Osteoarthritis of the Knee. A radiographic investigation. Acta Radiol Diagn. (Suppl) 27:77-82

Ayers DC, Dennis DA, Johanson NA, Pellegrini VD (1997). Instructional Course Lectures. The American Academy of Orthopaedic Surgeons. Common Complication of Total Knee Arthroplasty. J. Bone Joint Surg; 79-A(22):278-331

Bayne O & Camero HV (1984). Total Knee Arthroplasty following patellectomy. Clin Orthop; 186:112

Brinkman JM, et al (2008). Osteotomies arround the Knee: patient selection, stability of fixation and bone healing in high tibial osteotomies. J. Bone Joint Surg; 90-B:1548-57

Brown TD, et al (2006). Post-traumatic osteoarthritis. A first estímate of incidence, prevalence and burden of disease. J Orthop Trauma; 30:739-44

Brundtland GH (2007). The Bone and Joint Decade WHO Scientific Group meeting on burden musculoskeletal disease. Geneva. http://www.who.int/generaldirector/speeches/2000/english/...accessed

Callahan CM, Drake BG, Heck DA, Dittus RS (1994). Patients outcomes following tricompartimental total knee replacement. JAMA; 271:1349-57

Clark CR, Rorabech CH, MacDonald S, et al. (2001). Posterior-stabilized and cruciate-retaining total knee replacement: a randomized study. Clin Orthop; 392:208-12

Colizza WA, Insall JN & Scuderi GR (1995). The posterior stabilized total knee prosthesis. Assessment of polyethilene damage and osteolisis after a ten-year minimun follow-up. J Bone Joint Surg; 77-A:1713-20

Crockarell Jr. JR, and Guyton JL (2003). Arthroplasty of ankle and knee Chapter 6. Pp 245-313. In: Terry Canale S. Campell's Operative Orthopaedics Vol. One. Tenth Edition, Mosby, ISBN 0-323-01240-X. St. Louis

De Cárdenas OM, Álvarez RJ, Croas FA, et al (2008). Presentation of a protocol for Total Knee Arthroplasty. Rev Cubana Ortop Traumatol (on line), Vol 22 No. 2 pp. 0-0 ISSN 0864-215-X

De Cárdenas OM et al (2008). Revisión Knee replacement in an unusual case. Rev Cubana Ortop Traumatol (on line), Vol 22 No. 1 pp. 0-0 ISSN 0864-215-X

De Cárdenas OM (2010). Specials situations in Total Knee Arthroplasty. Proceeding of Cuban Orthopedic Congress ISBN 978-959-7158-95-0. Villa Clara, Sept.

De Cárdenas OM, Álvarez RJ, Croas FA, et al (2010). Kalisté Total Knee Arthroplasty System in patients with Rheumatoid Arthritis. Proceeding of Cuban Orthopedic Congress ISBN 978-959-7158-95-0. Villa Clara, Sept

Dennis DA, Kouistek RD, Strehl JB, et al (1998). Patients with PS-TKA demostrated greater flexion that patients with PCR-TKA when measured in weight bearing. J Arthroplasty; 13(7):748-52

Diduch DR et al (1977). Total Knee replacement in young active patients. J Bone Joint Surg; 79-A:571-82

Dorr LD (1993). Management of Bone Defects. Chapter 18, pp. 309-17. In: *Rand JA.* Total Knee Arthroplasty. *Raven Press.* New York. ISBN 0-88167-930-5

Dunbar MJ, Howard A, Bogoch EA, et al (2009). Orthopedics in 2020. Predictor of Musculoskeletal Need. An OAA-COA Symposium The Orthopaedic Forum. J Bone Joint Surg; 91:2276-86

El-Azab H, Halawa A, Anetzberger H, et al (2008). The effect of closed- and open- wedge high tibial osteotomy on the tibial slope: a retrospective radiological review of 120 cases. J Bone Joint Surg; 90-B:1193-7

Engh GA, & Parks NL (1994). The use a bone defect classification system in revisión Total Knee Arthroplasty. Orthop trans; 18:1138-9

Ensini A, Catani, Leardini A, et al (2007). Alignments and clinical results in conventional and navigated Total Knee Arthroplasty. Clin Orthop; 457:156-62

Ewald FC (1989). The Knee Society Total Knee Arthroplasty roentgenographic evaluation and Scoring system. Clin Orthop; 248:9-12

Giffin JR, Stabile K, Zantop T, et al (2007). Importancs of tibial slope for stability of the posterior cruciate ligament deficient Knee. Am J Sports Med; 35;1443-9

Hung CLW, Pan YW, Yuen CK, et al (2009). Interobserver and intraobserver error in distal femur transepicondylar axis measurement with computed tomography. J Arthroplasty; 26:96-100

Hungerford DS (1995). Malalignment, erosion and patella abscense. Chapter 11. Pp. 161- 75. In: Lotke PA. Master Technique in Orthopaedic Surgery Knee Arthroplasty. Lippincott Raven Publisher. Philadelphia. ISBN 0-7817-0032-9

Insall JN, Dorr LD, Scott RD, Scott WN (1989). Rationale of the Knee Society Clinical Rating System. Clin Orthop; 248:13-14

Jacobs WCH, Clement DJ, Wimenga AB (2008). Conservación del sacrificio del ligamento cruzado posterior en el reemplazo total de rodilla para el tratamiento de la Osteoartritis y la Artritis Reumatoide. (Revisión Cochrane traducida). Biblioteca Cochrane Plus; Número 2, Oxford, Update Software. Disponible en http://www.update-sofware.com. (Translated from the Cochrane Library, Issue. Chicester, UK, John Wiley & Sons. Ltd.

Dawson J., Fitzpatrick R, Murray D., Carr A (1998). Questionnaire on the perceptions of patients about total Knee replacement QPPTKR. J Bone Joint Surg; 80-B(1):63-69

Insall JN, Lachiewicz PF, Burnstein AH (1982). The posterior stabilized condylar prosthesis: A modification of the total condylar design. Two to four year clinical experience. J Bone Joint Surg; 64-A:1317-23

Johnson BP and Dorr LD (1999). Total Knee Arthroplasty after high tibial osteotomy. Chapter 12, pp. 178-92. In: Lotke PA. Master Technique in Orthopaedic Surgery Knee Arthroplasty. Lippincott-Raven Publisher. Philadelphia. ISBN 0-7817-0032- 9-1995

Katz MM et al (1987). Results of Total Knee Artroplasty after failed proximal tibial osteotomy for osteoarthritis; J Bone Joint Surg 69-A:225

Katz JN et al (2007). Association of hospital and surgeon procedure volumen with patient centered outcomes of total Knee replacement in a populatio-based cohort of patient age 65 years and older. Arthritis Rheum; 56:568-74

Leunox D, Hungerford D. & Krackow K (1987). Total Knee Arthroplasty following patellectomy. Clin Orthop; 223:220

Lingard EA, Berven S, Katz JN (2000). Management and care of patients undergoing Total Knee Arthroplasy: variations across different health care settings. Arthritis Care Res; 13:129-36

Lombardi Jr. AV, Mallory T, Fade RA, et al (2001). An algorithm for posterior cruciate ligament in Total Knee Arthroplasty. Clin Orthop; 392:75-87

Lombardi AV, Nett MP, Scott WN, et al (2009). Primary Total Knee Artrhoplasty. J Bone Joint Surg; 91 Suppl 5:52-5

Lotke PA (1999). Master Technique in Orthopaedic Surgery Knee Arthroplasty. Lippincott-Raven Publisher Philadelphia. ISBN 0-7817-0032-9-1995

Minns CJ, Baker KL, Dewey M, et al (2007). Effectiveness of phisiotherapy exercise after Knee Arthroplasty for Osteoarthritis: Systematic review and meta-analysis of randomised conrolled trials. BMJ; 335:812-5

Paletta GA & Laskin RS (1995). Total Knee Arthroplasty after a previus patellectomy. J Bone Joint Surg; 77-A:1708-12

Parvizi J. et al (2006). Management of stiffness following Total Knee Arthroplasty. J Bone Joint Surg *Am;* 88:175-181

Ranawat CS, Aglietti P, Shine J. (1976). A comparison of four model of Total Knee replacement prostheses. J Bone Joint Surg; 58-A:754-65

Ranawat CS, Padgett DE, Osashi Y (1989). Total Knee Arthroplasty for patients younger than 55 years. Clin Ortop; 248:27

Ranawat CS and Flynn Jr. WF (1999). Stiff Knee. Ankylosis and flexion. Chapter 10 pp. 141-59. In: Lotke PA. Master Technique in Orthopaedic Surgery. Knee Arthroplasty. Lippincott-Raven Publiser. Philadelphia. ISBN 0-7817-0032-9-1995

Ranawat ChS, Ranawat AS, Metha A (2003). Total Knee Arthroplasty rehabilitation protocol. What makes the difference? J. Arthroplasty; 18:27-30

Rand JA, Trousdale RT, Ilstrup DM et al (2009. Factors affecting the durability of Primary Total Knee Prosthesis. J Bone Joint Surg; 85-A:259-65

Rakin EA, Alarcon GS, Chang RW, et al (2004). NIH Consensus Statements on Total Knee Replacement. J. Bone Joint Surg; 86(6):1328-35

Robertsson O, Knutson K, Lewold S, et al (1997). Knee Arthroplasty in rheumatoid arthritis: a report from the Swedish Knee arthroplasty register on 4,381 primary operation 1985-1995. Acta Orthop Scand; 68:545-53

Rodríguez JA, Saddler S, Edelman S & Ranawat CH (1996). Long term results of Total Knee Arthroplasty in class 3 and 4 rheumatoid arthritis. J Arthroplasty; 11:141-15

Rubino LJ, Schoderhek RJ, Raymond Golish S et al (2008). The effect of plate position and size on tibial slope in high tibial osteotomy: a cadaveric study. J Knee Surg; 21:75-9

Shakespeare D., Kinsel V (2005). Rehabilitation after Total Knee Replacement. Time to go home? Knee; 12:185-9

Stuard MJ and Rand JA (1988). Total Knee Arthroplasty in young adults who have rheumatoid arthritis. J Bone Joint Surg; 70-A:84-7

Scott WN, Booth RE, Dalury DF et al (2009). Efficiency and economics in Joint Arthroplasty. J Bone Joint Surg; 91 Suppl 5:36-3

Scuderi GR, Insall JN (1989). The posterior stabilized Knee Prosthesis. Orthop Clin North Am; 20(1):71-8

Scuderi GR and Insall JN (1999). Varus and valgus fixed deformities. Chapter 8 pp. 111- 127 In: Lotke PA. Master Technique in Orthopaedic Surgery Knee Arthroplasty. Lippincott-Raven Publisher Philadelphia. ISBN 0-7817-0032-9-1995

Sculco TP (1999). Bone graft. Chapter 9, pp. 132-40 In: Lotke PA. Master Technique in Orthopaedic Surgery. Knee Arthroplasty. Lippincott-Raven Publisher. Philadelphia. ISBN 0-7817-0032-9.-1995

Stern S (2002). Cost considerations. An historical perspective. In: Scuderi GR & Tria Jr. AJ. Eds Surgical techniques in Total Knee Artroplasty. Springer-Verlag. New York

Whiteside, LA and Ohl MD (1990). Tibial tubercle osteotomy for exposure of the difficult Total Knee Arthroplasty. Clin Orthop; 260:6-9

Windsor RE, Insall JN, & Vincent KG (1988). Technical consideations of Total Knee Arthroplasty after proximal tibial osteotomy. J Bone Joint Surg; 70-A:547-555

Yan WP, Leung A, Lin KG, et al(2007). Interobserver and intraobserver errors in obtaining visually selected anatomical landmarks during registration process in non- image-based navigation assisted total Knee. J. Arthroplasty; 22:1050-61

22

Patient-Specific Patellofemoral Arthroplasty

Domenick J. Sisto[1], Ronald P. Grelsamer[2] and Vineet K. Sarin[3]
[1]*Los Angeles Orthopaedic Institute, Sherman Oaks, California*
[2]*Mount Sinai Medical Center, New York, New York*
[3]*Kinamed Incorporated, Camarillo, California*
USA

1. Introduction

In this chapter we review the topic of patellofemoral arthroplasty from a historical, technical, and clinical perspective. Emphasis is placed on the design rationale, surgical technique, and clinical results of so-called "patient-matched" or "patient-specific" patellofemoral arthroplasty in which the trochlear implant is matched to the anatomy of the individual patient through the use of pre-operative computerized imaging scans (Fig 1).

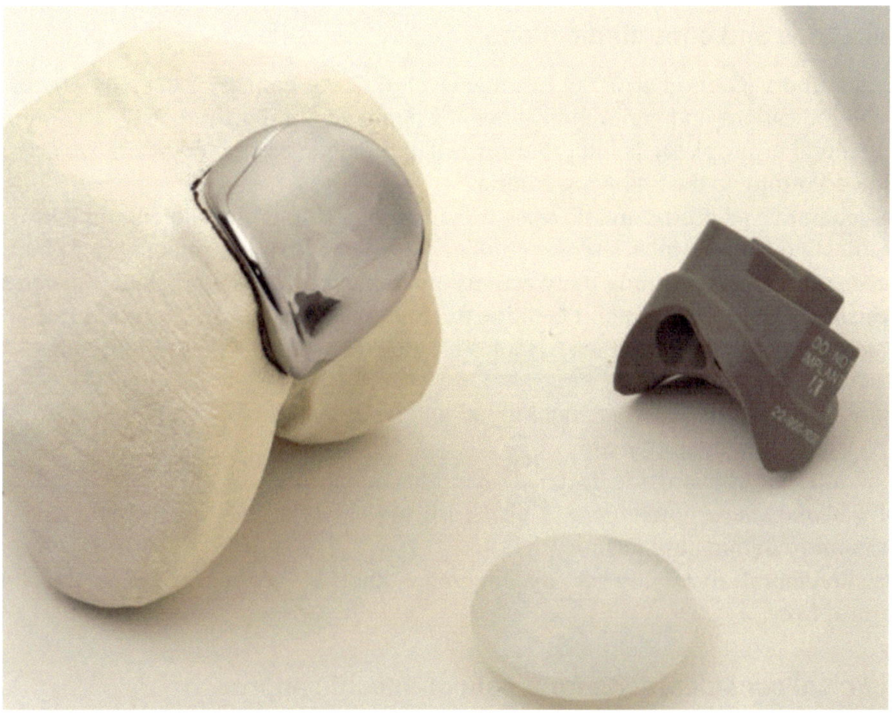

Fig. 1. Patient-specific patellofemoral implant mounted on patient-specific physical bone model, alongside a companion patient-specific drill guide & marking template and all-polyethylene patella button. Collectively these items constitute the patient-specific patellofemoral arthroplasty system described in this chapter.

The implants are inlayed into the articular cartilage without any intra-operative femoral bone resection. Clinical results involving patient-matched patellofemoral arthroplasty are presented with an average follow-up of 11 years. Case studies reviewing our collective experience with patient-matched trochlear implants in the setting of femoral trochlear dysplasia are also presented.

2. Historical perspective

The origins of patellofemoral arthroplasty (PFA or PFR) can be traced to 1955 with the introduction of the McKeever prosthesis (McKeever, 1955). This prosthesis consisted of a Vitallium® shell used to resurface only the patella. The procedure was eventually abandoned because of concerns regarding trochlear wear (Leadbetter et al, 2006). Blazina et al (1979) reported on the use of a patellofemoral prosthesis. In the decades that followed, a number of different patellofemoral prostheses were developed and studied (Lonner, 2004; Leadbetter et al, 2005; Lonner, 2007; Sisto & Sarin, 2008; Gupta et al, 2010). The clinical results with these designs have been highly variable, which has led to skepticism about the success of the procedure. A consensus view has emerged that appropriate patient selection and prosthesis design are the two most critical elements for achieving successful outcomes after patellofemoral arthroplasty (Arnbjornsson and Ryd, 1998; Kooijman et al, 2003; Lonner, 2004; Ackroyd et al, 2007; Lonner, 2007; Gupta et al, 2010).

3. Indications and contraindications

Previous authors (Grelsamer, 2006; Leadbetter et al, 2006; Lonner, 2007) have discussed in detail the indications and contraindications for patellofemoral arthroplasty. To summarize, patellofemoral arthroplasty is indicated for isolated patellofemoral degenerative arthritis of the knee, according to the following criteria:

- Degenerative or posttraumatic osteoarthritis limited to the patellofemoral joint, so that medial and lateral Ahlback scores (Ahlback, 1968) are less than or equal to 1 point;
- Severe symptoms affecting daily activity referable to patellofemoral joint degeneration unresponsive to lengthy non-operative treatment and conservative procedures;
- Patellofemoral malalignment/dysplasia induced degeneration with or without instability.

Contraindications include but are not limited to the following criteria:

- The lack of non-operative care;
- Pain referred from outside the patellofemoral compartment or even outside the knee;
- Medial and lateral tibiofemoral Ahlback scores (Ahlback, 1968) greater than 1 point;
- Systemic inflammatory arthropathy;
- Patellofemoral instability or malalignment that is uncorrectable at the time of arthroplasty.

4. Technical considerations for a patient-specific approach

4.1 Motivation

The shape and alignment of the human patellar trochlear groove is highly variable (Feinstein et al, 1996). Such variability presents a challenge for so-called "off-the-shelf" patellofemoral prostheses that feature a fixed geometry and a finite number of sizes. For patellofemoral compartments that deviate from an off-the-shelf implant's design paradigm, there exists an inherent tradeoff between fit and alignment that must be addressed intra-operatively. Many reported off-the-shelf implant failures are thought to be due to design deficiencies related to fit and alignment within the patellofemoral compartment (Lonner, 2004; Lonner, 2007; Gupta et al, 2010). The patient-specific approach to patellofemoral arthroplasty described in this chapter was conceived and developed in light of these challenges (Fig 2).

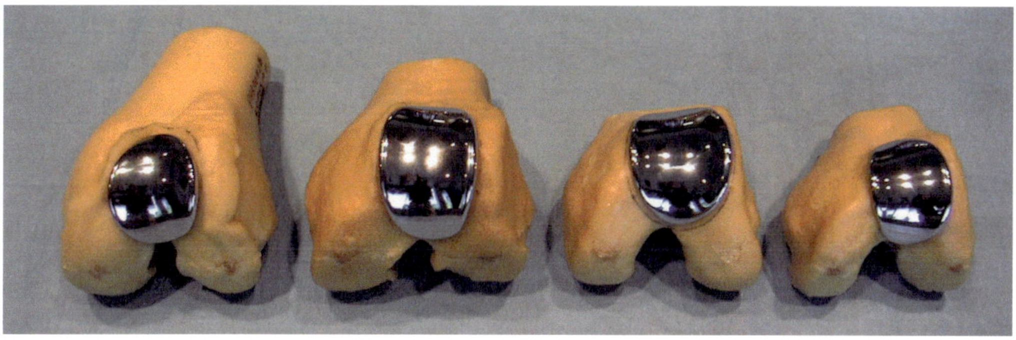

Fig. 2. Physical distal femur models from four patients treated with patient-specific patellofemoral arthroplasty (cartilage not shown). Note the substantial variation in trochlear groove geometry across this group, consistent with previously published findings. The patient-specific approach provides for a precise fit without bone resection or sculpting.

4.2 Design rationale

The design goal of patient-specific patellofemoral arthroplasty is to restore the mechanics of the patellofemoral compartment and maintain the native mechanics of the tibiofemoral compartments (Sisto & Sarin, 2006; Sisto & Sarin, 2008). Progression of arthritic disease into the medial and lateral knee compartments often contributes to the need for patellofemoral arthroplasty revision (Grelsamer, 2006). Poorly fitting off-the-shelf prostheses can detrimentally affect the mechanics of the knee joint (including the medial and lateral compartments), leading to disease progression into these compartments. Further, installing off-the-shelf prostheses can be a time-consuming process; and poorly fitting prostheses may require significant cement support. Patient-specific patellofemoral arthroplasty effectively addresses the design deficiencies and difficulties in surgical technique associated with off-the-shelf patellofemoral prostheses.

The patient-specific patellofemoral arthroplasty prosthesis described in this chapter is designed to custom-fit the bony anatomy; its bony contact surface is designed to conform to the bony anatomy of the patient's femoral trochlea using computed tomographic (CT) modeling (Fig 3). This approach allows for a precise fit of the implant to the trochlea without resection of subchondral femoral bone, as is necessary for so-called "onlay" off-the-shelf prostheses. Only removal of the overlying cartilage is necessary to obtain a precise fit with a patient-specific prosthesis. The trochlear prosthesis is designed to approximate normal patellofemoral kinematics by re-establishing a trochlear groove.

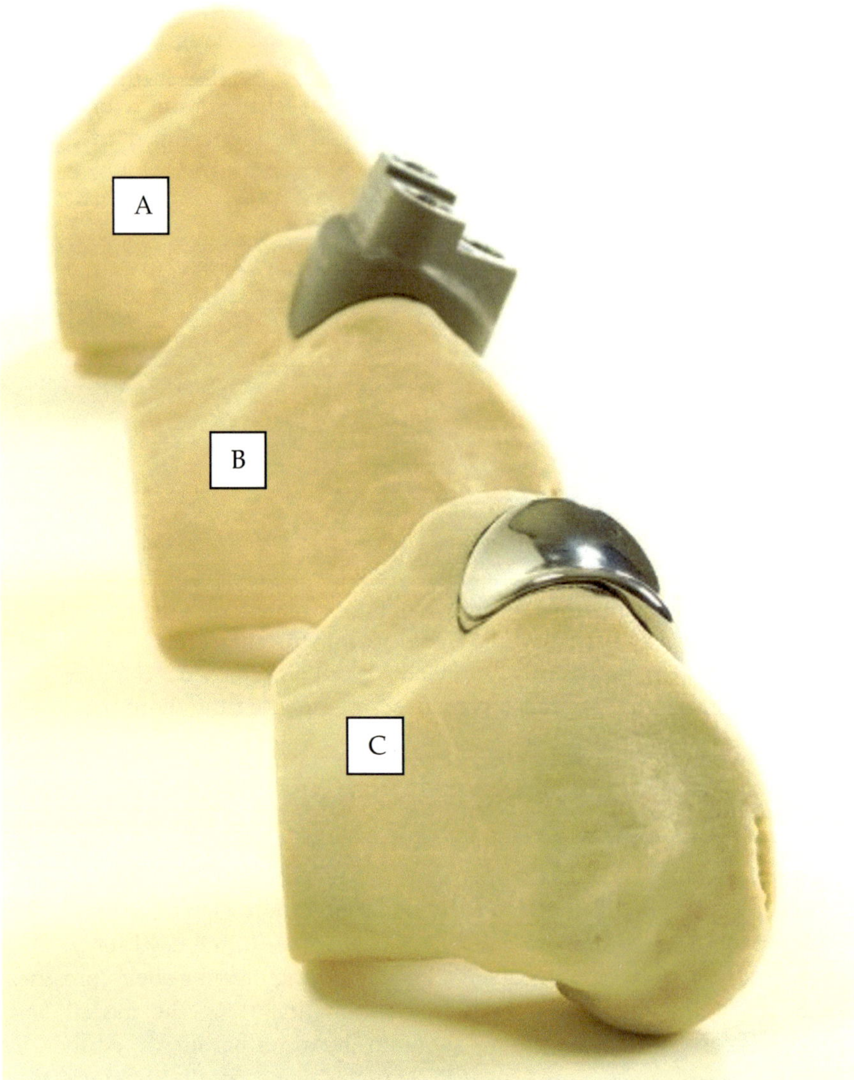

Fig. 3. Native patient-specific physical bone model (A), patient-specific bone model with companion patient-specific drill guide & marking template (B), and patient-specific bone model with companion patient-specific trochlear implant (C). Note the precise fit between patient-specific components and native unresected trochlear bone.

The distal margin of the patient-specific trochlear prosthesis is designed to rest 3 to 5 mm from the apex of the intercondylar notch. The prosthesis has a thickened lateral border to compensate for bone loss along the lateral edge of the trochlear groove and to provide congruency and tracking stability with the matching patellar implant. The thickened implant border does not anteriorize ("stuff") the patella relative to its pre-operative state because the anterior position of a given patella is defined by the thickness of the femoral implant's trochlear groove. The patient-specific femoral prosthesis may seem thick on lateral radiographs, but only because the radiograph is a 2-dimensional projection of a saddle-shaped structure.

The articular side of the patellofemoral implant has a radius of curvature matched to the curvature of a standard dome patellar implant. It is designed to constrain the patellar implant medially and laterally as it tracks along the trochlear groove. This design is, therefore, able to compensate for a deficient or dysplastic trochlear groove, which is often present in patellofemoral surgery candidates.

The bony-contact surface and the articulating surface of the patient-specific trochlear implant are "decoupled." The bony-contact surface is customized to fit the bony anatomy, while the articulating surface is designed to mate with a patella button prosthesis and provide medial-lateral constraint to the patella. The medial and lateral borders of the articular surface are thickened by a few millimeters to provide stability and congruency for the patella button.

The design rationale of patient-specific patellofemoral arthroplasty therefore eliminates the trade-off between fit and alignment that is inherent to off-the-shelf, particularly inlay, patellofemoral implants.

4.3 Stuffing

Overstuffing of the patellofemoral compartment has been cited (Lonner, 2007) as a concern over the use of patient-specific patellofemoral arthroplasty. Although this may be a theoretical concern, it has not been borne out by the clinical results. Moreover, the concept of patellofemoral overstuffing has been challenged. Merchant and colleagues (2008) state the following:

> The concept of overstuffing the patellofemoral joint has been simply and uncritically transferred from the femorotibial joint with no confirmatory studies. Because the capsule and inelastic ligaments secure the femorotibial joint, it is extremely important to balance these ligaments carefully during TKA and avoid a tibial insert that is too large. This will certainly overstuff this joint and lead to a poor result with decreased range of motion. The patellofemoral joint is a totally different articulation. Although the patellar ligament is inelastic, the quadriceps muscles are elastic and stretchable. This explains why the investigation by Bengs and Scott (2006) failed to support the claim of overstuffing by Conley et al (2007). More recently, Pierson et al (2007) reviewed 830 primary TKAs to determine the effects of so-called overstuffing the patellofemoral joint. Their findings did "not support the widely held belief that stuffing of the patellofemoral joint results in adverse outcomes after total knee arthroplasty."

The trochlear prosthesis is designed to restore the anterior position of the non-degenerated patella. The thickness of normal articular cartilage is approximately 5 to 7 mm on the patella and 2 to 3 mm in the trochlea, yielding a combined total cartilage thickness of 7 to 10 mm (Grelsamer, 2000). The trochlear prosthesis typically is 2 to 5 mm thick along its center arc, the tracking arc of the patella. This thickness is a function of native trochlear groove depth (i.e., thinner implants are created for shallower grooves). The thinner implants are designed specifically to avoid overstuffing the more dysplastic trochleas. Coupled with an anatomic restoration of the patella, the extensor lever arm is intended to be unchanged or improved from the pre-operative condition (see Fig 6, described later in this chapter). If concerns about overstuffing still persist, accommodations can be made by resecting more bone on the patellar side or by selecting a thinner patellar implant.

5. Peri-operative technique

The peri-operative technique for patient-specific patellofemoral arthroplasty has been previously described (Sisto & Sarin, 2007; Sisto et al, 2010; Lombardi, 2011) and consists of pre-operative planning, intra-operative technique, and post-operative management.

5.1 Pre-operative planning

A CT scan of the patient's knee is obtained using the following settings as specified by the manufacturer of the prosthesis (Kinamed Incorporated, Camarillo, California, USA):

- Voltage: 120 to 140 kV;
- Amperage: 200 to 300 mA;
- Scan Region: 5mm distal to the femoral condyles to 10mm proximal to the patella.

Computer modeling is then used to create a 3-dimensional physical model of the patient's distal femoral bone, which is sent to the surgeon. The manufacturer identifies the perimeter of coverage of the trochlear implant on this model. If deemed necessary based on the presence of significant osteophytes or bony defects in or near the native trochlea, the surgeon may physically remove osteophytes from the model and communicate these changes by returning the model to the implant manufacturer. The final design for the trochlear implant is then created after surgeon approval.

If changes are made during the design review, during surgery the surgeon will modify the real trochlear groove in the same manner as was done on the physical model. For this reason, it is imperative that the physical model be available for visual examination in the operating theatre.

It must be noted that patellofemoral arthroplasty is not a substitute for a patellar realignment procedure. Patella tracking must be evaluated for instability and soft tissue imbalance (Lonner, 2004; Grelsamer, 2000). Malalignment of the patella is determined through physical examination and standard radiographic evaluation. Assessment of patellar tracking is important in pre-operative planning, as patellar instability is the most often reported cause of dysfunction after patellofemoral arthroplasty. Tightness of the lateral retinaculum is often associated with lateralization and patellar tilt, which may be determined upon physical examination. Examination of medial structures for deficiency should also be carried out, as well as assessment of the tibial tuberosity (Q angle). Axial and lateral radiographs are often sufficient to quantify measures of patellar malalignment, including patella alta or baja, medial-lateral displacement and patellar tilt. Treatments are generally customized to each patient, although it remains to be determined if there are one or more standard procedures that will be optimal for most patients (Grelsamer, 2000).

5.2 Intra-operative technique

A standard midline incision is made to expose the patellofemoral joint, and the patella is everted or tilted 90°. The length of the incision is typically two-thirds the length of a standard total knee incision because tibial exposure is not necessary. The margin of cartilage to be removed is determined by placing the patient-specific drill guide onto the trochlea. Because the cartilage remnants on the trochlea will initially not permit a proper fit of the patient-specific custom drill guide, the surgeon first approximates the proper position of the drill guide (using the CT-created physical bone model as a template). The surgeon outlines the drill guide with methylene blue and by way of a ring curette removes the cartilage inside that outline. Osteophytes are removed as necessary. The patient-specific drill guide is then placed on the subchondral bone of the trochlea and moved slightly back and forth until it seats in its intended position as determined by the CT scan. Two headless nails are then used to secure the drill guide and the three holes are drilled. The holes are then thoroughly irrigated to remove any debris that may be present.

The trochlear prosthesis is designed to be used in conjunction with a standard off-the-shelf all-polyethylene patellar button of onlay design with a 25 mm radius of curvature. The residual patellar thickness is the same as with total knee arthroplasty.

During trialing, particular attention is paid to potential subluxation or catching within the limitations of a patient under anesthesia (Lonner, 2004). If realignment is necessary, balancing is carried out in the same manner as a non-prosthetic or total knee arthroplasty. To correct patellar tilt or lateral displacement of the patella, a proximal realignment procedure such as a lateral retinacular release, medial plication, vastus medialis obliquus advancement, and/or medial patellofemoral ligament repair may be carried out (Grelsamer, 2000). In the presence of a high Q angle, a distal realignment procedure such as transfer of the tibial tuberosity may be carried out to correct alignment of the extensor mechanism (Grelsamer, 2000). Any realignment or soft-tissue balancing strategy should be oriented toward addressing specific identifiable pathology (Grelsamer, 2000).

Cementing is carried out in standard knee arthroplasty fashion. Particular care needs to be taken to avoid cement seepage into the notch or other compartments. The cartilage of the other compartments must be kept moist throughout the procedure to avoid deterioration. Patellofemoral tracking is again evaluated and soft tissue corrections are carried out as necessary to ensure optimal patellar tracking.

5.3 Post-operative management

The need for prophylaxis against deep venous thrombosis has not been shown for patellofemoral replacement surgery. Postoperative rehabilitation consists of range of motion exercises as with any knee arthroplasty. As a rule, though, progress will be much quicker than with total knee arthroplasty patients. Immediate full-weight bearing is allowed. Physical therapy to restore quadriceps strength is encouraged. Twisting activities are discouraged, but no additional specific activity modifications are recommended.

6. Clinical results

Previous investigators have reported on clinical results obtained with off-the-shelf and patient-specific patellofemoral arthroplasty.

6.1 Results with off-the-shelf implants

Published clinical results with off-the-shelf patellofemoral implants have been previously reviewed in detail (Lonner, 2007; Sisto & Sarin, 2008; Gupta et al, 2010; Charalambous et al, 2011). These references cover twenty one studies that each involved from 14 to 306 patients who received 8 different off-the-shelf designs, with follow-up ranging from 6 months to 21 years. These reports demonstrate that clinical results with off-the-shelf patellofemoral implant designs have been highly variable.

The Australian national joint replacement registry reports that the cumulative revision rate at five and seven years for off-the-shelf patellofemoral implants used in the setting of primary osteoarthritis is 15.2% and 22.4%, respectively (Australian Orthopaedic Association, 2010).

6.2 Results with patient-matched Implants

6.2.1 Prior investigation

In an earlier published investigation (Sisto and Sarin, 2006), 100% survivorship with excellent or good Knee Society scores was reported at a mean duration of follow-up of 73 (range, 32 to 119) months. The study was a retrospective review of a consecutive single-surgeon series of patient-specific patellofemoral arthroplasties performed between March 1995 and August 2002. There were 25 patellofemoral arthroplasties performed in 22 patients (three staged bilaterals), 16 of whom were female. Mean age at the time of index arthroplasty was 45 (range, 23 to 51) years.

Only patients whose medial and lateral compartments scored less than or equal to 1 point on the Ahlback scale were indicated for patellofemoral arthroplasty. The patellofemoral compartments for all knees scored at least 4 points. The mean pre-operative Knee Society functional score was 49 points, and the mean pre-operative Knee Society objective score was 52 points.

There were 18 excellent and 7 good results at 73 months of follow-up. The mean post-operative Knee Society objective score was 91 (range, 82 to 96) points, and the mean post-operative Knee Society functional score was 89 (range, 81 to 94) points. All patients exhibited good to excellent Knee Society Score status and no patient had required additional surgery or had component loosening.

6.2.2 Eleven year follow-up

The objective of the eleven year follow-up study was to evaluate the longer-term success of patient-specific patellofemoral arthroplasty in the original patient cohort. For assessment of

Question	Answer
Has your custom PFA been replaced?	No: 25 out of 25 Yes: 0
Does your PFA keep you from doing anything that you would like to do?	No: 23 out of 25 Yes: 2 out of 25
How satisfied are you with your PFA?	Very Dissatisfied: 0 out of 25 Somewhat Satisfied: 0 out of 25 Very Satisfied: 25 out of 25
Have you had additional surgery on this knee since your PFA?	No: 25 out of 25 Yes: 0
How often do you take pain medication because of pain in this knee?	Never: 25 out of 25 Sometimes (1-2x per week): 0 Often (>1 per day): 0
If you have pain, where is the pain coming from?	Inside of Knee: 3 out of 25 Kneecap area: 21 out of 25 Outside of Knee: 1 out of 25
Does this knee feel weak or unstable?	No: 25 out of 25 Yes: 0
Would you undergo PFA with this custom implant again?	No: 0 Yes: 25 out of 25

Table 1. The original cohort included 25 patellofemoral arthroplasties (PFAs) in 22 patients. Each patient from the original cohort answered via telephone the above-listed questions, which were selected and adapted from the validated "Total Knee Function Questionnaire" (Weiss et al, 2002). All patients were successfully contacted and no knees were lost. Average time from index patellofemoral arthroplasty to completion of the questionnaire was 11.3 years (range, 7.8 to 14.9 years).

longer-term follow-up, the validated "Total Knee Function Questionnaire" (Weiss et al, 2002) was adapted and administered via telephone to each patient from the above-mentioned prior study. The questions were designed to assess the status of each patient's patellofemoral arthroplasty as well as their degree of knee function.
The questionnaire was completed for all 25 knees (Table 1). No knees from the original study were lost to follow-up. At a mean duration of 11.3 years (range, 7.8 to 14.9 years) from the index arthroplasty, all 25 patellofemoral arthroplasties were still in place and all patients reported themselves as being very satisfied. There were no reports of weakness, instability, or additional surgery. Two patients reported that despite their patellofemoral arthroplasty, they were not participating in sports activities. All patients experienced some pain, but not enough to warrant medication. All 22 patients said they would undergo the procedure again.
This 11 year follow-up study demonstrates that patient-specific patellofemoral arthroplasty is a safe and effective treatment for patients with isolated patellofemoral arthritis of the knee. These results compare favorably with those involving off-the-shelf patellofemoral arthroplasties that have been reported on over the past 30 years (Leadbetter et al, 2005; Leadbetter et al, 2006; Lonner, 2007; Sisto and Sarin, 2008; Gupta et al, 2010).

6.3 Complications

Progression of arthritis into the tibiofemoral compartment is a recognized complication of patellofemoral replacement; when symptomatic, this scenario leads to conversion to a total knee arthroplasty. Progression is more likely to develop when the disease patellofemoral arthritis does not have a clear origin, such as idiopathic arthritis (Grelsamer, 2006). Despite attempts to balance the extensor mechanism, patellar maltracking after patellofemoral arthroplasty can occur, especially when the patient pre-operatively demonstrates high level malalignment and/or dysplasia.

7. Case studies

Our (DJS and RPG) collective experience with patient-specific patellofemoral arthroplasty dates back to 1995 and consists of 91 cases in 79 patients through May 2011. Patients in our cohort generally fall into one of two categories: those having a "normal" femoral trochlear sulcus angle, with or without patellar tilt; and those having a femoral sulcus angle greater than 145°, i.e. a shallow or even convex trochlea – dysplastic trochleas will exhibit a crossing sign on a true lateral radiograph (Bollier and Fulkerson, 2011). The following case studies serve as illustrative examples.

7.1 Normal trochlear anatomy

Patient J.O. is a 49 year old male who initially presented with severe anterior knee pain 14 years ago after sustaining a twisting injury to his knee that was treated with arthroscopic surgery followed by a soft tissue realignment procedure two years later. During this time, he developed progressive and disabling anterior knee pain. He could not walk up or down stairs without assistance and could not kneel, squat or climb without severe pain.
Physical examination revealed severe anterior knee tenderness with severe crepitus and grinding in the retro-patellar space. He had no ligament instability and no medial or lateral joint line tenderness. All provocative tests for meniscal and ligamentous injury were

negative. The radiographs revealed severe patellofemoral arthritis and no medial or lateral joint line abnormalities (Fig 4).

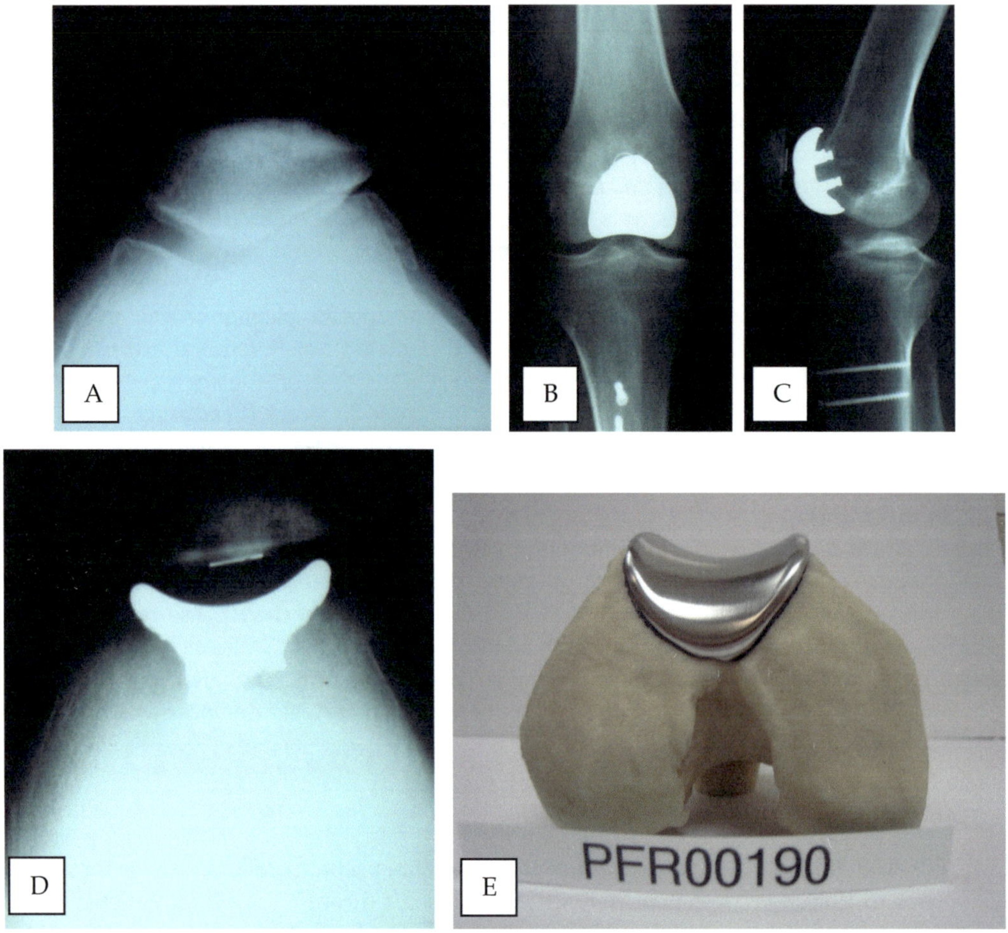

Fig. 4. A 49 year old male with isolated end-stage patellofemoral arthritis, without evidence of trochlear dysplasia as seen in pre-operative Merchant view (A), treated with a patient-matched patellofemoral prosthesis and all-polyethylene patella button. Post-operative anterior-posterior (B), lateral (C), and Merchant (D) views demonstrate proper orientation of patellofemoral prosthesis. Placement, fit, and alignment of the patient-specific trochlear implant was confirmed by the manufacturer using the patient-specific CT bone model prior to final polishing (E). See section 7.1 for additional case details.

The patient was initially treated with medications, heat, physical therapy and hyalgan injections without relief, and he remained symptomatic and disabled. In October 2009, he underwent a patient-matched custom patellofemoral arthroplasty of the right knee (Fig 4). Post-operatively, he has done remarkably well and has returned to his previous employment at the Los Angeles County Sheriff's Department. He currently has no pain and does not require any medications. He can ambulate up and down stairs without assistance and can kneel, squat and climb without pain.

7.2 Trochlear dysplasia

Patient D.B. is a 56 year old woman with anterior knee pain since her teenage years. Non-operative treatments had included activity modification, prescription and over-the-counter

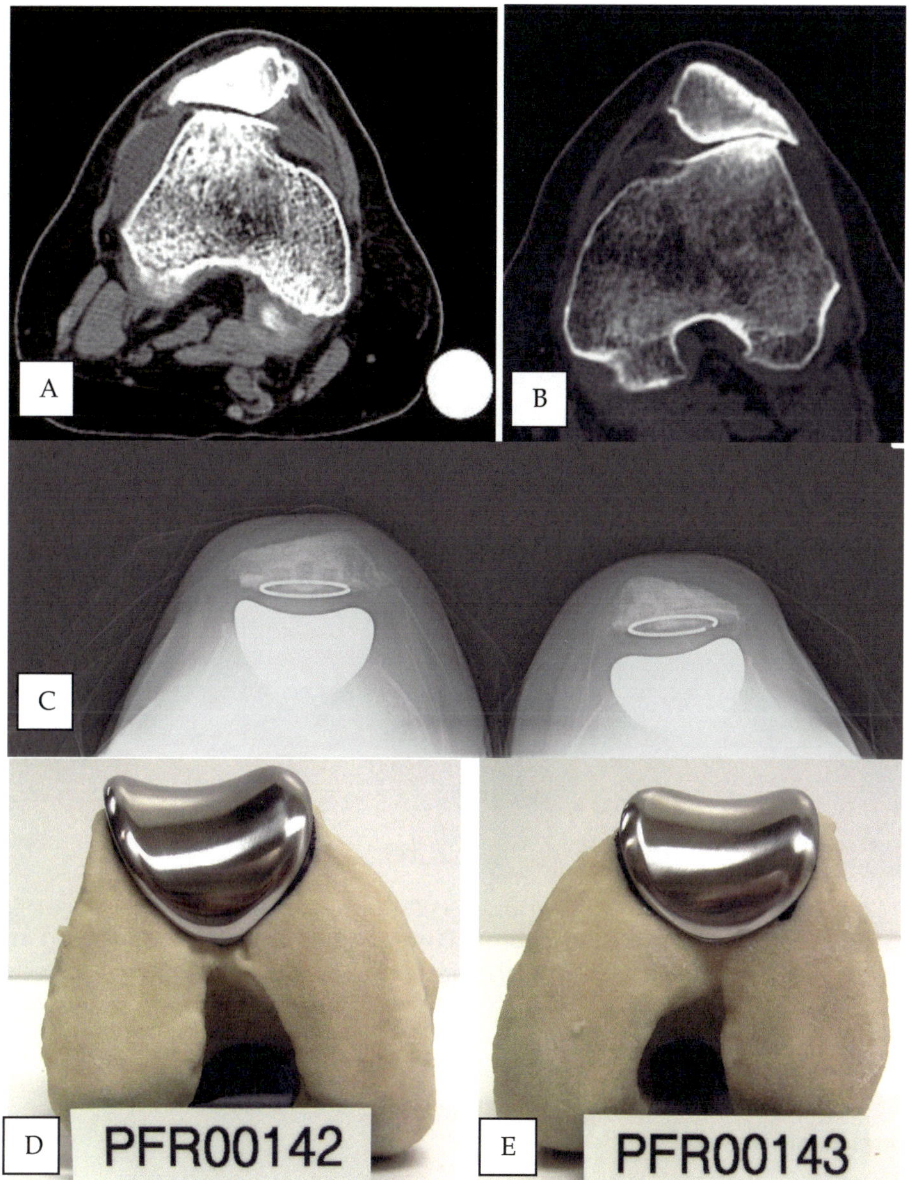

Fig. 5. A 56 year old female with bilateral isolated end-stage patellofemoral arthritis, with bilateral trochlear dysplasia (A, B), treated with patient-matched patellofemoral prostheses. Post-operative Merchant views (C) demonstrate proper orientation of patellofemoral implant components. Placement, fit, and alignment of both patient-specific trochlear implants were confirmed by the manufacturer using the patient-specific CT bone models prior to final polishing (D, E). See section 7.2 for additional case details.

pain medications, steroid and visco-supplementation injections, nutritional supplements, and physical therapy. Serum laboratory studies had not been suggestive of inflammatory arthritis.

Imaging studies demonstrated severe patellofemoral dysplasia and an absence of arthritis outside the patellofemoral compartment (Fig 5). She had undergone arthroscopies of both knees. She underwent patient-matched custom patellofemoral arthroplasty in September 2008 for her right knee and in December 2008 for her left knee.

Despite the chronically subluxed position of her patellae pre-operatively, an extensive intra-operative lateral release and medial plication have been sufficient to maintain her patellae centered within the patient-matched custom trochlear implant (Fig 5). She flexes easily to at least 120 degrees. The patient considers the procedure a success.

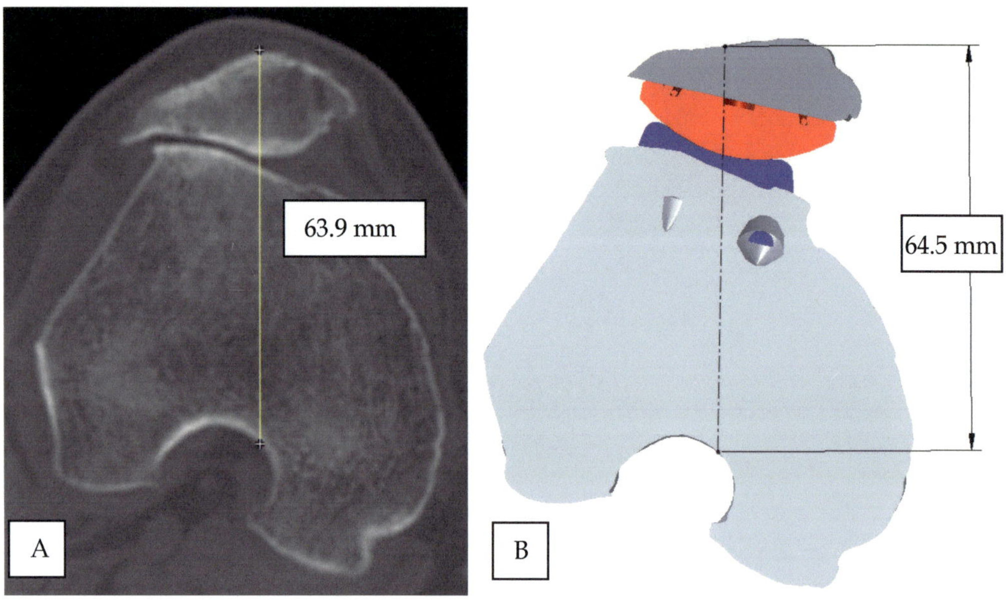

Fig. 6. Comparison of (A) pre-operative and (B) post-operative anterior-posterior patellar offset for the right knee described in Figure 5. Post-operative measurements were based on the known geometry of the patient-matched patellofemoral implant and the all-polyethylene patella selected at the time of surgery. In the presence of pronounced trochlear dysplasia (Figures 5A and 6A), treatment with a patient-specific patellofemoral arthroplasty prosthesis resulted in an insignificant net change in patellar offset (0.6 mm).

8. Conclusion

In this chapter we have reviewed the topic of patellofemoral arthroplasty from historical, technical, and clinical perspectives. The design rationale, peri-operative techniques, and 11 year clinical results of patient-matched patellofemoral arthroplasty have been reviewed and discussed. Experience with patient-matched trochlear implants in the setting of normal and dysplastic femoral trochleas have also been presented.

Patient-specific patellofemoral arthroplasty is a safe and effective treatment for patients with isolated patellofemoral arthritis. The results compare favorably with off-the-shelf patellofemoral arthroplasties that have been reported on over the past thirty years (Leadbetter et al, 2005; Leadbetter et al, 2006; Lonner, 2007; Sisto and Sarin, 2008; Gupta et al, 2010) and can be carried out more efficiently.

We believe the key elements that contribute to the success of patient-specific patellofemoral arthroplasty are as follows: (a) a strict inclusion criteria based on pre-operative radiographic evaluation; (b) a meticulous attention to soft-tissue balance and patellofemoral tracking at the time of arthroplasty; and (c) a patient-specific design and manufacturing methodology that ensures accurate and precise anatomic fit while simultaneously providing proper patellofemoral alignment and medial-lateral constraint.

9. References

Ackroyd CE, Newman JH, Evans R, Eldridge JD, Joslin CC (2007) The Avon patellofemoral arthroplasty: five-year survivorship and functional results. . *J Bone Joint Surg,* Vol. 89-B, pp. 310-5.

Ahlback S (1968) Osteoarthritis of the Knee. A Radiologic Investigation. *Acta Radiol Diagn (Stockh),* Vol. 277, pp. 7-72.

Arnebjornsson AH and Ryd L (1998) The use of isolated patellar prostheses in Sweden 1977-1986. *Int Orthop,* Vol. 22, No. 3, pp. 141-4.

National Joint Replacement Registry of Australia, Annual Report (2010).

Bengs BC and Scott RD (2006) The effect of patellar thickness on intraoperative knee flexion and patellar tracking in total knee arthroplasty. *J Arthroplasty,* Vol. 21, pp. 650–655.

Blazina ME, Fox JM, Del Pizzo W (1979) Patellofemoral replacement. *Clin Orthop Rel Res,* Vol. 144, pp. 98–102.

Bollier M and Fulkerson JP (2011) The role of trochlear dysplasia in patellofemoral instability. *J Am Acad Orthop Surg,* Vol. 19, No. 1, pp. 8-16.

Charalambous CP, Abiddin Z, Mills SP, Rogers S, Sutton P, Parkinson R (2011) The low contact stress patellofemoral replacement: High early failure rate. *J Bone Joint Surg,* Vol. 93-B, pp. 484-9.

Conley S, Rosenberg A, Crowninshield R (2007) The female knee: anatomic variations. *J Am Acad Orthop Surg,* Vol. 15 (suppl 1), pp. S31–S36.

Feinstein WK, Noble PC, Kamaric E, Tullos HS (1996) Anatomic alignment of the patellar groove. *Clin Orthop Rel Res,* Vol. *331,* pp. 64–73.

Fulkerson JP (2004) *Disorders of the Patellofemoral Joint.* 4th Edition. Philadelphia, PA. Lippincott Williams & Wilkins.

Grelsamer RP (2000) Current concepts review. Patellar malalignment. *J Bone Joint Surg,* Vol. 82-A, pp. 1639–1650.

Grelsamer RP (2006) Current concepts review. Patellofemoral Arthritis. *J Bone Joint Surg,* Vol. 88-A, pp. 1849–1860.

Gupta RR, Zywiel MG, Leadbetter WB, Bonutti P, Mont MA (2010) Scientific Evidence for the Use of Modern Patellofemoral Arthroplasty. *Expert Rev Med Devices,* Vol. 7, No. 1, pp. 51-66.

Kooijman HJ, Driessen AP, van Horn JR (2003) Long-term results of patellofemoral arthroplasty. A report of 56 arthroplasties with 17 years of follow-up. . *J Bone Joint Surg,* Vol. 85-B, pp. 836–40

Leadbetter WB, Ragland PS, Mont MA (2005) The appropriate use of patellofemoral arthroplasty. *Clin Orthop Rel Res,* Vol. 436, pp. 91–99.

Leadbetter WB, Seyler TM, Ragland PS (2006) Indications, Contraindications, and Pitfalls of Patellofemoral Arthroplasty. *J Bone Jt Surg*, Vol. 88-A(Suppl 4), pp. 122-137.

Lombardi AV (2011) Patellofemoral Arthroplasty: Custom Inlay Technique Offers a Patient Specific Approach. *Annual Meeting of the American Academy of Orthopaedic Surgeons*, pp. 142-144, San Diego, California, USA.

Lonner JH (2004) Patellofemoral Arthroplasty. Pros, Cons, and Design Considerations. *Clin Orthop Rel Res*, Vol. 428, pp. 158–165.

Lonner JH (2007) Patellofemoral Arthroplasty. *J Am Acad Orthop Surg*, Vol. 15, No. 8, pp. 495-506.

McKeever DC (1955) Patellar prosthesis. *J Bone Joint Surg*, Vol. 37-A, pp. 1074–1084.

Merchant AC, Arendt EA, Dye SF, Fredericson N, Grelsamer RP, Leadbetter WB, Post WR, Teitge RA (2008) The Female Knee. Anatomic Variations and the Female-Specific Total Knee Design. *Clin Orthop Rel Research*, Vol. 466, pp. 3059-3065.

Pierson JL, Ritter MA, Keating EM, Faris PM, Meding JB, Berend ME, Davis KE (2007) The effect of stuffing the patellofemoral compartment on the outcome of total knee arthroplasty. *J Bone Joint Surg*, Vol. 89-A, pp. 2195–2203.

Sisto DJ and Sarin VK (2006) Custom Patellofemoral Arthroplasty of the Knee. *J Bone Jt Surg*, Vol. 88-A, No. 7, pp. 1475-1480.

Sisto DJ and Sarin VK (2007) Custom Patellofemoral Arthroplasty of the Knee. Surgical Technique. *J Bone Jt Surg*, Vol. 89-A(Suppl 2), pp. 214-225.

Sisto DJ and Sarin VK (2008) Patellofemoral Arthroplasty with a Customized Trochlear Prosthesis. *Orthopedic Clinics of North America*, Vol. 39, No. 3, pp. 355-62.

Sisto DJ, Henry J, Sisto M, Sarin VK (2010) Patient-Specific Patellofemoral Arthroplasty. *Techniques in Knee Surgery*, Vol. 9, pp. 188-192.

Sisto DJ and Sarin VK (2011) Custom Patellofemoral Arthroplasty of the Knee: An Eleven Year Follow-Up. *Transactions of the Orthopaedic Research Society*, p. 1239, Long Beach, California, USA.

Weiss JM, Noble PC, Conditt MA, Kohl HW, Roberts S, Cook KF, Gordon MJ, Mathis KB (2002) What functional activities are important to patients with knee replacements? *Clin Orthop Rel Res*. Vol. 404. pp. 172-188.

Fixation of Periprosthetic Supracondylar Femur Fractures Above Total Knee Arthroplasty – The Indirect Reduction Technique with the Condylar Blade Plate and the Minimally Invasive Technique with the LISS

K. Kolb[1], P.A. Grützner[2], F. Marx[3] and W. Kolb[4]
[1]*Department of Trauma Surgery Klinikum am Steinenberg, Reutlingen*
[2]*Department of Trauma Surgery Unfallklinik Ludwigshafen*
[3]*Department of Trauma Surgery, Friedrich-Schiller-University, Jena*
[4]*Department of Trauma and Orthopaedic Surgery, Bethesda Hospital, Stuttgart*
Germany

1. Introduction

Supracondylar fractures of the femur after total knee arthroplasty are an uncommon but highly challenging injury (Streubel et al., 2010). The management of distal femoral fractures following a total knee replacement can be complex and requires the equipment, perioperative support and surgical skills of both trauma and revision arthroplasty services (Johnston et al., 2011, Nauth et al., 2011). The incidence of periprosthetic supracondylar femur fractures after total knee arthroplasties ranges from 0.3% to 2.5%. A patient with revision total knee arthroplasty has a significantly higher risk of supracondylar fracture above the prosthesis (2-4%) (Merkel & Johnson, 1986; Berry, 1999). Interprosthetic femoral fractures tend to occur more frequently in the supracondylar region above total knee arthroplasty components (Mamczak et al., 2010). Predisposing factors are female gender, poor bone stock, rotationally constrained implants, stress risers such as screw holes around the knee, malalignment of the prosthesis, endosteal ischaemia (bone cement, spongiosa preparation), anterior femoral notching, arthrofibrosis, chronic steroid use, rheumatoid arthritis, revision total knee arthroplasties, poliomyelitis and Parkinson's disease (Table 1, Aaron & Scott, 1987; Ayers, 1997; Berry, 1999; Bogoch et al., 1987; Cain et al., 1986; Cordeiro et al., 1990; Culp et al., 1987; Diehl et al., 2006; DiGioa et al., 1991; Figgie et al., 1990; Haddad et al., 1999; Hirsh et al., 1981; Lesh et al., 2000; Merkel et al., 1986; Moran et al., 1996; Ritter et al., 1988; Roscoe et al., 1989; Shawen et al., 2003; Short et al., 1981; Sisto et al., 1985; Wick et al., 2004; Zehntner & Ganz, 1993). A biomechanical study has shown that notching of the anterior cortex significantly lessens the load to failure by decreasing the bending strength by 18% and the torsional strength by approximately 40% (Lesh et al., 2000). In a retrospective study, the clinical results of 1089 consecutive total knee replacements demonstrated no difference in knees managed with or without anterior femoral notching (Ritter et al., 2005). This finding emphasises the potential for osseous remodelling to decrease the risk of

fracture should an anterior notch occur (Dennis, 2001). Additionally, should an anterior notch of the distal part of the femur occur, the surgeon should consider implantation of a femoral component with an attached diaphysis-engaging stem to support the weakened distal part of the femur (Dennis, 2001).
Motions of stiff knees under anaesthesia have a high risk of periprosthetic supracondylar femur fractures (Diehl et al., 2006).

General	Femur
Patient depending factors	
Osteoporosis	Female gender
Bone disease (M. Paget)	
Rheumatoid arthritis	Arthrofibrosis
Steroid abuse	
Neurologic abnormalities	
Malalignment	
Infections	
Surgery dependant factors	
Revision total knee arthroplasty	Malalignment of the prosthesis
Removal of cement	Implantation error
Screw holes around the knee	Anterior femoral notching
Osteolysis due to wear	
Stress shielding	
Motion under anaesthesia	Endosteal ischemia
Prosthesis dependant factors	
	Intramedullary stems
	Constrained prosthesis

Table 1. Risk factors for periprosthetic supracondylar femur fractures above total knee arthroplasty modified according to (Diehl et al., 2006 ; Nauth et al., 2011)

Most periprosthetic femur fractures occur between two and four years after a total knee arthroplasty (Ehrhardt & Kuster, 2010). The number of these cases may rise quickly, given the projection that, by the year 2030, the implantation of total knee arthroplasties will increase to 3.48 million in the United States, an increase of 673% compared with 2005. The most frequent mechanism of injury is a low-velocity fall onto the knee in combination with torsion or axial compression, with a smaller proportion resulting from high-energy trauma (e.g., motor vehicle accidents) (Su et al., 2004)
The complication rate of these fractures is between 25% and 75%. Conservative treatment of displaced fractures with casting results in malalignment (25-100%), non-union (20-35%), loss of motion of the knee, and inability to maintain reduction of the fracture (Kolb et al., 2009). Surgical treatment provides the best restoration of mechanical alignment to the limb, permits early mobilisation to avoid the complications of prolonged bed rest, and may maximise healing potential in a region where blood supply is already compromised by providing stable fixation (Rorabeck & Taylor, 1999). In 1970, the AO (Arbeitsgemeinschaft für Osteosynthesefragen) published the first results of 112 supracondylar femoral fractures treated according to their principles using a condylar plate, a fixed angle device, with 74% good or excellent results (Wenzl et al., 1970).

The reported complications of operative treatment included deep infection (3%), fixation failure (4%), non-union (9%), and revision surgery (13%) (Herrera et al., 2008). The treatment of periprosthetic fractures around the knee can be challenging for a number of reasons (Healy et al., 1993; Kim et al., 2006; Rhinelander, 1972): (1) these fractures occur in patients with poor bone stock that can compromise potential fixation; (2) the majority of these patients are elderly and, because of their age may have retarded fracture healing; (3) the epiphyseal and frequently the intramedullary blood supplies of the distal femur are interrupted after total knee arthroplasty; (4) after a fracture of the distal part of the femur immediate reduction of total bone blood flow by nearly 50% through the physiological vasoconstriction in both the periosteal and intramedullary vessels further impairs blood supply; (5) the attachment of the ligamentous structures to the fracture fragment may predispose these knees to potential instability, necessitating the use of a constrained prosthesis with all their potential problems. The wide metaphyseal and diaphyseal spaces, osteopenia, and distal extension of the fracture often associated with these elderly patients can result in suboptimal internal fixation (Ricci et al., 2006). Fractures with stable prostheses are best treated with some meeans of internal fixation and without stem revision (Dennis, 2001).

Ideally, the treatment of a supracondylar femoral fracture above a total knee arthroplasty would be characterised as follows (Kregor et al., 2001):

- The ability of the patient to return to pre-accident function,
- A surgical technique that is minimally invasive,
- Capability of immediate motion,
- No need for bone-grafting,
- Low risk of infection, and
- Adaptability to various total knee designs.

In practice, flexible intramedullary nails, rigid retrograde IM nails, angled blade plates, cobra plates, dynamic condylar screws and Ilizarov external fixators have been used (Althausen et al., 2003; Beris et al., 2010; Chettiar et al., 2009; Gliatis et al., 2005; Maniar et al., 1996; McLaren et al., 1994; Rorabeck & Taylor, 1999; Zehntner & Ganz, 1993).

Fixation with conventional compression plates, though for the most part successful, has its limitations (Kubiak et al., 2006). Conventional plate osteosynthesis (CPO) with rigid fixation has shown a high complication rate that includes delayed or non-union, infection, hardware failure and re-fracture after plate removal (Bostman, 1983; Claes et al., 1999; Finsen & Benum, 1986; Hidaka & Gustilo, 1984; Kenwright & Goodship, 1989; Kessler et al., 1992; Mulier et al., 1997; Noorda & Wuisman, 2002; Riemer et al., 1992; Stoffel et al., 2003).

(Mast et al., 1989) pioneered the indirect reduction technique without disturbance of the soft tissue envelope around the fracture itself.

The concept of the indirect reduction technique is to provide reduction of the fracture through traction across the intact soft tissues and decreased surgical dissection of the fracture site (Mast et al., 1989). Minimally invasive plate osteosynthesis (MIPO) have been introduced to go one step further (Krettek et al., 1997). Locked plate fixators improved the stability of plate osteosynthesis significantly (Streubel et al., 2010; Kolb et al., 2010). The combination of locked plate fixators and the MIPO technique allows for plate osteosynthesis without bone grafts (Streubel et al., 2010; Kolb et al., 2010).

The aim of this report is to describe new planning methods and new techniques of internal fixation for supracondylar femur fractures above total knee arthroplasty.

2. Preoperative assessment

Preoperative clinical evaluation involves questions related to general factors that include smoking, peripheral vascular and neurological status, nutritional status, comorbidities such as diabetes, alignment of the injured leg, pre-injury range of motion of the knee, knee extensor mechanism, signs of loosening of the prosthesis (weight dependant pain, knee instability, reduced walking distance), infection and activity level. Radiographic assessment includes anterior posterior (a.p.), lateral and oblique radiographs of the knee and femur including the hip and former radiographs if available (Diehl et al. 2006; Ehrhardt & Kuster, 2010). Specifically, the lateral radiograph is used to assess (Kregor et al., 2001) the following: 1. the integrity of the femoral component-bone interface to assess potential loosening, 2. the bone block attached to the femoral component, and 3. the position of the cement mantle and flange for the femoral component. Modern CT scans provide more information concerning the integrity of the femoral-bone interface to assess potential loosening of the prosthesis (Kregor et al., 2001; Ehrhardt & Kuster, 2010). Both the type and classification of fractures and the type of prosthesis should be known preoperatively because this information is very important for choosing the right treatment option (Ehrhardt & Kuster 2010). The operative report should be available whenever possible (Ehrhardt & Kuster, 2010).

2.1 Classification

The classification system that is the most valuable to management was created by Rorabeck & Young (Fig. 1, Rorabeck & Taylor, 1999; Dennis, 2001). Their classification system takes

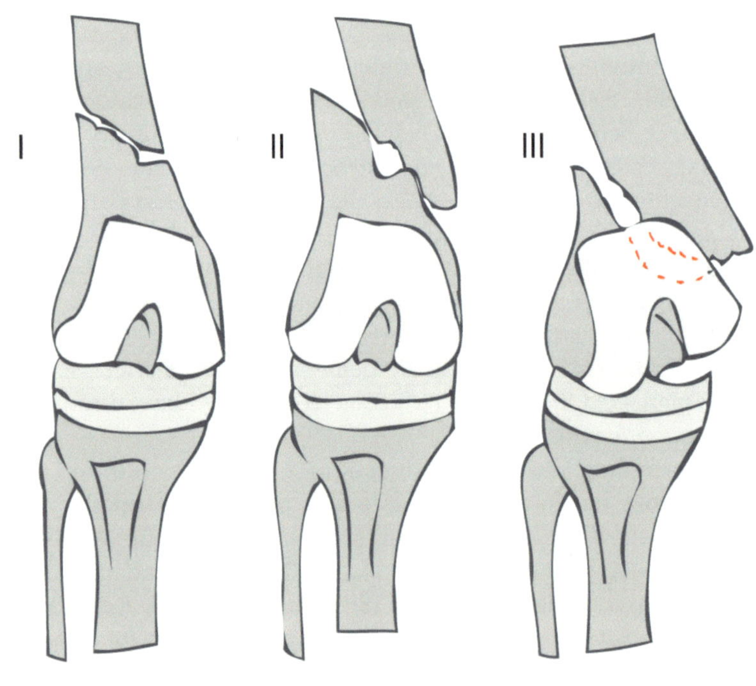

Fig. 1. The Classification system of supracondylar femoral fractures above total knee arthroplasties created by (Rorabeck & Young, 1999)

into account both the status of the prosthesis (that is, whether it is intact or failing) and the displacement of the fracture (Dennis, 2001).
(Su et al., 2004) developed their classification system because patients are increasingly being treated operatively and the bone stock of the distal segment continues to be considered a key limiting factor to obtaining adequate fixation (Herrera et al., 2008). Their classification system takes into account the height of the fractures (Table 2, Su et al., 2004).

Fracture Type	Fracture Height
I	Fracture above the femoral component
II	Fracture above the femoral component, fracture reaching the tip of the femoral component
III	Fractures below the tip of the femoral component

Table 2. Classification system of supracondylar femoral fractures above total knee arthroplasties created by (Su et al., 2004)

3. Treatment options

The goals of treating supracondylar femoral fractures above total knee arthroplasties are to obtain and maintain good postfracture alignment and stability to allow an early range of motion and bone healing (Culp et al., 1987; Rorabeck & Taylor, 1999; Dennis, 1998; Ehrhardt & Kuster, 2010). Acceptable alignments exhibit translations that are less than 5 mm, angulations that are less than 5°-10°, minimal rotations, less than 1 cm of femoral shortening, and proper tibiofemoral prosthetic joint alignments (DiGioia & Rubash, 1991). High malunion rates are common in association with varus, flexion, and internal rotation deformities typically seen as a result of forces exerted by the adductor and gastrocnemius muscle groups (Figgie et al., 1990; Dennis, 2001).

3.1 Non-operative treatment

The non-operative options include skeletal traction, application of a cast, pins and plaster, and cast bracing (Dennis et al., 2001). Traction has a high complication rate and is no longer an option. According to Rorabeck & Young, only fracture type I can be treated conservatively, 4-6 weeks with a cast and 6 weeks of mobilisation with a brace (Chen et al., 1994). However, this treatment may be associated with difficulty in maintaining the reduction, a prolonged period of immobilisation, reduced knee functions, malunion and non-union (McGraw, P.; & Kumar, A., 2010). Conservative treatment was followed by non-union in 20% and mal-union in 23% of the cases evaluated (Culp et al., 1987). Casting resulted in an average loss of motion of 26° (Culp et al., 1987). Of these fractures, 29% eventually required operative care (Harlow & Hofmann, 1994; Dennis, 2001).

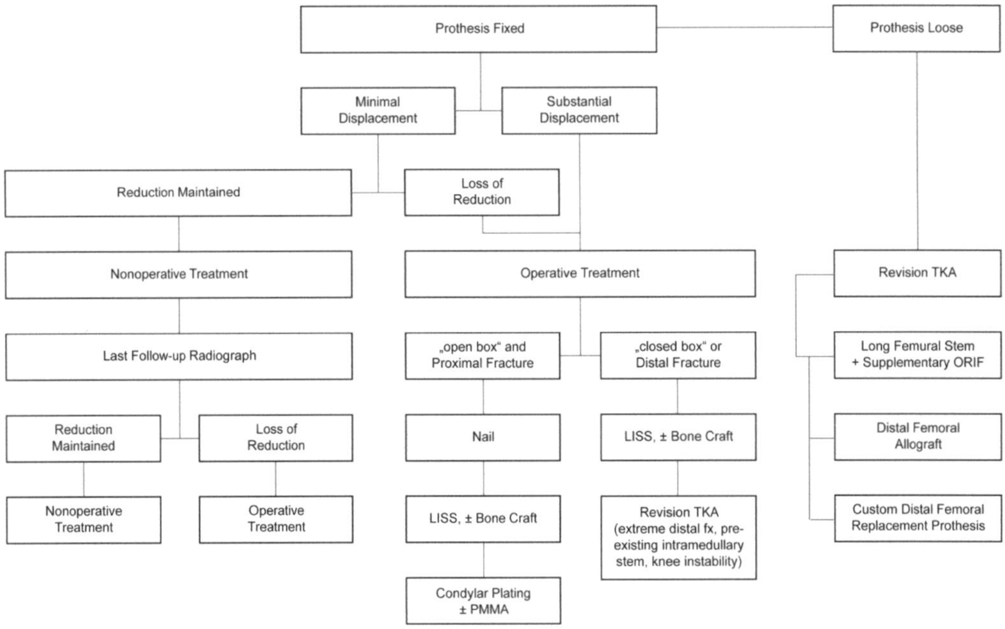

Fig. 2. Schematic of treatment options for supracondylar femoral fractures above total knee arthroplasties. TKA=total knee arthroplasty, PMMA=polymethylmethacrylate

3.2 Operative treatment

Several options are available to provide secure internal fixation of supracondylar fractures of the distal femur (Fig. 2, Ayers, 1997; Kolb et al., 2009). Many factors must be considered in choosing the most appropriate management method for these fractures including the patients general health, prefracture ambulatory status, fracture pattern, location, displacement, and type of implant (Su et al., 2004). Periprosthetic fractures above total knee arthroplasties have particular risks for failure, including wide metaphyseal and diaphyseal spaces, osteoporosis, small distal femoral fragments, and prosthetic anchorage pegs reducing the sites for fixation (Kolb et al., 2010). Surgical options include intramedullary devices, condylar buttress plates and, - more recently, – locking plates (internal fixators) that are typically placed in a submuscular manner (Herrera et al., 2008).

3.3 Coventional plate osteosynthesis

The two basic types of fixed angle devices are the condylar screw plate and the 95° condylar blade plate. They work best for more proximal fractures and when there is minimal comminution of the distal fragments (Ayers, 1997; Su et al., 2004). The advantages of the 95° condylar plate are that no bone has to be removed from the distal fragment when this device is inserted and that the blade is relatively thin (Healy et al., 1993). The blade can therefore, be placed closed to the lugs of the femoral component and close to the anterior femoral flange (Healy et al., 1993). Usually, the entry site for the blade chisel is at a height of 2.5-3 cm above the prosthetic joint line, depending on the configuration of the fracture and the prosthetic design (Moran et al., 1996). However, the angled 95° condylar blade plates do not provide sufficient stability in osteoporotic bone and might interfere with the fixation lugs of the femoral component, and the polymethylmethacrylate (Zehntner & Ganz 1993, Chen et al. 1994). Of the total numbers of conventional plate osteosynthese an average of 32% (range, 0-75%) primary bone grafts were used. A mean of 10% (range, 0-50%) of those with conventional plate osteosynthesis (CPO) had an implant failure and developed a non-union (Table 3, Kolb et al., 2009).

Authors, year of publication	Bone graft (n, % early/later	Infection	Implant failure	Non-union (n, %)	Results of fixation
Sisto et al., 1985	0	0	0	0	Valgus 3° 1 (33%) Valgus 5° 2 (66%)
Merkel et al., 1986	2 (40%)	1 (20%)	0	0	Normal alignment
Figgie et al., 1990	4 (40%)	0	5 (50%)	5 (50%)	Varus 7° 5 (23%)?
Healy et al., 1993	15/3 (75%/15%)	0	0	0	Normal alignment
Zehntner et al., 1993	2 (30%)	0	0	0	Valgus 5° (range, 0-10°)
Moran et al., 1996	6/2 (40%/13%)	0	3 (20%)	3 (20%)	Shortening 2 cm 3 (20%) Valgus 17° 1 (7%) Varus 2° 1 (7%)
Ochsner et al., 1999	0	0	0	0	Varus

Table 3. Complications of conventional plate osteosynthesis (CPO) of fractures above fixed total knee arthroplasties (from Kolb et al., 2009).

The indirect reduction technique allows for the use of longer plates with less pullout force acting on the screws due to improvement of the working leverage and significant stress reduction in the plate (50%-85%) (Kolb et al., 2009; Gautier & Sommer, 2003; Stoffel et al., 2003). Various methods have been used to enhance fixation using internal fixation (McGraw, P.; & Kumar, A., 2010). In severely osteoporotic bone, polymethylmethacrylate can be used to enhance screw fixation (Zehentner & Ganz, 1993). An intramedullary autograft is another option to help restore bone stock and achieve quadric-cortical fixation of the screws (Tani et al., 1998). However, this technique has not been widely used because of donor-site morbidity, particularly in elderly patients (McGraw, P.; & Kumar, A., 2010).

Combining medial strut allografts with compression plates allows for fixation of severe osteoporotic fractures and failures of initial open reduction and internal fixation (Wang & Wang, 2002). Three patients with very low and comminuted fractures exhibited good results using intramedullary fibular strut allografts without donor-site morbidities(Kumar et al., 2008).

The epiphyseal and frequently the intramedullary blood supplies of the distal femur are interrupted after total knee arthroplasty (Healy et al., 1993). Immediate reduction of total bone blood flow after a fracture of the distal part of the femur through physiological vasoconstriction in both the periosteal and intramedullary vessels by nearly 50% further impairs blood supply (Rhinelander, 1972). Fractures above total knee arthroplasties may have greater tendencies to non-unions than do distal femoral fractures not associated with arthoplasties (Moran et al., 1996). Microangiographic studies have demonstrated that much of the vascular supply to the callus area derives from the surrounding soft tissue (Rhinelander, 1972). Conventional plate osteosynthesis produces compression between the implant and the bone and probably further impairs the blood supply (Fig 3 Healy et al., 1993; Wagner, 2003). Plates interfere significantly with the periosteal blood supply, resulting in bone necrosis (Perren et al., 1988). Direct manipulation of bone fragments in conventional plate osteosynthesis is a major cause of devitalisation of the bone fragments (Leunig et al., 2000). Medial dissection of soft tissue can disrupt this important blood supply and is, thus, to be avoided (Mast et al., 1989).

The extreme difference in healing time between conservative treatment (3 months) and compression fixation (15 months) indicates that the circumstances can be improved (Perren, 2003). Bone union depends on respecting the capacity of the soft tissues to maintain vascular supply to the bone, on the reduction of the fracture, and on applying the technique that best provides the necessary stability for union to occur (Wagner & Frigg, 2006). Surgical treatment should take biological, biomechanical and surgical aspects into account (Table 4, Korner et al., 2003).

AO principles THEN (Müller et al., 1970)	Influences through clinical experiences and experimental investigations	AO principles NOW (Wagner & Frigg, 2006)
1. Anatomical precise reduction	Applied science concerning: - bone healings, - blood supply through soft tissues and bone, - biological shortcommings of ORIF in multifragmentary shaft fractures lead to a new way of thinking. As a consequence, indirect reduction techniques were developed	Fracture reduction and fixation to restore anatomical relationships. Reductions need not be anatomical but only axially aligned in the diaphysis and the metaphysis. Anatomical reduction is required for intra-articular reductions. The principles of articular fracture care: - atraumatic anatomical reduction of the articular surfaces, stable fixation of the articular fragments, and - metaphyseal reconstruction with bone grafting and buttressing apply as they did at the beginning

2. Rigid fixation, absolute stability	The most notable change in the treatment of diaphysael fractures has been the shift from the mechanical to the biological aspects of internal fixation. The preservation of the viability and integrity of the soft tissue envelope of the metaphysis has been recognized as the key to success. Today the dominant theme in the fixation of fractures of the diaphysis is the biology of bone and the preservation of the blood supply to bony fragments, and no longer the quest for absolute stability. Major changes have occurred in the timing of the different steps of metaphyseal reconstruction, as well as in the fixation methods and techniques. The comprehensive classification of long bones has helped predict treatment and outcome.	Stabilisation with different grades of stability, from high (absolute stability) to low (relative stability). Appropriate construct stability. Stability by compression or splinting, as the fracture pattern and the injury require. The joint surfaces require anatomical reduction with absolute stability. The majority of diaphyseal fractures are treated with relative stability methods (eg. intramedullary or extramedullary splinting).
3. Preserving blood supply	The present concept still emphasises that the blood supply through the soft tissues and bone is the most important aspect in fracture care. - atraumatic soft tissue technique through the appropriate surgical approaches, - atraumatic reduction and fixation techniques are mandatory, - implants with new bone-implant interface	Preservation of the blood supply to soft tissues and bone by careful handling and gentle reduction techniques and a newly designed bone-implant interface
4. Early protective motion for rehabilitation because pain was abolished and union assured		Early and safe mobilisation of the part and the patient. Early active motion can also be carried out because splint fixation is stable enough to allow postoperative functional care

Table 4. Comparison of AO principles from 1970 and 2006 (from Wagner and Frigg, 2006).

3.4 Plate osteosynthesis with the indirect reduction technique

The concept of biological internal fixation entails preserving the biologic reactivity of the tissue as much as possible (Rozbruch et al., 1998). This process includes careful tissue dissection, epiperiosteal bone dissection, and indirect reduction of the fracture to avoid the stripping and de-vascularisation of bone fragments (Rozbruch et al., 1998). (Mast et al., 1989) pioneered the indirect reduction of fractures without disturbance of the soft tissue envelope around the fracture and reduced blood loss. One example of an indirect reduction method is the distraction of fragments using a distractor, an external fixator, a plate or traction applied to a limb (Wagner & Frigg, 2006). The fragments are reduced using ligamentotaxis, minimising the extent to which they are manipulated and preserving their blood supply (Babst et al., 2001; Rüedi et al., 1998; Wagner & Frigg, 2006; Vidal et al., 1979). Primary grafting, which is often used in CPO is not necessary (Kolb et al., 2009; Ricci et al., 2005; Ricci et al., 2006). Minimally invasive techniques (i.e., MIPO) go one step further (Krettek et al., 1997). The bridging plate is one of the early developments of an internal fixator (Brunner & Weber, 1982). Recent developments are the Schuhli nut developed by Mast (Kolodziej et al., 1998), the Zespol plate (Ramotowski & Granowski, 1991), the point contact fixator (PC-Fix) (Tepic et al., 1997), the less invasive stabilisation system (LISS) (Frigg et al., 2001), and the locking compression plate (LCP) (Frigg, 2003). Healing has been accelerated with the PC-Fix, so that it removal is possible after only 3 months (Wagner & Frigg, 2006). Local infection resistance has been improved, such that 750 times more Staphylococcus aureus were required to produce the same incidence of infection with the PC-Fix as with the dynamic compression plate (Arens et al., 1999).

3.5 Minimally invasive osteosynthesis with internal fixators and retrograde nails

Internal fixators and retrograde nails have advantages in minimally invasive osteosynthesis (MIO) compared to the condylar plate (Ehrhardt & Kuster, 2010). Numerous studies (Chettiar et al., 2009; Gliatis et al., 2005; Henry, 1995; Mittlmeier et al., 2005; Murrell & Nunley, 1995; Platzer et al., 2010; Rolston et al., 1995; Smith et al., 1996) recommend nailing in the posterior cruciate ligament retaining femoral component with an open box. The supracondylar nail preserves the fracture haematoma, does not require extensive soft-tissue stripping, and provides fair stability to the fracture (Figgie et al., 1990; Gardner et al., 2004; Gliatis et al., 2005; Kolb et al., 2008; Mittlmeier & Beck 2005; Stedtfeld et al., 2004). Problems associated with the use of a retrograde nail include malalignment due to a poor starting point, flexion malalignment as a result of the knee flexion required for access to the joint during reaming and nail placement, and insufficient distal stability (Horwitz & Kubiak, 2010). The intercondylar distance must be at least 11mm or 12 mm to accommodate the nail, and the knee flexion must be at least 60° (Diehl et al., 2006; Kolb et al., 2010; Rolston et al., 1995). Small distal fragments should have enough space for at least two screws (Diehl et al., 2006, Kolb et al., 2010; Mittlmeier et al., 2005). Many systems include an interference screw that can be placed in the most distal screw hole to convert the nail to a fixed-angle device (Horwitz & Kubiak, 2010). However, these systems still fail because the osteoporotic cancellous bone is inadequate, and it is not uncommon for a distal femoral fracture to drift into valgus at the site of the nail fixation (Horwitz & Kubiak, 2010). Angular correction and additional stability can be achieved bx placing blocking screws in the distal fragment (Stedtfeld et al., 2004). In a retrospective study, 14 supracondylar periprosthetic fractures obtained good functional outcomes, a low complication rate and 100% fracture unions (Chettiar et al., 2009).

3.6 Minimally invasive osteosynthesis with the Less Invasive Stabilisation System (LISS)

The LISS has theoretical advantages for the treatment of supracondylar femoral fractures above well-fixed total knee arthroplasties (Kolb et al., 2010). Broadly, the advantages of the LISS fixator are attributable to three factors (Kregor et al., 2001):

1. The ability to place multiple fixed-angled locked screws, offering improved stability of the distal fragment,
2. the ability to place percutaneous screws in the proximal femur without dissection of the metaphyseal/diaphyseal component of the fracture,
3. the ability to place 3 or 4 screws even in small distal fragments.

The bridge-plating technique produces minimal biological damage with locked flexible fixation (Ehinger et al., 2011; Thielemann et al., 1988; Rozbruch et al., 1998; Perren, 2002; Gautier & Jakob, 2004). The minimally invasive plate-osteosynthesis technique leaves the blood supply largely intact and reduces blood loss compared with the conventional plate osteosynthesis using a standard approach (Mast et al., 1989; Krettek et al., 1997; Grützner et al., 1997; Farouk et al., 1998; Krettek et al., 2001; Althausen et al., 2003; Kolb et al., 2003). It avoids the need for precise reduction and exposure of the bone, thus reducing surgical trauma (Thielemann et al., 1988; Gerber et al., 1990; Ganz et al., 1991; Rozbruch et al., 1998; Perren, 2002). The locked plates provided significantly greater fixation stability than the standard plate, blade plate, condylar buttress plate, dynamic condylar screws, or the retrograde nail in biomechanical studies involving axial loading with mild to moderate osteoporotic femurs (Egol et al., 2004; Ganz et al., 1991; Koval et al., 1997; Marti et al., 2001; Salas et al., 2011; Zlowodzki et al., 2004). The probability of periprosthetic fracture of the locking plate compared to the retrograde IM nail (in a deterministic finite element model of each construct type) was higher under the applied loading conditions (locking plate 21.8% versus IM nail 0.019%) (Salas et al., 2011). By using an internal fixator with locked screw heads, the screw loading is primarily bending and not pullout (Gautier & Sommer, 2003; Wagner & Frigg, 2006). Locked screws provide improved anchorage and safety and they cannot be stripped during their insertion because they limit the torque applied to the screw thread (Perren, 2003, Fig 3a and 3b). The pull out resistance of the LISS is increased with convergent screws in the femoral condyle. These plates are particularly useful in the presence of a proximal femur implant as they allow unicortical screw fixation that overlap the distal part of the proximal implant, thereby avoiding a stress riser between the two implants (McGraw & Kumar, 2010). Blood supply to the bone is preserved, and no contact between the fixator and the bone required (Kolb et al., 2010).

3.7 Osteosynthesis with the locking compression plate (LCP) and polyaxial locking plates

In September 1998, Professor Michael Wagner (of the Wilhelminen Hospital in Vienna) questioned whether it was possible to make the LISS screw-head hole compatible with conventional bone screws (Frigg, 2003). As a result the locking compression plate (LCP) was developed. It has a combined plate hole, which allows for the use of conventional bone screws or locked screws. The possibility of using the LCP as a compression plate (> primary fracture healing), an internal fixator (> secondary fracture healing) or in a specific combination (hybrid fixation) allows for ideal plate anchorage that is adapted to the bone (Frigg, 2003; Wagner, 2003).

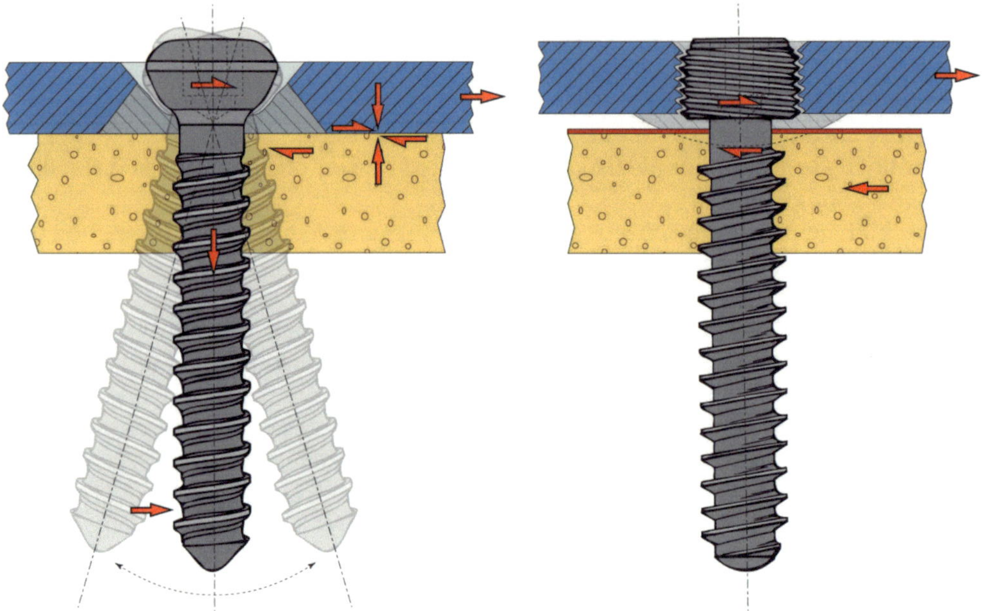

a) b)

Fig. 3. a left - Longitudinal section through the screw hole of a conventional plate screw. The inclination of the screw is not locked. The screw is tightened with an axial traction of 2000 to 3000 N, the plate is compressed onto the bone producing friction which resists a tangential load of 1000 N (friction = 0.4 x 2500 = 1000 N). Fig. 3. b right - Longirudinal section through the locked screw of an internal fixator. Because of the steep conical surfaces ("Morse cone") the screw locks upon application of minimal torque. Therefore absence of compression between the plate and bone allows either point contact or no contact thus enabling reduction of the contact damage to the blood supply. This type of forece transmission does not depend on axial preloading of the screw (from Perren, 2002).

Polyaxial locking plates (POLYAX Locked Plating Systemt, DePuy, Warsaw, IN, USA), which allow screw angulation within a maximum 40-degree cone, are now available (Haydukewych et al., 2007). As the conical threaded head engages the bushing, the bushing expands, placing hoop stresses on the surrounding hole and effectively locking the screw (Haydukewych et al., 2007). Polyaxial locking plates offer more fixation versatility without an apparent increase in mechanical complications related to loss of reduction (Haydukewych et al., 2007). The non-contact bridging plate for distal femurs (NCB DF, Zimmer, Warsaw, IN, USA) combines conventional plating techniques with polyaxial screw placement and angular stability (Ehrhardt et al., 2008). Results of this combination technique show promise with regard to union and malunion rates in periprosthetic fractures in elderly and osteoporotic patients (Ehrhardt et al., 2008; El-Zayat et al., 2010). In a biomechanical study, the POLYAX supported smaller loads compared with the LISS and NCB while under axial loading (Otto et al., 2009). In addition, the mode of failure of the NCB plate, creating an intra-articular fracture propagating from the distal posterior screw hole, may be of some concern (Otto et al., 2009).

4. Preoperative planning

Indirect reduction and closed fixation techniques are technically much more demanding than an open procedure; thus, accurate preoperative planning is needed to choose the appropriate implant size and length, shape of the plate and the number, position and order of insertion of the screws (Mast et al., 1989). The common issues related to the use of locked supracondylar plates for extraarticular distal femoral fractures are appropriate plate length, malalignment, and interference with total knee arthroplasty pegs (Horwitz & Kubiak, 2010). Plate length is important in patients with osteoporosis, both for fixation of the condylar fragment and to avoid creation of stress risers in the femoral shaft (Horwitz & Kubiak, 2010). Use of a long plate, while leaving some screw holes without screws, provides better fixation with less chance of failure at the proximal part of the diaphysis due to either pullout of the screws or a fracture at the tip of the plate (Sanders et al., 2002). The newer techniques

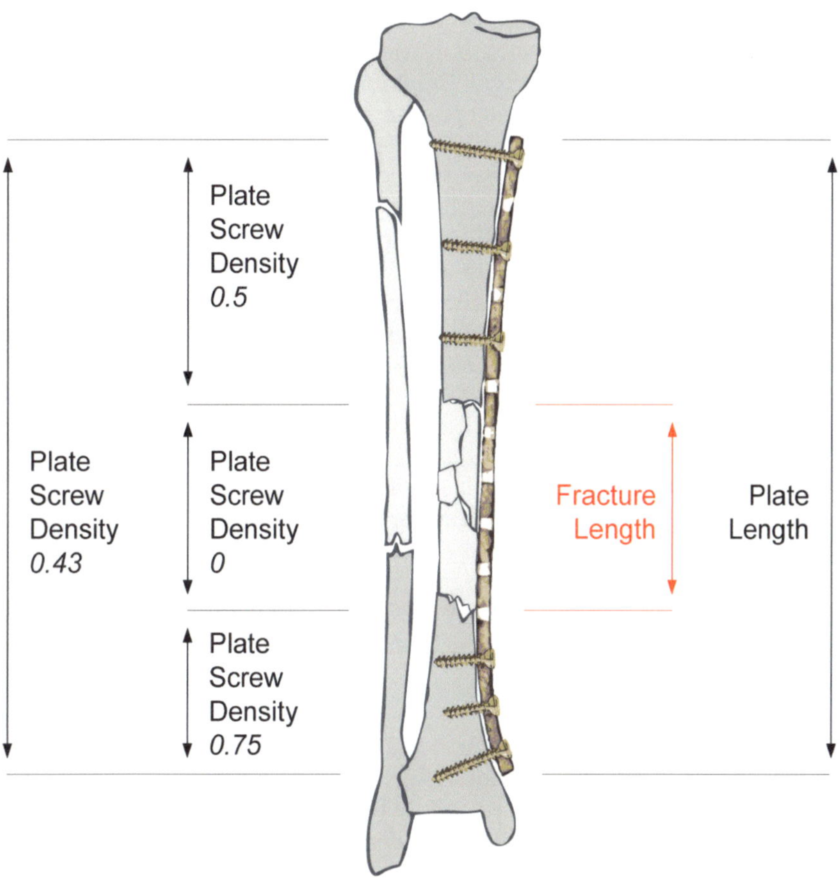

Fig. 4. The importance of plate-span ratio and plate-screw density in the bridge-plating technique. The schematic drawing shows a mechanically sound fixation of a comminuted diaphyseal fracture of the lower leg. The plate-span ratio is approximately 3, indicating that the plate is three times longer than the overall fracture area. The overall plate-screw density of the construct in this example is 0.43 & screws for a 14-hole plate (from Gautier and Sommer, 2003).

of indirect reduction and subcutaneous or submuscular implant insertion allow for increasing the plate length without additional soft tissue dissection (Gautier & Sommer, 2003). The plate length can be chosen according to the pure mechanical demands of the specific fracture that requires stabilisation (Gautier & Sommer, 2003). The working length has been shown to be the most important factor affecting axial stiffness and torsional rigidity (Stoffel et al., 2003). Increasing the working and plate lengths reduces considerably the von Mises stress in the LISS plate (Duda et al., 2002). In osteoporotic femurs, the use of self-tapping bicortical locking head screws with at least four or five screws in each fragment is recommended (Frigg & Wagner, 2006; Kregor et al., 2001).

As has been shown in total hip replacement, the LISS can be combined with periprosthetic screws, a locking attachment plate, or a cable system. The omission of one screw hole near the fracture site has been shown to significantly decrease, axial stiffness and torsional rigidity (by 64% and 36%, respectively (Stoffel et al., 2003).The number of screws has greater influence over shorter versus longer working lengths (Stoffel et al., 2003). Further more, more than three screws on either side of the fracture did little to increase axial stiffness; likewise, four screws did not increase torsional rigidity (Stoffel et al., 2003). In a biomechanical study locked and hybrid (combining of locked and unlocked) constructs demonstrated similar behaviour in osteoporotic bone; no differences between the locked and hybrid specimens were found at any cyclic interval (Gardner et al., 2006).

The plate-span ratio and the plate-screw density determine the ideal lengthof the internal fixator (Gautier & Sommer, 2003; Rozbruchet al., 1998). The plate-span ratio is the quotient of plate-length and fracture-length, while the plate-screw density is the quotient of the number of screws inserted into the plate and the number of plate holes (Rozbruch et al., 1998).The plate-span ratio should be higher than 2-3 in comminuted fractures and higher than 8-10 in simple fractures (Gautier & Sommer, 2003). The plate-screw densitiy should be below 0.5-0.4 (Fig. 4, Gautier & Sommer, 2003).

5. Surgical technique

The length of the 95° condylar blade plate and the LISS, positioning, and length of the screws are selected using the Association for Osteosynthesis/ASIF templates (Synthes Corporation). Leg length and axial alignment of the contralateral extremity are determined as described by (Kolb et al., 2009). Surgical procedures involved the tool preOp plan, developed by Siemens, to support osteosynthesis planning with regard to the 95° condylar blade plate and the LISS (Less Invasive Stabilisation System) (Synthes, West Chester, Pennsylvania) (Koudela et al., 2010).

5.1 Indirect reduction technique with the condylar blade plate

The indirect reduction technique is performed with the 95° condylar blade plate (Kolb et al., 2009; Müller et al., 1979; Ostrum & Geel, 1995). The surgical technique includes a standard lateral approach to the distal femur with the patient in a supine position. Hyperextension of the distal femoral fragment is corrected with the knee flexed to 60° over a supracondylar towel bump. After opening the fascia lata, the vastus lateralis muscle is elevated from the linea aspera, and the perforating vessels are preserved when possible. The lateral and anterior aspects of the femur are exposed. The posterior and medial soft tissues are not violated. The blade of the 95° condylar blade plate is inserted along the track previously made by the seating chisel parallel to a k-wire that marks the joint line. The window of the seating chisel is in the middle third of the anterior half of the distal femur, 2.5 cm above the prosthetic joint line and, if possible, anterior to the anchorage pegs of the prosthesis (Mast et al., 1989). Indirect reduction is obtained through manual traction or a compression-distraction device to obtain the appropriate axis, rotation and length of the femur. The plate is then attached to the proximal shaft with a Verbrugge clamp and fixed with screws. At least four divergent plate screws are used for proximal plate fixation. In three patients with severely osteoporotic bone, fractures were stabilised in combination with bone cement to enhance screw fixation. The screws are fully inserted into the cement while it is still soft after the plate is provisionally fixed to the femur, and the screws are tightened after the cement has set. Only one knee had a plate-bone interface failure after 4 weeks. Bone graft was required in only four patients with severely osteoporotic bone with comminution and in three in combination with bone cement.

5.1.1 Postoperative considerations

Postoperatively, patients are allowed toe-touch weight bearing for 6-8 weeks, except for one patient who has an associated tibial fracture. Two patients are mobilised with a glider cane. After removal of the suction drains on the second postoperative day, continuous passive motion is initiated.

6. Minimally invasive technique with the LISS

The standard anterolateral approach to the distal femur is performed on a radiolucent table with the patient in a supine position (Kolb et al., 2010). Hyperextension of the distal femoral fragment is corrected with the knee flexed over a supracondylar towel bump. Closed indirect reduction through manual traction with control of the axis, rotation and length, and temporary retention of the articular block on the shaft are attained. A 4 cm to 5 cm lateral incision is made over the distal femur. After sharp dissection through the skin and subcutaneous tissue, the iliotibial band is divided in line with its fibres. Atraumatic entry into the area between the vastus lateralis and the lateral femoral condyle (without visualising the metaphyseal part of the fracture) is performed. The perforating vessels are kept intact. The plate is placed slightly more distally than the recommended 1.0-1.5 cm, often directly adjacent to the femoral component to achieve maximal screw purchase (Kregor et al., 2001). The plate is used as an internal fixator and not as a reduction aid. The LISS was temporarily fixated using the aiming device with two 2.0 mm Kirschner wires (Fig. 5). At least four self-drilling monocortical locked screws are used for the articular block, and at least four self-tapping bicortical locked screws are used for the shaft. When interference occurs with an intercondylar box of the femoral component (in four patients), we use shorter self-tapping or periprosthetic screws. In two patients with interference from total hip replacements, periprosthetic locked screws were used in the proximal femoral fragment when the LISS overlapped a hip prosthesis. After a proximal screw pull-out due to malpositioning of the fixator, we obtain a true lateral view of the proximal shaft to ensure that the plate is centred on the bone in the lateral view before inserting the proximal screws, and we perform a mini-open approach over the proximal three holes of the fixator, facilitating the exact positioning of the fixator.
We require no intraoperative blood transfusion and no bone graft or soft tissue procedure.

6.1 Postoperative considerations

Active physiotherapy and continuous passive motion are initiated on day 2 after removal of the drains. Patients are allowed to partially bear weight (up to 20 kg) for 6 to 8 weeks.

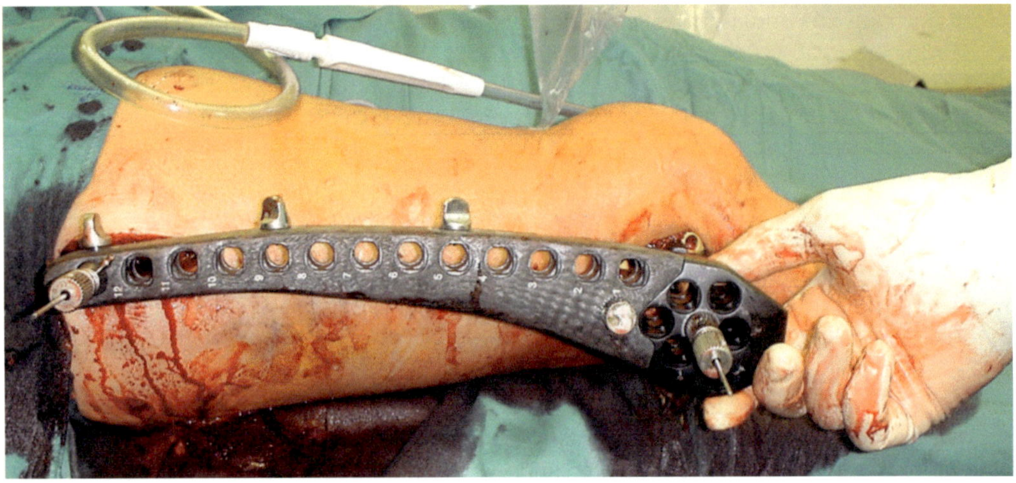

Fig. 5. Temporary fixation of the LISS with the aiming device with two 2.0 mm Kirschner wires.

7. Results and conclusions

The incidence of periprosthetic fractures is increasing as ageing populations throughout the world live longer (Kolb et al., 2010). Despite the increased risk of many of our patients all knees treated with the angled 95° condylar blade plate in indirect reduction technique healed without complications (Kolb et al., 2009). The angled 95° condylar plate in indirect reduction technique is still a good implant with good long-term results (Kolb et al., 2009). It works best in proximal fractures when there is minimal comminution of the distal fragment in the hands of a surgeon experienced with this device (Kolb et al., 2009). A minimally invasive, locked plating system permits stable fixation, early knee motion with good short- to mid-term results, and minimal complications (Kolb et al., 2010, Tables 5 and 6).

Authors Year of publication	Patients (n) for Follow-up (n, %)	Internal Fixation CPO/MIPO Nailing	Fracture Healing (weeks)	Mean Follow-up (years)	Good/Excellent Results (%) Scoring System
Sisto et al., 1985	3/3 (100%)	CPO (CP)	16 (12-20)	1.1	86 HSS knee score
Merkel et al., 1986	5/3 (60%)	CPO 4 (80%) Screws 1 (20%)	ND	3.0	76.3 KSS score
Cain et al., 1986	4/4	CPO 1 (25%) Rush pins 3 (75%)	Non-union 2 (50%)	2.5	25 Own rating system
Culp et al., 1987	30/22 (73%)	CPO (67%) Rush pins 2 (7%)	Non-union 1 (3%)	3.7	ND
Figgie et al., 1990	22/12	CPO 10 (45%) CP 5 (23%), Dual plating 2 (9%), CPB 2 (9%), Barr bolt and AO screws 1 (4%)	32 (16-64) Non-union 5 (23%)	ND	64 University knee score
Healy et al., 1993	20	CPO (CP/DCS 7/7, 35%, CBP 6, 30%)	16 (6-40)	2.2	84 KSS score

Zehntner et al., 1993	7/6 (86%)	CPO (CPB 6, 86%)	14 (12-16)	1.4	50 Cain rating system
McLaren et al., 1994	7/7 (100%)	Intramedullary supracondylar rod 7 (100%)	12	1.3	ND
Moran et al., 1996	15/15 (100%)	CPO (CP 9 60%, CBP 3 20% (2 with double plating)	12 (4-16), non-union 3 (20%)	2.5	KSS score
Ochsner et al., 1999	6/5 (83%)	CPO (Fork Plate) 6 (100%)	9	ND	ND
Wick et al., 2001)	6/6 (100%)	GSH nail 8 (100%)	12.4	1.4	69 Freeman score
Kregor et al., 2001	13	LISS 13/13 (100%)	ND	ND	ND
Althausen et al., 2003	11	LISS 5 (45%) Rush rod 4 (36%) CPO 2 (18%) Retrograde nail 1 (9%)	ND	ND	ND
Wick et al., 2004	18/18 (100%)	DFN (44%), GSH nail 1 (6%), LISS 9 (50%)		2.5	ND
Gliatis et al., 2005	10/10 (100%)	GSH 10 (100%)	12	2.9	59 WOMAC score
Ricci et al., 2006	24/22 (92%)	LCP 24 (100%)	12 (8-20), Non-union 3 (13%)	1.0	ND
O'Toole et al., 2006	14/11 (79%)	LISS 14 (100%)	ND	1.0	71 own score
Fulkerson et al., 2007	18	LISS 18	6.2 (3-19) months Delayed union 2 (11%) Non-union 3 (17%)	2.3	ND
Kolb et al., 2009	21/15 (71%)	CP	14 (12-16)	9 (712)	77 KSS score
Streubel et al., 2010	89/61 (69%) Group A (n=28), Group B (n=33)	Peri-Loc Distal Lateral Femur locking plate, Locking Condylar Plate, LISS	Delayed union 5 (18%), non-union 3 (11%) group A, delayed union 2 (6%), non-union 5 (15%) group B	Minimum follow-up 0.5	ND
Kolb et al., 2010	23/19 (83%)	LISS 23 (1005)	14 (9-21) Delayed union 2 (11%)	3.8 (2.2-5.6)	81 KSS score

Table 5. Results of surgically treated periprosthetic femur fractures above total knee arthroplasties

Authors Year	Malalignment	Bone graft (n, % early/late)	Infection (n, %)	Implant Failure	Scondary Surgical Procedure
Sisto et al., 1985	Valgus 3/5° ½ (33/66%)	0	0	0	0
Merkel et al., 1986	0	2 (40%), 1 (20%)	0	Intraoperative 1 Death	1 Above knee amputation
Cain et al., 1986	Valgus 10° 2 (25%)	0	0	0	0
Culp et al., 1987	3 (10%)	0	2 (7%)	0	2 Above knee amputations
Figgie et al., 1990	Varus 7° 5 (23%)	4 (18%)	0	5 (23%)	4 Revision osteosynthesis with bone grafting, 1 Revision TKA,
Healy et al., 1993	0	15/3 (75%)/(15%)	0	0	3 Revision osteosynthesis
Zehntner et al., 1993	Valgus 5° (0-10°)	2 (30%)	0	0	0
McLaren et al., 1994	0	0	0	0	1 Stress fracture at the proximal locking screw
Moran et al., 1996	Shortening 2 cm 3 (20%), Valgus 17° 1 (7%), Varus 2° 1 (7%)	6/2 (40%)/(13%)	0	3 (20%)	3 Revision osteosynthesis, 2 with bone graft
Ochsner et al., 1999	Varus 1 (17%)	0	0	0	1 Valgus osteotomy
Wick et al., 2001	Valgus 10° 1 (17%), Shortening 1 (17%)	0	0	0	0
Althausen et al., 2003	Rush rod valgus 13° 2 (50%), 10° 1 (25%),	0	0	0	ND

	Retrograde Nail varus 3° 1 (100%), Shortening >2 cm 1 (25%), CPO varus 4° 1 (50%)				
Kregor et al., 2001	0	0/1 (8%)	0	0	1 Revision osteosynthesis
Wick et al., 2004	Valgus 18° retrograde	0	1 (6%)	1 (6%) retrograde nail	1 Revision osteosynthesis 1 Hematoma
Gliatis et al., 2005	Valgus 35° 1 (11%)	0	0	0	ND
Ricci et al., 2006	Varus 6° 1 (4%), Valgus 7°/9°/13° 1/1/1 (4%)	0	2 (8%)	4 (17%) proximal screw failure	1 Above knee amputation 1 Debridement
O'Toole et al., 2006	0	0	0	0	0
Fulkerson et al., 2007	<5° Varus/Valgus angulation	0/1 (6%)	1 (6%)	1 (6%)	1 Revision to DCS and Dall-Miles cables, 2 Revision TKA, 1 Excision plasty
Kolb et al., 2009	Varus 5° 1 (5%)	4/1 (19%)/(5%)	0	1 (5%)	1 Revision osteosynthesis with bone graft and bone cement, 2 Hematomas
Streubel et al., 2010		2 (7%) Group A, 4 (12%) Group B	1 (4%) Group A, 1 (3%) Group B	0	8 Debridments, 6 Revision osteosynthesis
Kolb et al., 2010	Varus 7 1 (5%)	0	0	1 (5%)	1 Revision osteosynthesis

Table 6. Complications of surgically treated periprosthetic femur fractures above total knee arthroplasties

8. References

Aaron, R.K.; & Scott, R. (1987) Supracondylar fracture of the femur after total knee arthroplasty, Clin Orthop Relat Res, Vol.219, (June 1987), pp.136-139.

Althausen, P.L.; Lee, M.A.; Finkemeier, C.G.; Meehan, J.P.; & Rodrigo, J.J. (2003). Operative stabilization of supracondylar femur fractures above total knee arthroplasty: a comparison of four treatment methods, J Arthoplasty, Vol.18, No.7, (October 2003), pp.834-839.

Arens, S.; Eijer, H.; Schlegel, U.; Printzen, G.; Perren, S.M.; & Hansis, M. (1999). Influence of the design for fixation implants on local infection: experimental study of dynamic compression plates versus contact fixateurs in rabbits, J Orthop Trauma, Vol.13, No.7, (September-October 1999), pp.470-476.

Ayers, D.C. (1997). Supracondylar fracture of the distal femur proximal to a total knee replacement, Instruct Course Lect, Vol.46, pp.197-203.

Babst, R.; Hehli, M.; & Regazzoni, P. (2001). [LISS tractor. Combination of the "less invasive stabilization system" (LISS) with the AO distractor for the distal femur and proximal tibial fractures], Unfallchirurg, Vol.104, No.6, (June 2001), pp.530-535. German.

Beris AE, Lykissas MG, Sioros V, Mavrodonitis AN, Korompilias AV. (2010). Femoral periprosthetic fracture in osteoporotic bone after total knee replacement: treatment with external Ilizarov fixation, J Arthroplasty, Vol.25, No.7, (October 2010), pp.1168.e9-12.

Berry, D.J. (1999) Epidemiology: hip and knee, Orthop Clin North Am, Vol.30, No.2, (April 1999), pp.183-190. Review.

Böstman, O.M. (1983). Rotational refracture of the shaft of the adult tibia, Injury, Vol.15, No.2, (September 1983), pp.93-98.

Bogoch, E.; Hastings, D.; Gross, A.; & Gschwend, N. (1988). Supracondylar fractures of the femur adjacent to resurfacing and MacIntosh arthroplasties of the knee in patients with rheumatoid arthritis, Clin Orthop Relat Res, (April 1988), Vol.229, pp.213-220.

Brunner, C.; & Weber, B.G. (1982). Special Techniques in Internal Fixation, Springer, Berlin, Germany.

Cain, P.R.; Rubash, H.E.; Wissinger, H.A.; & McClain, E.J. (1986). Periprosthetic femoral fractures following total knee arthroplasty, Clin Orthop Relat Res, Vol.208, (July 1986), pp.205-214.

Chen, F.; Mont, M.A.; & Bachner, R.S. (1994). Management of ipsilateral supracondylar femur fractures following total knee arthroplasty, J Arthroplasty, Vol.9, No.5, (October 1994), pp.521-526.

Chettiar, K.; Jackson, M.P.; Brewin, J.; Dass, D.; & Butler-Manuel, P.A. (2009). Supracondylar periprosthetic femoral fractures following total knee arthroplasty: treatment with a retrograde intramedullary nail, Int Orthop, Vol.33, No.4, (August 2009), pp.981-985.

Claes, L.; Heitemeyer, U.; Krischak, G.; Braun, H.; & Hierholzer, G. (1999). Fixation technique influences osteogenesis of comminuted fractures, Clin Orthop Relat Res, Vol.365, (August 1999), pp.221-229.

Cordeiro, E.N.; Costa, R.C.; Carazzato, J.G.; & Silva Jdos, S. (1990). Periprosthetic fractures in patients with total knee arthroplasties, Clin Orthop Relat Res, Vol.252, (March 1990), pp.182-189.

Culp, R.W.; Schmidt, R.G.; Hanks, G.; Mak, A.; Esterhai, J.L.; & Heppenstall, R.B. (1987). Supracondylar fracture of the femur following prosthetic knee arthroplasty. Clin Orthop Relat Res, Vol.222, (September 1987), pp.212-222.

Dennis, D.A. (1998). Periprosthetic fractures following total knee arthroplasty: the good, bad, & ugly, Orthopedics, Vol.21, No.9, (September, 1998), pp.1048-1050. Review.

Dennis D.A. Periprosthetic fractures following total knee arthroplasty. (2001). J Bone Joint Surg Am, Vol.83, pp.120-130.

Diehl, P.; Burgkart, R.; Klier, T.; Glowalla, C.; & Gollwitzer, H. (2006) [Periprosthetic fractures after total knee arthroplasty, Orthopäde, Vol.35, No.9, (September 2006), pp.972-974. Review. German.

DiGioia, A.M.3rd.; & Rubash, H.E. (1991) Periprosthetic fractures of the femur after total knee arthroplasty. A literature review and treatment algorithm, Clin Orthop Relat Res, Vol.271, (October 1991), pp.135-142.

Duda, G.N.; Mandruzzato, F.; Heller, M.; Kassi, J.P.; Khodadadyan, C.; & Hass, N.P. (2002). Mechanical conditions in the internal stabilization of proximal tibial defects, Clin Biomech (Bristol, Avon), Vol.17, No.1, (January 2002), pp.64-72.

Egol, K.A.; Kubiak, E.N.; Fulkerson, E.; Kummer, F.J.; & Koval, K.J. (2004). Biomechanics of locked plates and screws, J Orthop Trauma, Vol.18, No.8, (September 2004), pp.488-493.

Ehinger, M.; Adam, P.; Abane, L.; Rahme, M.; Moor, B.K.; Arlettaz, Y.; & Bonnormet, F. (2011). Treatment of periprosthetic femoral fractures of the knee, Knee Surg Sports Traumatol Arthrosc, Mar 23. [Epub ahead of print].

Erhardt, J.B.; Grob, K.; Roderer, G.; Hoffmann, A.; Forster, T.N.; & Kuster, M.S. (2008). Treatment of periprosthetic femur fractures with the non-contact bridging plate: a new angular stable implant, Arch Orthop Trauma Surg, Vol.128, No.4, (April 2008), pp.409-416.

Erhardt JB, Kuster MS. (2010). [Periprosthetic fractures of the knee joint]. Orthopäde 2010;39:97-108.

El-Zayat, B.F.; Zettl, R.; Efe, T.; Krüger, A.; Eisenberg, F.; & Ruchholtz, S. (2010) [Minimally invasive treatment of geriatric and osteoporotic femur fractures with polyaxial locking implants (NCB-DF).], Unfallchirurg, (November 18, 2010), [Epub ahead of print].

Farouk, O.; Krettek, C.; Miclau, T.; Schandelmaier, P.; & Tscherne, H. (1998). Effects of percutaneous and conventional plating techniques on the blood supply to the femur, Arch Orthop Trauma Surg, Vol.117, No.8, pp.438-441.

Figgie, M.P.; Goldberg, V.M.; Figgie, H.E. 3rd.; & Sobel, M. (1990) The results of treatment of supracondylar fracture above total knee arthroplasty, J Arthroplasty, Vol.5, No.3, (September 1990), pp.267-276.

Finsen, V.; & Benum, P. (1986). Refracture of the hip rare after removal of fixation device, Acta Orthop Scand, Vol.57, No.5, (October 1986), pp.434-435.

Frigg, R.; Appenzeller, A.; Christensen, R.; Frenk, A.; Gilbert, S.; & Schavan, R. (2001). The development of the distal femur Less Invasive Stabilization System (LISS), Injury, Vol.32, Suppl 3, (December 2001), pp.SC24-31. Review.

Frigg, R. (2003). Development of the Locking Compression Plate, Injury, Vo.34, Suppl 2, pp.B6-10. Review.

Fulkerson, E.; Tejwani, N.; Stuchin, S.; & Egol, K. (2007). Management of periprosthetic femur fractures with a first generation locking plate, Injury, Vol.38, No.8, (August 2007), pp.965-972.

Ganz, R.; Mast, J.; Weber, B.; & Perren, S.M. (1991). Clinical aspects of „bio-logical" plating, Injury, Vol.22, pp.4-5.

Gardner, M.J.; Helfet, D.L.; & Lorich D.G. (2004). Has locked plating completely replaced conventional plating, Am J Orthop, Vol.33, No. 9, (September 2004), pp.439-446. Review.

Gardner, M.J.; Griffith, M.H.; Demetrakopoulos, D.; Brophy, R.H.; Grose, A.; Helfet, D.L.; Lorich, D.G. (2006). Hybrid locked plating of osteoporotic fractures of the humerus, J Bone Joint Surg Am, Vol.88, No.9, (September 2006, pp.1962-1967.

Gautier, E.; & Sommer, C. (2003) Guidelines for the clinical application of the LCP, Injury, Vol.34, Suppl 2, pp.B63-76. Review.

Gautier, E.; & Jakob, R.P. (2004). Biomechanics of osteosynthesis by screwed plates. In Biomechanics and biomaterials in orthopedics, D.G. Poitout (Ed.), pp.330-350, Springer, New York, USA.

Gerber, C.; Mast, J.; & Ganz, R. (1990). Biological internal fixation of fractures. Arch Orthop Trauma Surg, Vol.109, No.6, pp.295-303.

Gliatis, J.; Megas, P.; Panagiotpoulos, E.; & Lambiris, E. (2005). Midterm results of treatment with a retrograde nail for supracondylar periprosthetic fractures ofm the femur following total knee arthroplasty, J Orthop Trauma, Vol.19, No.3, (March 2005), pp.164-170.

Grützner, P.; Winkler, H.; & Wentzensen, A. (1997). [New aspects and developments of plate osteosynthesis. Point Contact Fixateur-PC Fix-Indication-technology-experiences, OPJ, Vol.3, pp.332-338.

Haddad, F.S.; Masri, B.A.; Garbuz, D.S.; & Duncan, C.P. (1999). The prevention of periprosthetic fractures in total hip and knee arthroplasty, Orthop Clin North Am, Vol.30, No.2, (April 1999), pp.191-207. Review.

Haidukewych, G.; Sems, S.A.; Huebner, D.; Horwitz, D.; & Levy, B. (2007). Results of polyaxial locked-plate fixation of periarticular fractures of the knee, J Bone Joint Surg Am, Vol.89, No.3, (March 2007), pp.614-620.

Harlow, M.L.; & Hofmann, A.A. (1994). Periprosthetic fractures. In The knee, W.N. Scott (Ed.), pp.1405-1417, CV Mosby, St. Louis, USA.

Healy, W.L.; Siliski, J.M.; & Incavo, S.J. (1993). Operative treatment of distal femoral fractures proximal to total knee replacements, J Bone Joint Surg Am, Vol.75, No.1, pp.27-34.

Henry, S.L. (1995). Management of supracondylar fractures proximal to total knee arthroplasty with the GSH supracondylar nail, Contemp Orthop, Vol.31, No.4, (October 1995), pp.231-238.

Herrera, D.A.; Kregor, P.J.; Cole, P.A.; Levy, B.A.; Jönsson, A.; & Zlowodzki, M. (2008). Treatment of acute distal femur fractures above total knee arthroplasty: a systematic review of 415 cases (1981-2006), Acta Orthop, Vol.79, No.1, (February 2006), pp.22-27.

Hidaka, S.; & Gustilo, R.B. (1984). Refracture of bones of the forearm after plate removal, J Bone Joint Surg Am, Vol.66, No.8, (October 1984), pp.1241-1243.

Hirsh, D.M.; Bhalla, S.; & Roffman, M. (1981) Supracondylar fracture of the femur following total knee replacement. Report of four cases, J Bone Joint Surg Am, Vol.63, No.1, (January 1981), pp.162-163.

Horwitz, D.S. & Kubiak, E.N. (2010). Surgical treatment of osteoporotic fractures about the knee, Instr Course Lect, Vol.59, pp.511-523. Review.

Johnston, A.T.; Tsiridis, E.; Eyres, K.S.; & Toms, A.D. (2011). Periprosthetic fractures in the distal femur following total knee replacement: A review and guide to management, Knee, Jul 7. [Epub ahead of print].

Kenwright, J.; & Goodship, A.E. (1989). Controlled mechanical stimulation in the treatment of tibial fractures, Clin Orthop Relat Res, Vol.241, (April 1989), pp.36-47.

Kim, K.I.; Egol, K.A.; Hozak, W.J.; & Parvizi J. (2006). Periprosthetic fractures after total knee arthroplasties, Clin Orthop Relat Res, Vol.446, (May 2006), pp.167-175.

Kessler, S.B.; Deiler, S.; Schiffl.Deiler, M.; Uhthoff, H.K.; & Schweiberer, L. (1992). Refractures: a consequence of impaired local bone viability, Arch Orthop Trauma Surg, Vol.111, No.2, pp.96-101.

Kolb, K.; Koller, H.; Lorenz, I.; Holz, U.; Marx, F.; Grützner, P.; & Kolb, W. (2009). Operative treatment of distal femoral fractures above total knee arthroplasty with the indirect reduction technique: a long-term follow-up study, Injury, Vol.40, No.4, (April 2009), pp.433-439.

Kolb, K.; Grützner, P.; Koller, H.; Windisch, C.; Marx, F.; & Kolb, W. (2009). The condylar plate for treatment of distal femoral fractures: a long-term follow-up study, Injury, Vol.40, No.4, (April 2009), pp.440-448.

Kolb, W.; Guhlmann, H.; Friedel, R.; & Nestmann, H. (2003). [Fixation of periprosthetic femur fractures with the less invasive stabilization system (LISS)-a new minimally invasive treatment with locked fixed-angle screws], Zentralbl Chir, Vol.218, No.1, (January 2003), pp.53-59. German.

Kolb, W.; Guhlmann, H.; Windisch, C.; Marx, F.; kolb, K.; & Koller, H. (2008). Fixation of distal femoral fractures with the Less Invasive Stabilization Sytems: a minimally invasive treatment with locked fixed-angled screws, J Trauma, Vol.65, No.6, (December 2008), pp.1425-1434.

Kolb, W.; Guhlmann, H.; Windisch, C.; Marx, F.; Koller, H.; & Kolb, K. (2010). Fixation of periprosthetic femur fracture above total knee arthroplasty with the less invasive stabilization system: a midterm follow-up stady, J Trauma, Vol.69, No.3, (September 2010), pp.670-676.

Kolodziej, P.; Lee, F.S.; Patel, A.; Kassab, S.S.; Shen, K.L.; Yang, K.H.; & Mast, J.W. (1998). Biomechnical evaluation of the schuhli nut, Clin Orthop Relat Res, Vol.347, (February 1998), pp.79-85.

Korner, J.; Lill, H.; Müller, L.P.; Rommens, P.M.; Schneider, E. & Linke, B. (2003). The LCP-concept in the operative treatment of distal humerus fractures - biological, biomechanical and surgical aspects, Injury, Vol.34, Suppl 2, (November 2003), pp.B20-30. Review.

Koudela, K. Jr.; Koudelová, J.; Koudela, K. Sr.; Kunesova. M.; Kren, J.; & Pokorny, J. (2010). [Radiographic measurements in total knee arthroplasty and their role in clinical practice], Acta Chir Orthop Traumatol Cech, Vol.77, Vol.4, (August 2010), pp.304-311.

Koval, K.J.; Hoehl, J.J.; Kummer, F.J.; & Simon, J.A. (1997). Distal femoral fixation: a biomechanical comparison of the standard condylar buttress plate, a locked buttress plate, and the 95-degree blade plate, J Orthop Trauma, Vol.11, No.7, (October 1997), pp.521-524.

Kregor, P.J.; Hughes, J.L.; & Cole, P.A. (2001). Fixation of distal femoral fractures above total knee arthroplasty utilizing the Less Invasive Stabilizations System (L.I.S.S.), Injury, Vol.32, Suppl 3, pp.SC64-75:

Krettek, C.; Schandelmaier, P.; Miclau, T.; & Tscherne, H. (1997). Minimally invasive percutaneous plate osteosynthesis (MIPPO) using DCS in proximal and distal femoral fractures, Injury, Vol.28, (Suppl 1), pp.S-A20-30.

Krettek, C.; Müller, M.; & Miclau, T. (2001). Evolution of minimally invasive plate osteosynthesis (MIPO) in the femur, Injury, Vol.32, Suppl 3, pp.S-C14-S-C23.

Kubiak, E.N.; Fulkerson, E.; Strauss, E.; & Egol. K.A. (2006). The evolution of locked plates, J Bone Joint Surg Am, Vol.88, Suppl 4, (December 2006), pp.189-200. Review.

Kumar, A.; & Chambers, I. (2008). Management of periprosthetic fracture above total knee arthroplasty using intramedullary fibular allograft and plate fixation, J Arthroplasty, Vol.23, No.4, (June 2008), pp.554-558.

Lesh, M.L.; Schneider, D.J.; Deol, G.; Davis, B.; Jacobs, C.R.; & Pellegrini, V.D. Jr. (2000). The consequence of anterior femoral notching in total knee arthroplasty. A biomechanical study, J Bone Joint Surg Am, Vol.82, No.8, (August 2000), pp.1096-1101.

Leunig, M.; Hertel, R,; Siebenrock, K.A.; Ballmer, F.T.; Mast, J.W.; & Ganz, R. (2000). The evolution of indirect reduction techniques for the treatment of fractures, Clin Orthop Relat Res, Vol.375; (June 2000), pp.7-14. Review.

Mamczak, C.N.; Gardner, M.J.; Bolhofner, B.; Borelli, J. Jr.; Streubel, P.N.; & Ricci, W.M. (2010). Interprosthetic femoral fractures, J Orthop Trauma, Vol.24, No.12, (December 2010), pp.740-744.

Maniar, R.N.; Umlas, M.E.; Rodriguez, J.A.; & Ranawat, C.S. (1996). Supracondylar femoral fracture above a PFC posterior cruciate-substituting total knee arthroplasty treated with supracondylar nailing. A unique technical problem, J Arthroplasty, Vol.11, No.5, (August 1996), pp.637-639.

Marti, A.; Fankhauser, C.; Frenk, A.; Cordey, J.; & Gasser, B. (2001). Biomechanical evalutation evaluation of the less invasive stabilization system for the internal fixation of distal femur fractures, J Orthop Trauma, Vol.15, No.7, (September-October 2001), pp.482-487.

Mast, J.; Jacob, R.; & Ganz, R. (1989). Planning and reduction techniques in fracture surgery, Springer, New York, USA. .

http://www.medical.siemens.com/webapp/wcs/stores/servlet/ProductDisplay~q_catalogId~e_-3~a_catTree~e_100010,1007665,12760,1032265~a_langId~e_-3~a_productId~e_202741~a_storeId~e_10001.htm

McGraw, P.; & Kumar, A. (2010). Periprosthetic fractures of the femur after total knee arthroplasty, J Orthop Traumatol, Vol.11, No.3, (September 2010), pp.135-141. Review.

McLaren, A.C.; Dupont, J.A.; & Schroeber, D.C. (1994). Open reduction internal fixation of supracondylar fractures above total knee arthroplasties using the intramedullary rod, Clin Orthop Relat Res, Vol.302, (May 1994), pp.194-198.

Merkel, K.D.; & Johnson E.W.jr. (1986). Supracondylar fracture of the femur after total knee arthtoplasty, J Bone Joint Surg Am, Vol.68, No.1, (January 1986), pp.29-43.

Stedtfeld, H.W.; Mittlmeier, T.; Landgraf, P.; & Ewert, A. (2004). The logic and clinical applications of blocking screws, J Bone Joint Surg Am, Vol.86, Suppl 2, pp.17-25.

Mittlmeier, T.; Stöckle, U.; Perka, C.; & Schaser, K.D. (2005). [Periprosthetic fractures after total knee joint arthroplasty, Unfallchirurg, Vol.108, No.6, (June 2005), pp.481-495; quiz 496. Review. German.

Mittlmeier, T.; & Beck, M. (2005). [Retrograde medullary locking in periprosthetic distal femoral fracture after condylar knee joint replacement], Unfallchirurg, Vol.108, No.6, (June 2005), pp.497-501. Review. German.

Moran, M.C.; Brick, G.W.; Sledge, C.B.; Dysart, S.H.; & Chien, E.P. (1996). Supracondylra femoral fracture following total knee arthroplasty, Clin Orthop Relat Res, Vol.324, (March 1996), pp.196-209.

Mulier, T.; Seligson, D.; Sioen, W.; van den Bergh, J.; & Reynaert, P. (1997). Operative treatment of humeral shaft fractures, Acta Orthop Belg, Vol.63, No.3, pp.170-177.

Müller, M.E.; Allgöwer, M.; & Willenegger, H. (1970). Manual of Internal Fixation, first ed., Springer, New York, USA.

Müller, M.E.; Allgöwer, M.; Schneider, R.; & Willenegger, H. (1979). Manual of Internal Fixation, 2nd ed., Springer, New York, USA.

Murrell, G.A.; & Nunley, J.A. (1995). Interlocked supracondylar intramedullary nails for supracondylar fractures after total knee arthroplasty. A new treatment method, J Arthoplasty, Vol.10, No.1, (February 1995), pp.37-42.

Nauth, A.; Ristevski, B.; Begué, T.; & Schemitsch, E.H. (2011). Periprosthetic distal femur fractures: current concepts, J Orthop Trauma, Vol.25, Suppl 1, (June 2011), pp.S82-85.

Noorda, R.J,; & Wuisman, P.I. (2002). Mennen plate fixation for the treatment of periprosthetic femoral fracture: a multicenter study of thirty-six fractures, J Bone Joint Surg Am, Vol.84, No.12, (December 2002), pp.2211-2215.

Ochsner, P.E.; & Pfister, A. (1999). Use of the fork plate for internal fixation of periprosthetic fractures and osteotomies in connection with total knee replacement, Orthopedics, Vol.22, No.5, (May 1999), pp.517-521.

Ostrum, R.F.; & Geel, C. (1995). Indirect reduction and internal fixation of supracondylar femur fractures without bone graft, J Orthop Trauma, Vol.9, No.4, pp.278-284.

O'Toole, R.V.; Gobezie, R.; Hwang, R.; Chandler, A.R.; Smith, R.M.; Estok, D.M.2nd.; &Vrahas, M.S. (2006). Low complication rate of LISS for femur fractures adjacent to stable hip or knee arthroplasty, Clin Orthop Relat Res, Vol.450, (September 2006), pp.203-210.

Otto, R.J.; Moed, B.R.; & Bledsoe, J.G. (2009). Biomechanical comparison of polyaxial locking plates and a fixed-angle locking plate for internal fixation of distal femurs, J Orthop Trauma, Vol.23, No.9, (October 2009), pp.645-652.

Perren, S.M.; Coredy, J.; Rahn, B.A.; Gautier, E.; & Schneider, E. (1988). Early temporary porosis of bone induced by internal fixation implants. A reaction to necrosis, not to stress protection? Clin Orthop Relat Res, Vol.232, (Juliy 1988), pp.139-151. Review.

Perren, S.M. (2002). Evolution of the internal fixation of long bone fractures, J Bone Joint Surg Br, Vol.84, No.8, (November 2002), pp.1093-1110. Review.

Perren, S.M. (2003) Backgrounds of the technology of internal fixators, Injury, Vol.34, Suppl 2, pp.B1-3.

Platzer, P.; Schuster, R.; Aldrian, S.; Prosquill, S.; Krumboeck, A.; Zehetgruber, I.; Kovar, F.; Schwarmeis, K.; & Vecsei, V. (2010). Management and outcome of periprosthetic fractures after total knee arthroplasty, J Trauma, Vol.68, No.6, (June 2010), pp.1464-1470.

Ramotowski, W.; & Granowski, R. (1991). Zespol. An original method of stable osteosynthesis, Clin Orthop Relat Res, Vol.272, (November 1991), pp.67-75.

Rhinelander, F.W. (1972). Circulation in bone. In: Bourne GH, editor. 2nd ed., The biochemistry and physiology of bone, vol 2, 2nd ed. New York: Academic Press, p. 1-77.

Ricci, W.M.; Bolhofner, B.R.; Loftus, T.; Cox, C.; Mitchell, S.; & Borelli, J. Jr. (2005). Indirect reduction and plate fixation, without grafting, for periprosthetic femoral shaft fractures about a stable intramedullary implant, J Bone Joint Surg Am, Vol.87, No.10, (October 2005), pp.2240-2245.

Ricci, W.M. ; Loftus, T.; Cox, C.; & Borelli, J. (2006). Locked plates with minimally invasive insertion techniques for the treatment of periprosthetic supracondylar femur fractures above total knee arthroplasty J Orthop Trauma, Vol.20, No.3, (March 2006), pp.190-196.

Ricci, W.M.; Bolnhofner, B.R.; Loftus, T.; Cox, C.; Mitchell, S.; & Borrelli, J. Jr. (2006). Indirect reduction and plate fixation without grafting, for periprosthetic femoral shaft fractures about a stable intramedullary implant. Surgical technique, J Bone Joint Surg Am, Vol.88, Suppl 1 Pt2, (September 2006), pp.275-282.

Riemer, B.L.; Butterfield, S.L.; Burke, C.J 3rd.; & Mathews, D. (1992). Immediate plate fixation of highly comminuted femoral diaphyseal fractures in blunt polytrauma patients, Orthopedics, Vol.15, No.8, (August 1992), pp.907-916.

Ritter, M.A.; Faris, P.M.; & Keating, E.M. (1988) Anterior femoral notching and ipsilateral supracondylar femur fracture in total knee arthroplasty, J Arthroplasty, Vol.3, No.2, pp.185-187.

Ritter, M.A.; Thong, A.E.; Keating, E.M.; Faris, P.M.; Meding, J.B.; Berend, M.E.; Pierson, J.L.; & Davis, K.E. (2005). The effect of femoral notching during total knee arthroplasty on the prevalence of postoperative femoral fractures and on clinical outcome, J Bone Joint Surg Am, Vol.87, No.11, (November 2005), pp.2411-2414.

Rolston, L.R.; Christ, D.J.; Halpern, A.; O'Connor, P.L.; Ryan, T.G.; & Uggen, W.M. (1995). Treatment of supracondylar fractures of the femur proximal to a total knee arthroplasty, J Bone Joint Surg Am, Vol.77, No.6, (June 1995), pp.924-931.

Rorabeck CH, Taylor JW. Periprosthetic fractures of the femur complicating total knee arthroplasty. Orthop Clin North Am 1999;30:265-277.

Roscoe, M.W.; Goodman, S.B.; & Schatzker, J. (1989) Supracondylar fracture of the femur after GUERPAR total knee arthroplasty, Clin Orthop Relat Res, Vol.241, (April 1989), pp.221-223.

Rozbruch, S.R.; Müller, U.; Gautier, E.; & Ganz, R. (1998). The evolution of femoral shaft plating technique, Clin Orthop Relat Res, Vol.354, (September 1998), pp.195-208.

Rüedi, T.P.; Sommer,C.; & Leutenegger, A. (1998). New techniques in indirect reduction of long bone fractures, Clin Orthop Relat Res, Vol.347, (February 1998), pp.27-34. Review.

Salas, C.; Mercer, D.; DeCoster, T.A.; & Reda Taha, M.M. (2011) Experimental and probahilistic analysis of distal femoral periprosthetic fracture: a comparison of locking plate and intramedullary nail fixation. Part A: experimental investigation, Comput Methods Biomech Biomed Engin, Vol.12, No.2, (February 2011), pp.157-164.

Sanders, R.; Haidukewych, G.J.; Milne, T.; Dennis, J.; & Latta, L.L. (2002). Minimal versus maximal plate fixation techniques of the ulna: the biomechanical effect of number of screws and plate length, J Orthop Trauma, Vol.16, No.3, (March 2002), pp.166-171.

Shawen, S.B.; Belmont, P.J.Jr.; Klemme, W.R.; Topoleski, L.D.; Xenos, J.S.; & Orchowski, J.R. (2003) Osteoporosis and anterior femoral notching in periprosthetic supracondylar femoral fractures: a biomechanical analysis, J Bone Joint Surg Am, Vol.85, No.1, (January 2003), pp.115-121.

Short, W.H.; Hootnick, D.R.; & Murray, D.G. (1981). Ipsilateral supracondylar femur fractures following knee arthroplasty, Clin Orthop Relar Res, Vol.158, (July-August 1981), pp.111-116.

Sisto, D.J.; Lachiewicz, P.F.; & Insall, J.N. (1985). Treatment of supracondylar fractures following prosthetic arthroplasty of the knee, Clin Orthop Relat Res, Vol.196, (June 1985), pp.265-272.

Smith, W.J.; Martin, S.L.; & Mabrey, J.D. (1996). Use of supracondylar nail for treatment of a supracondylar fracture of the femur following total knee arthroplasty, J Arthroplasty, Vol.11, No.2, (February 1996), pp.210-213.

Streubel, P.N.; Gardner, M.J.; Morshed, S.; Collinge, C.A.; Gallagher, B.; & Ricci, W.M. (2010). Are extreme distal periprosthetic supracondylar fractures of the femur too distal to fix using a lateral locked plate? J Bone Joint Surg Br, Vol.92, Vol.4, (April 2010), pp.527-534.

Stoffel, K.; Dieter, U.; Stachowiak, G.; Gächter, A.; & Kuster, M.S. (2003) Biomechanical testing of the LCP – how can stability in locked internal fixators be controlled? Injury, Vol.34, Suppl 2, pp.B11-19.

Su, E.T.; Dewal, H.; & Di Cesare, P.E. (2004) Perisprosthetic femoral fractures above total knee replacements, Am J Acad Orthop Surg, Vol.12, No.1, (January-February 2004), pp.12-20. Review.

Tani, Y.; Inoue, K.; Kanecko, H.; Nishioka, J.; & Hukuda, S. (1998). Intramedullary fibular graft for supracondylar fracture of the femur following total knee arthroplasty, Arch Orthop Trauma Surg, Vol.117, No.1-2, pp.103-104.

Tepic, S.; Remiger, A.R.; Morikawa, K.; Predieri, M.; & Perren, S.M. (1997). Strength recovery in fractured sheep tibia treated with a plate or an internal fixator: an experimental study with a two-year follow-up, J Orthop Trauma, Vol.11, No.1, (January 1997), pp.14-23.

Thielemann, F.W.; Blersch, E.; & Holz, U. (1988). [Plate osteosynthesis of femoral shaft fracture with reference to biological aspects], Unfallchirurg, Vol.91, No.9, (September 1988), pp.389-394. German.

Vidal, J.; Buscayret, C.; Fischbach, C.; Brahin, B.; Paran, M.; & Escare, P. (1977). [New method of treatment of comminuted fractures of the lower end of the radius: „ligamentary taxis"], Acta Orthop Belg, Vol.43, No.6, pp.781-789. French.

Wagner, M. (2003). General principles for the clinical use of the LCP, Injury, Vol.34, Suppl 2, (November 2003), pp.B31-42. Review.

Wagner, M. & Frigg, R. (2006). Manual of Fracture Management, Internal Fixators, Concepts and Cases using LCP and LISS, Thieme, New York, USA.

Wang, J.W.; & Wang, C.J. (2002). Supracobdylar fractures of the femur above total knee arthroplasties with cortical allograft struts, J Arthroplasty, Vo.17, No.3, (April 2002), pp.365-372.

Wenzl, H.; Casey, P.A.; Hérbert, P.; & Bellin, J. (1970). Die operative Behandlung der distalen Femurfraktur. AO Bulletin, Chur AO: Arbeitsgemeinschaft für Osteosynthesefragen.

Wick, M, Müller, E.J.; & Muhr, G. (2001). [Supracondylar femoral fractures in knee endoprosthesis. Stabilizing with retrograde interlocking nail], Unfallchirurg, Vol.104, No.5, (May 2001), pp.410-413. German.

Wick, M.; Müller, E.J.; Kutscha-Lissberg, F.; Hopf, F.; & Muhr, G. (2004). [Periprosthetic supracondylar femoral farctures: LISS or retrogarde intramedullary nailing? Problems with use of minimally invasive technique], Unfallchirurg, Vol.107, No.3, (March 2004), pp.181-188. German.

Zehntner, M.K.; & Ganz, R. (1993). Internal fixation of supracondylar fractures after condylar total knee arthroplasty. Clin Orthop Relat Res, Vol.293, (August 1993), pp.219-224.

Zlowodzki, M.; Williamson, S.; Cole, P.A.; Zardiackas, L.D.; & Kregor, P.J. (2004). Biomechanical evaluation of the less invasive stabilization system, angled blade plate, and retrograde intramedullary nail for the internal fixation of distal femur fractures, J Orthop Trauma, Vol.18, No.8, (September 2004), pp.494-502.

24

Knee Arthrodesis with the Ilizarov External Fixator as Treatment for Septic Failure of Knee Arthroplasty

M. Spina[1], G. Gualdrini[2], M. Fosco[2] and A. Giunti[2]
[1]*Department of Orthopaedics and Traumatology Surgery, Ospedale Borgo Trento, Azienda Universitaria Integrata, Verona*
[2]*First Department of Orthopaedics and Traumatology Surgery, Istituto Ortopedico Rizzoli, Bologna*
Italy

1. Introduction

Femoral-tibial fusion remains one of the last treatment choices for recurrent septic failure of knee prostheses. It can be achieved by different surgical techniques, such as intramedullary nailing, mono/biaxial or circular external fixators, and fixation with long plates and screws.
In other studies, the rate of knee fusion following septic prosthetic loosening has been reported to range from 27% [1] up to 31-33% [2, 3] and even 41-42% [4, 5]. However, authors often do not report the way that fusion is achieved; others use an unspecified external fixation with a success rate ranging from 67 to 90% [6-9], and with a mean fusion time that ranges from 4.4 to 6 months.
More precisely, other authors report that fusion rates with the Ilizarov circular external fixator range from 64-75% [10, 11] to 83-93% [12, 13] and even up to 100% [14]. Mean fusion times range from 6.8 to 13 months.
Among our series of 58 septic knee prostheses treated in our ward from 1990 to 2007, 17 (29.3%) underwent femoral-tibial fusion. The fusions were attempted in all cases with the Ilizarov circular external fixator. The choice of fusion was dictated by bad local conditions of the knee (Fig. 1), the precarious general health status of the patient, and his determination to

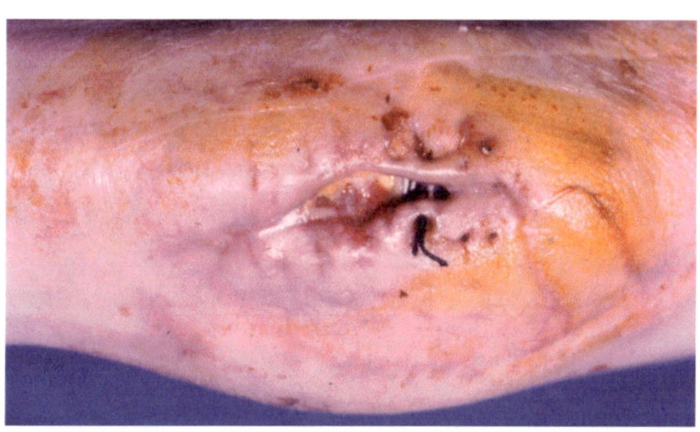

Fig. 1. Precarious local condition of the right knee in a septic prosthesis loosening

find a definitive solution to the problem. Another important factor was the number of failed prosthetic revision procedures due to septic loosening (Fig. 2).

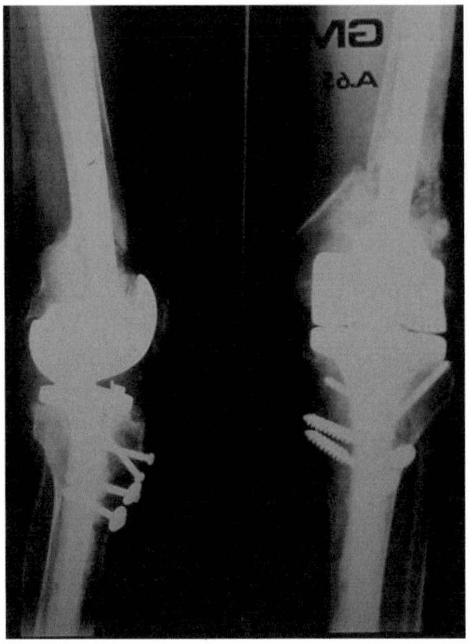

Fig. 2. A/P and L X-ray of a septic knee revision prosthesis loosening

The objective of our study was to evaluate the reliability of the Ilizarov circular external fixator as a surgical technique for knee arthrodesis, and to compare it to other fusion procedures.

2. Materials and methods

The data for this investigation were collected and analyzed in compliance with the procedures and policies set forth by the Helsinki Declaration, and all patients gave their informed consent. The study was authorized by the local ethical committee.

The series included 17 femoral-tibial fusions, representing 29.3% of all septic knee prosthetic loosenings (58) treated on the First Ward of the Rizzoli Orthopedic Institute from 1990 to 2007 (Table 1). Nine patients were women (53%) and eight were men (47%); the mean age at the time of fusion was 62.9 years (women 68.3 and men 56.8), ranging from 26 to 80 years. Eleven patients had a secreting fistula. The microbiological culture examination was positive for Staphylococcus epidermidis in eight cases, Staphylococcus aureus in four cases, Enterococcus in four cases, and other bacterial species to lesser degrees (Fig. 3). The culture examination was negative in four patients (23.5%), even when there were local conditions, and laboratory (ESR and CRP elevated) and radiological (locally increased uptake in total body scintigraphy with marked granulocytes) evaluations were positive for infection. Ten patients had previously been surgically treated for primary arthritis (58.8%), four for posttraumatic arthritis (23.5%), one for sequelae of tuberculous arthritis (5.9%), one for rheumatic arthropathy (5.9%), and one for arthropathy following pigmented villonodular synovitis (5.9%). Five patients were treated at our institute from the implantation of the primary prosthesis, whereas the remaining 12 patients were initially treated at other institutes. The Cierny-Mader classification was used for clinical and anatomopathological assessment [15], while the Engh classification was used to evaluate bone defects [16]. According to the Cierny-Mader system, ten patients (58.8%) belonged to group IV Bls, four patients (23.6%) to group IV Bs, and the remaining patients (17.6%) to group IV Bl.

A	B	C	D	E	F	G	H	I	L	M	N	O	P	Q
67	F	Rheumatoid Arthritis	SX	NO	Staphylococcus Aureous	YES	4B L-S	2	NO	3	Healed	8	None	-4 cm
57	F	Osteoarthritis	DX	YES (one revision TKA)	Staphylococcus Epidermidis and Aureous. Enterococcus	YES	4B L-S	2	NO	8	Healed	24	Small fistula (after 16 months)	-6 cm
51	M	Tubercular arthropathy	SX	YES (one revision TKA)	Staphylococcus Agalactiae, Epidermidis, Haemoliticus	NO	4B L-S	2	NO	8	Healed	6	Thrombo-phlebitis	-2 cm
80	F	Osteoarthritis	DX	YES (one revision TKA)	Pseudomonas Aeruginosa	NO	4B S	2	NO	3	Healed	50	None	-4 cm
55	M	Osteoarthritis	DX	NO	Not isolated	NO	4B S	2	NO	5	Not healed	6	Intolerance	/
70	F	Osteoarthritis	SX	NO	Staphylococcus Epidermidis	YES	4B L-S	3	YES	7	Not healed	†	Nonunion	/
64	F	Posttraumatic osteoarthritis	DX	NO	Staphylococcus Aureous	YES	4B L-S	2	NO	5	Healed	8	None	-4 cm
48	M	Posttraumatic osteoarthritis	SX	NO	Staphylococcus Epidermidis	YES	4B L	2	NO	8	Healed	28	None	-3 cm
70	F	Osteoarthritis	SX	YES (one revision TKA)	Not isolated	NO	4B S	2	NO	2	Not healed	6	Intolerance	/
74	M	Osteoarthritis	DX	NO	Not isolated	YES	4B L-S	3	YES	16	Healed	15	None	-3 cm
70	F	Osteoarthritis	DX	NO	Not isolated	YES	4B L-S	3	YES	6	Healed	66	None	-5 cm
65	M	Posttraumatic osteoarthritis	DX	NO	Staphylococcus Epidermidis, Pseudomonas Aeruginosa	YES	4B L-S	3	YES	14	Healed	101	None	-6 cm
64	F	Osteoarthritis	SX	NO	Enterococcus Fecalis	YES	4B L	3	YES	12	Healed	17	None	-6 cm
73	F	Osteoarthritis	DX	YES (two revisions TKA)	Streptococcus, Staphylococcus Epidermidis	YES	4B L-S	3	YES	20 (2 attempt)	Not healed	24	Nonunion	/
26	M	Posttraumatic osteoarthritis	SX	NO	Staphylococcus Epidermidis	NO	4B L	3	NO	18	Healed	32	None	0 cm
66	M	Osteoarthritis	SX	NO	Enterococcus, Pseudomonas Aeruginosa	NO	4B S	2	NO	4	Healed	8	None	-3 cm
70	M	Pigmented villinodular synovitis arthropathy	SX	NO	Staphylococcus Aureous, Epidermidis, Enterococcus	YES	4B L-S	2	NO	16	Healed	82	None	-4 cm

A Age at fusion, B Sex, C Initial diagnosis, D Side, E Revision, F Bacteria, G Fistula, H Cierny-Mader Classification, I Engh Classification, L Cement spacer, M Mean Time to Fusion (months), N Result, O Follow up (months), P Problems/Obstacles/Complications, Q Limb shortness (centimeters)

Table 1. Summary of the data on the patients included in this study

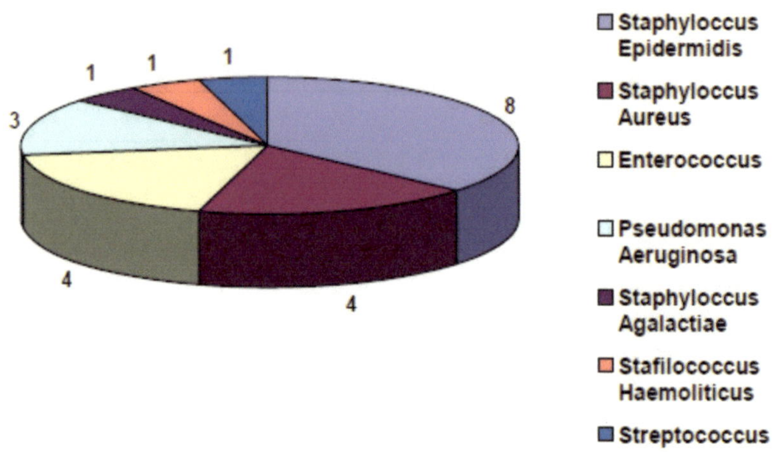

Fig. 3. Type and distribution of the isolated microbes

According to the Engh classification, ten patients (58.8%) were considered type II, and the remaining (41.2%) were considered type III. Different surgical treatments were performed depending on the Engh classification.

For type II Engh patients the treatment involved:

- Injection of the fistulous tract, when present, with methylene blue dye;
- Removal of prosthetic components and cement mantle, samples taken for microbiological culture testing, than surgical debridement and regularization of the femoral and tibial bone surfaces;
- Femoral–tibial stabilization under compression with the Ilizarov external fixator, applying 5–6 mm diameter percutaneous half-pins with a hydroxyapatite coating for femoral arches, a distal femoral ring, and a pair of tibial rings stabilized with Kirschner wires;
- Specific or wide-ranging antibiotic therapy for four/six weeks.

For Engh type III patients (except in one case) the treatment involved:

- Injection of the fistulous tract, when present, with methylene blue dye
- Removal of prosthetic components cement mantle, samples taken for microbiological
- culture testing, than surgical debridement and regularization of the femoral and tibial bone surfaces
- Application of antibiotic-loaded cement spacer stained with methylene blue (Fig. 4)
- Hinged brace and specific or wide-ranging antibiotic therapy for four/six weeks
- Assessment of infection indices and clinical condition, then further surgical debridement followed by femoral–tibial fusion with the external fixator
- Specific or wide-ranging antibiotic therapy for four/six weeks if the culture exam is positive at the time of fusion.

An additional surgical stage with the application of an antibiotic-loaded cement spacer is used for 4–6 weeks in patients belonging to Engh group III, because in our experience surgical debridement alone may not be sufficient to eradicate the infection in cases with large bone defects.

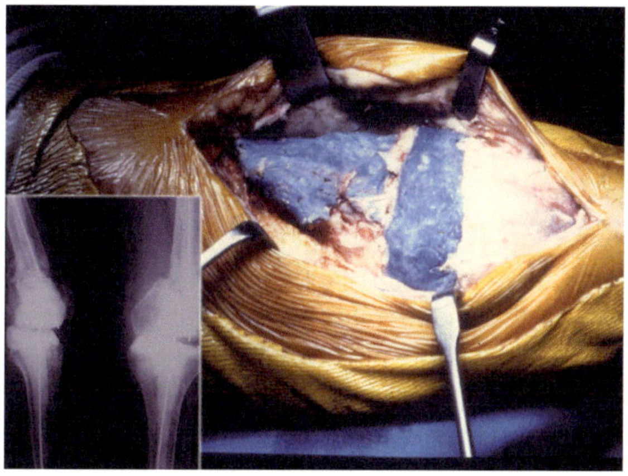

Fig. 4. a Antibiotic-loaded cement spacer stained with methylene blue following knee prosthesis removal. b A/P and L X-ray of a knee with cement spacer in situ

The type of antibiotic used in the spacer depended on the result of the microbiological test performed previously. In our series, in most cases we used vancomycin at a dose of 2-4 g of antibiotic per 40 g of cement.

In a 26-year-old patient with a final limb shortening of 11 cm, femoral and tibial lengthening were performed at same time as the fusion.

Patients who were considered healed showed a continuous cancellous trabecular pattern from femur to tibia at standard radiographs (Fig. 5) and no clinical and instrumental signs of an active infection. Stability at the fusion site was evaluated with the varus-valgus stress test. The femoral-tibial fusion was assessed both radiographically and clinically.

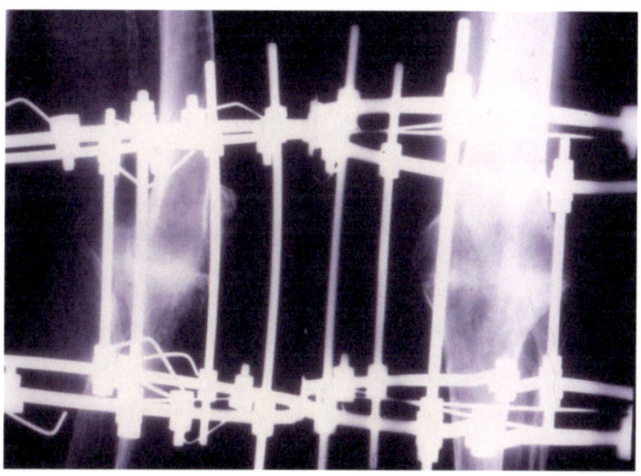

Fig. 5. A/P and L X-ray showing continuity of the trabecular-medullary pattern in a patient treated with Ilizarov's external fixator

3. Technical notes for assembling the external fixator

3.1 Femoral component

The fixator is anchored to the femoral diaphysis by three or four 5-6-mm percutaneous half-pins coated in hydroxyapatite and fixed to two Ilizarov arches of the same diameter but different lengths (the distal one is longer). The arches are positioned perpendicular to the long axis of the femur. Four screws are recommended for patients over 60 kg in body weight. The distal arch is connected to a ring with a size proportional to the diameter of the knee and anchored to the distal femur by two Ilizarov wires.

3.2 Tibial component

The femoral distal ring is connected by three hinged rods to two rings of the same diameter that are anchored to the proximal tibial diaphysis by Ilizarov wires. For good fusion it is important that the fixator is connected to bone by Ilizarov wires on both sides of the subsequent fusion. In this setup the circular external fixator is bulky but effective. The hinged connection allows compression at the fusion site with deviations in flexion, external rotation and valgus of the tibia with respect to the femur. Proximal percutaneous screws and Ilizarov wires often cause local swelling of the skin. This is the most uncomfortable aspect for the patient (Figs. 6, 7).

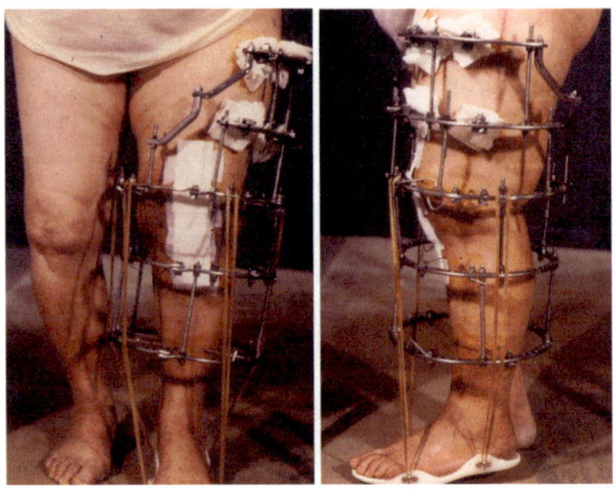

Fig. 6. Left knee in a patient treated by fusion using an Ilizarov circular external fixator. A splint is present to support the foot

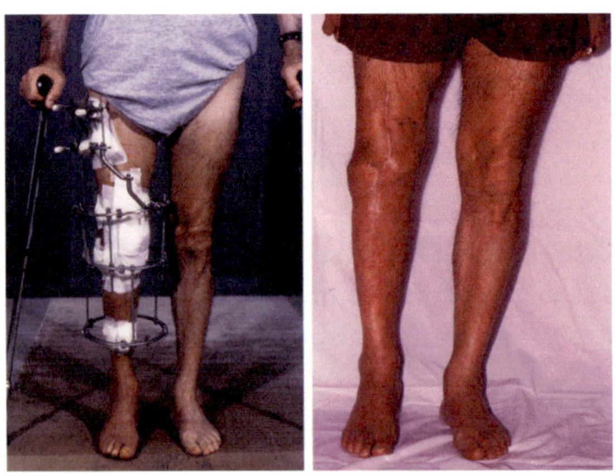

Fig. 7. Type IV Bls patient treated using an Ilizarov external fixator for left knee fusion. Functional stable limb bearing was achieved after 101 months

4. Results

Among the 17 patients, 13 fusions were achieved at the first surgical attempt in a mean time of 9.3 months (range 3–18 months) (Figs. 8, ,9) the mean follow-up was 30 months (range 6–101 months) (Table 1).

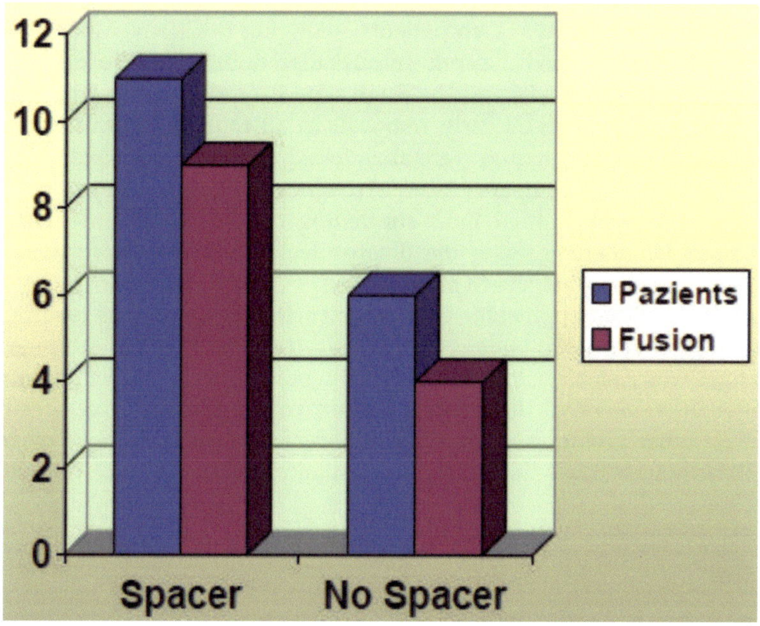

Fig. 8. Comparison of patients according to treatment and fusion rate

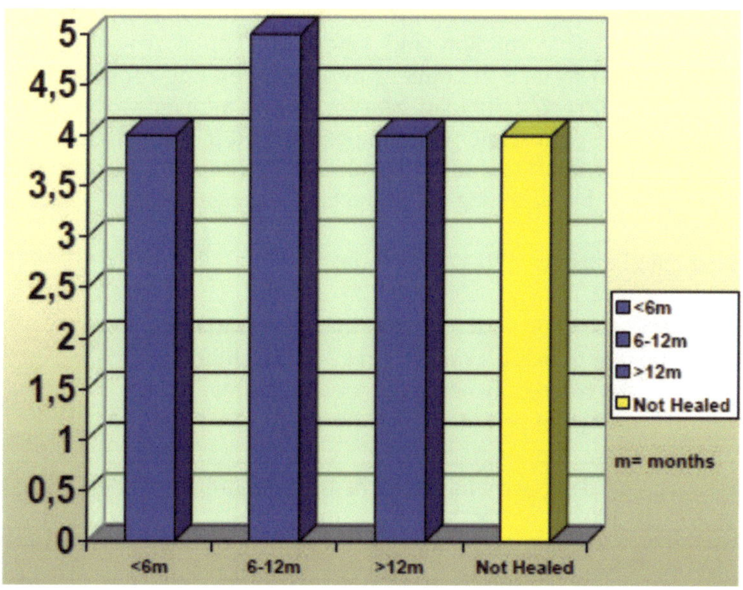

Fig. 9. Duration of treatment with Ilizarov fixator in healed patients

To assess difficulties that occur during treatment with the Ilizarov external fixator, Paley's classification was used [17] to distinguish problems, obstacles and complications. Problems represent difficulties that require no operative intervention to resolve, while obstacles represent difficulties that require an operative intervention. All intraoperative injuries and all problems that are not resolved before the end of treatment are considered true complications. In our cohort there were four complications (23.5%) that were responsible for treatment failure in four patients. Two patients belonging to Cierny-Mader IV Bls and the Engh type III group developed a septic intrarticular nonunion. The other two patients belonging to Cierny-Mader IV Bs and the Engh type II group developed an intolerance to the external fixator that led to its early removal. In all four patients, further attempts at fusion with other surgical techniques were abandoned and a hinged brace was applied. The mean residual limb length discrepancy was 3.8 cm (range 0-6 cm). One obstacle occurred in a 26-year-old patient with a final limb shortening of 11 cm; femoral-tibial fusion and femoral and tibial lengthening using the Ilizarov technique were performed at the same time, thus restoring the original length of the limb.
Problems included a thrombophlebitis in a patient with severe venous insufficiency of the lower limbs and previous deep venous thrombosis; this was treated with pharmacological therapy. Another was a small fistula at a surgical wound that developed in another patient 16 months after the removal of the external fixator, which resolved after specific antibiotic therapy. Among other problems, there were superficial wound infections of percutaneous screws and Ilizarov wire tracts that were never quantified but which always resolved with local disinfection.

5. Discussion

Femoral-tibial fusion is a valid alternative upon septic failure of primary and revision total knee arthroplasty, and is usually well tolerated by patients.
This treatment restores good limb loading, decreasing pain and eliminating infection.
Circular external fixation provides stability at the fusion site and correct femoral-tibial alignment in flexion, external rotation and valgus deviation. Any type of correction is possible without the need to take the patient into the operating room. The circular fixator provides very good stability, so daily load-bearing may be allowed without limitation. It is a low-cost option from a hospital economics perspective, and it ensures a low risk of infection. In particular cases during treatment for femoral-tibial fusion, the fixator can restore severe limb-length discrepancy by applying a distraction osteogenesis technique on the tibial and/or femoral side.
Disadvantages of circular external fixator include:

- A long learning curve
- Objective discomfort for the patient due to the wide field of the device
- Nonrigid fixation due to flexible metal wires and percutaneous screws
- Cutaneous infections frequently occur at wire entry sites
- Loosening and breakage of percutaneous screws
- Long treatment times.

Knee arthrodesis achieved by various types of intramedullary nailing has a success rate ranging from 67 to 100% [6, 18-24] in a mean time of about six months. Using intramedullary nailing in a knee with a periprosthetic infection poses a number of problems, such as the risk of spreading the infection into the medullary canal, the difficulty involved in treating infection recurrence, the possibility of nail migration or breakage, and the

impossibility of performing a compression at the fusion site and clinically assessing its stability during treatment [23, 25].
The technique of femoral–tibial fusion with a monoaxial or biaxial external fixator has a success rate that ranges from 68 [26] to 89% [27] and up to 100% [28, 29]. These fixators, especially monoaxial ones, are fairly well tolerated by patients. However, they do not allow significant changes in the axis, and, due to their structural characteristics, they are rigid and not entirely reliable for complete load-bearing [30].
Finally, bone fusion with dual compression plates has a success rate ranging from 80 [31] to 100% [32]. The authors, however, report high rates of complications (18.2%) such as stress fractures and persistent infection. Healing in some cases was achieved after repeated surgical attempts. Bone fixation with plates and screws is rigid and enables axial

Author(s)	N° of Knees	Classification Used	Fusion rate	Mean Time to fusion (range) in months	Mean residual limb shortness	Complications	Mean FU in months
Johannsen HG et al (2005) [11]	8	none	75%	3,5 (3-4)	3,5 cm	12,5% (1 chronic osteomyelitis)	10
Manzotti A et al (2001) [12]	6	none	83%	6,8 (10,3-5,1)	-	None	34,2
Garberina MJ et al (2000) [10]	19	none	68%	4,6 (3-6,8)	-	26,3% (2 fractures, 2 valgus angulation, 1 wound infection)	32
Oostenbroek & van Roermund (2001) [13]	15	Mild/Moderate/Severe loss of bone	93%	12 (6-24,7)	4 cm	80% (2 femoral fractures 3 osteitis 3 frame instability 1 non-union 1 femoral angulation 1 heel decubitus 1 pneumonia infection)	52
David R et al (2001) [14]	13	none	100%	6,4 (4,6-8,4)	3,7 cm	7,7% (1 wound infection)	40,8
Spina M et al (2009)	17	Combined Engh/ Cierny-Mader	76,5%	9,3 (3-18)	3,8 cm	11,7% (1 Thrombophlebitis, 1 small fistula)	30

Table 2. Literature review of knee arthrodesis with an Ilizarov circular external fixator

compression [33]. It is, however, a complex procedure that is very invasive and at risk of infection. Nichols et al. [32] advise against this technique in the presence of widespread infection.

The existing literature on femoral-tibial fusion with an Ilizarov circular external fixator reports success rates that vary in different studies from 64 [10] to 100% [14] (Table 2). In our series, the rate of complete healing was 76.5% at the first surgical attempt in a mean time of 9.3 months. Failures consisted of four patients (23.5% of the entire group); two of these patients had bad general health conditions; one patient died a few months after removal of the external fixator; another did not heal despite a second attempt at fusion with an Ilizarov external fixator. The other two patients were affected by an anxious-depressive syndrome that contributed to severe intolerance to the external fixator, so its early removal was inevitable. This event accounted for 50% of the failures, so we believe in the importance of carefully assessing the patient's ability to cooperate before treatment.

Our selection of an Ilizarov circular external fixator was dictated by its low cost, versatility, stability under load, possibility to performing modifications during treatment, and low risk of septic dissemination. Nevertheless, in our opinion, careful patient selection is required, as old age and psychological intolerance are generally compromising factors. The treatment time is long and an experienced surgeon is needed to assemble the external fixator and manage it later.

6. References

[1] Husted H, Toftgaard Jensen T. Clinical outcome after treatment of infected primary total knee arthroplasty. Acta Orthop Belg. 2002;68(5):500–507. [PubMed]

[2] Blom AW, Brown J, Taylor AH, Pattison G, Whitehouse S, Bannister GC. Infection after total knee arthroplasty. J Bone Joint Surg Br. 2004;86(5):688–691. doi: 10.1302/0301-620X.86B5.14887. [PubMed] [Cross Ref]

[3] Weng X, Li L, Qui G, Li J, Tian Y, Hen J, Wang Y, Jin J, Ye Q, Zhao H. Treatment of infected total knee arthroplasty. Zhonghua Wai Ke Za Zhi. 2002;40(9):669–672. [PubMed]

[4] Bengston S, Knutson K, Lidgren L. Treatment of infected knee arthroplasty. Clin Orthop Relat Res. 1989;245:173–178. [PubMed]

[5] Hanssen AD, Trousdale RT, Osmon DR. Patient outcome with reinfection following reimplantation for the infected total knee arthroplasty. Clin Orthop Relat Res. 1995;321:55–67. [PubMed]

[6] Mabry TM, Jacofsky DJ, Haidukewych GJ, Hanssen AD. Comparison of intramedullary nailing and external fixation knee arthrodesis for the infected knee replacement. Clin Orthop Relat Res. 2007;464:11–15. [PubMed]

[7] Figgie HE, III, Brody GA, Inglis AE, Sculco TP, Goldberg VM, Figgie MP. Knee arthrodesis following total knee arthroplasty in rheumatoid arthritis. Clin Orthop. 1987;224:237–243. [PubMed]

[8] Klinger HM, Spahn G, Schultz W, Baums MH. Arthrodesis of the knee after failed infected total knee arthroplasty. Knee Surg Sports Traumatol Arthrosc. 2006;14(5):447–453. doi: 10.1007/s00167-005-0664-3. [PubMed] [Cross Ref]

[9] Rudolph F, Fengler F, Hein W. Arthrodesis as an alternative in infected knee arthroplasty. Beitr Orthop Traumatol. 1989;36(8):374–380. [PubMed]

[10] Garberina MJ, Fitch RD, Hoffmann ED, Hardaker WT, Vail TP, Scully SP. Knee arthrodesis with circular external fixation. Clin Orthop. 2001;382:168–178. doi: 10.1097/00003086-200101000-00023. [PubMed] [Cross Ref]
[11] Johannsen HG, Skov O, Weeth ER. Knee arthrodesis with external fixator after infected knee arthroplasty. Ugeskr Laeger. 2005;167(35):3295–3296. [PubMed]
[12] Manzotti A, Pullen C, Deromedis B, Catagni MA. Knee arthrodesis after infected total knee arthroplasty using the Ilizarov method. Clin Orthop Relat Res. 2001;389:143–149. doi: 10.1097/00003086-200108000-00020. [PubMed] [Cross Ref]
[13] Oostenbroek HJ, Roermund PM. Arthrodesis of the knee after an infected arthroplasty using the Ilizarov method. J Bone Joint Surg Br. 2001;83:50–54. doi: 10.1302/0301-620X.83B1.10572. [PubMed] [Cross Ref]
[14] David R, Shtarker H, Horesh Z, Tsur A, Soudry M. Arthrodesis with Ilizarov device for failed knee arthroplasty. Orthopedics. 2001;24:33–36. [PubMed]
[15] Cierny G, Mader JT, Penninck JJ (1985) A clinical staging system for adult osteomyelitis. Contemp Orthop 10(5)
[16] Engh GA, Ammeen DJ. Bone loss with revision total knee arthroplasty: defect classification and alternatives for reconstruction. AAOS Instr Course Lect. 1999;48(22):167–175.
[17] Paley D. Problems, obstacles, and complications of limb lengthening by the Ilizarov technique. Clin Orthop Relat Res. 1990;250:81–104. [PubMed]
[18] Wilde AH, Stearns KL. Intramedullary fixation for arthrodesis of the knee after infected total knee arthroplasty. Clin Orthop Relat Res. 1989;248:87–92. [PubMed]
[19] Bargiotas K, Wohlrab D, Sewecke JJ, Lavinge G, DeMeo PJ, Sotereanos GN. Arthrodesis of the knee with a long intramedullary nail following the failure of a total knee arthroplasty as the result of infection. Surgical technique. J Bone Joint Surg Am. 2006;89:103–110. doi: 10.2106/JBJS.F.01125. [PubMed] [Cross Ref]
[20] Senior CJ, Assuncao RE, Barlow IW. Knee arthrodesis for limb salvage with an intramedullary couplet nail. Arch Orthop Trauma Surg. 2007;128:683–687. doi: 10.1007/s00402-007-0386-8. [PubMed] [Cross Ref]
[21] Volpi R, Dehoux E, Touchard P, Mensa C, Segal P. Knee arthrodesis using a customized intramedullary nail: 14 cases. Rev Chir Orthop Reparatrice Appar Mot. 2004;90(1):58–64. [PubMed]
[22] Lai KA, Shen WJ, Yang CY. Arthrodesis with a short Huckstep nail as a salvage procedure for failed total knee arthroplasty. J Bone Joint Surg. 1998;80(3):380–388. [PubMed]
[23] Waldman BJ, Mont MA, Payman KR, Freiberg AA, Windsor RE, Sculco TP, Hungerford DS. Infected knee arthroplasty treated with arthrodesis using a modular nail. Clin Orthop Relat Res. 1999;367:230–237. doi: 10.1097/00003086-199910000-00029. [PubMed] [Cross Ref]
[24] Jorgensen PS, Torholm C. Arthrodesis after infected knee arthroplasty using long arthrodesis nail. A report of five cases. Am J Knee Surg. 1995;8(3):110–113. [PubMed]
[25] Donley BG, Matthews LS, Kaufer H. Arthrodesis of the knee with an intramedullary nail. J Bone Joint Surg Am. 1991;73(6):907–913. [PubMed]
[26] Rand J, Bryan R, Chao E (1987) Failed total knee arthroplasty treated by arthrodesis of the knee using the Ace-Fisher apparatus. J Bone J Surg 69:39.

[27] Parratte S, Madougou S, Villaba M, Stein A, Rochwerger A, Curvale G. Knee arthrodesis with a double mono-bar external fixators to salvage infected knee arthroplasty: retrospective analysis of 18 knees with mean seven-year follow-up. Rev Chir Orthop Reparatrice Appar Mot. 2007;93(4):373–380. [PubMed]

[28] Fidler MW. Knee arthrodesis following prosthesis removal: use of the Wagner apparatus. J Bone Joint Surg. 1983;65B:29–31.

[29] Wade PJ, Denham RA. Arthrodesis of the knee after failed knee replacement. J Bone Joint Surg Br. 1984;66:362–366. [PubMed]

[30] Hak DJ, Lieberman JR, Finerman GA. Single plane and biplane external fixators for knee arthrodesis. Clin Orthop Relat Res. 1995;316:134–144. [PubMed]

[31] Munzinger U, Knessl J, Gschwend N. Arthrodesis following knee arthroplasty. Orthopade. 1987;16(4):301–309. [PubMed]

[32] Nichols SJ, Landon GC, Tullos HS. Arthrodesis with dual plates after failed total knee arthroplasty. J Bone Joint Surg Am. 1991;73(7):1020–1024. [PubMed]

[33] Christie MJ, Boer DK, McQueen DA, Cooke FW, et al. Salvage procedures for failed total knee arthroplasty. J Bone J Surg Am. 2003;85:S58–S62.

Part 5

Computer Assisted Total Knee Arthroplasty

25

Strategies to Improve the Function, Kinematic and Implants' Positioning of a TKA with Minimally Invasive Computer-Assisted Navigation

Nicola Biasca[1] and Matthias Bungartz[2]
[1]*Orthopedic Clinic Luzern AG, Hirslanden Clinic St. Anna, Luzern*
[2]*Klinik für Orthopädie und Unfallchirurgie, Lehrstuhl für Orthopädie der Friedrich-Schiller-Universität Jena, Waldkrankenhaus „Rudolf Elle" Eisenberg*
[1]*Switzerland*
[2]*Germany*

1. Introduction

Total Knee Arthroplasty (TKA) is a well established, highly successful procedure, with numerous long-term follow-up studies reporting clinical success rates of 72-100% at 10-20 years in terms of pain reduction, functional improvement and overall patient satisfaction [1-5]. Although TKA is generally successful, and despite the advances in surgical techniques, instrumentation and implant designs, between 5 to 8% of all patients still develop complications such as anterior knee pain, loosening, instability, malpositioning, infection or fractures [6-8]. Imperfection in the coronar, sagittal and axial alignments of the femoral and/ or of tibial components, improper ligament balancing and incorrect joint line restoration can lead to soft tissue imbalance and inability to re-establish optimal kinematics and the overall biomechanics of the joint, with persistent anterior knee pain, patellar maltracking, instability or limitation of movement [9-14, 15].

Several investigators have demonstrated on the basis of conventional radiography and computer-tomography that TKA, implanted with computer-assisted navigation and conventional approach, has more accurate component alignment than TKA implanted conventionally [9, 15-29].

The introduction of minimally invasive surgery (MIS) has gained in importance in orthopedics and especially in TKA. Patient`s demand for high activity level after TKA, concerns about postoperative pain, fast rehabilitation process, possible reduction in duration of hospitalization and costs in connection with the necessity of health care savings have led to the rapid advancement of less invasive surgical approaches and techniques as well as the development of new instrumentation by the orthopedic implant industry.

Regardless of the numerous advantages of minimal-invasive TKA, concern is driven about loss of accuracy for implant placement and increased complications related to skin slough and infection when a minimally invasive approach is used [30, 31]. Furthermore reduced operative visualization, a steep learning curve, an increased risk of complications, excessive skin trauma and compromised implant fixation and alignment are topic of objection. In addition few surgeons have expressed concern about minimally invasive surgery and its relevance to TKA as well as the safety of operations performed "through a keyhole" and are convinced that at present there is no credible evidence that smaller incisions significantly benefit the patient receiving MIS TKA. By contrast, proponents of MIS TKA report that MIS patients, compared to patients undergoing conventional TKA, Experience shortened hospital stay, less pain-control medications, faster recovery of knee range of motion and decreased blood loss all without compromise of accuracy or short-term outcome [32-34].

2. Computer-assisted navigated orthopedic surgery

The principle of computer-assisted surgery in orthopedics is based on the creation of a digital map for the different steps during operation. Using this map, the surgeon is guided through the operating process. The development of the digital image is based on three different basic ideas.

One system uses anatomical information which is achieved from pre-operatively performed CT- or MRI-scans, the second system is "peri-operatively-imaged" in which anatomical imaging occurs in the operating suite at the time of surgery. This requires a specially modified fluoroscopy unit, which entails the presence of a relatively bulky and expensive apparatus during surgery. These two systems display the "image-based systems". The third group on the contrary is "image-free" and relies on information acquired during surgery. This "image-free" navigation allows the surgeon to quantify data, receive real-time dynamic intra-operative maneuvering feedback and to obtain more reproducible results.

A very important feature of this navigation system is its ability to provide instant feedback regarding *in vivo* kinematics of the joint at different stages of the operation. Alignment and ligament stability can be assessed with the trials in place to ensure proper function. Furthermore, this system allows the surgeon to measure the coronal, sagittal and axial deformities, the alignments and the stability of the joint before, during and after the implantation of a TKA. These characteristics of the navigation system provide the unique opportunity to assess *in vivo* the kinematics of the knee during surgery and implement beneficial changes of the components or alteration in components selection.

We were using at the Orthopedic Clinic at the Hospital Oberengadin in Samedan an "image-free" navigation system (Stryker® Leibinger Knee Navigation System, Stryker® Leibinger, precisioN Knee Navigation Software V 4.0). This system is available in an active wireless PC-based guidance system, which is based on an image-free navigation method, and thus does not require pre-operative computer tomography or intra-operative fluoroscopy. It comprises a module for analyzing the alignment of the leg, the alignment of the resection planes and thus of the prosthetic components. The system also allows the surgeon to quantify the kinematics of the knee and the balancing of the soft tissue (Further details on the Stryker® Knee Navigation System are available on http://www.europe.stryker.com/).

2.1.1 Surgical procedure

The patient is placed supine on a standard operating table. A tourniquet is applied after exsanguination of the limb, and standard skin preparation and draping are undertaken. To obtain best exposition of all structures during the procedure, two distally positioned leg holders are fixed on the operating table to allow full flexion and extension of the leg. Flexing the knee thereby exposes the posterior structures whereas extension facilitates access to the anterior anatomy of the knee.

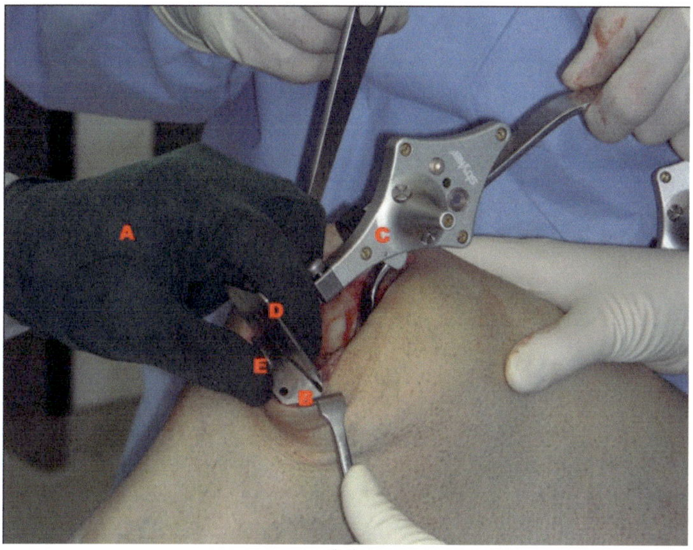

1A

Fig. 1A. The proximal tibial resection requires the surgeon to position the MIS Cutting Guide in relation to the three axes of freedom controlling the varus/ valgus, the depth and the posterior slope, with a freehand technique (A). The cutting guide block/ tracker construct (B-C-D) is then hold by the surgeon with a "tripod grip" (A). The universal tracker (C) is attached to the resection plane probe (D), which in turn is placed into the captured slot of the cutting guide block (B). The cutting guide block (B) is pinned into place with three pins (E).

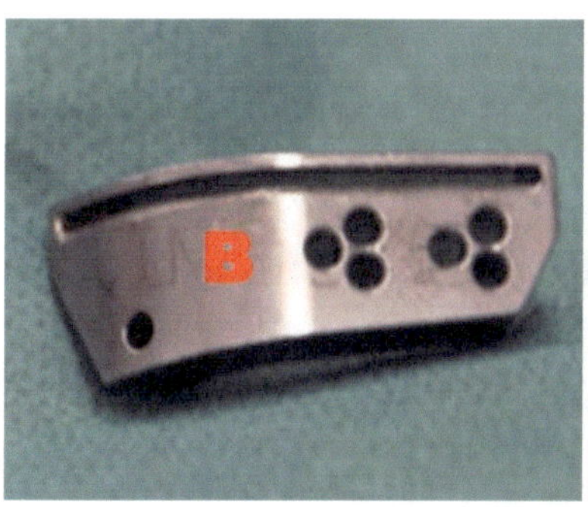

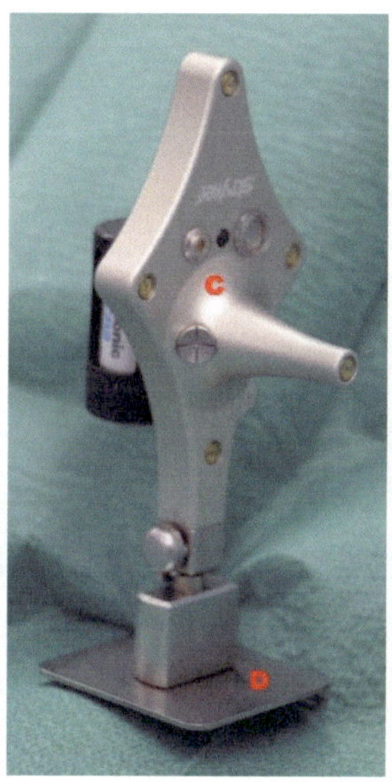

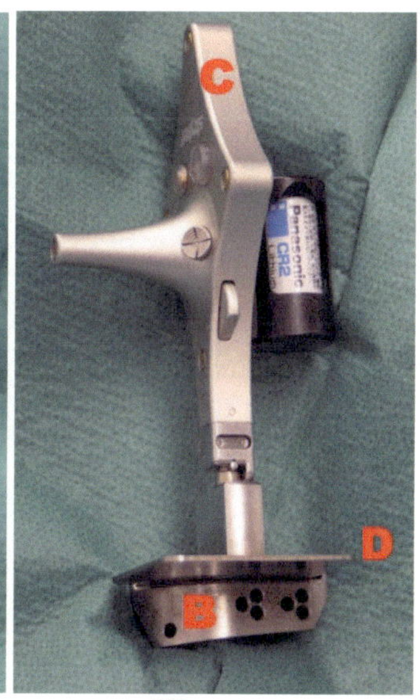

1B 1C 1D

Fig. 1B-D. MIS TKA must be performed with accurate instruments:
Fig. 1B. The cutting guide block (B).
Fig. 1C. The universal tracker (C) is attached to the resection plane probe (D).
Fig. 1D. The universal tracker (C) is attached to the resection plane probe (D), which in turn is placed into the captured slot of the cutting guide block (B).

Fig. 1A-D. Proximal tibial resection

As standard approach we used a mid-vastus approach [35-38]. To enable a better exposure and visibility of the lateral compartment the patella was osteotomized freehand to 12-14 mm bone thickness for later resurfacing in order to reconstruct preoperative thickness. All interventions were performed by a single surgeon (NB), who is a high volume arthroplasty surgeon and uses computer-navigation routinely for over six years.

Two pin trackers need to be fixed rigidly at the beginning of the operation on the lateral distal femur and on the ventral proximal tibia, both within the surgical access zone (For further details information's please see the references 24 and 25).

The digitizing pointer is now used to mark the key anatomical landmarks. After that procedure the surgeon is able to reproduce the correct joint kinematics at any time of the operation in any position of the leg with the Knee Navigation System software. After analyzing the kinematics curves and axis, bone cuts are performed using the information obtained from the navigation system.

We usually prefer starting with tibial cut first. The proximal tibial cut is made in a one-step procedure, controlling the desired posterior slope, varus/ valgus and depth. The degree of posterior slope of the tibial cut is aimed to match the original posterior slope of the tibial plateau as measured in the pre-operative lateral x-ray [16]. Using freehand technique, the position of the probe is adjusted according to the image and data shown on the computer. MIS TKA must be performed with accurate instruments that are coordinated with the procedure. The guide is held with a "tripod grip" technique (Figures 1A-D), and the visual movements of the guide can be monitored in real time on the screen (Figure 2).

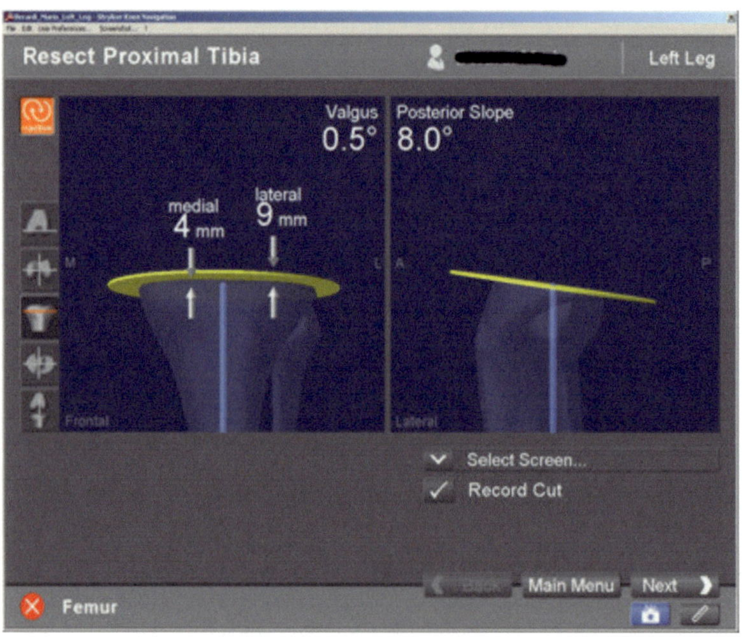

Fig. 2. The virtual position of cutting guide/ tracker construct is now an active tool, which can be monitored (i.e. the varus/ valgus angle, the slope angel and the depth) on the computer navigation screen.

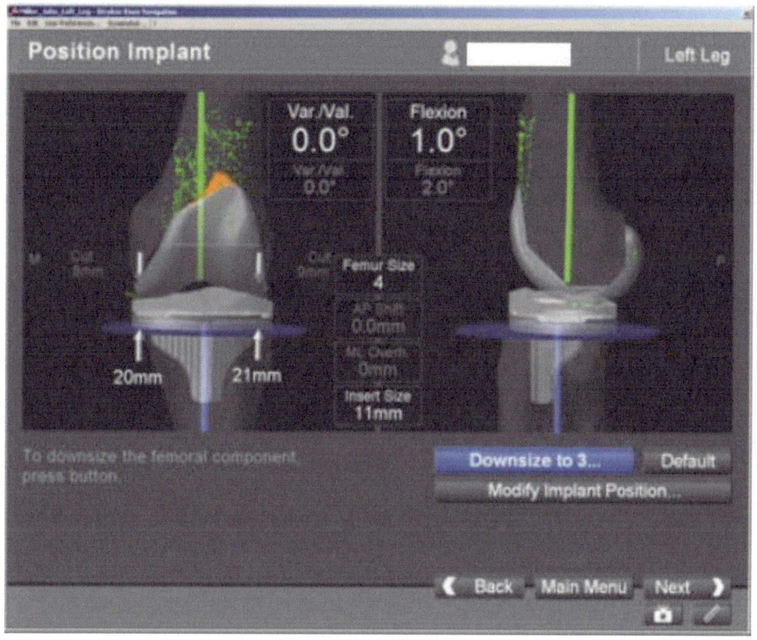

3A

Fig. 3A. "Implant Position": The system allows the surgeon to check the position of the implant.

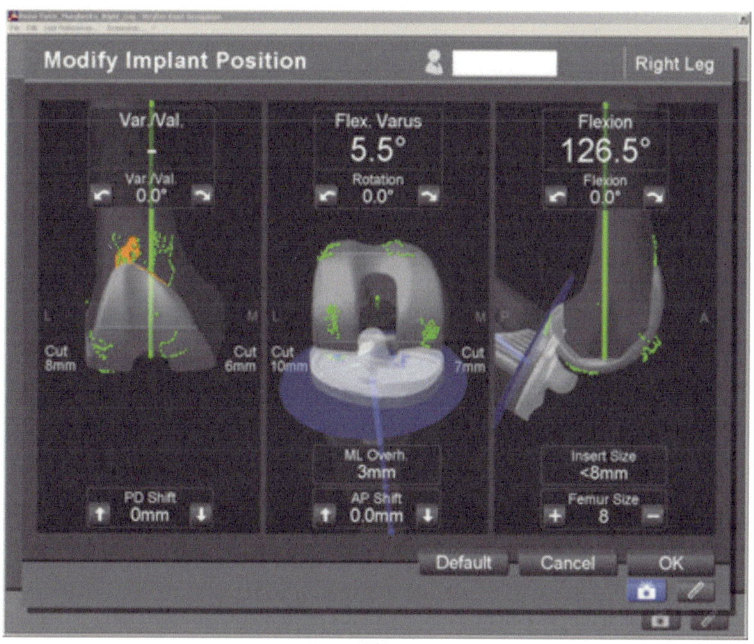

3B

Fig. 3B. "Modify Implant Position": This system allows the surgeon to modify the flexion/ extension, varus/ valgus, internal/ external rotation, anterior/ posterior shift, proximal/ distal shift of the femoral implant and to adjust its implant size relative to femur.

Fig. 3A. and 3B. Implant Position and Modify Implant Position:

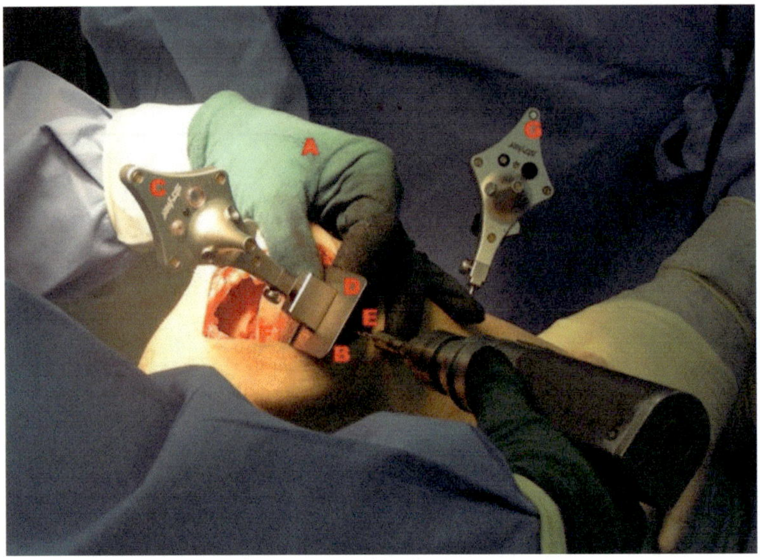

4A

Fig. 4A. With the freehand technique (A) the same cutting guide block (B) is used with the universal tracker (C) and with the resection plane probe (D) in the captured slot (E) and placed on the external border of the medial distal femur condyle (F). Similar to tibial cutting, a freehand technique with the cutting guide block (B-C-D) is used for the distal femoral resection. The block is pinned into place with three pins (E). The femoral tracker (G) is visible in this picture.

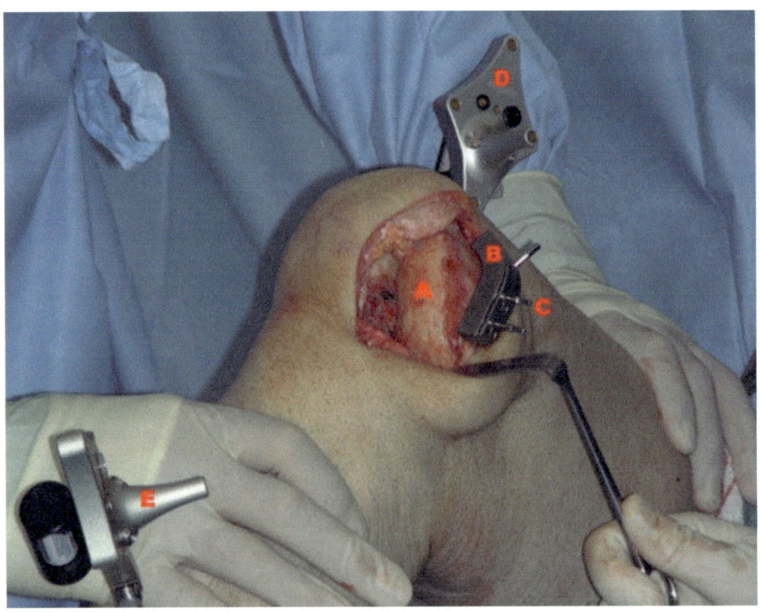

4B

Fig. 4B. The distal femoral resection (A) is done with the cutting guide block (B), which is fixed with three pins (C) and the surgeon can now use a saw blade to cut the desired distal femoral (A) resection. The femoral tracker (D) and tibial trackers (E) are visible in this picture. Now the distal femoral bone resection can be done with the saw through the cutting guide block.

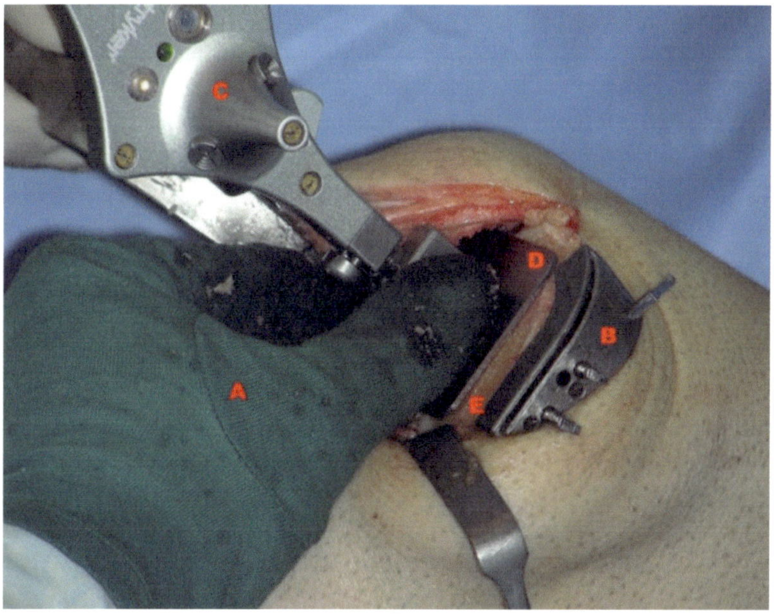

4C

Fig. 4C. Control of the corrected resection of the distal femoral bone with the freehand technique (A): After resection with the cutting guide block (B), the universal tracker (C) in connection with the resection plane probe (D) can verify the accuracy of the cut of the distal femoral bone surface (E), re-correct the resection if it is necessary and finally record the distal femoral cut on the screen. In this picture the resection plane probe (D) is hold on the distal femoral bone cut surface (E) to record the resection result.

Fig. 4A-C. Distal femoral resection

Afterwards, the surgeon has the possibility to continue with the bone resection of the distal femur. In a two-step process, using two femoral cutting blocks, the cutting guide and the femoral alignment guide and the resection plane probe, the cuts are performed. Distal femoral resection requires control of the flexion/extension, varus/ valgus and depth of bone resection, based on our decision of the implant positioning and sizing (Figures 4A-C).

The rotational alignment is subsequently established with the femoral alignment guide and resection plane probe. The femoral component rotation is aimed to be 0° in relation to the special algorithm of surgical transepicondylar axis and the Whiteside line as provided by the computer software. Care is taken to avoid notching the ventral femoral cortex. We finally finish the femur preparation with the femoral resection guide and the femoral trochlea with the corresponding resection guide. Hereby care is taken to release any flexion contracture and to remove all the posterior femoral osteophytes. The femoral component is then inserted and, once correctly seated, the fixation lugholes are drilled.

Subsequently the tibial bone resection is finalized: The appropriately sized tibial baseplate is inserted and its rotation is determined through self-adjustment by flexing and extending the knee with the trial femoral and inlay components implanted. The tibial component rotation is marked, and later the component is implanted with the desired rotation [39, 40].

2.1.2 Trial component insertion

Before the insertion of the trial components, the tibial and femoral bone cuts are again verified with a small resection plane probe, which is directly applied on the resection planes of the affected bone. Every cut is recorded and stored by the system, and can be used for post-operative evaluation and quality control. After completion and digital check of the tibial, femoral and soft tissue preparation, the trial components are inserted and once again the correct position of the trial components is checked with a small resection plane probe for position. Subsequently, the patella preparation is finished and patellar tracking is checked with the implant trials in place.

2.1.3 Trial components soft tissue assessment

After the insertion of the trial components, limb alignment and soft tissue balancing are assessed with the intra-operative kinematics by moving the limb from extension to full flexion under neutral, varus and valgus stress, manually applied through the heel of the foot, carefully keeping the same rotation. Using this information, the surgeon can simulate changes of polyethylene insert and soft tissue release by repeating the assessment. In this way one can obtain a constant dynamic feedback in the process of balancing the knee (Figures 5A and B).

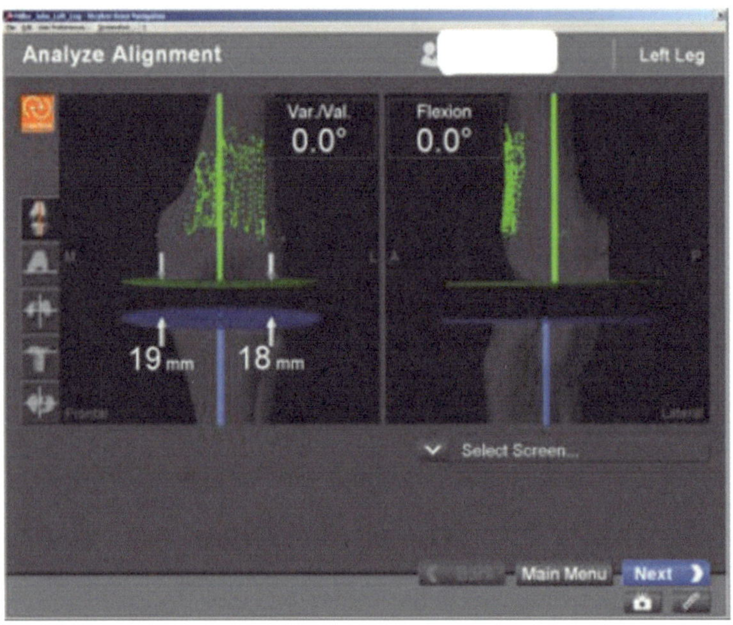

5A

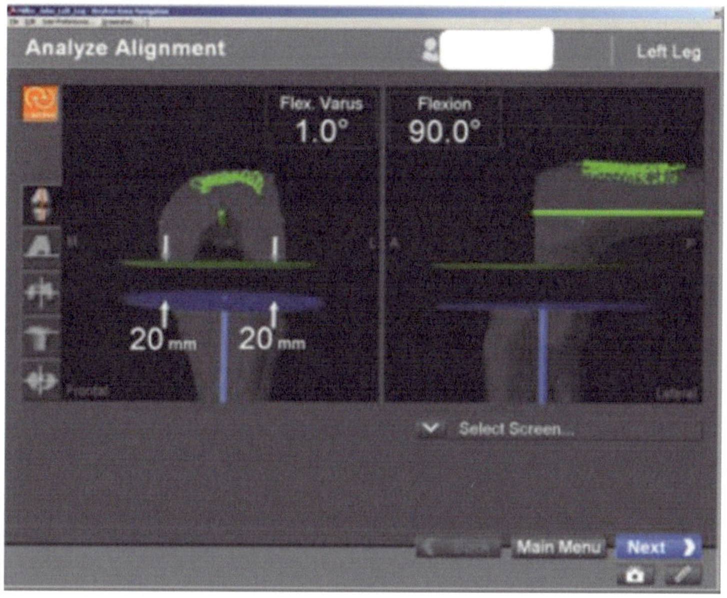

5B

Fig. 5A. and B. The Gap monitoring enables the surgeon to analyze varus/valgus, extension/flexion as well as the gap in extension (A) and flexion (B) upon performance of all cuts with a mechanical tensioner to ensure equal medial and lateral tension in both flexion and extension. This maneuver can also be done through the all ROM under neutral, varus and valgus stress.

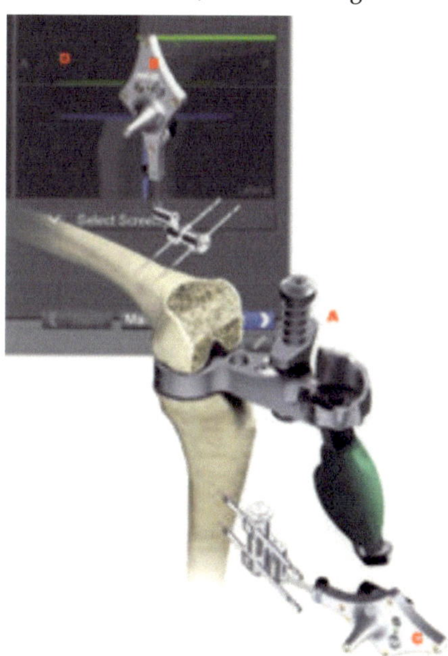

5C

Fig. 5C. Schematic view of the gap monitoring in flexion with a mechanical tensioner (A). The femoral tracker (B), the tibial tracker (C) and the screen (D) are visible in this picture.

Fig. 5A-C. Gap monitoring

2.1.4 Definite component insertion

All our patients received a posterior-stabilized "Scorpio" total knee prosthesis (Stryker® Howmedica Osteonics, Freiburg, Germany). After jet-lavage (approx. 3 L of Ringer Solution) of the resection planes the femoral and tibial components are cemented with the Stryker® Compact Vacuum Cement Mixing System. It is still possible to control the position of the tibial and femoral components with the resection plane probe and, if necessary, improve (Figures 6A and B). Then again the definitive position is documented with the navigation system.

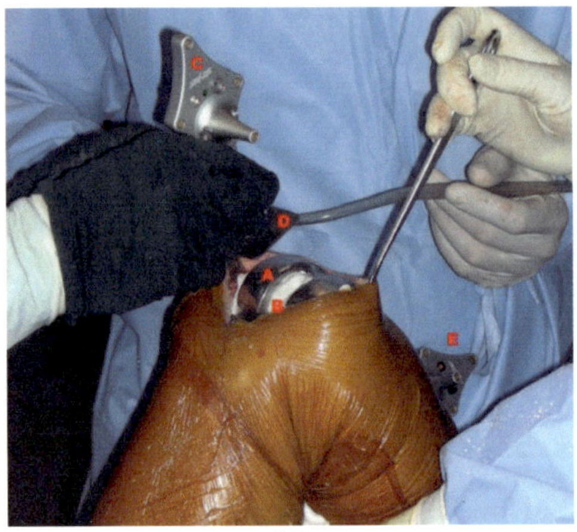

6A

Fig. 6A. After insertion of the femoral component (A) with cement (B), the surgeon has the possibility to check the position of the femoral component with the universal tracker (C) and the resection plane probe (D) and if necessary to improve its position before the cement is fully polymerized. The femoral tracker (E) is visible in this picture.

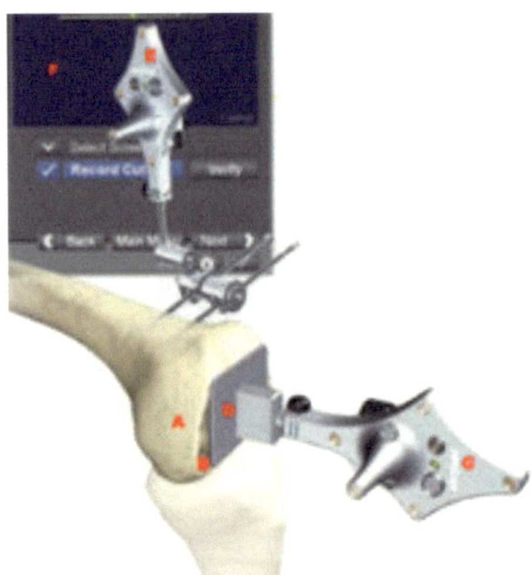

6B

Fig. 6B. Schematic view to check the position of the femoral component with the universal tracker (C) and the resection plane probe (D). In this schematic view, without a Prosthetic component, the distal femoral condyle (A), the distal femoral cut surface (B), the femoral tracker (E) and the screen (F) are visible.

Fig. 6A. and B. Final control of the position the femoral component

Any excessive cement is removed under direct vision. In the same way the femoral component is cemented, a polyethylene inlay trial is then inserted and thereafter the patellar component is embedded with cement. After the cement is fully polymerized, the tourniquet is released and subtle hemostasis performed. Before the final choice of the inlay size is made, it is still possible to assess the joint and soft tissue balance using different size of polyethylene inlay trials and to show the resulting kinematics analysis on screen.

2.1.5 Wound closure

The joint is accurately irrigated and an intraarticular drain is inserted. The arthrotomy is closed with interrupted absorbable sutures (Vicryl 2.0) with the knee at 90° of flexion. After putting a second, subcutaneous drain, the subcutaneous layer is closed with Vicryl 2.0, and the skin is closed with Ethycrin 4.0.

Subsequently the final outcome and the kinematics are documented, recorded and compared to the initial data to assess the success of any correction (Figures 7A and 7B).

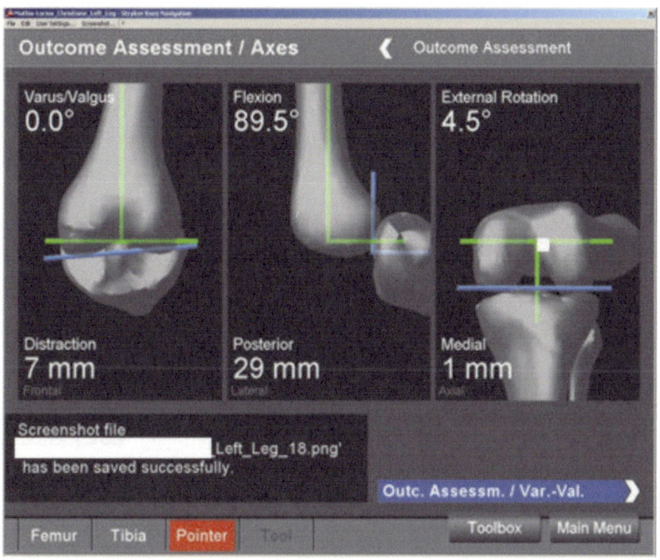

7A

Actual	min					+96°	max
+ Flexion - Hyperextension	-0.5°	+0.0°	+30.0°	+45.0°	+60.0°	+90.0°	+129.0°
+ Valgus - Varus	-1.5°	-1.0°	+0.5°	+0.5°	+1.0°	+0.0°	-0.5°
+ Internal - External	-8.0°	-8.0°	-5.0°	-5.0°	-5.0°	-3.0°	+4.0°
+ Compression - Distraction	-10	-10	-13	-11	-7	+0	+12
+ Medial - Lateral	+6	+6	+5	+5	+6	+7	+8
+ Anterior - Posterior	+10	+10	-8	-15	-22	-30	-38

7B

Fig. 7A. and B. The final outcome of the 3-dimensional axis (A) is documented on the screen as a value with a chart (B).

2.2 Postoperative treatment

For post-operative pain control, our patients first receive a "one-off sciatic nerve block (SB)" and then a continuous femoral nerve block (FB) [41, 42], combined with oral analgesics for both groups. Physical therapy is started as early as 4 to 6 hours post-operatively (continuous passive motion) and consequently intensified under supervision of an experienced physiotherapist (i.e. continuous passive motion 3 times a day, early ambulation, walking exercises, active bending and extending exercises, active knee stretching exercises, walking up and down stairs, leg press, ergometer-bike riding, coordination exercises, getting up from a seated position, strengthen exercises, etc.). Patients are allowed to full weight bearing as tolerated. Patients are discharged from the hospital once they are able to flex the knee joint to 120°, to perform an unassisted straight-leg raise, to walk independently with or without crutches, to rise from a chair to standing and sit from standing without support, and to ascend and descend a full flight of stairs. All patients receive Low Molecular Weight Heparin (LMWH, i.e. Fraxiparine®, Nadroparin) or a direct oral Factor Xa inhibitor (i.e. Xarelto®, Rivaroxaban) for deep venous thrombosis prophylaxis for 6 weeks. Outpatient physical therapy is started immediately after discharge. The Patients are evaluated clinically and radiographically in the office at 6 weeks, 3 months and 6 months.

2.3 Radiographic follow-up

All patients received full-length standing antero-posterior radiographs pre-operatively, at 6 weeks as well as 6 and 12 months post-operatively ("Philips® Multidiagnost 3"). Pre- and post-operative mechanical axes (i.e. the coronal mechanical axis of the limb, the Hip-Knee-Angle) were determined from radiographs. A mechanical axis of more than 3° varus/ valgus was determined as outlier as defined previously [17, 18]. Conventional radiographic assessment involved short-leg-length weight-bearing antero-posterior (AP) radiographs, as well as non-rotated short-leg-length lateral radiographs at 30° of knee flexion and patella axial radiographs. The alignment of the prosthetic components was evaluated on the short-length standard radiographs. Radiographic parameters, including the coronal femoral component angle, the sagittal femoral component angle, the coronal tibial component angle and the sagittal tibial component angle (i.e. tibial slope angle) were evaluated to determine the correct position of the femoral and tibial components [43, 44]. The coronal alignment of the femoral component was measured in relation to the anatomical femoral axis (ideal value = 96°) and of the tibial component in relation to the anatomical tibial axis (ideal value = 90°). To determine the sagittal angle of the femoral and tibial components, a perpendicular line, drawn from the midline of the femoral respectively tibial components, was compared with the midline of the distal segment of the femur and of the proximal segment of the tibia using the Knee Score reference lines [45]. Although little consensus on the ideal reference for defining the slope of the tibia on the lateral radiograph is reached, we used the technique described by Catani et al. and Yoo et al., measuring the slope of the tibial component on conventional short-length sagittal view radiographs with reference to the proximal anatomic axis [16, 46]. Pre- and post-operative sagittal tibial component angles (i.e. tibial slope angle) were compared on conventional short-length lateral radiographs in 30° of knee flexion. All patients also received standardized CT-scans of both knees 6 weeks postoperatively to evaluate rotational alignment of the components according to the technique described by Berger et al. for our follow-up study [47].

3. Results and discussion

3.1 CN TKA versus MIS CN TKA

In a previous study we compared two groups of patients either with a standard medial parapatellar approach (CN-TKA group) or with a minimal invasive mid-vastus approach (MIS CN-TKA group) [For further detailed information please see the references 48]. No inaccuracies of the Knee Navigation System (i.e. dirty reflectors, camera or rounding errors), or of the references pin itself (i.e. loosening of the reference pin intraoperatively and consequent inaccuracies in reference readings) were found. No switch to the conventional implantation method was necessary. Postoperative recovery of the patients was uneventful, there were no infections or wound healing disorders in both groups. No patients were lost to follow-up.

3.1.1 Clinical outcome

The mean postoperative range of motion (ROM) after 3 months was significantly higher in MIS CN-TKA (125° MIS CN-TKA group vs. 118° CN-TKA group) ($p = 0.037$). However, 6 months after operation there was no statistical relevant difference in range of motion between the two groups (125° vs. 122°) to be found. The Knee Society Clinical Rating Score (i.e. the knee and function scores) had improved in both groups to almost identical values 6 months after the operation. The mean length of hospital stay was significantly reduced in the MIS CN-TKA group ($p < 0.0005$) resulting in a total duration of 8 days (range 6 - 9 days) versus 17 days (range: 8 - 31 days) in the CN-TKA group. We found no statistically difference between operation time and blood loss in the computer-assisted MIS TKA compared to the conventional CN-TKA group [For further detailed information please see the reference 48].

3.1.2 Radiological outcome

The radiographic coronal mechanical axis of the limb (i.e. the Hip-Knee-Angle) improved to an orthograde level in both groups (CN TKA 0.5° versus MIS CN-TKA 0.7 °). We found no outliers in both groups regarding alignment .
The tibial slope was significantly reconstructed to match the preoperative value not only in the conventional CN-TKA group (CN-TKA: mean value 1.6°) but also in the minimally invasive CN-TKA group (MIS CN-TKA: mean value 1.4°). The same accuracy was found for the implantation of the tibial component in the coronal alignment with no statistically significant difference between the conventional CN-TKA group (CN-TKA: mean value 91.3°) and the minimally invasive CN-TKA group (MIS CN-TKA: mean value 91.4°).
With regard to the accuracy of the coronal alignment of the femoral component we found a correct implantation of the femoral component in all cases and there was no statistically significant difference between both groups (CN-TKA (96.2°) vs. MIS CN-TK (95.2°)). The post-operative radiological analysis of the sagittal alignment of the femoral component in relation to the anatomical femoral axis revealed slight more flexion of the femoral components in both groups than planned pre-operatively (CN-TKA: mean value 6.9° versus MIS CN-TKA: mean value 7.8°). However, the intra-operative alignment of the sagittal femoral cut showed an accurate value closed to 1° of flexion not only in the conventional CN-TKA group (CN-TKA Group: mean value of 0.58°, standard deviation

0.44°, Range 0.00 - 1.50), but also in minimally invasive CN-TKA group (MIS CN-TKA Group: mean value of 1.03°, standard deviation 0.40°, Range 0.50 - 2.00). Moreover, the anterior flange of the femoral component was parallel to the dorsal femoral cortex in every patient of both groups.

3.1.3 Computed tomography outcome

The Analysis of the postoperative CT scans revealed a statistically significant reconstruction of the desired rotational alignment of the femoral component parallel to the transepicondylar axis not only in the conventional CN-TKA group (CN-TKA: mean value 0.7°) but also in the minimally invasive CN-TKA group (MIS CN-TKA: mean value 1.3°) ($p = 0.018$). No outliers in the rotational alignment of the femoral prosthesis could be documented [For further detailed information please see the reference 48].

3.2 Discussion

It is well known by now that malposition of TKA affects implant fixation and leads to an increased risk of loosening, instability and decreased survival of the prosthesis. Computer-assisted navigation systems have been designed to increase the precision of implantation of TKA allowing the surgeon to reproduce the mechanical axes measured on full-length standing radiographs of the lower limb and reduces the number of outliers in the alignment of the limb compared to traditional mechanical instrumented TKA [9, 15-19, 21, 22, 48-54]. Two recent meta-analysis comparing alignment outcomes for computer-assisted navigated versus conventional TKA indicate a significant improvement in component orientation and mechanical axis, when computer-assisted navigation is used [55, 56]. Our analysis demonstrated that it is possible to achieve straight mechanical axes not only in the conventional but also in the minimally invasive approaches by using a computer-assisted navigation. Additionally intra-operative alignment of the femoral and tibial bone resection was accurate in all three planes not only in the conventional but also in the minimally invasive computer navigated TKA group. Similar intra-operative results have been published and our results showed the same accuracy of the intra-operative bone resections with the navigation system as the above mentioned [9, 16-18, 22].

However, the solely measurement of mechanical axis alone appears too basic as an indicator of correct limb alignment and long-term outcome. Accurate angles of the individual components in the coronal and sagittal planes, correct axial alignment and proper ligament and soft tissue balancing contribute to the success of knee replacement surgery and should be taken in consideration as well. The results of these data were also accurate in both groups using the computer-assisted navigation technique.

Different studies have compared computer-assisted systems with traditional implantation for improvement of component orientation. Most authors showed that the coronal alignment (i.e. the varus/ valgus alignment) of the femoral component was improved with the use of navigation [9, 16-18, 57-59]. Only few studies did not report an improvement in component alignment between patients in who navigation was used [60, 61]. Despite the fact that in these studies the senior authors have more experience with conventional than navigated TKA, the reduction of outliers was greater in the navigation group. However, all these studies investigated TKA implanted using conventional approach.

We were also able to demonstrate that, by using a computer-assisted navigation system, it is possible to implant the femoral and tibial components in the desired coronal and sagittal planes not only with the conventional but also with a minimally invasive approach. The post-operative radiographic analyses of the coronal alignment of the femoral and tibial components showed reliable results in both groups without any outliers in either group [For further detailed information please see the references 48].

Few further studies found the same accurate reconstruction of the sagittal alignment of the femoral component by using the navigation system, however with a standard conventional approach [9, 16, 19, 24, 25, 49, 57, 58, 62].

Literature documents that the influence of computer-assisted navigation on the alignment of the tibial component remains unclear. Several authors confirmed that the coronal alignment of the tibial component (i.e. the varus/ valgus alignment) is improved with the use of navigation [9, 24, 62], whereas other authors did not find evidence for improvement in coronal alignment [19, 49]. We found the same preciseness for the implantation of the tibial component in the coronal plane in the conventional as well as in the minimally invasive approach. Furthermore, we could demonstrate that the sagittal tibial component angle (i.e. the tibial slope angle) can be accurately and reproducibly reconstructed to match the original value of the tibial plateau in both computer-assisted approaches. Although some studies disagree that the alignment in the sagittal plane of the tibial component can be improved with navigation, our result confirmed, as it has been reported by other authors, that the surgeon can use, in practical terms, computer-assisted navigation to accurately restore the tibial slope during TKA using minimally invasive approaches as well [19, 24, 25, 28, 48, 49, 58, 63-68].

Even small abnormalities of rotational alignment of the components have a considerable influence on patellar tracking, varus/ valgus stability and on the overall biomechanics of the joint. The accuracy to adjust the rotational alignment of the femoral component is a prerequisite to avoid malfunctioning TKAs. Debate still exists whether a navigation system does improve the rotational alignment of the femoral component or not [67]. Several reference axes have been proposed to establish proper rotational alignment of the femoral components [63]. Of these axes, the transepicondylar axis approximates the flexion-extension axis of the knee. Furthermore, although there is no consensus about the best landmarks to gauge femoral rotation, alignment according to the surgical epicondylar axis seems to come closest to allowing physiological biomechanics [7, 8, 10, 67]. Debate continues with regard to how accurately and easily the transepicondylar axis can be located intra-operatively. Siston et al. found high variability in rotational alignment of the femoral component in a cadaver study [63]. This variability may be explained by the higher or lower ability of the surgeon to identify intra-operatively the medial epicondyle with its bone ridge and sulcus and the attachment of the deep and superficial fibers of the medial ligament, by the learning curve of the surgeon associated with the use of navigation and finally by the individual surgeon's skills. The algorithm of the Knee Navigation Software to establish the proper femoral rotational alignment by averaging the angle subtended by the Whiteside's line and the transepicondylar axis, gives the surgeon the possibility to improve the accuracy of the femoral rotational alignment without excessively increasing operative time. The analysis of our post-operative rotational alignment of the femoral component by CT-scans revealed a statistically significant reconstruction of the desired rotational alignment of the prosthesis parallel to the transepicondylar axis not only in the conventional but also in the minimally invasive computer-assisted navigated approaches. These results are in agreement with other studies using standard approaches, computer-assisted navigation and an improved computer tomography protocol [16, 17, 24, 68].

Although it has been reported that the rotational mismatch between the femoral and tibial components is decreased with navigation, controversy still exists as to whether navigation systems do improve the rotational alignment of the tibial component in the axial plane [24, 68, 69]. We used the technique describe by Dalury and Eckhoff et al., whereby the orientation of the tibial tray was determined by allowing it to float into position with respect to the femoral component while the knee was placed through a full arc of flexion and extension [39, 40]. We were able to document an accurate alignment of the tibial component in the CT scan postoperatively in both computer-assisted navigated groups as well. However, we do believe that a navigation system that relies only on digitization of landmarks to establish the rotational alignment of the tibial component is not reliable enough. Further research is therefore necessary.

In addition to component malpositioning, tibiofemoral instability is another very important factor that might lead to implant failure and chronic pain. Some studies point out that 30% to 35% of the revision TKA were due to an uncorrected joint stability [20-21]. Tibiofemoral instability often represents a failure to correct the soft tissues balancing throughout the full range of motion and to adjust the flexion and extension gaps at the time of the primary arthroplasty. Furthermore, it is important to take the different behavior of involved ligaments on the medial and lateral aspects into consideration as well. This instability can be in extension, midflexion and/ or in flexion. Stability and function of TKA are strictly related to the interplay among the prosthetic component alignment, the articular surface geometry (flat or congruent polyethylene insert), the type and designs of prosthesis (cruciate-retaining versus cruciate-substituting prosthesis), as well as the balancing of the soft tissue and muscle action. Of all these factors, implant component alignments, joint line restoration and soft tissue balancing "can and must be" assessed and restored by the surgeon during the intervention. Calculation of the joint line height both at the femur and tibia is usually performed by measurements on pre- and post-operative radiographs using standard anatomical indices, which are very inaccurate and not reproducible. The computer assisted navigation system allows the surgeon to measure and restore accurately the alignments of the prosthetic components in all three geometrical planes, femoral joint height and the tibial joint line, as well as the desired soft tissue balancing [54].

An established concept is the preparation of a rectangular joint gap in TKA. With a posterior stabilized TKA, flexion and extension gaps can be different. This has been regarded as an important goal achieving good joint function. However, the lateral tibiofemoral joint is physiologically lax, and as consequence the flexion gap may not be rectangular. Van Damme et al. reported in a cadaveric study on normal non-arthritic knee joint an increased laxity lateral compared to medial in full extension, and an increased lateral laxity from 0° to 90° flexion [70]. Because of technical difficulties, only few data are available on the physiological laxity of the joint. Such analysis can only be performed if the flexed knee is imaged three-dimensionally both in neutral position and under a varus/ valgus stress. Tokuhara et al. analyzed quantitatively the stability of the medial and lateral tibiofemoral joint for normal knees in an open MRI [71]. Their results indicate that the flexion gap in a normal knee is not rectangular and that the lateral joint gap is significantly lax. Recent biomechanical studies have further shown that flexion of the knee is associated with a significant medial-pivot internal rotation of the tibia [72-75]. Thus, in rotation the medial condyle is immobile and the lateral condyle is mobile on the tibial surface.

Since 1977, several studies have investigated the relationship between soft tissue release and the resulting changes in the tibiofemoral gaps in TKA using optical encoders, pressure-sensitive film, fluoroscopy or knee analysis system [76-79]. Computer-assisted surgical technology enables the surgeon to measure and assess knee behavior during operation, allowing real-time monitoring of knee's behavior from extension to flexion and soft tissue balance. In a previous study, we measured the mechanical axis and the varus/ valgus stability of the joint at different time points with the computer-assisted navigation and we documented a similar increased lateral joint laxity before and after implantation of the components at 45° and 90° of knee flexion. We even found that the overall laxity was decreasing beyond 45°/ 60° of flexion to maximal flexion [80]. Therefore, knee navigation allows the surgeon to objectively quantify and monitor kinematics and stability of the TKA through the full ROM pre-, intra- and post-operatively. Leaving the knee too lax after TKA may theoretically lead to tibiofemoral instability and excessive tightness of the joint in different position may cause stiffness. However, differently from TKA alignment, no data are available to define what is a well-balanced knee intra- and/or post-operatively. We suggested as ideal laxity for TKA a varus/ valgus laxity of an approximately total joint-line opening between 1.5° to 2° to be achieved from maximal extension to 45°/ 60° flexion and decreasing to 0.5° to 1.0° by further increasing flexion [80]. These findings serve as a benchmark for future soft tissue laxity measurements and additional work should be performed to validate these proposed values. The computer navigation will help to correlate the collected data and clinical outcomes more objectively than in the past and enable the setting of more accurate limits for soft tissue management.

Despite some motivating factors, including a potential reduction in duration of hospitalization and costs, one should not discount that the patient-driven desires include their concerns about postoperative pain, prolonged rehabilitation, and less than- ideal functional outcomes associated with conventional TKA. Various authors have also reported superior clinical results and decreased cost using minimally invasive techniques for TKA [24, 32, 43, 51. 52]. Obtaining these results with standard approaches and conventional instruments seem to cause much more soft tissue damages leading to an arduous recovery period for the patients. Although the length of the skin incision is shorter in the MIS approach, MIS knee surgery should not be defined by the size of the skin incision, but rather by the method of soft tissue handling once the skin is incised. Therefore, we should better substitute the misnomer "minimally invasive surgery" (MIS) for "soft-tissue sparing" surgery. We believe that minimal trauma of the soft tissue and bone results in better post-operative function and accelerated rehabilitation.

In a previous study, we were able to demonstrate that minimally invasive computer-assisted navigated TKA is able to achieve these objectives. With the minimally invasive approach patients were mobilized more aggressively reaching full weight bearing and profit by earlier discharge. Postoperative ROM after 3 months was significantly higher in MIS CN-TKA, but after 6 months differences were minimal. Clinical scores were identical for both groups six months after surgery. However, these clinical scores have turned out not to be ideal for the evaluation of patient satisfaction immediately after a computer-assisted navigated TKA with a conventional or MIS approach [81-83]. It would have been more appropriate to use patients' self-reported measures of outcome, such as the WOMAC and the SF-36 score systems. In addition, a recent prospective randomized controlled study demonstrated a positive correlation between accurate mechanical alignment after TKA and functional and quality-of-life patients' outcomes [84]. At all post-operative follow-up intervals from 6 weeks to 12 months the total IKSS score were significantly better in patients with a mechanical axis within 3° of neutral compared to those greater than 3°. Moreover, the SF-12 physical scores at all intervals from 3 months were also significantly better for patients with a mechanical axis within 3° of neutral, and at 12 months these patients demonstrated better SF-12 mental-scores as well. Furthermore, another recent study showed, that TKA with good alignment lead to better function with quicker rehabilitation and earlier hospital discharge as well [85]. Therefore, the use of a computer-assisted navigation not only leads to reproducible accuracy of implant positioning in all three planes, but also to better functional outcomes with quicker rehabilitation and earlier hospital discharge due to the advantages of minimally invasive techniques.

3.3 Conclusion

Modern computerized knee navigation systems, appropriately used, aid surgeons to accurately optimize mechanical and axial alignments of the components in all three planes to avoid any malrotation and/ or any errors in coronal, sagittal and axial alignments. These advantages can be achieved not only in the conventional but also in minimally invasive approach without loss of accuracy. There is an increasing statistical evidence of a positive correlation between accurate mechanical alignment after TKA and a better functional as well as quality-of-life patient outcomes. Nevertheless the surgeon has to keep potential pitfalls in association with the computer-assisted procedures in mind. If used correctly, the system is very sophisticated and will improve accuracy. Therefore it will enhance the surgeon`s perspective, but should never replace it.

The use of a computer-assisted navigation leads to reproducible accuracy of implant positioning in all three planes not only in the conventional but also in minimally invasive approaches. In contrast to even the most elaborate mechanical instrumentation system, which relies on visual inspection to confirm the accuracy of the alignment and stability of the TKA, computer-assisted navigation allows the surgeon to objectify every operative osteotomy, the position of trials and finally of the implants. It is well known that there is a definite relationship between the accuracy of implant positioning and longevity and therefore it is imperative to reproduce the implant positioning after a TKA.

Despite the above mentioned advantages and excellent results that may be achieved with computer-assisted navigation, certain factors still cause concern and need to be optimized. As only the cutting guides are navigated, the surgeons may make less than optimal bone resections by bending the saw blade, especially when attempting to cut through sclerotic areas of bone. Differences in cement thickness may also potentially lead to malalignment, even though bone resection was accurate. These latter two problems, which can occur with conventional instrumentation as well, can be obviated only by using the verification

plate of the navigation system to verify the correct level and direction of the performed osteotomy.
Computer-assisted technology assists the surgeon to reliably measure kinematics of TKA alignment and stability of the TKA on a screen. Furthermore, surgeons have the opportunity to improve their surgical performance with a direct intra-operative documentation of alignment and orientation of instruments, trials and implants. Additionally computer-assisted navigation allows to verify the final alignment of the implants after component implantation and before the cement hardens to avoid or probably correct considerable error in alignment.
Incorrect positioning of the components may only be a co-factor together with tibiofemoral instability and soft tissue trauma with MIS approach, leading to suboptimal implant loading with early loosening and increased wear. The use of computer-assisted navigation alone will not empower the surgeon to accurately and reproducibly implant a TKA. This might be especially true for the minimally invasive technique. Much technical expertise in the conventional TKA, the skill of the surgeon and their familiarity with the instruments may also be necessary to obtain good results.

4. Competing interests

The authors declare that they have no competing interest.

5. Authors' contributions

We thank Prof. Fabio Catani, Dr. Andrea Ensini, and their collaborator of the Istituti Ortopedici Rizzoli of Bologna, Italy, for their great personal commitment and help with the statistical analysis.

6. Acknowledgements

We appreciate the contribution of Dr. M. Brouwer, Dr. F. Tichler and Dr. M. Stephan, chairmen of the Anesthesiology Department at the Hospital Oberengadin in Samedan, who have contributed to the anesthesiology part of this article, as well. We also acknowledge the great support of the operating room personnel for their cooperation and the Swiss Stryker Company for their permanent remarkable supervision.
No funding or external support was received by any of the authors in support of or in any relationship to the study.

7. References

[1] Callaghan JJ, O'Rourke MR, Iossi MF, Liu SS, Goetz DD, Vittetoe DA, et al. Cemented rotating-platform total knee replacement. A concise follow-up at a minimum of fifteen years. J Bone Joint Surg Am 2005; 87: 1995-1998.
[2] Gill GS, Joshi AB. Long-term results of kinematic condylar knee replacement: An analysis of 404 knees. J Bone Joint Surg Br 2001; 83: 335-358.
[3] Pavone V, Boettner F, Fickert S, Sculco TP. Total condylar knee arthroplasty: A long term follow-up. Clin Orthop Relat Res 2001; 388: 18-25.

[4] Ritter MA, Berend ME, Meding JB, Keating EM, Faris PM, Crites BM. Long-term follow-up of anatomic graduated components posterior cruciate-retaining total knee replacement. Clin Orthop Relat Res 2001; 388: 51-57.
[5] Rodrigues JA, Bhende H, Ranawat CS. Total condylar knee replacement: A 20-year follow-up study. Clin Orthop Relat Res 2001; 388: 10-17.
[6] Insall JN, Binazzi R, Soudry M, Mestriner L. Total knee arthroplasty. Clin Orthop Relat Res 1985; 192: 13-22.
[7] Insall JN, Scuderi GR, Komistek RD, Math K, Dennis D, Anderson DT. Correlation between condylar lift-off and femoral component alignment. Clin Orthop Relat Res 2002; 403: 143-152.
[8] Barrack RL, Schrader T, Bertot AJ, Wolfe MW, Myers L. Component rotation and anterior knee pain after total knee arthroplasty. Clin Orthop Relat Res 2001; 392: 46-55.
[9] Sparmann M, Wolke B, Czupalla H, Banzer D, Zink A. Positioning of total knee arthroplasty with and without navigation support. J Bone Joint Surg Br 2003; 85: 830-835.
[10] Miller MC, Berger RA, Petrella AJ, Karmas A, Rubash HE. Optimizing femoral component rotation in total knee arthroplasty. Clin Orthop Relat Res 2001; 392: 38-45.
[11] Nagamine R, White SE, McCarthy DS, Whiteside LA. Effect of rotational malposition of the femoral component on knee stability kinematics after total knee arthroplasty. J Arthroplasty 1995; 10: 265-270.
[12] Romero J, Duronio JF, Sohrabi A, Alexander N, MacWilliams BC, Jones L, Hungerford D. Varus and valgus flexion laxity of total knee alignment methods in loaded cadaveric knees. Clin Orthop Relat Res 2002; 394: 243-253.
[13] Figgie HE, Goldberg VM, Heiple KG, Moller HS, Gordon NH. The influence of tibial-patellofemoral location on function of the knee in patients with posterior stabilized condylar knee prosthesis. J Bone Joint Surg Am 1986; 68: 1035-40.
[14] Piazza SJ, Delp SL, Stulberg SD, Stern SH. Posterior tilting of the tibial component decreases femoral rollback in posterior-substituting knee replacement: a computer simulation study. J Orthop Res 1998; 16: 264-70.
[15] Ritter MA, Faris PM, Keating EM, Meding JB. Postoperative alignment of total knee replacement. Its effect on survival. Clin Orthop Relat Res 1994; 299: 153-156.
[16] Catani F, Leardini A, Ensini A, Cucca G, Bragonzoni L, Toksvig-Larsen S, Giannini S. The stability of cemented tibial component of total knee arthroplasty: Posterior cruciate-retaining versus posterior-stabilized design. J Arthroplasty 2004; 19(6): 775-782.
[17] Jeffery RS, Morris RW, Denham RA. Coronal alignment after total knee replacement. J Bone Joint Surg Br 1991; 73: 709–714.
[18] Rand JA, Coventry MB. Ten-year evaluation of geometric total knee arthroplasty. Clin Orthop Relat Res 1988; 232: 168–173.
[19] Matziolis G, Krocher D, Weiss U, Tohtz S, Perka C. A prospective, randomized study of computer-assisted and conventional total knee arthroplasty. J Bone Joint Surg Am 2007; 89:236-243.
[20] Lotke PA, Ecker ML. Influence of positioning of prosthesis in total knee replacement. J Bone Joint Surg Am 1977; 59: 77–79.

[21] Nabeyama R, Matsuda S, Miura H, Mawatari T, Kawano T, Iwamoto Y. The accuracy of image-guided knee replacement based on computed tomography. J Bone Joint Surg Br 2004; 86: 366–371.
[22] Sharkey PF, Hozack WJ, Rothman RH, Shastri S, Jacoby S. Insall Award paper: why are total knee arthroplasties failing today? Clin Orthop Relat Res 2002; 404: 7–13.
[23] Stulberg S, Loan P, Sarin V. Computer-assisted navigation in total knee replacement: Results of an initial experience in thirty-five patients. J Bone Joint Surg Am 2002; 84: 90-98.
[24] Chauhan SK, Scott RG, Breidahl W, Beaver RJ. Computer-assisted knee arthroplasty versus a conventional jig-based technique. A randomized, prospective trial. J Bone Joint Surg Br 2004 Apr; 86(3): 372-7.
[25] Stöckl B, Nogler M, Rosiek R, Fischer M, Kriesmer, Kessler O. Navigation improved accuracy of rotational alignment in total knee arthroplasty. Clin Orthop Relat Res 2004; 426: 180-186.
[26] Bäthis H, Perlick L, Tingart M, Luring C, Zurakowski D, Grifka J. Alignment in total knee arthroplasty: A comparison of computer-assisted surgery with conventional technique. J Bone Joint Surg Br 2004; 86: 682-687.
[27] Martin A, Wohlgenannt O, Prenn M, Oelsch C, Strempel A. Imageless navigation for TKA increased implant accuracy. Clin Orthop Relat Res 2007; 460: 178-184.
[28] Ensini A, Catani F, Leardini A, Romagnoli M, Giannini S. Alignments and clinical results in conventional and navigated total knee arthoplasty. Clin Orthop Relat Res 2007; 457:156-162.
[29] Mielke RK, Clemens U, Jens JH, Kershally S. Navigation in knee endoprosthesis implantation: Preliminary experience and prospective comparative study with conventional implantation technique. Z Orthop Ihre Grenzgeb 2001; 139: 109-116.
[30] Dalury DF and Dennis DA. Mini-incision total knee arthroplasty can increase risk of component malalignment. Clin Orthop Relat Res 2005; 440:77-81.
[31] Insall JN. Choises and compromises in total knee arthroplasty. Clin Orthop Relat Res 1988; 226:43-48.
[32] Bonutti PM, Mont MA, McMahon M, Ragland PS, Kester M. Minimally invasive total knee arthroplasty. J Bone Joint Surg Am 2004; 86: 26-32.
[33] Repicci JA. Mini-invasive knee unicompartmental arthroplasty: bone-sparing technique. Surg Technol Int. 2003; 11: 282-286.
[34] Tria AJ, Coon TM. Minimal incision total knee arthroplasty. Clin Orthop Relat Res 2003; 416: 185-190.
[35] Scuderi GR, Tenholder M, Capeci C. Surgical approaches in mini-incision Total Knee Arthroplsty. Clin Orthop Relat Res 2004; 428:61-67.
[36] Hofmann AA, Plaster RL, Murdock LE. Subvastus (southern) approach for primary total knee arthroplasty. Clin Orthop Relat Res 1991; 269:70-77.
[37] Engh GA, Holt BT, Parks NL. A midvastus muscle-splitting approach for the total knee arthroplasty. J Arthroplasty 1997; 12: 322.
[38] Berger TO, Aglietti P, Mondanelli N, Sensi L. Mini-subvastus versus parapatellar approach in total knee arthroplasty. Clin Orthop Relat Res 2005; 440: 82-87.
[39] Dalury DF. Observations of the proximal tibia in total knee arthroplasty. Clin Orthop Relat Res 2001; 389:150-155.

[40] Eckhoff DG, Metzger RG, Vandewalle MV. Malrotation associated with implant alignment technique in total knee arthroplasty. Clin Orthop Relat Res 1995; 3211: 28-31.
[41] Labat G. Its Technique and clinical applications: Regional Anesthesia. 2nd edition. Philadelphia, W.B. Saunders, 1924: 45-55.
[42] Winnie AP, Ramamurthy S, Durrani Z. The inguinal paravascular technic of lumbar plexus anesthesia: the '3-in-1 block'. Anesthesia and Analgesia 1973; 52: 989–96.
[43] Biasca N, Wirth S, Bungartz M. Mechanical accuracy of navigated minimally invasive total knee arthroplasty (MIS TKA). The Knee 2009;16 (1): 22–29.
[44] Chin PL, Yang KY, Yeo SJ, Lo NN. Randomized control trial comparing radiographic total knee arthroplasty implant placement using computer navigation versus conventional technique. J Arthroplasty 2005; 20:618-626.
[45] Ewald FC. The Knee Society Total Knee Arthroplasty roentgenographic evaluation and scoring system. Clin Orthop Relat Res 1989; 248: 9-12.
[46] Yoo JH, Chang CB, Shin KS, Seong SC, Kim TK. Anatomical references to assess the posterior tibial slope in total knee arthroplasty: A comparison of 5 anatomical axes. J Arthroplasty 2008; 23(4): 586-592.
[47] Berger RA, Rubash HE, Seel MJ, Thompson WH. Determining the rotational alignment of the femoral component in total knee arthroplasty using the epicondylar axis. Clin Orthop Relat Res 1993; 286: 40-47.
[48] Biasca, N., Bungartz, M.: New on Minimally invasive computer-assisted navigated Total Knee Arthroplasty (MIS TKA). Minerva Orthop Traumat 2010; 1:1-10.
[49] Jenny JY, Boeri C. Navigated implantation of total knee endoprosthesis: A comparative study with conventional instruments. Z Orthop Ihre Grenzgeb 2001; 139: 117-119.
[50] Laskin RS. New techniques and concepts in total knee replacement. Clin Orthop Relat Res 2003; 416:151-153.
[51] Bonutti PM, Neal DJ, Kestler MA. Minimal incision total knee arthroplasty using the suspended leg technique. Orthopedics 2003; 26: 899-903.
[52] Laskin RS. Minimally invasive total knee arthroplasty: The results justify its use. Clin Orthop Relat Res 2005; 440: 54-59.
[53] Karpman RR, Smith HL. Comparison of the early results of minimally invasive vs standard approaches to total knee arthroplasty: A prospective, randomized study. J Arthroplasty 2008, 24(5):681-8.
[54] Catani F, Biasca N, Ensini A, Leardini A, Belvedere C, Giannini S. Tibial and femoral joint line restoration after navigated total knee arthroplasty. J Bone Joint Surg Am 2010, in Review.
[55] Bauwens K, Matthes G, Wich M, Gebhard F, HansonB, Ekkernkamp A, et al. Navigated total knee replacement: A meta-analysis. J Bone Joint Surg Am 2007; 89:261-269.
[56] Mason JB, Fehring TK, Estok R, Banel D, Fahrbach K. Meta-analysis of alignment outcomes in computer-assisted total knee arthroplasty surgery. J Arthroplasty 2007; 22(8): 1097-1106.
[57] Jenny JY, Clemens U, Kohler S, Kiefer H, Konermann W, Miehlke RK. Consistency of implantation of a total knee arthroplasty with a non-image-based navigation system. J Arthroplasty 2005; 20(7): 832-839.

[58] Haaker RG, Stockheim M, Kamp M, Proff G, Breitenfelder J, Ottersbach A. Computer-assisted navigation increased precision of component placement in total knee arthroplasty. Clin Orthop Relat Res 2005; 433: 152-159.

[59] Molfetta L, Caldo D. Computer navigation versus conventional implantation for varus knee total arthroplasty: A case-control study at 5 years follow-up. The Knee 2008; 15: 75-79.

[60] Kim YH, Kim JS, Yoon SH. Alignment and orientation of the components in total knee replacement with and without navigation support. J Bone Joint Surg Br 2007; 89(4): 471-476.

[61] Malik MH, Wadia F, Porter ML. Preliminary radiological evaluation of the Vector Vision CT-free knee module for implantation of the LCS knee prosthesis. The Knee 2007; 14(1): 19-21.

[62] Decking R, Markmann Y, Fuchs J, Puhl W, Scharf HP. Leg axis after computer-navigated total knee arthroplasty: A randomized trial comparing computer-navigated and manual implantation. J Arthroplasty 2005; 20(3): 282-288.

[63] Siston RA, Patel JJ, Goodman SB, Delp SL, Giori NJ. The variability of femoral rotational alignment in total knee arthroplasty. J Bone Joint Surg Am 2005; 87: 2276-2280.

[64] Catani F, Biasca N, Ensini A, Leardini A, Bianchi L, Digennari V, et al. Alignment deviation between bone resection and final implant positioning in computer-navigated total knee arthroplasty. J Bone Joint Surg Am 2008: 90: 765-771.

[65] Hart R, Janecek M, Chaker A, Bucek P. Total knee arthroplasty implanted with and without kinematic navigation. Int Orthop 2003; 27: 366-369.

[66] Oberst M, Bertsch C, Wurstlin S, Holz U. CT analysis of leg alignment after conventional versus navigated knee prosthesis implantation. Unfallchirurg 2003; 106:941-948.

[67] Olcott CW, Scott RD. The Ranawat Award. Femoral component rotation during total knee arthroplasty. Clin Orthop Relat Res 1999; 367: 39–42.

[68] Chauhan SK, Clark GW, Lloyd S, Scott RG, Breidahl W, Sikorski JM. Computer-assisted total knee replacement: A controlled cadaver study using a multi-parameter quantitative ct assessment of alignment (the Perth CT Protocol). J Bone Joint Surg Br 2004; 86-B: 818-23.

[69] Siston RA, Giori NJ, Goodman SB, Delp SL. Surgical navigation for total knee arthroplasty: A perspective. J Biomech 2007; 40: 728-735.

[70] Van Damme G, Defoort K, Ducoulombier Y, Van Glabbeek F, Bellemans J, Victor J. What should the surgeon aim for when performing computer-assisted total knee arthroplasty? J Bone Joint Surg Am 2005; 87(Suppl 2): 52–58

[71] Tokuhara Y, Kadoya, Y, Nakagawa, S., et al. The flexion gap in normal knees: An MRI Study. J Bone Joint Surg [Br] 2004; 86B1: 1133-6

[72] Todo S, Kadoya Y, Moilanen T, et al. Anteroposterior and rotational movement of the femur during knee flexion. Clin Orthop 1999;362: 162-70.

[73] Hill PF, Vedi V, Williams A, et al. Tibiofemoral movement 2: the loaded and unloaded living knee studied by MRI. J Bone Joint Surg 2000;82-B: 1196-8.

[74] Iwaki H, Pinskerova V, Freeman MAR. Tibiofemoral movement 1: the shapes and relative movement of the femur and tibia in the unloaded cadaver knee. J Bone Joint Surg 2000;82-B: 1189-95.

[75] Nakagawa S, Kadoya Y, Todo S, et al. Tibiofemoral movement 3: full flexion in the living knee studied by MRI. J Bone Joint Surg [Br] 2000;82-B: 1199-200.
[76] Moore TH, Meyer MH. Apparatus to position knees for varus-valgus stress roentgenograms. J Bone J Surg Am 1977;59: 984.
[77] Takahashi T, Wada Y, Yamamoto H. Soft tissue balancing with pressure distribution during total knee arthroplasty. J Bone J Surg Br 1997;79: 235-239.
[78] Stahelin T, Kessler O, Pfirmann C, Jacob HAC, Romero J. Fluoroscopy assisted stress radiography for varus-valgus stability assessment in flexion after total knee arthroplasty. J Arthroplasty 2003;18: 513-515.
[79] Oliver JH, Coughlin LP. Objective knee evaluation using the Genucum knee analysis system: Clinical implications. Am J Sports Medicine 1987;15: 571-578.
[80] Wirth S, Biasca N. Joint laxity in navigated total knee arthroplasty. Presented at the 2006 CAOS Annual Meeting, Helsinki, 2006.
[81] Ranawat CS, Insall J, Shine J. Duo-Condylar knee arthroplasty: Hospital for Special Surgery design. Clin Orthop Relat Res 1976; 120: 76-82
[82] Insall JN, Dorr LD, Scott RD, Scott WN. Rationale of the Knee Society Clinical Rating System. Clin Orthop Relat Res 1989; 248: 13-14.
[83] Lingard EA, Katz JN, Wright RJ, Wright EA, Sledge CB. Validity and responsiveness of the Knee Society Clinical Rating System in comparison with the SF-36 and WOMAC. J Bone Joint Surg Am 2001; 83(12): 1856-1864.
[84] Choong PF, Dowsey MM, Stoney JD. Does accurate anatomical alignment result in better function and quality of life? A prospective randomized controlled trial comparing conventional and computer-assisted total knee arthroplasty. J Arthroplasty 2008, 24(4):560-9.
[85] Longstaff LM, Sloan K, Stamp N, Scaddan M, Beaver R. Good alignment after Total Knee Arthroplasty leads to faster rehabilitation and better function. J Arthroplasty 2008, 24(4):570-8.

26

Possibilities of Computer Application in Primary Knee Replacement

František Okál, Adel Safi, Martin Komzák and Radek Hart
Department of Orthopaedics & Traumatology
General Hospital Znojmo
Czech Republic

1. Introduction

Frequency of knee joint osteoarthritis has been growing over the last years. Range of degeneration involvement of the knee joint varies from unicompartmental to tricompartmental. The medial part of the knee is damaged most frequently. The solution of serious knee joint degeneration is a total replacement by endoprosthesis. It is indicated not only in the case of idiopathic gonarthrosis, but also in rheumatoid arthritis, osteonecrosis, post-traumatic arthritis or in different arthropathies. The fundamental condition for long term survival of a knee joint endoprosthesis (TKR) is the right position of femoral and tibial components with mechanical axis correction of a lower limb. Endoprosthesis implanted in wrong position can lead to acceleration of polyethylene wear and component release. Abnormal varus or valgus position have already been proved as a main cause of component failure. A malposition of femoral and tibial components has also a great influence on patella tracking during knee movement and on possible patellofemoral complications. That is why single bone resectiones must be performed with a great emphasis on the precision and in relation to the mechanical axis of the limb. Surgeons use a scale of different targeting equipments which serve preferably to the best possible matching of the bone cuts to the patient's geometry. The results show that even in cases of surgeon's great experience in TKR up to 30 % of operated cases have a four-degree and larger deviation of tibiofemoral angle from the ideal mechanical axis after bones resections. That is why computer navigation systems have been developed to eliminate the error of surgeon (Insall et al., 1985). The computer navigation systems were integrated into a routine orthopaedic practice more than thirteen years ago. After that the navigation became quickly a common tool at many working places for primary implantations of knee endoprosthesis. Instrumentation for mechanical targeting of resections described earlier have certain restrictions which cannot be exceeded. For example, it is a certain degree of freedom such as a rotation of a femoral and tibial components or impossibility to reach their perfectly accurate position with regard to the resected bones. It may be said that standard targeting deviced are constructed for the standard bone geometry.

The first study of navigation in orthopaedics reporting the use of infrared radiation was made by the group of Saragaglia (Grenoble, France) in years 1994 -1996 and in 1997 these surgeons implanted the first total endoprosthesis of a knee joint (Laskin, 1984; Bitter et al., 1994) under the assistance of the OrthoPilot navigation system (B.Braun-Aesculap,

Tuttlingen, Germany). In 1995 independently of the above mentioned group Krackow and Mihalko conducted a project of the development of a system for computer controlled TKR with the use of the Optitrack equipment (Northern Digital, Ontario, Canada). The first navigated implantation of TKR was made by this group in 1997 as well (Krackow, 1983). This project led to the creation of the Knee Track Module (Stryker Howmedica Osteonics, Allendale, NJ). Both systems - OrthoPilot and Knee Track Module represents first kinematic navigation systems.

We distinguish 4 basic types of navigation nowadays:

1. Kinematic navigation (imageless, CT-free) - is used for data registration through combination of physical palpation and kinematics. Data are transferred into a computer by means of infrared radiation. This type is the most often used way of navigation in orthopaedic surgery.
2. Fluoroscopy based navigation - it registers combined data obtained by physical palpation and kinematics but it uses C-arm at the beginning. Images are created by a computer on the basis of this information. Then surgeon operates on the radiologic replica of patient's anatomic area. The system is more frequently used in traumatology and in spine surgery.
3. CT-based navigation - it uses computer tomography for data collection. Today, it is used the mostly in a revision surgery and spine surgery.
4. MR-based navigation - it uses magnetic resonance for data collection. It is used mainly in neurosurgery.

The most simple and the most practical of these methods is the kinematic navigation. Anatomical structures are digitized by orientation palpation points with a portable "pointer". During bone resection computer shows surgeon the ideal position of instruments and optimal bone cuts. Computer equipped systems, which consist of standard resection patterns on the one hand and highly accurate navigation system on the other hand, are a natural consequence of current computer technology integration into surgery. Computer software reduces the risk of surgeon's error and enables fast and accurate placement of resection blocks (Hart & Janeček, 2003). It eliminates the use of intramedullary and extramedullary targeting devices and so reduces the risk of pulmonary embolism.

The aim of this chapter is to present the experience of authors with using of kinematic navigation systems and computer generally in the implantation of total and unicompartmental knee joint replacements. It points out to advantages and disadvantages of a navigation application during surgeries and to the importance of pre-operative planning by the help of digital images in connection with a surgical planning station. It also refers to special circumstances when the computer navigation technology can be the only one possibility of the implantation of the knee endoprosthesis.

2. Computer navigation in standard or minimally invasive total knee replacement

Authors of the article have been working with kinematic navigation systems routinely since the beginning of the year 2000. The study, which was published in the 2003 by the senior surgeon (Hart et al., 2003), was the third randomized study evaluating the use of navigation in a standard TKR surgery in world literature. Higher accuracy in case of the use of navigation in comparison with a standard instrumentarium in TKR has already been confirmed. Navigation system usually consists of five basic parts: 3D-camera with a control unit, infrared diodes, computer system, foot switch and mobile case with transformer (Fig. 1). A camera placed on a tracing bar localizes the position of diodes in an operative field. The camera is connected with the control unit and it enables to distinguish diode deviation already from the distance of tenths of one millimeter. Three diodes are needed at least during surgery. These are placed on nondeformable basis and they can be anchored by fastening mechanism on relevant bicortical screws, palpator or resection blocks. The computer system is formed by a computer itself and a keyboard with mouse. The computer gets information about diodes movement, it evaluates information and transfers it into a graphic form on a monitor. The foot switch has two pedals and it enables surgeon to control individual steps of the navigation system.

Before an operation we take standing weight bearing X-rays of the whole lower limb of a frontal plane and a standard X-rays of a sagittal plane. We evaluate relevant axis and angles, measure size of deformity and plan the size of endoprosthesis components in both planes in a way mentioned in the following subchapter by the help of PACS system with its application module. The patient's preparation before surgery does not differ from a standard procedure. The navigation system (camera) is being placed into the opposite side with regard to the surgeon into the distance of approximately 2 m.

Minimally invasive (MIS) or less invasive approach is an alternative to a common approach to the knee joint in TKR. Its use in connection with the navigation was published by the team of authors in 2006 (Hart et al., 2006). The procedure itself with the use of navigation does not differ from a standard parapatellar approach (Hart et al., 2005). In this case the navigation system serves as "the third eye" of the surgeon working in reducting operative field. The skin incision length is usually up to 12 cm. Subvastus approach does not disturb the extensor apparatus. M.vastus medialis is lifted and arthrotomy is made. It is followed by percutaneous insertion of original bicortical self drilling screw into the distal femur approximately 7 cm above the articular surface. We insert the second screw similarly into the proximal tibia about 10-12 cm below the articular surface. Then diodes are fastened on both screws. We fasten the third diode as a mobile one on a palpator (pointer).

Further step is to determine the real anatomy of a lower limb. A mechanical axis is determined by three points - by the center of hip, knee and ankle joints. First, we enter the information about the center of knee joint into the computer by a palpator with the fixed diode. Next, we determine the center of a hip joint. Movement of the femur in all planes has one fixed point which is the center of the femoral head. We determine the center of a hip joint by circular movements in a slight flexion. As the third, we localize the center of the ankle joint. We fasten an elastic tape on the area of tarsus during the surgery and the mobile diode on it. Then we enter data into the soft-ware by the movement in the ankle joint to the maximum extent of flexion and extension. Last we precisely determine the center of a knee joint. One of the possibilities how to determine the center of the knee is palpation of one anatomic point on each side of a joint. The second possibility is to use the same kinematic procedure as in the ankle joint: first is done of the determination rotation axis by tibial rotation round its longitudinal axis in flexion of 90° and second is to get the second transverse axis by movements of flexion - extension.

Then follows is the collection and saving of information relating to orientation points in the knee area which is necessary to do for an accurate placement of resection blocks and for the accurate size of the femoral component. A palpator with a fixed mobile diode is used for it.

The size of a femoral component is given by the distance of a dorsal condylar line and anterior femoral corticalis. We palpate medial and lateral epicondyles as well to determine the exact rotation of the femoral component. Next, we check orientation points in the area of the ankle joint. A malleolar line serves to an additional confirmation of the ankle joint center.

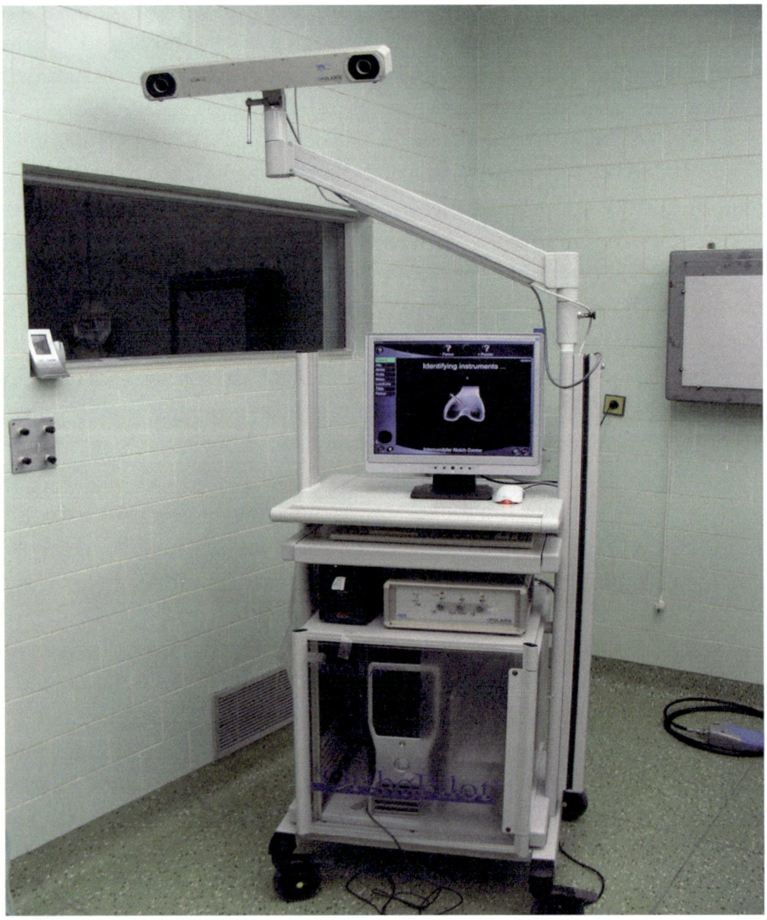

Fig. 1. Kinematic navigation system

After setting of all orientation points, an axis reconstruction of a lower limb appears on the monitor, both in a sagittal and frontal plane. Numeric data appear on the monitor as well besides the graphic illustration. In the frontal plane we get the information about the deformity in the sense of varus - valgus. The program will illustrate the degree of flexion contracture too. In this moment, it is necessary to compare computer specified values with preoperative measured values on X-ray photographs. If we find out (exceptionally) a difference greater than 5° in both planes, it is necessary to recheck fixation quality of both diodes and to repeat the whole procedure. First of all the proximal tibia is resected. A mobile diode is fasten to a resection block and we follow on the monitor the accuracy of its placement on proximal tibia. Both, the block orientation in a sagittal plane and frontal plane and the height of resection, are illustrated. We fix the block to the bone first by one pin to secure the zero deviation from the ideal position in a sagittal plane and the requested level of resection. Then, the resection block position in a frontal plane is corrected and after reaching the zero deviation in the frontal plane, the resection block is fixated by the second pin.

After the proximal tibia resection the balancement of collateral ligaments is being found out. After balancing of the collateral ligaments, it is being approached to balancing of extension and flexion gaps. After that the femoral resection follows. First, we reach zero position (90° to the femoral mechanical axis) in a sagittal and then in a frontal plane. The block is fixed to the femur by two pins and articular surface is resected.

After the application of a relevant trying components including an polyethylene insert of suitable height, the collateral ligaments balance is checked again. Graphic and numeric expression of the real limb mechanical axis is being watched on a monitor and values shown are compared with actual clinical findings. If the result is satisfactory, original components are implanted. The mechanical axis of the limb is being checked again during hardening of the bone cement.

A prospective study has been accomplished in author's institution (Hart et al., 2006) in which results of knee joint replacements in 40 patients implanted by MIS approach were compared with 40 endoprosthesis implanted through a standard approach. Arthritis of 3rd and 4th degree was indication for all these surgeries. Less pain and faster rehabilitation was found early after surgery in MIS group. This difference was only found until 10th day after surgery. This difference was not obvious after 6 and 12 weeks after the surgery. TKR implantation accuracy was preserved with the use of the computer navigation system in cases with MIS approach in comparison with the standard approach.

3. Comparison of preoperative digital planning with computer navigation in TKR

The knowledge of mechanical and anatomical axis construction of lower limb and basic angles is necessary for a correct planning and also for a post-operative evaluation of obtained component position. The connecting line between the centre of the femoral head and the centre of the knee joint is called the mechanical axis of the femur, the connecting line between the centre of the knee and the ankle joint is called the mechanical axis of the tibia. The line between the femoral head centre and the ankle joint centre (the Mikulicz's line) constitutes the mechanical axis of the lower limb. If it runs through the centre of the knee joint, femoral and tibial mechanical axes are parallel. In case of a varus knee deformity the mechanical axis of lower limb runs medially from its centre and the medial angle between femoral and tibial mechanical axes is smaller than 180°. In case of a valgus deformity the mechanical axis of a lower limb runs laterally from the knee joint centre and the medial angle between femoral and tibial mechanical axes is greater than 180°.

The right position of a lower limb during of X-ray examination is important for an accurate preoperative planning. The AP X-ray is performed under the load in standing patient in such a position so that the patella aims forward. The rotation of the lower limb within 10° does not influence the result of axis measurement significantly (Whietside & Arima, 1995). Greater external rotation of the limb simulates a varus deformity, the internal rotation simulates a valgus deviation. Severe gonarthrosis is usually connected with a flexional contracture which causes a possible mistake of measurement during the preoperative planning. The lateral X-ray of the knee is also taken in the standing patient with his knee in extension. Weight-bearing radiographs of the whole lower limb are necessary for an accurate determination of axial relations.

PACS (Picture Archiving and Communication System) system serves to the X-ray photographs storing. It is a storing and communication system of image data which supports both photos distribution and their description and arrangement. It serves to acceptance, storing, distribution and picture display. It is becoming an essential part of orthopaedic surgeon's everyday practice in connection with an orthopaedic planning station. Orthopaedic planning tools enable more accurate preoperative templating of TKRs than former standard templating (Fig. 2.).

It is possible to measure angles on the femoral and the tibial and the relation of femoral and tibial axis by means of a planning station on digitalized X-rays. It is possible to plan height of needed proximal tibial and distal femoral resection and to template femoral and tibial component sizes and polyethylene inlay height and their positions. Accuracy of TKR can be checked postoperatively in the same way. There was compared a lower limb axis deviation measured by PACS before and after a surgery with values gained by kinematic computer navigation preoperatively in the authors´ institution (Hart et al., 2010). There was also compared the size of components measured during the pre-operative planning by PACS, with sizes measured by the navigation during the surgery. There were 311 total knee endoprosthesis evaluated from January 2009 till September 2010 (21 months). All surgeries were done by experienced surgeons. Primary gonarthrosis was an indication for knee replacement in 278 cases. After proximal tibial osteotomy or fractures of the knee 33 TKR were done. Surgical technique was the same in all patients. In 253 cases was used the replacement with preservation of posterior cruciate ligament, in 58 cases with its resection. In all cases both components were fixated by bone cement.

Before and after surgery X-ray weight-bearing images of the whole lower limb were taken. By the help of PACS with the application of the orthopaedic planning station there was measured a lower limb axis before surgery (the angle between the mechanical femoral axis and the mechanical tibial axis) and components sizes and these values were compared with values measured by computer navigation during the surgery. The value of the deformity of lower limb axis measured by computer navigation before and after implantation was recorded during the surgery. The load during the surgery was imitated by axial pressure on a heel in the axis of operated lower limb. Postoperative radiological control was carried out on the seventh postoperative day with the full weight bearing. Agreement between components sizes planned by the orthopaedic planning station in PACS and really implanted components with the use of computer navigation was 73 % (in 227 endoprostheses) in the femoral component, 91 % (in 283 endoprostheses) in a tibial component and 48 % (in 149 endoprostheses) in polyethylene inserts.

In the majority of cases of disagreements smaller femoral (92 %) or tibial (90 %) component was implanted than which had been planned preoperativelly, in case of polyethylene inlay it was mostly necessary to use higher sizes (86 %). The cause of disagreement on the femoral component size in 84 total endoprostheses (27 %) was greater difference between a flexion and extension gap than 3 mm according to navigation. This is not possible to be found out

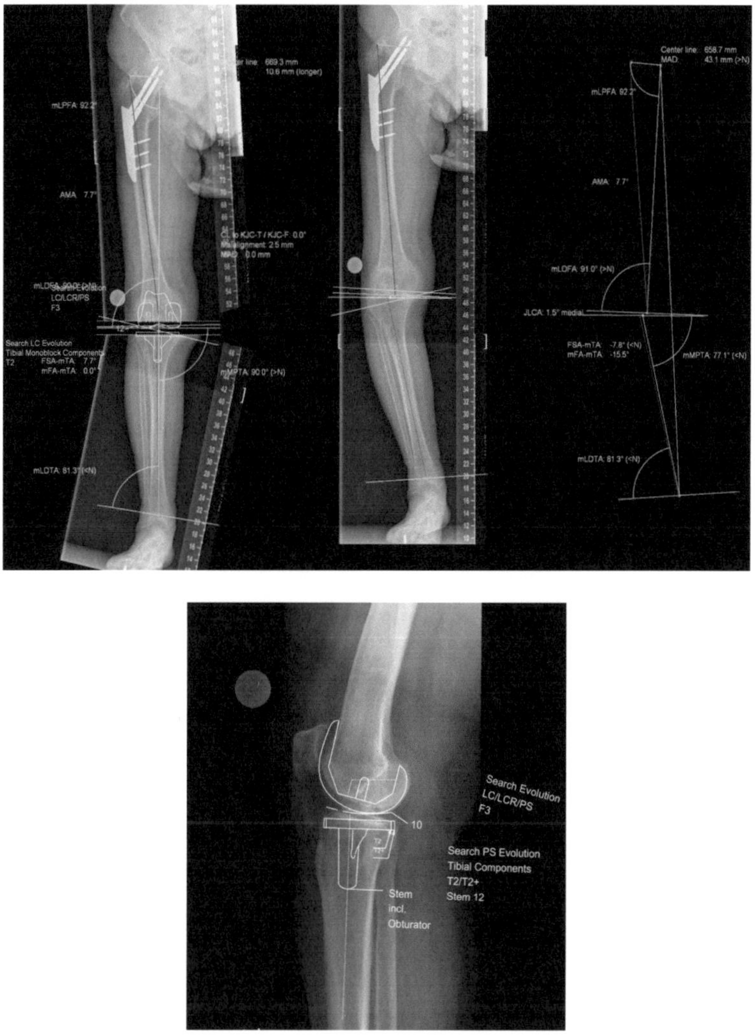

Fig. 2. The X-rays with preoperative templating by the orthopaedic planning station in PACS.

by the preoperative planning on X-ray photographs. Also a tibial component implantation of another size planned by PACS (9 %) had its cause in the size change of an implanted femoral component (the difference between both components would be larger than two sizes). In cases of 77 total replacements (92 %) there was the necessity to implant smaller femoral component by one size to balance tighter flexion gap. It was less frequent that the flexion gap was larger than extension one. This imbalance was solved by larger femoral component (8 %). Preoperative planning of the tibial component size by the help of PACS is relatively accurate because its size is determined only by AP and mediolateral dimensions of the tibial plate are and it is not influenced by flexional or extension gaps. The greatest disagreement was registered in polyethylene inlay planning - in 162 total endoprostheses (52 %). In 116 cases (72 %) there was implanted higher polyethylene insert by 2 mm than what had been planned preoperatively by PACS system. In 23 replacements (14 %) there was implanted higher polyethylene insert by 4 mm and in 23 cases (14 %) lower insert by 2 mm. The cause of this disagreement is usually knee joint balancing done by releasing of soft tissues on medial side in cases of varus deformity or on lateral side in cases of a valgus deformity.

These results show that the preoperative planning by digital templating estimates femoral component and polyethylene insert sizes only approximately, while tibial component sizes quite precisely. The computer navigation has its main significance in determination of the femoral component size depending on collected data accuracy and on flexional and extension gap balancing. The height of polyethylene inlay is determined by resection sizes of a proximal tibia and distal femur, by balancing of gaps and by knee joint stability during testing of trial inserts after cementing of original components.

The average mechanical axis measured preoperatively by PACS was 5.3° of varus (range 20.5° valgus to 16.9° varus). The mechanical axis measured by the navigation before endoprosthesis implantation was on the average 1.8° of varus (the range 13° valgus to 11° varus). Agreement in both measurements (with the difference less than 3°) was achieved only in 171 total replacements (55 %). The Table 1 shows an absolute value distribution of a lower limb mechanical axis deviation measured by PACS before surgery and by navigation at the beginning of the surgery.

In 190 patients (61 %), where the mechanical axis deviation measured by PACS was smaller than 10°, was an agreement with values measured by the navigation in 87 % of cases (165 endoprostheses). In 121 patients with the deviation of the mechanical axis preoperatively more than 10° (39 %) the agreement with values measured by the navigation was only in 5 % of cases (6 replacements). The reason for this difference is the relation between the force acting on the knee joint and the amount of lower limb deformity. In X-ray examination of the whole lower limb under the load the axial deformity of knee joint gets worse due to body weight. This deformity in ligaments is emphasized with a bigger axial deviation. The measurement of the mechanical axis deviation preoperatively by the navigation takes place only in a lying position with exclusion of the weight of the body. That is why the value is always smaller than the value measured during the preoperative planning. The bigger is the axis deviation measured by PACS, the bigger is the difference between values. Pressure on the heel in the axis of a lower limb during the navigation simulates the limb load insufficiently.

deviation (mFA - mTA)	number and % of the patients (MediCAD®2.06)	number and % of the patients (OrthoPilot)
0° - 5.0°	34 (11 %)	47 (15 %)
5.1° - 10.0°	156 (50 %)	255 (82 %)
> 10.0°	121 (39 %)	9 (3 %)

Table 1. The deviation of the axis of lower limb measured by orthopaedic planning system in PACS and by kinematic navigation system preoperatively.

The average mechanical axis measured by the navigation after the total endoprosthesis implantation was 0.4° varus (range, 3.0° valgus to 2.0° varus). The mechanical axis measured by PACS after the surgery was on average 0.5° varus (range, 3.5° valgus to 4.2° varus).

Agreement in both measurements (with the difference less than 3°) was achieved in 90 % of cases (280 endoprostheses). These results show the importance of navigation in total endoprosthesis implantations - the axis deviation within the range of 0° – 2.0° was measured post-operatively in 280 patients (90 %) by to the navigation and in 274 patients (88 %) by PACS. The axial deviation over 4° was not recorded by the navigation and only in 3 patients (1 %) by PACS. The Table 2 shows an absolute value distribution of the lower limb axis after endoprosthesis implantation measured by the navigation and PACS.

deviation (mFA - mTA)	number and % of the patients (MediCAD®2.06)	number and % of the patients (OrthoPilot)
0° - 2.0°	274 (88 %)	280 (90 %)
2.1° - 4.0°	34 (11 %)	31 (10 %)
> 4.0°	3 (1 %)	0

Table 2. The deviation of the axis of lower limb measured by orthopaedic planning system in PACS and by kinematic navigation system postoperatively

4. Computer navigation of valgus knee kinematics before TKR

Computer navigation technique can be used for a surgical approach choice in TKR implantation. Valgus deformity was analysed in the author's institutions in 50 patients. At the beginning of a surgery there were fixated navigation markers to the tibia and femur in these valgus limbs and data were collected for the navigation just before surgical approach was chosen. After data registration (software for correcting osteotomy) changes in values of a lower limb axis deformity in various of knee joint flexion (0°, 30°, 60°, 90°, 120°) were observed. In case of persistance of axis valgus deformity throughout the whole range of a knee movement it is called “right" valgus, in case of gradual transition of valgus deformity into varus during flexion it is called “false” valgus. In a „right“ valgus knee there is a mismatch between both condyles in both the vertical and anteroposterior dimensions, the lateral condyle is generally smaller. (Šváb et al., 2010). In a „false“ valgus knee there is no mismatch between anteroposterior dimensions of both condyles, the knee axis changes from valgus into varus with increased degree of flexion and lateral soft tissue structures are that´s why not so contracted as in „true“ valgus knee deformity, where the knee stays in valgus deviation during the whole range of motion.

In case of the “right” valgus deformity the lateral parapatellar approach according to Keblish is preferred because of an easier release of tight lateral structures. In case of the false deformities a standard medial parapatellar approach can be used. Valgus deformity of a lower limb was measured preoperatively by the navigation within the range from 4° to 13° (on average 7.8°). The right valgus deformity was observed during the knee joint passive flexion in 34 patients (68 %). The average value of the valgus knee joint deformity in extension in the group with the right valgus was 7.9° (range, 4° to 13°). Deviation value in this group decreased gradually during flexion in all cases. The difference in the degree of axis deviation between 0° and 120° of flexion in this group was on average 5.5° (range, 1° to 10°). Changes of the axial deviation depending on the degree of the knee joint flexion are illustrated in figure 3.

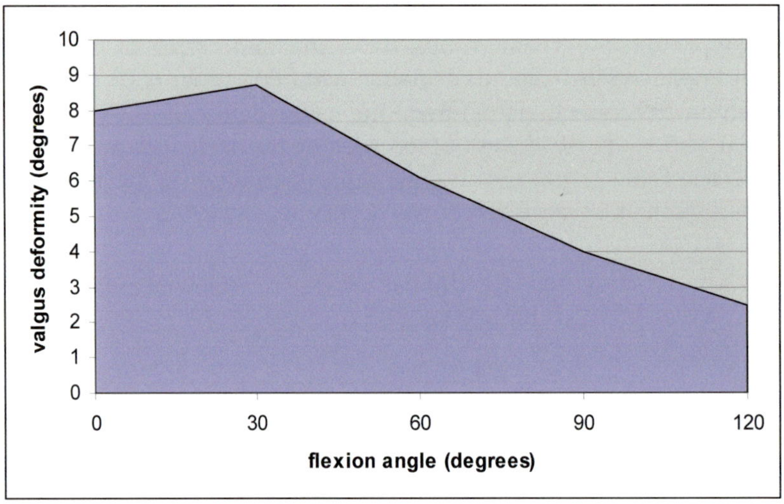

Fig. 3. The progress of the „true" valgosity during the flexion of the knee joint

The false valgus deformity of a knee joint was registered in 16 patients (32 %). In this group the average value of the valgus deformity was 7.5° (range, 6° to 9°). The varus deviation of the mechanical axis was already observed in 60° or 90° of flexion. The difference in the degree of the axis deviation of the limb between 0° and 120° of flexion in this group was on average 12.0° (range, 10° to 14°). Changes of the axial deviation depending on the degree of knee joint flexion with pseudovalgus are illustrated in figure 4.

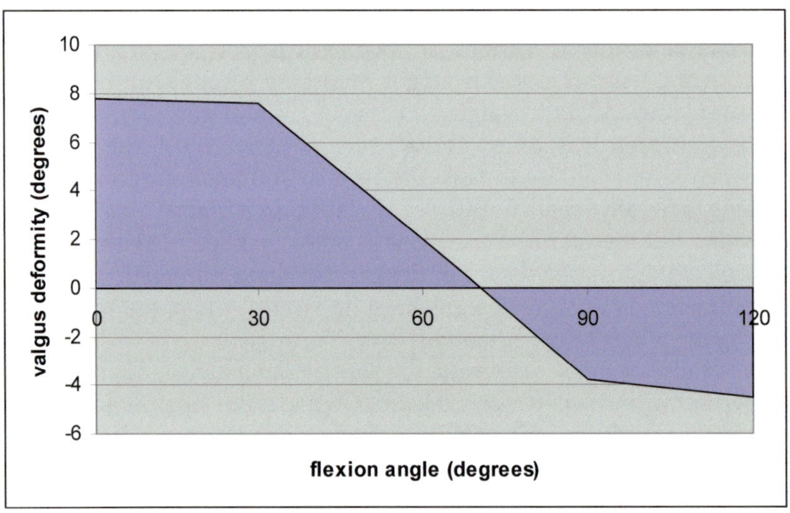

Fig. 4. The progress of the „false" valgosity during the flexion of the knee joint.

Because of the analysis of the knee joint valgus deformity by the computer navigation at the beginning of the surgery the operative time extended on average by 6 minutes (range, 4 to 11 minutes). The navigation was used consequently after the switch on the TKR a module for total endoprosthesis implantation.

5. Kinematic navigation in TKR with distal femoral disturbances

Kinematic navigation system is usually used to precise the knee endoprosthesis implantation. In cases of distal femoral deformity or in the presence of metal material in the distal femur is the navigation the best way how to solve this problem (Fig. 5).

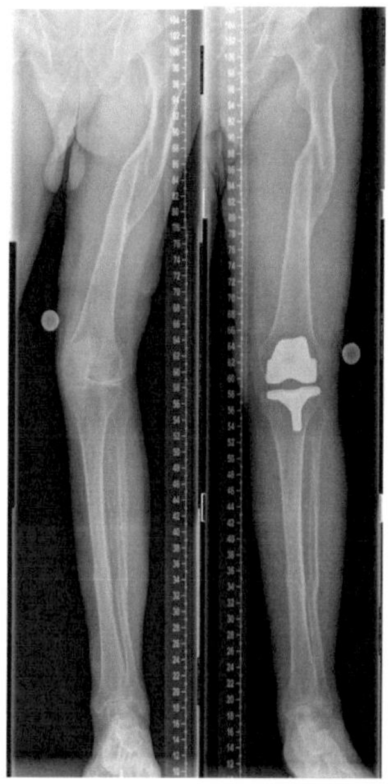

Fig. 5. The X-rays show the deformity of the femur, before and after implantation of TKR

The deformity can be caused by an injury or chronic osteopathy. Some metal material can be present after fracture osteosynthesis or after a revision implantation of hip joint total endoprosthesis. In these cases it is not possible to use standard intramedullary targeting devices and the kinematic navigation system is the best possibility how to implant the femoral component of the knee joint replacement correctly. 13 patients with the femoral deformity or presence of some metal material in the area of the distal femur have been operated in the authors´ institution. It was the condition after the distal femoral metaphyseal fracture with left plate in 4 patients. In 5 patients it was the condition after femoral diaphyseal fracture treated by an intramedullary nail (in one case the nail was broken). In 1 patient the femoral fracture was healed with an extended fragment malposition ad latus. In 3 patients the long stem femoral component of a hip replacement was present. In all these patients a standard implantation of a knee joint replacement was done with use of the computer navigation technique. The record lower limb axis has been restored in all these patients.

6. Kinematic navigation system for prevention of the hypocorrection or hypercorrection of the mechanical axis in UKA

The importance of kinematic navigation during the implantation of unicompartmental replacements is high. It can be used for knee surfaces resection but first of all for a simple control of the axial limb deviation during the implantation of the UKA. At the beginning of the surgery it is necessary to fix navigation markers percutaneuosly at the femur and tibia, to collect data (software for correction osteotomy) and to display the measured lower limb axis (Fig. 6).

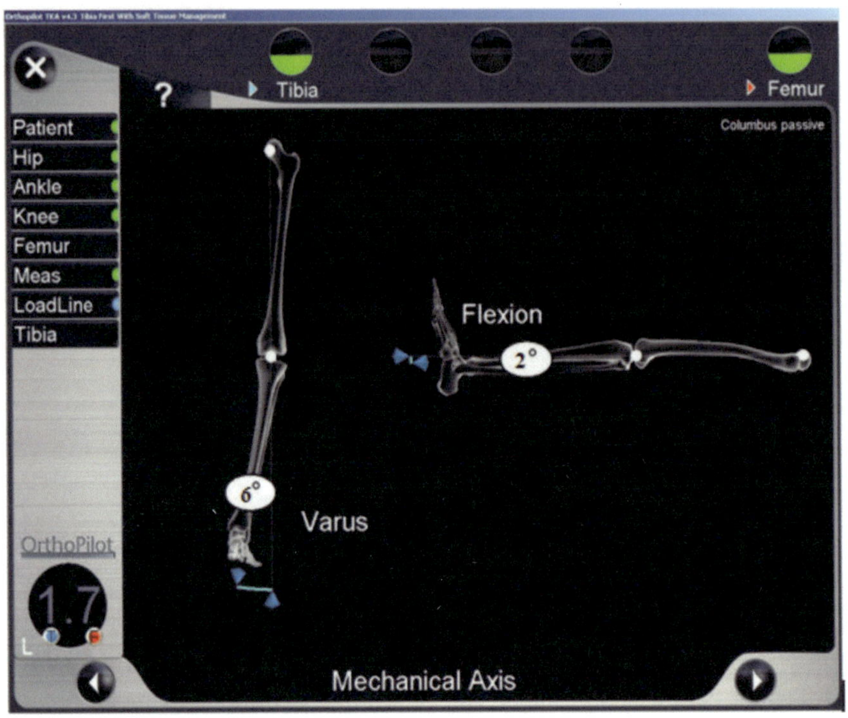

Fig. 6. The axis of the lower limb shown on the display of kinematic navigation system before UCA implantation

Then we implant the knee joint unicopartmental replacement throught a standard medial parapatellar approach and standard surgical technique. After the fixation of tibial and femoral components by bone cement the navigation is used for the right choice of polyethylene insert height with regard to its stability and especially the limb axis. The right size of the polyethylene insert is chosen so that the lower limb mechanical axis would be straight. There were implanted 67 unicompartmental replacements in the authors´ institution from April 2008 till September 2010 (30 months) (Fig. 7).

In 32 patients the replacement was made in a standard way without navigation, in 35 patients with the kinematic navigation. There were 20 men of average age 69.5 years (range, 54 to 82 years) and 47 women of average age 69.2 years (range, 49 to 85 years). In 29 cases a right knee was operated and in 38 cases a left knee. The medial compartmental replacement was done in all patients. All surgeries were made by experienced surgeons. In the group of patients operated without the use of navigation the average lower limb axial deviation was measured before the surgery was 5.1° varus (range, 1.0° to 12.6°). The average axial deviation measured radiologically in the long weight bearing X-rays after surgery was 2.1° of valgus (range, 8.5° valgus to 5.2° varus). The overcorrection of the lower limb mechanical axis into valgus without the use of navigation happened in 20 patients (63 %). The hypercorrection of axis into valgus > 2.0° happened in 12 patients (38 %). Varus deformity > 2.0° after surgery was recorded in 6 patients (18 %). The Table 3 shows the distribution of an absolute value of a lower limb mechanical axis after the unicompartmental endoprosthesis implantation measured by the planning station PACS.

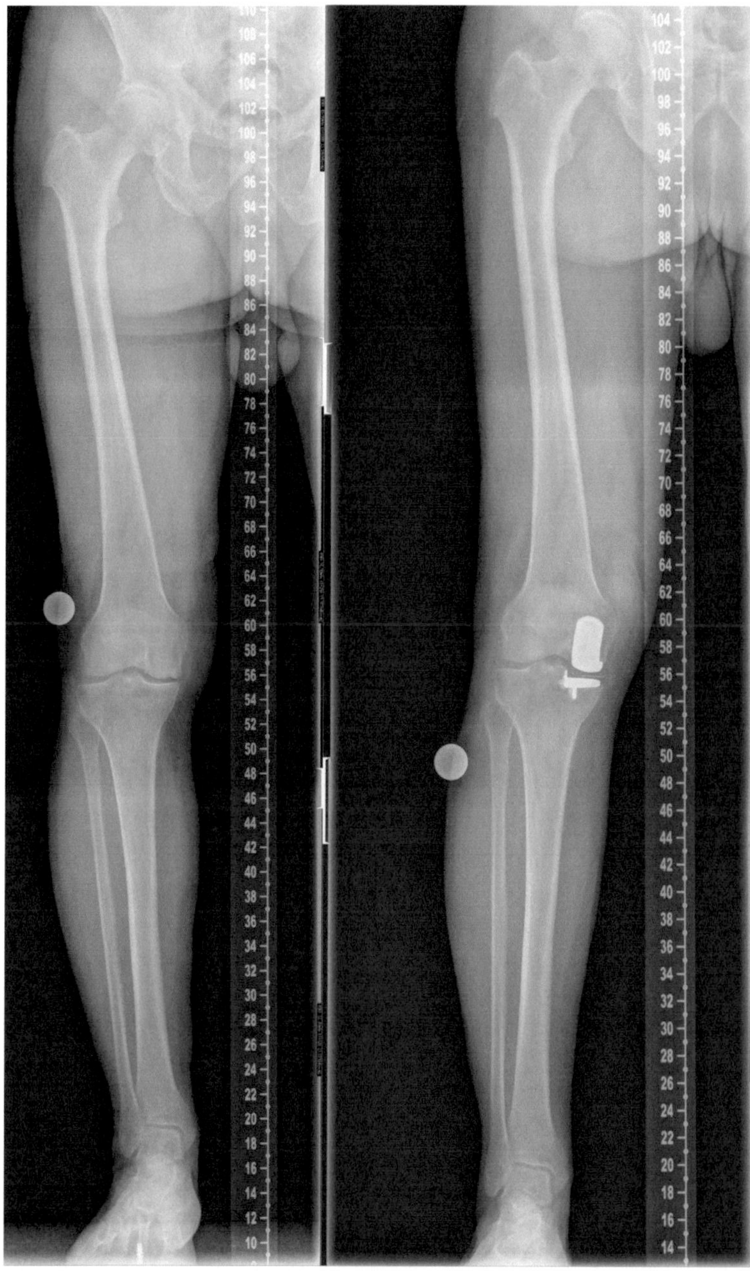

Fig. 7. The X-rays show the correction of the axis of lower limb before and after the surgery

valgus deformity	number of patients	varus deformity	number of patients
0.1° - 2.0°	8 (25 %)	0° - 2.0°	6 (19 %)
2.1° - 4.0°	8 (25 %)	2.1° - 4.0°	3 (9 %)
> 4.0°	4 (13 %)	> 4.0°	3 (9 %)

Table 3. This table shows the distribution of deformity of a lower limb mechanical axis after UCA implantation without navigation system

The average axis deviation of the lower limb was 4.1° varus (range, 1.0° to 9.0°) in the group of patients operated with the use of navigation (35 replacements). Axial deviations measured by navigation after the endoprosthesis implantation and by PACS 7 day after the surgery were the same (with the difference ≤ 2°) in 92 % of cases. The average axial deviation measured after the surgery was 0.5° varus (range, 5.1° valgus to 6.5°). The overcorrection of the lower limb mechanical axis into valgus happened only in 6 patients (17 %) with the use of the navigation. In these cases the hypercorrection was due to the prevention of mobile polyethylene core dislocation. The axis hypercorrection into valgus ≥ 2.0° happened in one patient (3 %). Varus deformity > 2.0° after the surgery was found in 4 patients (12 %). The Table 4 shows absolute value distribution of the lower limb mechanical axis after the unicompartmental endoprosthesis implantation measured by planning station PACS.

valgus deformity	number of patients	varus deformity	number of patients
0.1° - 2.0°	5 (14 %)	0° - 2.0°	25 (71 %)
2.1° - 4.0°	1 (3 %)	2.1° - 4.0°	3 (9 %)
4.0° <	0	4.0° <	1 (3 %)

Table 4. The table shows the distribution of deformity of a lower limb mechanical axis after UCA implantation with navigation system

The kinematic computer navigation represents significant help for the right choice of mobile polyethylene inlay height. An implant failure is threatening in cases of varus deformity reversing. In cases of more frequently observed hypercorrection into valgus lateral gonarthrosis usually develops. Both situations must be later solved by a conversion on TKR.

7. Conclusion

The importance of the kinematic computer navigation of knee endoprosthesis lies above all in the reduction of out-layers. This fact is important especially for beginning orthopaedic surgeons. The kinematic navigation should prevent from wrong resection of distal femur or proximal tibia. Navigation succeeds in 88 % cases (Hart et al, 2003) to reach the deviation from an ideal axial position of a lower limb less than 2°. Without the navigation it is observed in 70 % cases. However, it is not possible to rely on the kinematic navigation absolutely (as it is only auxiliary method). The key factor of the navigation system

successful use during the whole surgical procedure is to keep an unchanged position of femoral and tibial diodes. Change of their position can influence dramatically the result of the whole navigation process. It is possible to avoid this complication in osteoporotic skeleton by an accessory Kirschner wire which prevents from the screw rotation. The time waste during the surgery, which represents time less than 10 minutes in hands of experienced surgeons, is not significant with regard to the above mentioned navigation system advantages.
Another substantial benefit of the computer navigation in a total knee joint endoprosthesis implantation is incases after fractures of the femur, where osteosynthesis material is left or after bone healing in a malposition which makes impossible to carry out the distal femoral resection with the use of an intramedullary targeting device. The navigation helps routinely also at the beginning of the surgery to distinguish the right valgus deformity from the false one. According to it we choose the suitable surgical approach. In unicompartmental knee joint replacements it is possible to choose the right polyethylene inlay height by the help of the navigation so that the lower limb mechanical axis is restored as accurately as possible. In this way we avoid axis overcorrection into valgus in most cases and subsequent decompensation of the lateral compartment and later necessity of conversion on TKR.

8. References

Hart, R., Janeček, M., Chaker, A. & Bucek, P. (2003). Total knee arthroplasty implanted with and without kinematic navigation. *International orthopaedics,* 27, 6, 366-369, DOI: 10.1007/s00264-003-0501-6

Hart, R. & Janeček, M. (2003). *Osové postavení dolní končetiny a poloha komponent kolenní endoprotézy s přihlédnutím ke kinematické počítačové navigace,* Neptun, , ISBN 80-902896-5-7, Praque, Czech Republic

Hart, R., Krejzla, J., Janeček, M. & Mahel, P. (2005). Minimally invasive total knee replacement surgery with use of the kinematic navigation. El Mochel Movie.

Hart, R., Janeček, M., Čižmář, I., Štipčák, V., Kučera, B. & Filan, P. (2006). Minimal-invasive und navigierte implantation von knietotalendoprothesen, radiologische analyse und frühe klinische ergebnisse. *Der Orthopäde,* 35, 5, 552-557, ISSN: 0085-4530

Hart, R., Janeček, M., Safi, A. & Okál, F. (2010). Digital temlating compared with kinematic navigation in TKR, *Proceedings of 10th Annual Meeting of CAOS-International,* Paris, France, June 2010

Insall, J.N., Binazzi, R., Soudry, M. & Mestriner, L.A. (1985). Total knee arthroplasty. *Clinical orthopaedics,* 192, 13-22, ISSN 1528-1132

Krackow, K.A. (1983). Approaches to planning lower extremity alignment for total knee arthoplasty and osteotomy about the knee. *Advances in operative orthopaedics,* 7, 69-88

Laskin, R. S. (1984). Alignment of total knee components. *Orthopedics,* 7, 62-72

Ritter, A.M., Faris, M.P., Keating, E.M. & Meding, J.B. (1994). Postoperative alignment of total knee replacement, its effect on survival. *Clinical orthopaedics,* 299, 153-156 ISSN 1528-1132

Šváb, P., Hart, R., Bárta, R. & Šmíd, P. (2010). Computer navigation of valgus knee kinematice before TKR, *Proceedings of 14th National Conference of Orthopaedy*, Praque, Czech Republic, May 2010

Whietside, L.A & Arima, J. (1995). The Anteroposterior axis for femoral rotational alignment in valgus total knee arthroplasty. *Clinical orthopaedics*, 321, 168-172.

27

Concepts in Computer Assisted Total Knee Replacement Surgery

M. Fosco[1], R. Ben Ayad[1], R. Fantasia[1],
D. Dallari[1] and D. Tigani[2]
[1]*From First Ward of Orthopaedic Surgery, University of Bologna, Rizzoli Orthopaedic Institute, Bologna*
[2]*From Department of Orthopaedic Surgery, Santa Maria alle Scotte Hospital ,Siena*
Italy

1. Introduction

Total knee arthroplasty (TKA) is commonly considered to be a reliable procedure, with implant survival rates higher than 90% at 10 to 15 years of follow-up. The goal of total knee replacement surgery is to relieve pain and obtain better knee function, those achieved by correct patient selection, pre-operative deformity, implant design, correct surgical technique and patient participation in the rehabilitation protocol (Nizard et al, 2002).
Several technical requirements during TKA are important to obtain good results:

- correction of deformities;
- achievement of functional joint motion and stability;
- optimal balancing of soft tissues;
- satisfactory alignment in the frontal, sagittal and horizontal planes.

From literature data alignment in frontal plane must be into 2° or 3° range around a neutral alignment; this thought is demonstrated by Ritter at al who observed that prostheses implanted in varus position had a lower survival rate than prostheses implanted in a neutral or valgus position (Ritter et al, 1994); moreover Jeffery at al observed that when mechanical axis was in 3° valgus-varus range, the loosening rate was 3%, whereas it's 24% when the alignment was out of this range (Jeffery et al, 1991). The alignment in the horizontal plane is of particular importance for extensor mechanism stability, patellar wear, tilted patella, prostheses dislocation or loosening. In a study of Berger et al it was observed that patients with extensor mechanism problems have internal rotation of the femoral and tibial components (Berger et al, 1998).
Technically, there is a definite relationship between the accuracy of implant positioning and long-term durability (Jeffery et al, 1991; Stulberg et al, 2002): the position of prosthetic components and, consequently the alignment of mechanical axis, could be the cause of polyethylene wear due to overload stresses, ending finally by prosthetic loosening. The postoperative mechanical axis of the lower limb should be a straight line passing through the center of the hip, the center of the knee, and the center of the ankle; so that satisfactory

position of a TKA prosthesis is commonly accepted to be an alignment within 3° from this neutral axis (Fig. 1).

To improve precision of implant positioning, various mechanical alignment guides are used, both intramedullary and extramedullary, but technical errors with these conventional surgical techniques still occur. Moreover, mechanical alignment and sizing devices presume a standardized bone geometry that may not be applied to all patients. Even the most elaborate mechanical instrumentation systems rely on visual inspection to confirm the accuracy of stability and of limb and implant alignment at the conclusion of the TKA procedure.

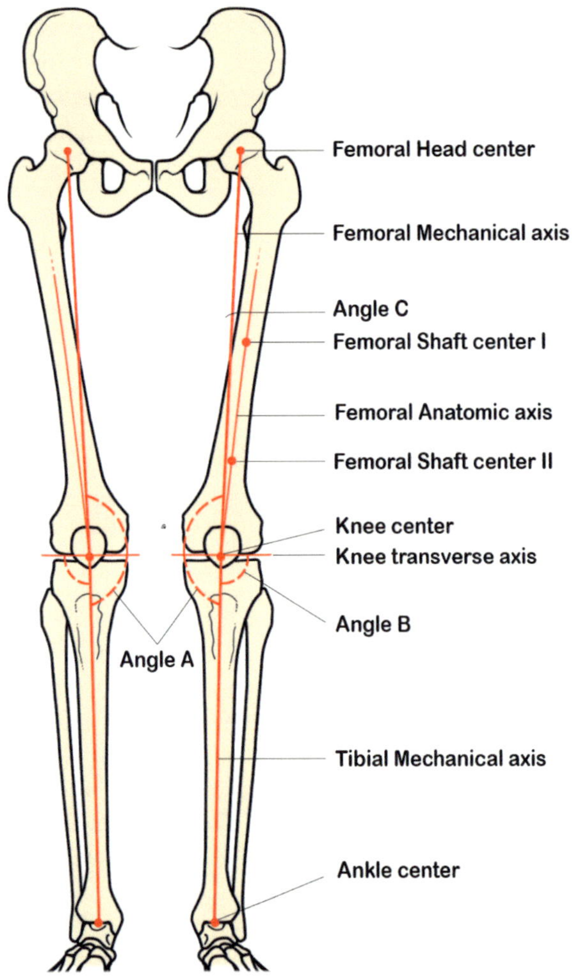

Fig. 1. Axes of the lower limb. Angle A represents knee mechanical physiologic valgus angle of 3°. Angle B represents tibia shaft angle, that is in 3° of varus from knee transverse axis. Angle C corresponds to angle between femoral anatomic and mechanical axis (6° of valgus). Femoral anatomic axis could be easily determined by two points located at the centre of the shaft. Mechanical axis of the lower limb passes near or through knee center and lies from femoral head center to ankle center.

Computer assisted surgery (CAS) for TKA was firstly introduced to improve the accuracy of alignment of the implanted prosthesis, thinking that it could make an inexperienced or occasional TKA surgeon performing more like an expert TKA surgeon, or to address the limitations inherent in mechanical instrumentation systems used for total knee replacement surgery (Jeffery et al, 1991; Stulberg et al, 2002).
During the last Decades CAS instrumentations have been improved in accuracy and various studies have been made to analyse results using this technique in TKA surgery. Advocates of this technique in total knee replacement claim benefits in terms of improving accuracy for alignment of the leg and orientation of the components, as well as a reduction in blood loss and a lower rate of intracranial micro emboli compared with traditional surgery.
The survival rate for modern total knee artroplasty is reported between 80% to 95% after 10 years of follow up (Buechel et al, 2002; Robertsson et al, 2001), and the most important factor of failure is malalignment of mechanical axis (Jeffery et al, 1991; Rand et al, 1988). Recently the introduction of CAS have gained up improvement in post operative mechanical alignment (Bathis et al, 2004; Chauhan et al, 2004; Chin et al, 2005; Decking et al, 2005; Haaker et al, 2005). However, no clear published results associated with superior clinical and patients perceived functional results and consequently longer survival rate (Stulberg et al, 2006).

2. History of CAS and review of literature

The history of CAS for total knee replacement was dated back to the middle nineties (Picard et al, 1997). Intraoperative navigation in total joint replacement began in 1992, when W. Barger, in Sacramento (California) performed the first computer assisted surgery in orthopaedics for total hip replacement, while the first total knee replacement began in France, in January 1997, by F. Picard and D. Saragaglia after a study on cadavers (Picard et al, 1997; Saragaglia et al, 2001; Delp et al; 1998) and then started a prospective randomized study comparing the computer assisted technique to the conventional surgery in 50 patients. The postoperative mechanical axis was 181.2° ± 2.72° in CAS group and 179.04° ± 2.53° in conventional group, with a statistical significant value in favor of CAS group and reduction of outliers. The mechanical axis was in fact between 177° and 183° in 75% of patients in conventional group and in 84% in CAS group (Saragaglia et al, 2001). The Authors concluded their paper saying that computer-assisted surgery for total knee arthroplasty provides remarkably reliable results and that "once the growing pains of this new material have been mastered, all surgeons should be able to expect an improvement in the positioning of prosthetic implantations".
Bathis et al. in a prospective study compared an imageless navigation system to conventional methods using an intramedullary femoral guide and an extra-medullary tibia jig. They reported the postoperative mechanical axis to be within 3° of varus or valgus in 96% of the navigation cases versus 78% of the conventional cases (Bathis et al, 2004).
Other study by Chauman et al. in which they compared a computer-assisted knee arthroplasty with the current conventional jig-based technique in 70 patients randomly allocated to receive either of the methods. All the patients were evaluated postoperatively with computer tomography imaging observing a significant improvement in the alignment

of the components using computer-assisted surgery with regard to femoral varus/valgus (p=0.032), femoral rotation (p=0.001), tibial varus/valgus (p=0.047) tibial posterior slope (p=0.0001), tibial rotation (p=0.011) and femoral-tibial mismatch (p=0.037). The Authors reported that computer-assisted surgery took longer time with a mean increase of 13 minutes regarding the conventional technique, but the blood loss was significantly lower (Chauchan et al, 2004).

A significant number of recent randomized controlled trial studies compared the use of imageless CAS with conventional methods; the results of these studies are shown in Table 1.

Authors	**Year of publication**	**M.A >3° (n/N)**		**M.A >2° (n/N)**	
		CAS	Conv	CAS	Conv
Saragaglia	2001	4/25	6/25	10/25	11/25
Sparmann	2003	0/120	16/120	3/120	27/120
Chauhan	2004	5/34	10/30	11/34	11/30
Bathis	2004	3/80	18/80	15/80	32/80
Stulberg	2006	21/38	19/40	30/38	30/40
Pang	2009	2/35	9/35	7/35	17/35
Choong	2009	7/57	21/54	\	\

Table 1. Different RCTs studies comparing post-operative mechanical angle in conventional and imageless CAS knee arthroplasty. CAS=Computer Assisted Surgery, Conv= conventional surgery, M.A= Mechanical Angle, n= number of knees, N= total number of knees.

Most of those meta-analysis studies of the best available evidence indicate significant improvement in component orientation and a better restoration of the mechanical limb alignment when CAS is used (Mason et al, 2007). In review of the past literature, there were only few papers which have indicated that there was no significant difference between computer-assisted navigated TKA and conventional TKA (Mielke et al, 2001).

In the report by Kim et al (Kim et al, 2007), bilateral sequential total knee replacements were carried out by one senior author in 160 patients (320 knees). One knee was replaced using a CT-free computer-assisted navigation system and the other side replaced conventionally without navigation. The Authors studied their cases with both standard radiological and CT imaging to determine the alignment of the components. The results of imaging and the number of outliers for all radiological parameters were not statistically different between the groups (p=0.109 to p=0.920). The post-operative limb alignment (femoral-tibial angle) exceeded 3° of varus/valgus deviation in only 18% (Sparman et al, 2003) of the patients operated by using the conventional technique, and in about 21%(Jenny et al, 2001) of the patients that were operated by navigation system.

3. Different computer navigation systems

Existing computer assisted surgery system must allow the accomplishment of the objectives above described: ensure optimal positioning of the prosthesis in the three planes (frontal, sagittal and horizontal); ensure optimization of the ligament balance; maintain joint stability (Nizard et al, 2002).

Firstly, computer-assisted navigation systems could be distinguished between active and passive computer systems as described by Picard at al. (Picard et al, 2001).

Active computer systems, also named robots, are able to realize the entire surgical procedure after the knee as been exposed through a conventional approach. The use of such complicated systems is viable only if the installation and functions during the surgical procedure can be performed within a reasonable time. The results of such systems have been presented in different studies (Tenbusch et al, 2001).

Passive computer systems do not perform any part of the surgical procedure which remains under direct control of the surgeon, that allowing him to apply and positioning the cutting guides.

Location systems for such CAS procedure crucially require a perfect and permanent fixation to the instrument. Two location systems are currently available, magnetic field detector and optical detector. Magnetic location systems are designed to generate a cylindrical field of about 80cm of diameter, received by collectors called dynamic reference frames (DRFs), which are fixed to the instruments or to the bone. This system does not require any particular position of the surgical team around the patient or between the system and the collectors, so no line of sight issues are present with EM tracking, but this system introduces the problem of metal influence. In fact, their failure is related to the use of ferromagnetic instrument in conventional technique like bone retractors, hammers and drill as well as mobile phones and hand watches. Lionberger (Lionberger et al, 2006) who studied the various problems of electromagnetic technology, pointed out the limited distortion of titanium, cobalt-chrome and some stainless steels. The software is furthermore designed with the possibility to induce an "off-signal" before the externally-generated source of instability or signal inaccuracy can be produced. Potentially, the collectors are linked to the computer system by wires, that could be troublesome during surgery.

Optical systems using infrared light are the most widely employed method of connection between the surgical field and the computer. These consist of two or three infrared camera sensors that detect the position of active or passive trackers implanted on the leg through rigid bodies or special shape instrument, which must all remain within the line of sight (Fig. 2).

The active leg trackers use systems that have light emitting diodes (LED) which sent out light pulsed to the optical localizer (Fig. 3). Opposite passive leg trackers use reflecting spheres mounted to the rigid body; recently new trackers are available consists of reflective discs connected together in angular arrangement (Fig. 4). Potential mistakes of data detection could be due to proximity of two localizers.

The advantage of optical systems is accurate detection without possible distorted information, while main disadvantages are usually due to reflecting spheres wear, the volume of infrared camera in the surgical room and also necessary adaptable positioning of surgical team personal to the system until the collectors have been located by the camera (Table 2).

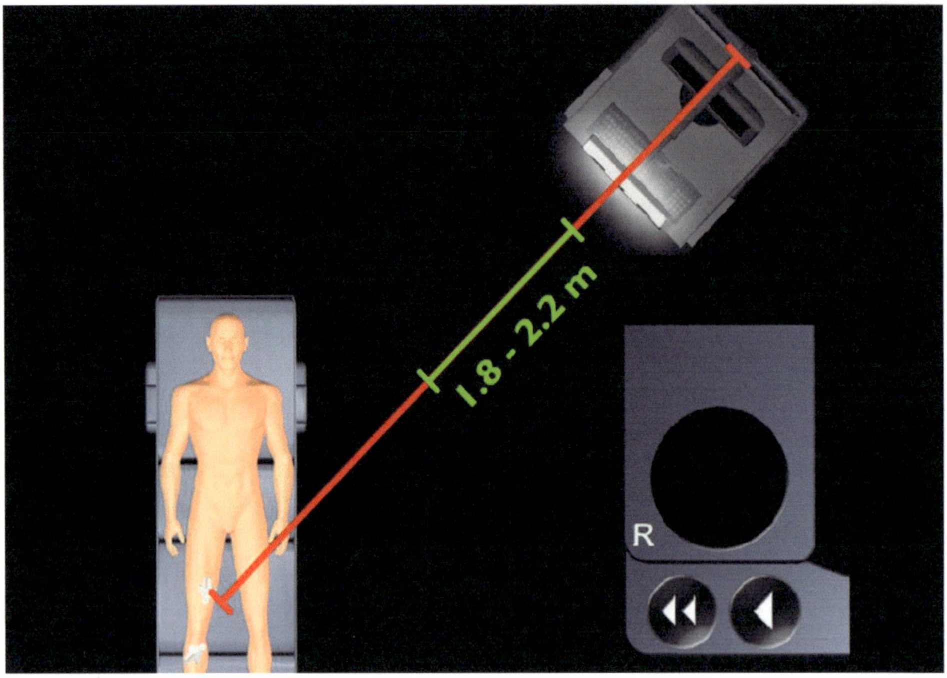

Fig. 2. Working station, consisting on display monitor and infra-red light camera sensors attached to stander, is positioned in a far position. Trackers have to be always within the line of sight with the camera. (Courtesy of B.Braun, Melsungen, D).

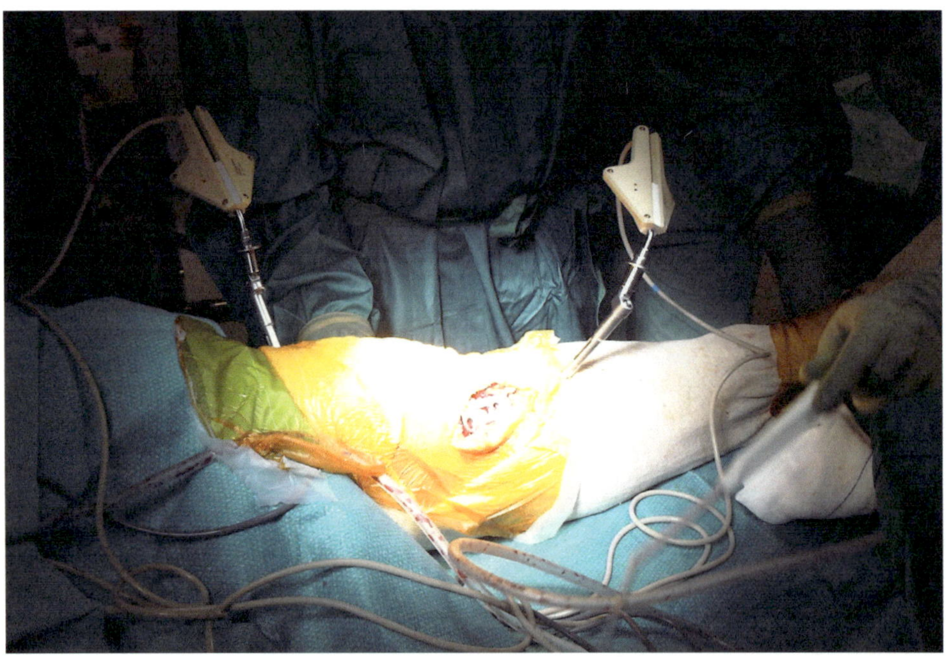

Fig. 3. Active optical trackers and intra-operative alignment of femoral and tibial parts

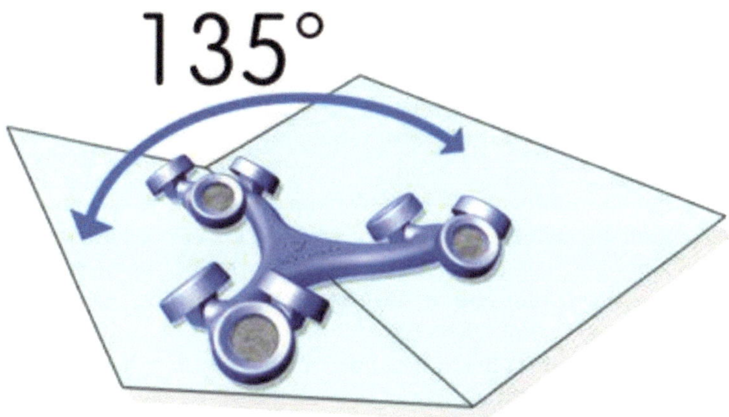

Fig. 4. Disc shape optical passive trackers connected in angular pattern (Courtesy of Zimmer, Warsaw, USA)

NAVIGATION SYSTEM		MAIN DISADVANTAGES
According to Picard et al, 2001	Active computer systems (robots)	Technically complicated and expensive system, very long surgical time
	Passive computer systems	Partially surgeon controlled-dependent results
According to Stulberg et al, 2002	Image-based (CT, MRI, fluoroscopic view)	Irradiation exposure of patient, adjunctive cost for peri-operative imaging procedure
	Image free	Additional surgical time, no clear information concerning the implants rotation
SIGNAL DETECTOR		**MAIN DISADVANTAGES**
Magnetic field detector		Metal influence needing specific-instrumentation, sometimes distorted information detected
Optical detector		Mistakes of data due to proximity of localizers, bulky camera, adaptable positioning of surgical team personal
TRACKER		**MAIN DISADVANTAGES**
Active optical trackers		Less detection accuracy due room light interferance
Passive optical trackers		Needing instrument calibration as first step, frequent cleaning of reflecting spheres/discs during surgery

Table 2. Different systems and components of navigation surgery.

3.1 Image-based navigation systems

According to Stulberg et al. CAS for joint replacement can be classified into two categories: image based and image-free navigation systems.

Using imaging devices the preoperative morphological data acquisition is necessary, which is gained by two different sources. The first one is preoperative imaging by a CT scan or MRI; second one is perioperative fluoroscopy imaging, performed in the operating room, during surgery. This imaging requires a specially modified fluoroscopy unit and entails the maneuvering of a relatively bulky and expensive apparatus during surgery.

CT-scan imaging modality which allow 3D reconstruction of bone morphology and bony landmarks, is probably the most time consuming step for the surgeon, while the MRI could be used in order to have information on soft tissue structure, but definition of bony landmarks is far inferior to that of CT-scan.

In such system, the registration and identification of special pointes process during the surgery is needed in order to match it with the image saved on the screen. Programmed software, using a mathematical algorithm, is able to help surgeon to identify these points during the matching process. Main advantage of image based systems is that it can be used in cases with extreme deformities, as seen in post fracture malunion and some bone disease, like Paget disease. It is possible to reconstruct 3D models when ipsilateral hip arthroplasty is present, and also in cases of revision of mono-compartemental knee prostheses or in two stage revision with temporary spacer in situ. However the main disadvantage is mandatory to obtain a preoperative CT-scan which is an additional hospital expense and a source of irradiation for the patients (Nizard et al, 2001).

Although potentially useful for knee reconstructive surgery imaging devices currently employed with CAS have been at present abandoned as requiring additional steps without providing significant benefits.

3.2 Image-free navigation systems

Image-free optical systems using infrared light are currently the most widely employed method of connection between the surgical field and the computer. These systems utilizes either optical (infra-red light), or electromagnetic devices that detect the position of active or passive markers implanted on the leg through rigid bodies or special shape instrument, which must all remain within the line of sight. The most important characteristic of this system is its ability to provide instant information regarding in vivo kinematics of the joint thus allowing the surgeon to quantify data, have dynamic intraoperative feedback or information and obtain more reproducible results..

First step is localization of important bony points: center of femoral head, knee center and ankle center are main points to identify (Fig. 5). Junction between these three points define the mechanical axis of lower limb. Several methods are available to define these points, which include:

- Center of femoral head localized by kinematic analysis of the hip joint; passive mobilization of the hip is needed to determine this center without reference point on the iliac crest.
- Knee center can be defined in two ways, one is based on kinematic analysis which requires passive mobilization of the knee, the other way is based on the definition of anatomic landmark (i.e. intercondylar trochlear notch, anterior tibial plateau eminence) (Yoshioka et al, 1989).

- Ankle center which is also determined by two methods, kinematic analysis of the ankle during passive motion, the other method is acquisition of anatomical points on the medial and lateral malleoli.

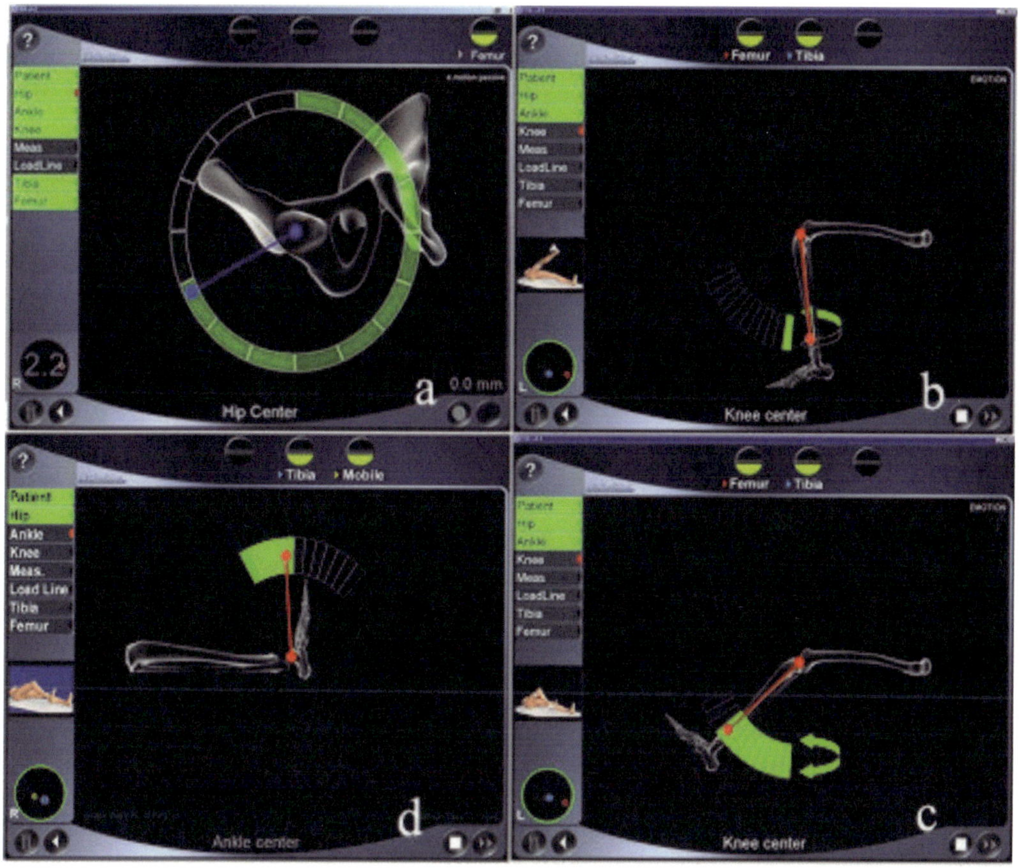

Fig. 5. Localization of hip (A), knee (B,C) and ankle (D) joint center.

Two types of information can be given by these image free systems, in two or three dimensions (3D). In two-dimensional systems, only the axes in frontal and sagittal planes are available. In 3D systems, digitization of anatomical structures allows reconstruction of an almost complete distal femur or proximal tibia using either statistically reshaped bony structures or completely redesigned bony structures from direct digitization.

The most important advantage of this system is avoidance of irradiation exposure, while their disadvantages are represented by additional time needed during the operation, and no clear information obtained concerning the rotational position of the implants (Arima et al,1995; Kats et al, 2001; Saragaglia et al, 2001).

The first results reported with these systems are encouraging (Saragaglia et al, 2001; Clemens et al, 2001; Jenny et al, 2001; Kiefer et al, 2001). In a randomized study Saragaglia et al. have compared 25 knees operated with a conventional technique and 25 knees operated with the Orthopilot® navigation system; a satisfactory alignment in the frontal plane, defined as a mechanical axis between 3° varus and 3° valgus alignment, was observed more often with the navigation system (84% versus 75% conventional technique). In a case-control study, Jenny et al. compared 60 prostheses implanted with the Orthopilot® system to 60 prostheses implanted using a conventional technique. With the navigation system 53 out of 60 prostheses were in the 3° valgus-3° varus range, whereas only 43 out of 60 were in this range with conventional system ($p<0.05$). Tigani et al. analysing 123 patients who underwent TKA with CAS, have retrospectively compared two different techniques of total knee arthroplasty (gap balancing and measured resection) utilizing different computer navigation systems; using inter class correlation ICC and paired *t*-test, they reported that no difference regarding the joint line level, and significant improvement in the ability to create mechanical alignment at 180°±3° in frontal plane in 95% of the operated patients (Tigani et al, 2010).

4. Indication for CAS in knee surgery

Computer-assisted navigation seems to be helpful in those difficult situations where accurate alignment remains crucial but traditional instrumentation is not applicable. Traditional cutting guides during knee arthroplasty relies on intramedullary (IM) femoral instruments and either intramedullary or extramedullary (EM) tibial instruments to obtain proper axial alignment.

Intramedullary instruments cannot be used in patients with:

- Retained hardware that would be difficult or inadvisable to remove (Fig. 6) or long-stemmed hip implants (Fig. 7) that could obstruct introduction of long IM instruments;
- Severe posttraumatic extrarticular femoral deformity when one is unable to pass an IM guide to accurately make a distal femoral cut (Fig. 8);
- IM guides may increase the infection risk in patients with history of focal diaphyseal osteomyelitis around the knee joint (Fehring et al, 2006);
- Patients with severe cardiopulmonary disease or a history of foramen ovale who may be at risk for embolic dissemination because of femoral IM instrumentation (Berman et al, 1998).

These problems can be avoided with extramedullary jigs on the tibial side, but EM instrumentation is cumbersome on the femoral side, which requires radiographically identifying the femoral head and a freehand technique of pinning the distal femoral resection guide. In cases with retained hardware or prosthesis, the distance from the articular surface is a topic question to take into consideration. The surgeon should be aware that in addition to the 9 to 11 mm of usual resection amount on distal femur a supplementary distance of at least 12 to 17 mm of femoral bone, according to the size and type of prosthesis, is necessary for the central box housing of posterior stabilized prosthesis (Haas et al, 2000).

In cases of extrarticular deformity, simultaneous or staged corrective osteotomy and total knee arthroplasty has been advocated to achieve normal alignment of the long bones and better ligament balancing. However, this technique may be associated with substantial complications, including nonunion at the osteotomy site and arthrofibrosis (Engh et al, 1990; Lonner et al, 2000).

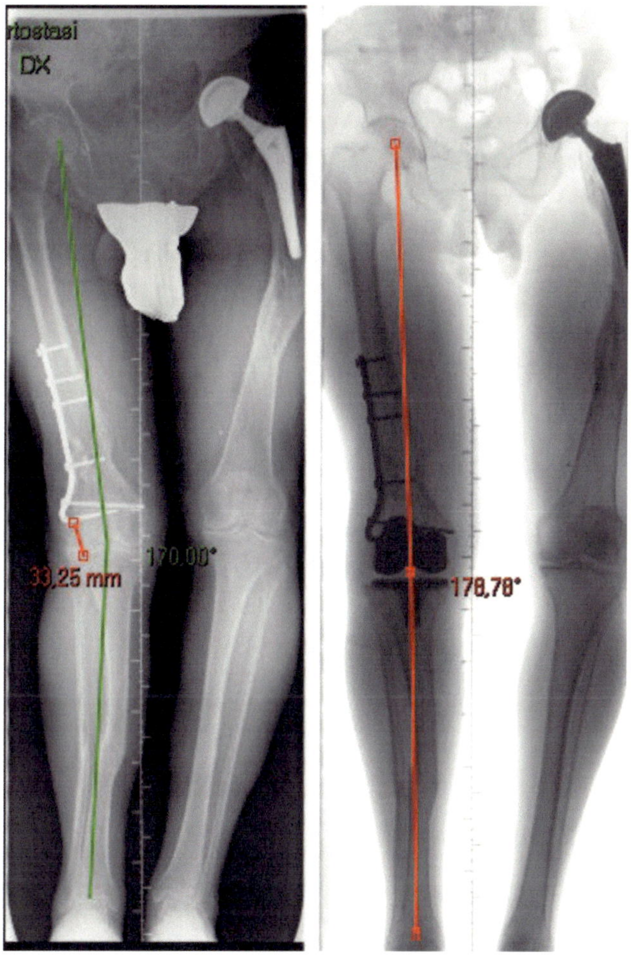

Fig. 6. Patient with blade-plate on distal right femur that prevent use of intramedullary guides. CAS during TKA surgery allow to correct mechanical axis and good positioning of prosthetic components.

An alternative to the combined osteotomy/TKA approach is to perform intraarticular bone resection and soft-tissue balancing. This procedure may be appropriate when the insertion of the collateral ligaments of the knee would not be jeopardized by the intra-articular bone resection (Wolff et al, 1991). The limits of intra-articular correction of an extrarticular deformity have been elucidated by Wang (Wang et al; 2001), who found that intraarticular resection without osteotomy was successful for patients with an average of 20° of coronal plane deformity in the tibia and femur. So that CAS facilitates correction of the deformity and helps avoid massive intra-articular soft tissue release.

Obese patients are another challenging subgroup undergoing TKA. In these cases CAS helps to accurately estimate the center of the femoral head and the overall limb and component alignment, otherwise difficult to be clinically judged with conventional technique. Various authors (Berend et al, 2004; Choong et al, 2009) reported higher incidence of revision when body mass index was more than 30, with only 56% of knees having a final mechanical axis aligned within 3° of neutral using conventional technique, compared to 93% of knees in the navigated group.

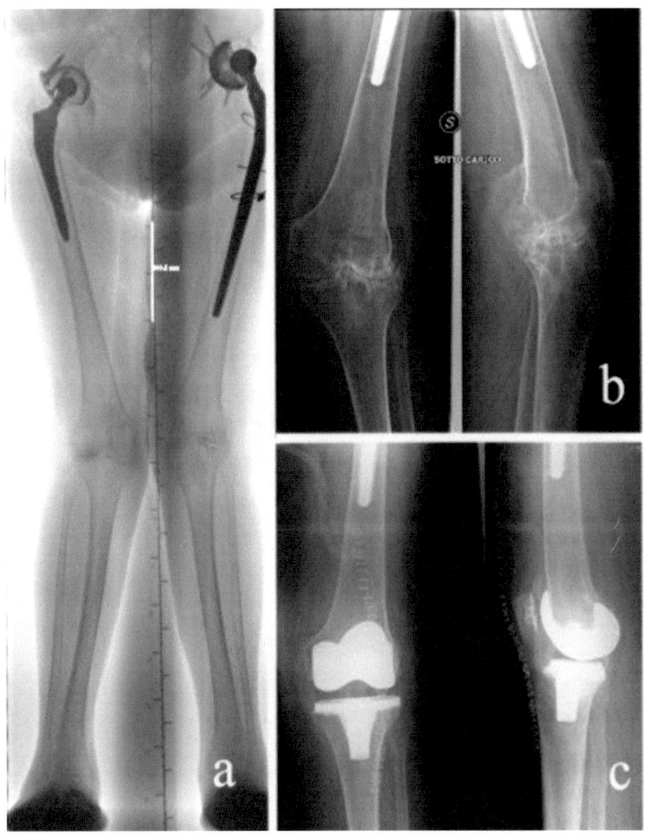

Fig. 7. Valgus osteoarthric knees in patient with long stemmed arthroplasty at left hip. Computer-assisted surgery allow to implant knee prosthesis without use of intramedullary femoral guide.

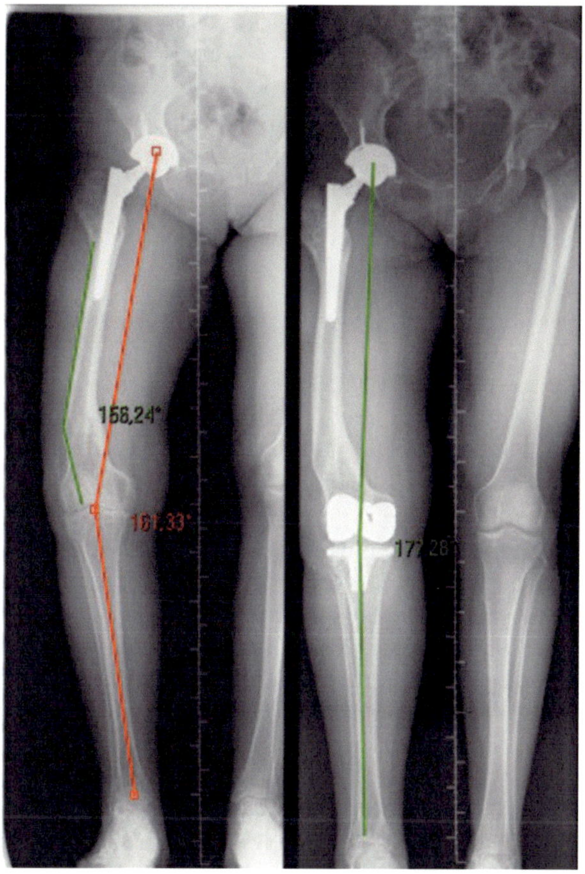

Fig. 8. Knee osteoarthritis with extrarticular femoral post-traumatic deformity(malunion). TKA was performed using computer-assisted technique with intrarticular correction of the deformity.

5. Advantages and disadvantages of CAS

Computer-assisted surgery in TKA offers several advantages against traditional surgery, that can be resumed as follow:

- Better accuracy in bone cutting and positioning of prosthetic components (Martin et al, 2007; Bathis et al, 2004; Aravind et al, 2011). In a study of Martin et al, they found that the mechanical axis of the limb was within 3° varus/valgus in 92% of the patients who had navigated procedures versus 76% of patients who had conventional surgery. The tibial slope showed a rate of inaccuracy of 3° or less for 98 % of the patients in the navigated TKA group versus 80% of the patients in the conventional group (Martin et al, 2007);
- The possibility to do a three-dimensional planning and alignment of the prothesis (Stockl et al, 2004);
- Dynamic assessment of deformity at any angle as opposed to conventional technique where tensioning devices can be used in 0° extension and 90° flexion (Aravind et al, 2011);

- Assessment of soft tissue and collateral tension when gap balancing technique applied (Chauhan et al, 2004);
- Intra-operative range of motion analysis to achieve maximum function, as confirmed by some reports like that of Austin et al, who observed as navigation could be a reliable tool for performing in vivo assessment of range of motion (Austin et al, 2008);
- Decreased incidence of pulmonary embolism in knee surgery, due to using of only extra-medullary guidance (Kalairajah et al, 2005);
- Minimally invasive surgery, which allows lesser blood loss during and after operation, reduces risks at transfusion and decreased hospital admission duration, those gives financial saving (Kalairajah et al, 2005);
- Early rehabilitation and shorter hospital stay, due to improved accuracy in limb alignment and soft tissue balance obtained with computer-assisted TKA (Choong et al, 2009).

Nevertheless, there are some disadvantages by using navigation:

- The surgical time was longer for navigated TKA than for the conventional procedure (Martin et al, 2007);
- Additional incisions for reference pins;
- Increased incidence of fractures or infections related to the pins sites (less than 1% reported complication rate) (Wysocki et al, 2008; Chi-Huan et al, 2008; Manzotti et al, 2008; Bonutti et al, 2008; Jung et al, 2007; Ossendorf et al, 2006). According to literature, larger pins diameter (5 mm), eccentric or repeated drilling and diaphyseal placement may be at greater risk of such complication (Wysocki et al, 2008; Chi-Huan et al, 2008);
- Financial saving by low hospital duration cost effective in health care however is still not realized. Solver et al. applying Moarkov decision model to evaluate the impact of hospital volume on the cost-effectiveness of CAS arthroplasty, have revealed that CAS is less likely to be cost-effective investment in health care improvement in centers with low volume of joint replacements, where its benefit is most likely to be realized; anyway it may be effective in centers with high volume of joint replacements (Solver et al, 2008).

Computer system is very sophisticated and, if used correctly, will improve accuracy. The system enhances the surgeon's perspective but should never replace it. Some pitfalls that can arise by using this technique include:

- Malfunctioning of the navigation system due to: dirty reflectors, camera or rounding errors or dislodgement of the reference pins (low rate of about 0.5%) which is likely due to less secure fixation afforded by unicortical fixation (Richard et al, 2010);
- Stretching against the extensor mechanism by reference pins;
- Inaccurate identification of the anatomic bone landmarks (Robinson et al, 2006);
- Avulsion of the patellae tendon by excessive traction on the patella;
- Inappropriate tibia rotation could be a less frequent pitfall when using imageless systems;
- Data registration inaccuracy; nevertheless causes to this problem must be understood by surgeons who use these devices. At least three potential causes of registration inaccuracy were identified when this image-free navigation system was applied to total knee replacement surgery:

1. Preoperative deformity and instability related to the original pathology of arthritic knee.
2. Computer hardware and software inaccuracy.
3. Surgical technique.

Additional updates of the computer software and surgical hardware are important because they appear to have substantially reduced the registration variations that result from all three causes of this type of inaccuracy in computer-assisted orthopaedic applications.

6. Surgical strategies with CAS

As for standard conventional surgery, two surgical strategies are possible in TKA with CAS (Hungerford et al, 1982): a measured resection approach (Fig. 9), in which bone landmarks are used to guide resections equal to the distal and posterior thickness of the femoral component, or a gap-balancing approach (Fig. 10), in which equal collateral ligament tension in extension and flexion is sought before and as a guide to definitive bone cuts. Both techniques aim to have symmetric flexion and extension gaps in terms of gap size and angular alignment.

In computer aided technique, after the first step of registration and identification of the key anatomic landmarks the computer system will identify the bone position in the space, the pre-requisite for the registration are the trackers which are attached to the bone, thus commonly considered the most fundamental aspect of registration accuracy. After registration process, the computer system kinematically gathers the information regarding joint anatomy, limb alignment, level of bone to be resected and matches knee anatomy with the size and type of the implant. The following implementation and verification step determine cutting blocks position, component to component position and soft tissue balance (Aravind et al, 2011).

Surgical steps in imageless CAS knee arthroplasty, do not require any preoperative plane or image. The initial step is the instrument calibration in passive rigid body systems (Orthosoft- Zimmer®) (Fig. 11), or without calibration in active rigid body systems (Orthopilot®- Aesculap/B-Braun).

This followed by the placement of the femoral and tibial trackers or rigid bodies that should be fixed to bone with precaution, to avoid any injury of adjucent neurovascular structures and the interference with surgical tools. The trackers should be in the field of the infrared camera to remain detectable throughout the procedure. Trackers fixation should be positioned with an angle of almost 90° with respect to diaphysis and on vertical axis 30-45° medially in femur and 45°-60° medially in tibia.

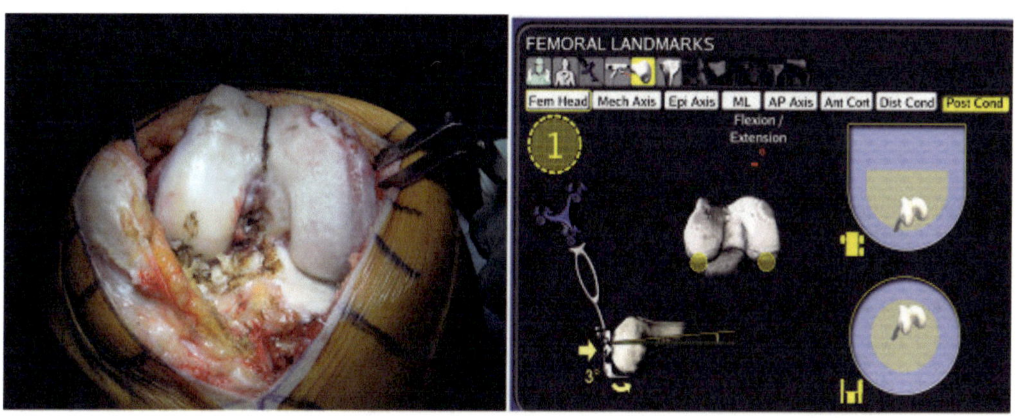

Fig. 9. The measured resection approach, in which bone landmarks are used to guide resections equal to the distal and posterior thickness of the femoral component

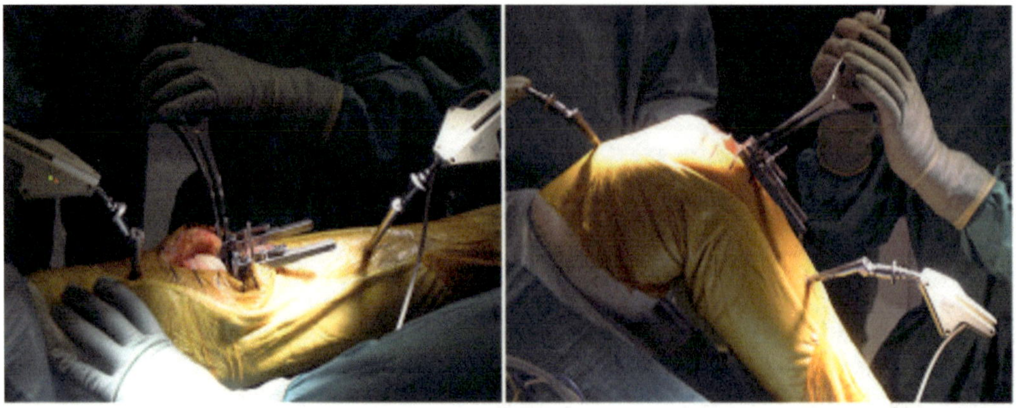

Fig. 10. The gap balancing approach, in which identical collateral ligament tension in extension and flexion is sought before and as a guide to final bone cuts

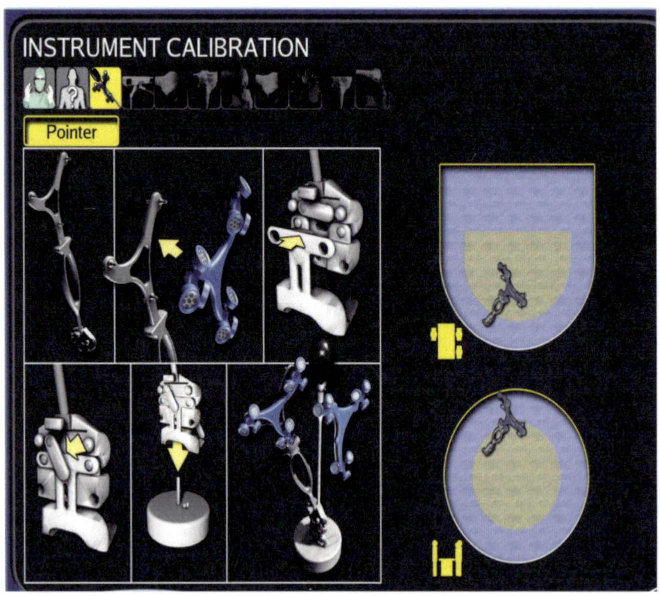

Fig. 11. Passive rigid bodies trackers calibration.

Once the knee is exposed next step consists on registration of the anatomical axis through the localization of the center of the knee, the center of the hip, and the center of the ankle joint using kinematic registration, those visualized on the computer screen (Fig 5).
The other anatomical landmarks located with the pointer or special paddle and necessary for the virtual reconstruction of the lower limb axis are the distal, posterior femoral condyles, medial/lateral tibial plateau and anterior tibial eminence. When soft tissues balance technique is used, it can be performed before or after bone resections with the trial spacer in place or using mechanical retractors both in extension and 90° flexion (Fig. 12).

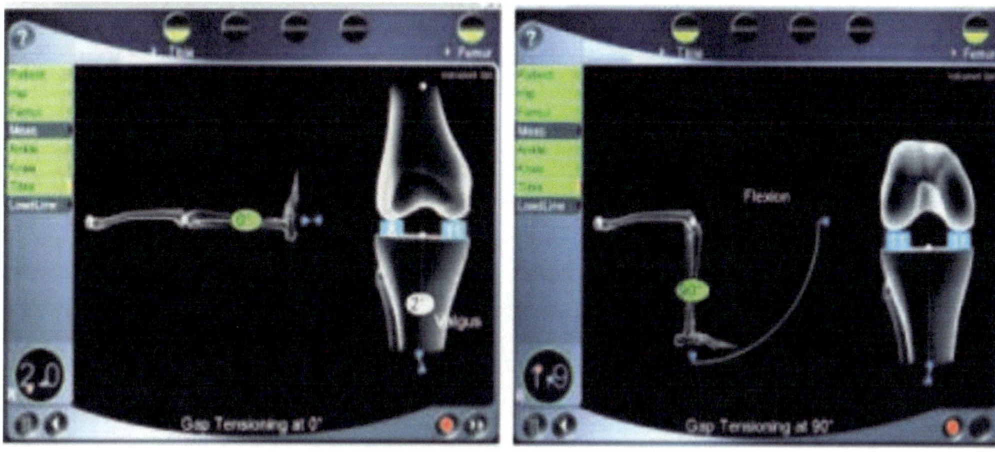

Fig. 12. Visualization of gap after tensioning of soft tissue in extention and flexion.

Now the initial lower limb mechanical axis can be visualized on the screen and in different angles of flexion; in addiction the degree of deformity to be corrected by bone cuts, and the initial knee range of motion can be registered. The most important surgical step in navigating TKA is the planning for 3D reconstruction for bone cuts and prosthesis orientation, through the working screen visible on the monitor (Fig. 13).
During this step, the surgeon by moving the virtual pointer tip, can target any value on the screen, except for the measured gaps. So that, through this procedure all femur cuts and sizes of the components to be implanted can be planned step by step, as well as the notching and the implant rotation.

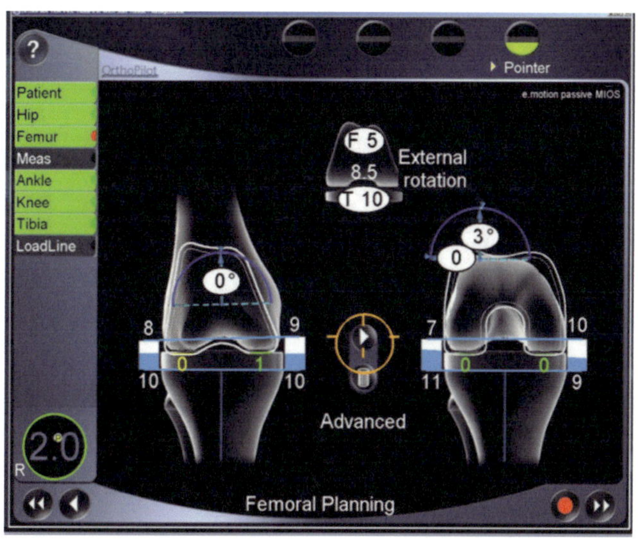

Fig. 13. Planning screen guided by surgeon.

The varus/valgus angle display, resection height display and femoral rotation display can be modified during this step before starting femoral cuts and to achieve equal rectangular gap spaces in both flexion and extention. The tibia display on the screen indicates the gap remaining after all cuts and after the implantation of all components, assuming possible additional soft tissue release will be carried out. Computer-based alignment systems have been developed to address the limitations inherent in mechanical instrumentation, so that it is recommended that before definitive prosthetic components implantation, the limb axis and the knee range of motion be controlled by CAS monitoring with the trail component in place (Fig. 14).

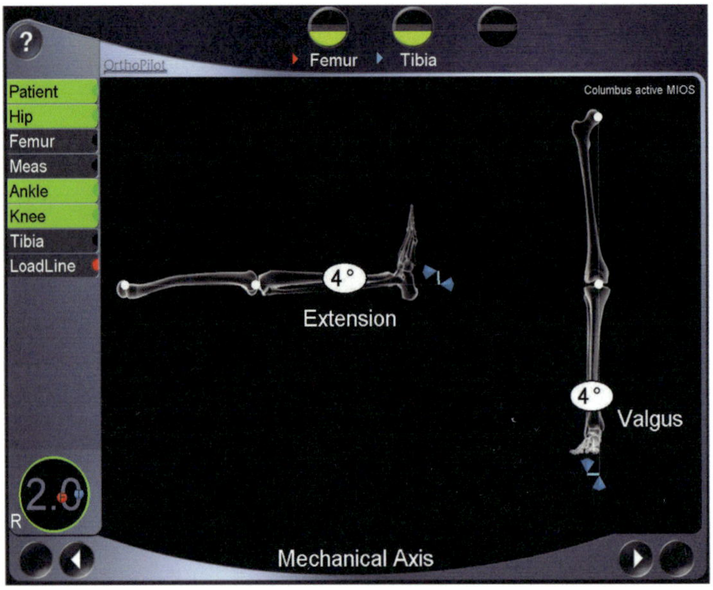

Fig. 14. Limb axis and range of motion controller before component implantation.

7. Conclusions

Total knee prosthetic component implantation using computer aided navigation allows the surgeon to reproduce the mechanical axis measured on full-length of the lower limb radiographs, thus reducing the number of outliers in the alignment of the limb compared with traditional instrument techniques.

Although analysis of alignment and prosthetic component orientation after computer-navigated and conventional implantation shows different results, three recent statistical studies of alignment outcome for computer-assisted knee surgery indicate significant improvement in accuracy of component orientation and mechanical axis restoration (Bauwens et al, 2007; Mason et al, 2007; Tigani et al, 2011).

Furthermore, regarding tibial component orientation, some authors have demonstrated notable improvement in sagittal-tibial component angle (i.e., the tibial slope angle) which can be reconstructed accurately and reproducibly to match the original value of the tibial plateau, although some studies did not find that the alignment in the sagittal plane of the tibial component was improved with navigation guidance (Biasca et al, 2009; Chauhan et al, 2004; Ensini et al, 2007; Matziolis et al, 2007; Sto¨ckl et al, 2004).

Debate about whether a CAS system improves the rotational alignment of the femoral component still exists and as described in the text, several femoral reference landmarks have been proposed to establish proper rotational alignment of the femoral components, although there is no consensus about the best landmarks to gauge that. Siston et al (Siston et al, 2005), in a cadaver study, they found high variability in the rotational alignment of the femoral component. This variability may be explained by the surgeon's greater or lesser ability to identify the medial epicondyle intraoperatively and by the ascending learning curve for the surgeon associated with habitual use of navigation devices, they can minimize the errors in the femoral landmark acquisition.

Although, the rotational mismatch between the tibial and femoral components is decreased with the role of CAS in knee replacement, controversy still exists as to whether navigation systems improve the rotational alignment of the tibial component in the axial plane (Chauhan et al, 2004; Siston et al, 2007). One solution to avoid such complication is the technique describe by Dalury (Dalury et al, 2001) and Eckhoff (Eckhoff et al, 1995) in which the orientation of the tibial tray was determined by allowing it to float into position with respect to the femoral component while the knee was placed through a full arc of motion and in a CT scan postoperative study it was documented an accurate alignment of the tibial component (Biasca et al, 2009).

Other certain factors to be faced intraoperatively, even by experienced surgeon is the patient bone status: in severe osteopenic bone the pins placed to hold the trackers may become loose, making all further measurements inaccurate. Therefore, the surgeon must be very careful when handling pins and trackers. Moreover, attempts to cut through sclerotic areas of bone might create resection errors due to forced bending of the saw blade which can occur with conventional instrumentation as well. Such pitfall can be recognized with the computed-assisted navigation only by using the verification plate of the knee computer system, which allows the surgeon to check-out every cutting procedure during the operation and to verify the correct resection level and also of the programmed joint line level.

Although someone argued that CAS is advised for use for inexperienced surgeons, last researches did not support the assumption of an automatic advantage (Yau et al, 2008). The use of computer navigation technology improve the accuracy in recreation of mechanical alignment in TKA when compared with the conventional jig-based technique. Nevertheless the volume of the operations performed by the surgeon, the experience in using computer navigation technology and severity of the preoperative deformity seems to be major contributing factors.

Knee navigation systems are not yet universally accepted, and their cost/benefit ratio remains a matter for further discussion. In fact, there is an absence of high quality studies demonstrating a longer implant survival rate, better clinical outcome, or enhanced postoperative function.

However CAS has an important value and could be more useful in those particular cases in which standard mechanical instrumentation cannot be used: presence of angular deformities, IM sclerosis, long-stemmed hip implants, or hardware within the femoral canal.

8. Acknowledgment

The authors did not receive any outside funding or grants in support of their research for or preparation of this work.

9. References

Arima J., Whiteside L. A., McCarthy D. S., White S. E. 1995. Femoral rotational alignment, based on the anteroposterior axis, in total knee arthroplasty in a valgus knee. A technical note. *J Bone Joint Surg Am*, Vol.77, No.9 (September 1995), pp. 1331-34, ISSN 1535-1386

Austin, MD Elie Ghanem, MD Ashish Joshi, MD Rachel Trappler, BS Javad Parvizi, MD, FRCS William J. Hozack, MD. (2008). The Assessment of Intraoperative Prosthetic Knee Range of Motion Using Two Methods. *J Arthroplasty*. Vol.23, No.4, (June 2008), pp.515-21, ISSN:0883-5403

Bäthis H, Perlick L, Tingart M, Lüring C, Zurakowski D, Grifka J. (2004). Alignment in total knee arthroplasty. A comparison of computer-assisted surgery with the conventional technique. *J Bone Joint Surg Br*, Vol.86, No.5, (July 2004), pp.682-7, ISSN:0301-620X

Bauwens K, Matthes G, Wich M, Gebhard F, Hanson B, Ekkernkamp A, Stengel D. (2007). Navigated total knee replacement. A meta-analysis. *J Bone Joint Surg Am*, Vol.89, No.2, (February 2007), pp.261-9, ISSN 1535-1386

Berend ME, Ritter MA, Meding JB, Faris PM, Keating EM, Redelman R, Faris GW, Davis KE. (2004). Tibial component failure mechanisms in total knee arthroplasty. *Clin Orthop Relat Res*, Vol.428, (November 2004), pp.26-34, ISSN 1528-1132

Berger RA, Crossett L.S, Jacobs J.J, Rubash H.E. Malrotation causing patellofemoral complications after total knee arthroplasty. *Clin Orthop Relat Res*, Vol.356, (November 1998), pp.144-53, ISSN 1528-1132

Berman AT, Parmet JL, Harding SP, Israelite CL, Chandrasekaran K. (1998). Emboli observed with use of transesophageal echocardiography immediately after tourniquet release during total knee arthroplasty with cement. *J Bone Joint Surg Am*, Vol.80, No.3, (March 1998), pp.389–94, ISSN 1535-1386

Biasca N, Schneider TO, Bungartez M. (2009). Minimally invasive computer-navigated total knee arthroplasty. *Orthop Clin N Am*, Vol.40, No.4, (October 2009), pp.537–63, ISSN 1059-1516

Bonutti P, Dethmers D, Stiehl JB. (2008). Femoral shaft fracture resulting from femoral tracker placement in navigated TKA. *Clin Orthop Relat Res*, Vol.466, No.6, (June 2008), pp.1499-502

Buechel FF. (2002). Long term follow up after mobile-bearing total knee replacement. *Clin Orthop Relat Res*, Vol.404, (November 2002), pp.404:40, ISSN 1528-1132

Chauchan, RG Scott, W Breidhal. (2004). Computer-assisted knee arthroplasty versus a conventional jig-based technique. A randomised, prospective trial. *J Bone Joint Surg Br*, Vol.86, No.3, (April 2004), pp.372-7, ISSN:0301-620X

Chauhan SK, Clark GW, Lioyd S, Scott RG, Breidahl W, Sikorski JM. (2004). Computer assisted total knee replacement. A controlled cadaver study using multi-parametrer quantitative CT assessment of alignment (the Perth CT protocol). *J Bone Joint Surgery Br*, Vol.86, No.6, (August 2004), pp.818-23, ISSN:0301-620X

Chi-Huan L, Tain-Hsiung C, Yu-Ping S, Po-Chou S, Kung-Sheng L, Wei-Ming C. (2008). Periprosthetic femoral supracondylar fracture after total knee arthroplasty with navigation system. *J Arthroplasty*, Vol.23, No.2, (February 2008), pp.304-7, ISSN:0883-5403

Chin PL, Yang KY, Yeo SJ, Lo NN. (2005). Randomized control trial comparing radiographic total knee arthroplasty implant placement using computer navigation versus conventional technique. *J Arthroplasty*, Vol.20, No.5, (August 2005), pp.618-26, ISSN:0883-5403

Choong PF, Dowsey MM, Stoney JD. (2009). Does accurate anatomical alignment result in better function and quality of life? Comparing conventional and computer-assisted total knee arthroplasty. *J Arthroplasty*, Vol.24, No.4, (June 2009), pp.560-569, ISSN:0883-5403

Clemens U., Miehlke R., Jens J. (2001). Computer integrated instrumentation in knee arthroplasty-the first 100 cases with the orthopilot knee navigation system. Poster 6. In: *International CAOS-Symposium*, Davos, 2001

Dalury DF. (2001). Observations of the proximal tibia in total knee arthroplasty. *Clin Orthop Relat Res*, Vol.389, (August 2001), pp.150–5, ISSN 1528-1132

Decking R, Markmann Y, Fuchs J, Puhl W, Scharf HP. (2005). Leg axis after computer-navigated total knee arthroplasty: a prospective randomized trial comparing computer-navigated and manual implantation. *J Arthroplasty*, Vol.20, No.3, (April 2005), pp.282-8, ISSN:0883-5403

Delp SL, Stulberg SD, Davies B, Picard F, Leitner F. (1998). Computer assisted knee replacement. *Clin Orthop Relat Res*, Vol.354, (September 1998), pp.49-56, ISSN 1528-1132

Desai, Asterios Dramis, Danile Kendoff, Tim N. Board. (2011). Critical review of the current practice for computer assisted navigation in total knee replacement surgery: cost-effectiveness and clinical outcome. *Curr Rev Musculoskelet Med*, Vol.4, No.1, (March 2011), pp.11-15, ISSN 1935-9748

Eckhoff DG, Metzger RG, Vandewalle MV. (1995). Malrotation associated with implant alignment technique in total knee arthroplasty. *Clin Orthop Relat Res*,Vol.321, (December 1995), pp.28–31, ISSN 1528-1132

Engh GA,Petersen TL. (1990). Comparative Experience With Intrarnedullary and Extramedullary Alignment in Total Knee Arthroplasty. *J Arthroplasty*, Vol.5, No.1, (March 1990), pp.1-8, ISSN:0883-5403

Ensini A, Catani F, Leardini A, Romagnoli M, Giannini S. (2007). Alignments and clinical results in conventional and navigated total knee arthroplasty. *Clin Orthop Relat Res*, Vol.457, (April 2007), pp.156–62, ISSN 1528-1132

Fehring TK, Mason JB, Moskal J, Pollock DC, Mann J, Williams VJ. (2006). When computer-assisted knee replacement is the best alternative. *Clin Orthop Relat Res*. Vol.452, (November 2006), pp.132-6, ISSN 1528-1132

Haaker RG, Stockheim M, Hamp M, Proff G, Breitenfelder J, Ottersbach A. (2005). Computer assisted navigation increases precision of component placement in total knee arthroplasty. *Clin Orthop Relat Res*, Vol.433, (April 2005), pp.152-9, ISSN 1528-1132

Haas S, C Nelson, R Laskin. (2000). Posterior stabilized knee arthroplasty: an assessment of the bone resection. *Knee*, Vol.7, No.1 (January 2000), pp.25-9, ISSN 1873-5800

Hungerford DS, Kenna RV, Krackow KA. (1982). The porous coated anatomic total knee. *Orthop Clin North Am*, Vol.13, No.1, (January 1982), pp.103–122, ISSN 1558-1373

Jeffery R, Morris R, Denham R. (1991). Coronal alignment after total knee replacement. *J Bone Joint Surg Br*, Vol.73, No.5, September 1991, pp.709-14, ISSN:0301-620X

Jenny J, Boeri C. (2001). Image-free computer-assisted total knee prosthesis implantation: A radiological matched-paired comparison with surgeon-controlled instrumentation. Poster 431. In: *American Academy of Orthopaedic Surgeons*, San Francisco, 2001

Jenny JY, Boeri C. (2001). Navigated implantation of total knee endoprosthesis: a comparative study with conventional instrument. *Z Orthop Ihre Grenzgeb*, Vol.139, No.2, (March-April 2001), pp.117-9, ISSN 0044-3220

Jung HJ, Jung YB, Song KS, Park SJ, Lee JS. (2007). Fractures associated with computer-navigated total knee arthroplasty. A report of two cases. *J Bone Joint Surg Am*, Vol.89, No.10, (October 2007), pp.2280-4, ISSN 1535-1386

Kalairajah Y, Simpson D, Cossey AJ, Verrall GM, Spriggins AJ. (2006). Are systemic emboli reduced in computer-assisted knee surgery? A prospective, randomized, clinical trial. *J Bone Joint Surg Br*,Vol.88, No.2, (February 2006), pp.198-202, ISSN:0301-620X

Katz MA, Beck TD, Silber JS, Seldes RM, Lotke PA (2001). Determining femoral rotational alignment in total knee arthroplasty. Reliability of techniques. *J Arthroplasty*, Vol.16, No.3, (April 2001), pp.301-5, ISSN:0883-5403

Kiefer H, Langemeyer D, Schmerwitz U, Krause F. (2001). Computer aided knee arthroplasty versus conventional technique. First results. Poster 132. In : *International CAOS-Symposium*, Davos, 2001

Kim Y.-H, MD, Kim J.-S, MD and Yoon S.-H, MD. (2007). Alignment and orientation of the components in total knee replacement with and without navigation support. *J Bone Joint Surg Br*, Vol.89, No.4, (April 2007), pp.471-476, ISSN:0301-620X

Lionberger DR. (2006). The attraction of electromagnetic computer-assisted navigation in orthopedic surgery. In: *Navigation and MIS in orthopedic surgery*, Stiehl J, Konermann W, Haaker R, Di Gioia A, (Eds.). pp.44-53, ISBN 978-3-540-36690-4, Springer, Heidelberg

Lonner JH, Siliski JM, Lotke PA. (2000). Simultaneous femoral osteotomy and total knee arthroplasty for treatment of osteoarthritis associated with severe extra-articular deformity. *J Bone Joint Surg Am*, Vol.82, No.3, (March 2000), pp.342-8, ISSN 1535-1386

Manzotti A, Confalonieri N, Pullen C. (2008). Intra-operative tibial fracture during computer assisted total knee replacement: A case report. *Knee Surg Sports Traumatol Arthrosc*, Vol.16, No.5, (May 2008), pp.493-6, ISSN 1433-7347

Martin A, Wohlgenannt O, Prenn M, Prenn M, Oelsch C, von Strempel A. (2007). Imageless navigation for TKA increased implant accuracy. *Clin Orthop Relat Res*, Vol.460, (July 2007), pp.178–84, ISSN 1528-1132

Mason, TK Fehring, R Estok, YD Banel and K Fahrbach. (2007). Meta-Analysis of Alignment Outcomes in Computer-Assisted Total Knee Arthroplasty Surgery. *J Arthroplasty*, Vol.22, No.8, (December 2007), pp.1097-106, ISSN:0883-5403

Matziolis G, Krocher D, Weiss U, Tohtz S, Perka C. (2007). A prospective,randomized study of computer-assisted and conventional total knee arthroplasty. *J Bone Joint Surg Am*, Vol.89, No.2, (February 2007), pp.236-43, ISSN 1535-1386

Mielke. U Clemens, JH Jens, S Kershally. (2001). Navigation in knee endoprosthesis implantation: preliminary experiences and prospective comparative study with conventional implantation technique. *Z Orthop Ihre Grenzgeb*, Vol.139, No.2, (March-April 2001), pp.109-16, ISSN 0044-3220

Nizard R. (2002). Computer assisted surgery for total knee arthroplasty. *Acta Orthopaedica Belgica,* Vol.68, No.3, (June 2002), pp.215-30, ISSN 0001-6462

Nizard R. First experience with a computer-assisted surgery system for total knee arthroplasty. In : *Proceedings of the 5th EFORT Meeting,* Rhodes, 2001

Ossendorf C, Fuchs B, Koch P. (2006). Femoral stress fracture after computer navigated total knee arthroplasty. *Knee* Vol.13, No.5, (October 2006), pp.397-9, ISSN 1873-5800

Picard F., Moody J., Jaramax B., DiGioia A.,Nikou C., LaBarca R. (2001). A classification proposal for computer assisted knee systems. Poster 93. In: *International CAOS-Symposium,* Davos, 2001

Picard, F Leitner, D Saragaglia, P Cinquin. (1997). Mise en place d'une prothèse totale du genou assistée par ordinateur: A propos de 7 implantations sur cadavre. *Rev Chir Orthop Reparatrice Appar Mot.* Vol.83, Suppl.II, (1997), pp.31, ISSN 1776-2553

Rand JA, Coventry MB. (1988). Ten years evaluation of geometric total knee arthroplasty. *Clin Orthop Relat Res,* Vol.232, (July 1988), pp.168-73, ISSN 1528-1132

Richard F., Owens Jr, MD, and Michael L. Swank. (2010). Low incidence of postoperative complications due to pin placement in computer-navigated total knee arthroplasty. *J Arthroplasty,* Vol.25, No.7, (October 2010), pp.1096-1098, ISSN:0883-5403

Ritter M. A, Faris P.M, Keating E.M, Meding J.B. (1994). Postoperative alignment of total knee replacement. It's effect on survival. *Clin Orthop Relat Res,* Vol.299, (February 1994), pp.153-156, ISSN 1528-1132

Robertsson O, Knutson K, lewold S, et al. (2001). The Swedish knee arthroplasty register 1975-1997: an update with special emphasis on 41,223 Knees operated on in 1988-1997. *Acta Orthop Scand ,* Vol.72, No.5, (October 2001), pp.503-13, ISSN 0001-6470

Robinson M, Eckhoff DG, Reinig KD, Bagur MM, Bach JM. (2006). Variability of landmark identification in total knee arthroplasty. *Clin Orthop Relat Res,* Vol.442, (January 2006), pp.57-62, ISSN 1528-1132

Saragaglia D, Picard F, Chaussard C, Montbarbon E, Leitner F, Cinquin P. (2001). Computer assisted knee arthropalsty: comparison with a conventional procedure. Results of 50 cases in a prospective randomized study. *Rev Chir Orthop Reparatrice Appar Mot,* Vol.87, No.1, (February 2001), pp.18-28, ISSN 1776-2553

Siston RA, Patel JJ, Goodman SB, Delp SL, Giori NJ. (2005). The variability of femoral rotational alignment in total knee arthroplasty. *J Bone Joint Surg Am,* Vol.87, No.10, (October 2005), pp.2276–80, ISSN 1535-1386

Siston RA, Giori NJ, Goodman SB, Delp SL. (2007). Surgical navigation for total knee arthroplasty: a perspective. *J Biomech,* Vol.40, No.4, (2007), pp.728–35, ISSN 1873-2380

Solver JM, Anna N, Tosteson A, Bozic KJ, Rubash HE, Malchau H. (2008). Impact of the hospital valume on economic value of the computer navigation for total knee replacement. *J Bone Joint Surg Am,* Vol.90, No.7, (July 2008), pp.1492-500, ISSN 1535-1386

Stöckl B, Nogler M, Rosiek R, Fischer M, Krismer M, Kessler O. (2004). Navigation improved accuracy of rotational alignment in total knee arthroplasty. *Clin Orthop Relat Res,* Vol.426, (September 2004), pp.180–6, ISSN 1528-1132

Stulberg SD, Loan P, Sarin B, Sarin V. Computer-assisted navigation in total knee replacement: Results of an initial experience in thirty-five patients. *J Bone Joint Surg Am,* Vol.84, Suppl 2, (2002), pp.90-8, ISSN 1535-1386

Stulberg SD, Yaffe MA, Koo SS. (2006). Computer-Assisted Surgery versus Manual Total Knee Arthroplasty: A Case-Controlled Study. *J Bone Joint Surg Am*, Vol.88, Suppl.4, (December 2006), pp.47-54, ISSN 1535-1386

Tenbusch M., Lahmer A., Wiesel U., Borner M. First results using the Robodoc® system for total knee replacement. Poster 13. In : *International CAOS-Symposium*, Davos, 2001

Tigani D, Sabbioni G, Ben Ayad R, Filanti M, Rani N, Del Piccolo N. (2010). Comparison between two computer-assisted total knee arthroplasty: gap-balancing versus measured resection technique. *Knee Surg Sports Traumatol Arthrosc*, Vol.18, No.10, (October 2010), pp.1304–1310, ISSN 1433-7347

Wang JW, Wang CJ. (2002). Total knee arthroplasty for arthritis of the knee with extra-articular deformity. *J Bone Joint Surg Am*, Vol.84-A, No.10, (October 2002), pp.1769-74, ISSN 1535-1386

Wolff AM, Hungerford DS, Pepe CL. (1991). The effect of extraarticular varus and valgus deformity on total knee arthroplasty. *Clin Orthop Relat Res*, Vol.271, (October 1991), pp.35-51, ISSN 1528-1132

Wysocki WR, Sheinkop B, Virkus WW, Della Valle CJ. (2008). Femoral fracture through a previous pin site after computer-assisted total knee arthroplasty. *J Arthroplasty*, Vol.23, No.3, (April 2008), pp.462-5, ISSN:0883-5403

Yau WP, Chiu KY. Cutting errors in total knee replacement: assessment by computer assisted surgery. (2008). *Knee Surg Sports Traumatol Arthrosc*, Vol.16, No.7, (July 2008), pp.670-3, ISSN 1433-7347

Yau WP, Chiu KY, Zuo JL, Tang WM, and Ng TP. (2008). Computer Navigation Did Not Improve Alignment in a Lower-volume Total Knee Practice. *Clin Orthop Relat Res*, Vol.466, No.4, (April 2008), pp.935–945, ISSN 1528-1132

Yoshioka Y., Siu D., Scudamore R., Cooke T. (1989). Tibial anatomy and functional axes. *J Orthop Res*, Vol.7, No.1, (1989), pp.132-137, ISSN 1554-527X

28

Computer Assisted Orthopedic Surgery in TKA

Eun Kyoo Song and Jong Keun Seon
Chonnam National University Hwasun Hospital
Korea

1. Introduction

Since Campbell and Boyd first developed a mold hemiarthroplasty in 1940, the procedure for a total knee arthroplasty has advanced greatly with the development of new materials and the increasing understanding of the knee joint biomechanics. And accurate alignment of the component and soft tissue balancing has been cited as the essential for the success of total knee arthroplasty. Although mechanical alignment guides have been designed to improve alignment accuracy, there are several fundamental limitations of this technology that will inhibit additional improvements. The long-term survival rate of a total knee arthroplasty after a 10-year follow up was reported to be 80% to 95% (Knutson et al., 1986; Ranawat et al., 1993; Scuderi et al., 1989). Various factors affect this long-term survival, the most closely related factor being the physiologic recovery of the leg alignment (Laskin, 1984; Ritter et al., 1994). Upon a follow-up study of more than 8 years, the loosening rate was only 3% in those patients with a correctly recovered leg alignment, but was 24% in those with an incomplete recovery of the leg alignment(Stulberg et al., 2002). There are limits on improving the alignment accuracy using a conventional total knee arthroplasty. Teter et al. (Teter et al., 1995) found that when a tibial extramedullary alignment guide was used, approximately 8% of the cuts were deviated 4 degrees of the ideal 90 degrees cut (perpendicular to the mechanical axis). However, this finding was based on coronal imaging, and the rate of malalignment may be considerably greater when the sagittal imaging is considered. Computer-assisted surgery(CAS) was introduced to overcome these difficulties and errors. Computer-assisted total knee arthroplasty has gained increasing acceptance among orthopedic surgeons as a technique to improve surgical precision and patient outcomes.

2. The history of computer assisted TKA

Computer-assisted surgery was first introduced in the neurosurgical field in 1980s to find surgical sites in the brain or spinal cord accurately. In orthopedic surgery, the American veterinarian Howard Paul and the orthopedic surgeon William Bargar first sought to improve femoral stem incorporation during total hip arthroplasty(THA), and devised a new drill to achieve a precise match for femoral prostheses. In fact, this concept was the basic idea that drove the development of medical robot. In 1986, Davis started a joint project between IBM(International Business Machine Corp.) and the University of California to develop the ROBODOC®(Integrated Surgical Systems, Davis, CA) system. As a resultant, Integrated Surgical Systems (ISS) was founded by IBM in 1990, and subsequently, the first robot-assisted THA was performed on a human in 1992 in California using the ROBODOC system, which was later approved by the European Union in 1994. In 1997, Saragaglia developed a navigation system called Orthopilot®(Aesculap, Tuttlingen, Germany), which allows surgeons to perform surgery without any other imaging technique.

These Computer-assisted Orthopedic Surgery (CAOS) techniques were developed to minimize errors due to malalignment and inappropriate prosthesis insertion. The navigation system produced good results clinically and radiologically, but other factors, such as, the subtle movements of cutting blocks and the vibration of oscillating saws were then focused on as potential causes of inaccurate bone cutting, and these efforts resulted in the developments of robot systems. The ROBODOC and CASPAR systems were introduced almost simultaneously in Germany in 2000, and used to conduct the first robotic TKA in the same year. In 2007, ISS was purchased by the South Korean company Curexo, and in 2008 the FDA approved ROBODOC for THA. However, the FDA has not yet to approve ROBODOC for TKA. Nevertheless, 10 institutions in South Korea and 60 institutions worldwide use the ROBODOC system for TKA.

3. Navigation-assisted TKA

3.1 Classification

Many manufacturers produce navigation-assisted surgery systems and it is difficult to classify. However they can be divided into two groups based on their dependence to imaging; image based systems and image free systems.

3.1.1 Image based system

Image based navigation systems use the data acquired from computed tomography or fluoroscopy to determine operating factors, such as, joint centers, the movement tracks of surgical tools, and the alignments of prostheses. These systems require the registration of a CT image acquired prior to surgery, or the registration of fluoroscopic data during surgery, where registration means not only inputting CT or fluoroscopic data, but also matching imaging data to joint kinematic information acquired during surgery and bone dimensional information acquired using indexes and calipers. By using kinematic and surface registration data, the system determines in real-time the location of the bone resection site, placement and alignment of the cutting block, and joint alignment for the prosthesis concerned. Surgery is then performed according to the data produced.

Accordingly, the registration process is perhaps the most critical for image based systems. The accuracy of registration can be detrimentally affected when border lines on CT images are blurred or segmented, cortical fixation screws are loose, or when computer hardware or software is defective. All image based systems can perform fluoroscopic registration automatically during surgery. However, this can be inconvenient because the fluoroscope is needed during operation.

3.1.2 Image free system

Although image based systems are useful during preoperative planning and postoperative evaluation, the image-acquiring process can be time-consuming and troublesome, and consequently, image free systems are becoming more popular. These systems track the sizes, shapes, locations, and alignments of musculoskeletal structure based on a standard human frame in real-time during surgery, and then register and guide bone resection using navigation. Image free systems need tracking cameras and markers, the latter of which are referred to as rigid bodies, because they are fixed onto bones (at least four sites) with a pin or clamp. In addition, the tools and calipers used also have tracing markers that used by the system to guide the operative procedure. Optical systems use infrared lights and electromagnetic systems use electromagnets to detect markers. Systems based on the use of ultrasound are also under development, and have been reported to have errors of < 1mm or 1° of error range.

3.1.2.1 Optical systems

Both active and passive optical systems are available. Active systems have an LED (light-emitting diode) attached to each rigid body that emits infrared signals that are captured by a camera, whereas passive systems have a reflecting sphere attached to each rigid body, and the system senses the reflection of light emitted from an LED source mounted on the camera. It should be noted that signal interpretation depends on the amount of light detected, and thus, the active type requires a cable type or a battery type probe, and the passive type requires that the reflecting spheres are meticulously cleaned. For the active type, surgery starts with the attachment of a rigid body to the tibia and femur; the infrared LEDs are then attached using a cortical screw. When the hip, knee, and ankle joint are moved in sequence, LEDs emit infrared and the optical localizer monitors and calculates the joint centers and the movement ranges of the three joints 3-dimensionally to determine the location of the mechanical axis (kinematic registration). During surgery, the surgeon uses a pointer to mark the bony and articular landmarks and notes useful surgical information, such as, the locations and orientations of the femur and tibia. Using this information, the surgeon can promptly identify the optimal bone cutting line, and decide on its direction and position.

The ligament tensioner can be used to balance the ligament by tensioning the internal and external lateral ligament, and the internal and external knee joint gaps can then be measured in extension and flexion, which allows the external rotation range to be adjusted in accordance with flexion and extension intervals during distal femur anterior and posterior side dissections. In addition, It can assess implant size and location, which enables the surgeon to consider individual joint properties.

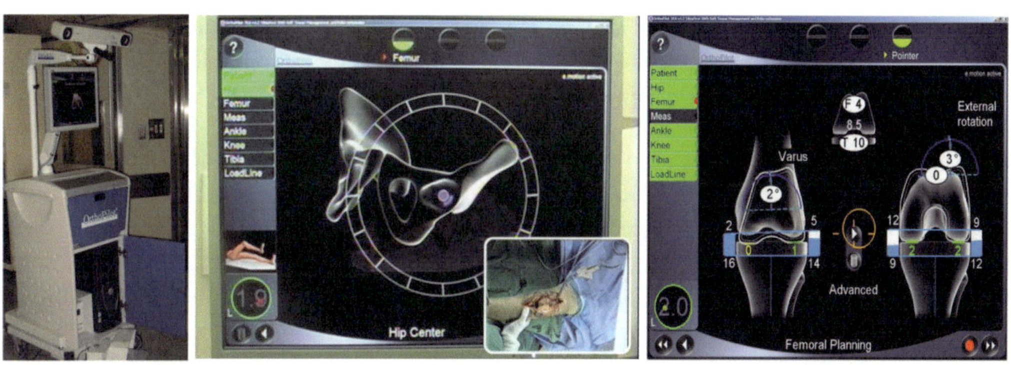

(A) (B) (C)

Fig. 1. Optical navigation system. (A) Appearance, (B) and (C) Different monitor views.

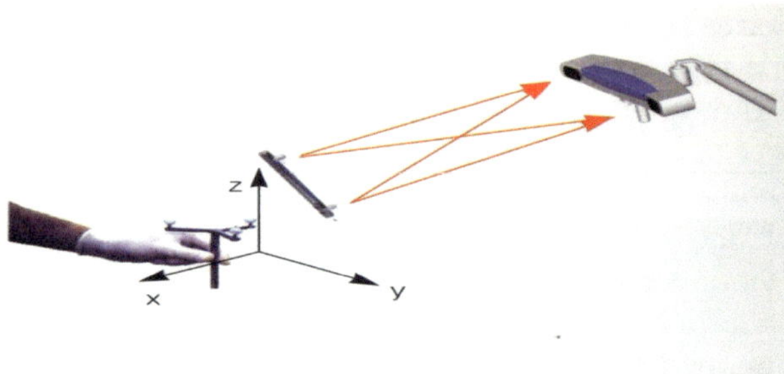

Fig. 2. Optical camera

The optical system of image free systems is fast and highly accurate, but operators should be careful about individual positioning to ensure visualization of the surgical field. The field can also be influenced by illumination intensity, and according to Tria(Tria et al, 2006), this system uses a large transmitter, which requires additional skin incision and a larger drill hole to hold the transmitter.

3.1.2.2 Electromagnetic Computer System (EMC)

As its name implies the EMC system is based on the detection of a weak magnetic field by sensors, transformed to digitalized voltage by receivers, and then transmitted to a computer. The magnetic field is produced by a localizer using direct or variable currents, although direct currents operation provides a more stable magnetic field. The localizer contains at least three generator coils and the coil numbers to a large extent dictate the performance of system because precision is dependent on the coil number. On the other hand, larger capacity computers are required for high coil numbers. EMC systems use dynamic reference frames(DRFs), which function as trackers, and resulting movement information can be used during surgery.

The early computer-based navigation systems had some disadvantages, such as, limited camera field of view, the requirement for sterilization, damage and tethering of soft tissue, and disruption of the surgical field by large surgical instruments. To avoid these disadvantages, researchers attempted to use non-line-of sight signals, which represented the beginning of EMC.

The EMC system was first applied in the pediatric neurologic surgical and ENT fields. In the orthopedic field, it was used secondary to conventional navigation due to signal instabilities, metallic interference, and its slower speed, which was caused by positional changes. However, after the coil number was increased and by enabling it to be attached to soft tissue, it has been more widely used.

The EMC system has the advantage of convenience during surgery, because it is not affected by the surgeon's position. Furthermore, gap balance is easily matched because the real shape of bone and dimensional data can be seen simultaneously. In addition, when a bone excision is incorrect, it can be corrected promptly, and because surgical instruments were small, it can easily be used during 'Minimal Invasive Surgery'. However, the EMC system suffers from distortion and low speed, and its safety has not been proven in humans. Furthermore, costs are high because the coil can only be used once.

Distortions can be classified as being due to conduction distortions and ferrous interference. When distortions are present, data may be incorrect or the monitor screen freezes or displays 'no reading'. Conduction distortions can be caused by most metals, including aluminum, and carbon based materials, although titanium causes less distortion. Metal disturbances are more problematic when the ferrous content is high, and thus, efforts must be made to eliminate ferrous content from the proximity of the unit system, for example, a 'fluoroscopy-possible' operating table should be used and EMC instruments should be located near the surgical field. In addition, it should be added that surgeons require training and experience of the EMC system.

However, EMC represents advancement over other navigation systems because gap balance can be easily adjusted, incorrect bone dissection can be corrected promptly, and because its small size is useful for minimally invasive surgery.

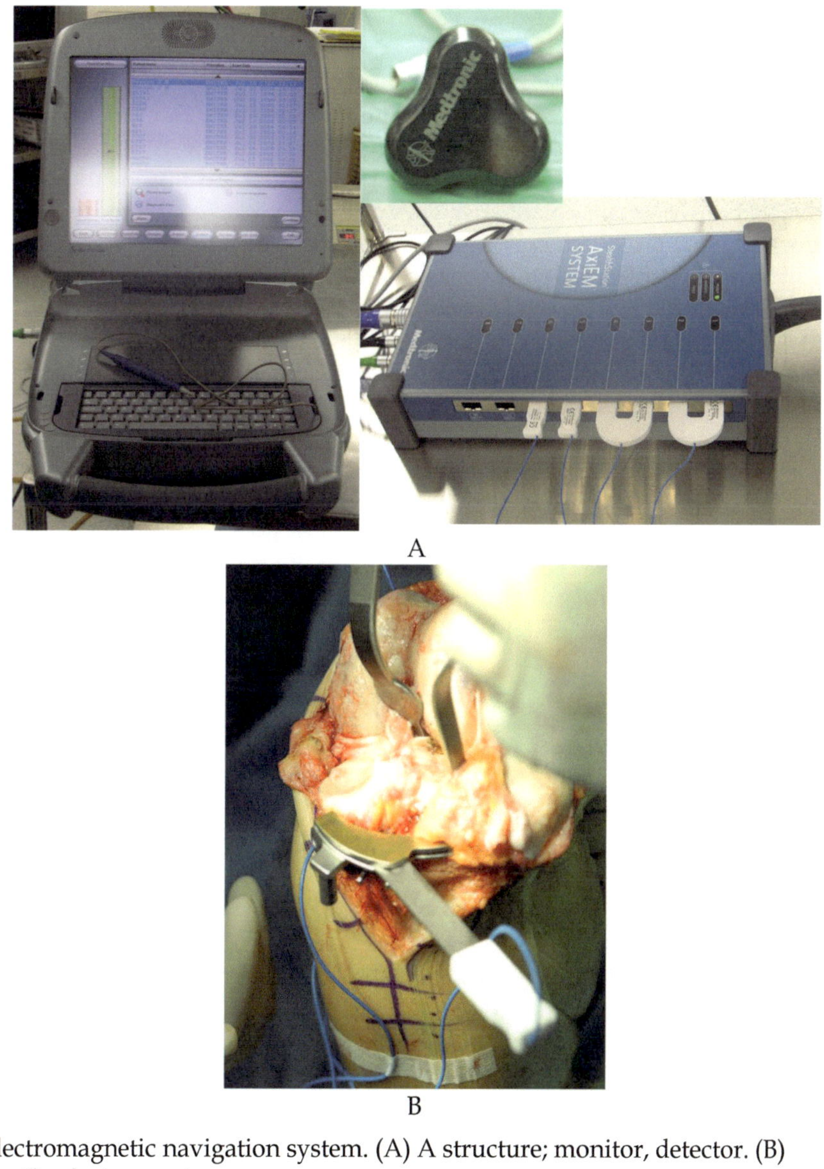

A

B

Fig. 3. Electromagnetic navigation system. (A) A structure; monitor, detector. (B) Intraoperative instrument.

According to Seon and Song(Seon and Song, 2004), the above two navigation systems showed more than a 3° malalignment in 15% of patients. It was suggested that this was caused by anatomical point ambiguity in real patients and registration failure. Furthermore, when registration failure occurs, EMS determined mechanical axis are more affected, and thus, these two authors concluded that EMS is more inaccurate than optical system.

3.2 Advantages and disadvantages navigation-assisted TKA

3.2.1 Advantages

3.2.1.1 Limb alignment

Many researchers have demonstrated the accuracy of lower leg alignment and the excellent implantation offered by navigation systems for TKA. Bathis et al.(Bathis et al., 2004) prospectively compared 80 TKAs performed using a navigation system with 80 TKAs performed using a conventional method, and found that varus and valgus angles of the mechanical axis and femur implantation in the coronal plane were more precise in the navigation group. Sterlbug et al. (Sterlbug et al., 2002) evaluated the precision of implantation and lower leg alignment after TKA using a conventional intramedullary guide. Their findings suggested that femoral implants tend to be varus, flex, internally rotate, and that tibia implants tend to be placed in varus position . There was no misalignment of more than 3°, and only 4 of 20 cases showed less than 3° alignment in the coronal or axial plane.
This result supports the previously reported argument that conventional TKA tends to cause varus, and that the margin of error between femur and tibia implantation could be less than 1°, which reduces the overall alignment error and can enhance surgical accuracy. According to comparative studies on navigation and conventional surgery groups, navigation systems showed statistically better results in terms of mechanical axis recovery, far fewer outliers, and more precise femur implantation in the coronal and axial planes.
The following features of navigation system can lead to precise lower leg alignment. The surgeon obtains thickness and angle of bone excision information in real time, and patients with an abnormal anatomical structure can be operated on correctly. During operation of total knee joint arthroplasty, matching flexion and extension intervals and ligament

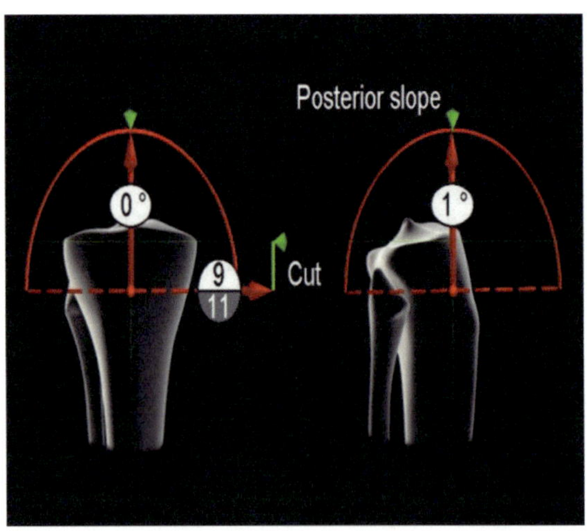

Fig. 4. Real-time monitoring

balancing are difficult due to damaged soft tissue, but navigation system can check flexion and extension intervals and ligament balancing instantly. Haaker et al.(Haaker et al., 2005) reported that real-time correction is possible after evaluating and collecting exact osteotomy data, implantation and soft tissue stability status promptly.

3.2.1.2 Functional results

The use of navigation systems during TKA produces accurate limb alignment, but the effect of this accuracy on functional outcome is still under dispute. However, Choong et al.(Choong et al., 2009) reported patients that underwent navigation assisted surgery showed precise limb alignment (<3°), and concluded that accuracy improved new knee function and quality of life. Lehnen et al. (Lehnen et al., 2010) reported, in a 1-year follow up study, that Western Ontario and McMaster University (WOMAC) scores and Knee Society scores of 43 navigation assisted surgery patients were notably higher than those of 122 patients that underwent conventional surgery. Patient satisfaction was 91% in the navigation assisted group, but only 70% in the conventional surgery group.

3.2.1.3 Bleeding

In navigation assisted total knee arthroplasty, the intramedullary jigs are not needed, and therefore, less bleeding can be expected as compared with conventional methods. Chauhan et al.(Chauhan et al., 2004) performed a randomized prospective study on 70 patients randomly allocated to computer-assisted surgery or conventional surgery. Mean amounts of bleeding were compared, and whereas the computer surgery group lost an average of 252mL (25-620), the conventional surgery group lost 446mL (100-1100). Furthermore, this low bleeding amount reduced the incidence of blood transfusions, and was useful when operating on patients in whom blood transfusion was problematic. Schnurr et al.(Schnurr et al., 2010) studied blood losses and transfusion amounts for 500 TKA operations. Average blood loss in their conventional and navigation groups were 1375mL and 1242mL, respectively. Furthermore, mean transfusion ratio was 0.23 in the conventional group and 0.12 in the navigation assisted group.

3.2.1.4 Embolisms

Conventional TKA uses intramedullary jigs, which increase intramedullary pressure and increase the risk of fat embolism. Chauhan et al.(Chauhan et al., 2004) compared navigation guided TKA and conventional TKA and reported that acute confusional states caused by transient fat embolisms occurred more frequently in conventional TKA patients. On the other hand, the risk of fat embolism in TKA patients is remarkably reduced when navigation systems or extramedullary alignment guides are used. Kalairajah et al. (Kalairajah et al., 2006) reporting on a study based on noninvasive monitoring, navigation assisted surgery stated fewer embolisms in the systemic circulation during operation than during conventional surgery.

3.2.1.5 Miscellaneous

Navigation assisted surgery, unlike conventional surgery, provides accurate records and comprehensive data on operations performed, which can be helpful during future investigations. Surgical wound healing characteristic are known to be similar for the two methods. Browne et al.(Browne et al., 2010) in a meta-analysis of 101,596 TKA patients, found that patients who underwent navigation guided surgery had a lower risk of cardiovascular complications than patient who underwent conventional surgery.

3.2.2 Disadvantages

3.2.2.1 Pin fixation

In a navigation assisted surgery, pins are fixed on to the bones to acquire real-time information of the limb alignment. Potential complications involving the pin fixations have been reported. Some investigators reported that additional 4cm of incision was needed for the pin fixations during navigation surgery, and this could cause delayed soft tissue healing and increased risk of infection. The additional incision of the quadriceps femoris muscle were needed in order to install the femoral tracking array can cause delayed healing of the muscle during the early stage of rehabilitation. The fracture of the pin fixation site for the reference array could also occur. Sikorski et al.(Sikorski et al., 2004) reported that the accuracy of the navigation assisted surgery can be impaired in osteoporotic patients due to the loosening of the pinning site. Song et al.(Song et al., 2006) reported that inappropriately registered data in navigation assisted surgery can change the outcome of the operation creating an incorrect mechanical axis.

3.2.2.2 Prolonged operation time

Operation time differ between authors, but generally, navigation assisted TKA takes 15 to 30 minutes longer than conventional TKA. The type of prosthesis used and the skills of the operator can affect operation time, it has been reported that the learning curve requires 10~20 procedures. Bauwen et al(Bauwen et al., 2004) reviewed computer-assisted TKA related articles between 1990 and 2008, and reported that the accuracy of mechanical axis alignment was the same as that of conventional TKA and that operation times were 23% longer.

3.2.2.3 Cost

Newer techniques require new equipment, and thus, costs inevitably increases. However, several authors have concluded that navigation assisted surgery extends the life spans of prostheses and reduces the potential risk of revision surgery, and that it is less costly in the long term.

3.2.2.4 Errors of the navigation system

Many investigators have reported that navigation assisted TKA produces more accurate results. Seon et al.(Seon et al., 2004) reported that the accuracies of optical and electromagnetic navigation systems are affected by the registration of anatomical locations. Mullaji et al.(Mullaji et al., 2007) reported in a comparative study of navigation assisted TKA and conventional TKA that the accuracies of navigation systems depends on joint deformity, instability, computer hardware, computer software, and the surgical techniques used. In addition, they found that patients with 20~30° of varus deformity before TKA had more varus mechanical axes after surgery than patients with 10~20°of varus deformity before operation. Furthermore, the former patients showed significantly higher rates of varus locations of femoral and tibial prostheses. These findings indicate that radiographs should be used to determine the degree of varus deformity when placing sensors.

3.3 Operative procedure (Orthopilot® Version 4.0 or 4.2)

The following text concerns that of the Orthopilot Version 4.0 or 4.2 (Aesculap, Tuttlingen, Germany) navigation system which is an image-free system.

Operation was performed using the gap technique with navigation. Using a medial parapatellar approach, the knee joint was exposed and the hip, knee, and ankle centers were navigated. Anatomical landmarks were registered by hand using a pointer to define the joint line and the mechanical axis of the leg. The mechanical axis was then restored to neutral (±2°) at full extension by stepwise meticulous medial soft tissue release and osteophyte removal (Fig. 5). Proximal tibial bone cutting was performed under real-time navigation system control and the posterior cruciate ligament was preserved and confirmed to be functionally intact. Flexion and extension gaps were measured at full extension and at 90° of flexion using a tensioning device (V-STAT tensor, Zimmer) and a special torque wrench set at 200N before femoral bone cutting (precutting flexion and extension gaps) (Fig. 6). Gap differences were classified as; balanced, tight in flexion, or tight in extension. A balanced gap was defined as one having a flexion/extension gap difference of within 3mm, a tight flexion gap as a gap with an extension gap of at least 3mm more that the corresponding flexion gap, and a tight extension gap as one with a flexion gap of at least 3mm more that the corresponding extension gap. Levels of distal and posterior femoral cuts and amounts of femoral component rotations were determined based on extension-flexion and medial-lateral gap differences (Fig. 7). Following final bone cuts and soft tissue release completion, flexion, and extension gaps were reassessed (final flexion and extension gaps) (Fig. 8). And if soft tissue balance is adequate, the prosthesis are inserted.

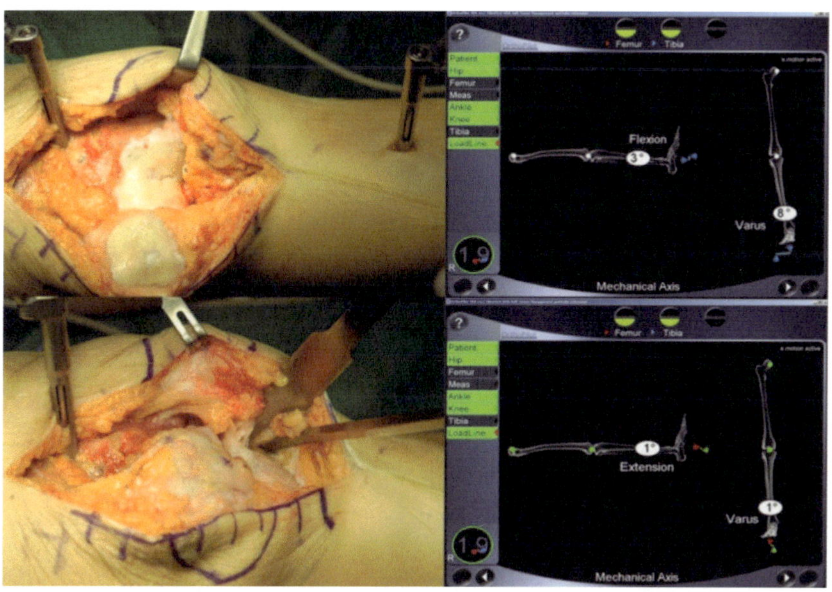

Fig. 5. After performing anatomical and kinematic registrations, the mechanical axis was restored to neutral (±2°) at full extension by incremental meticulous medial soft tissue release and osteophyte removal.

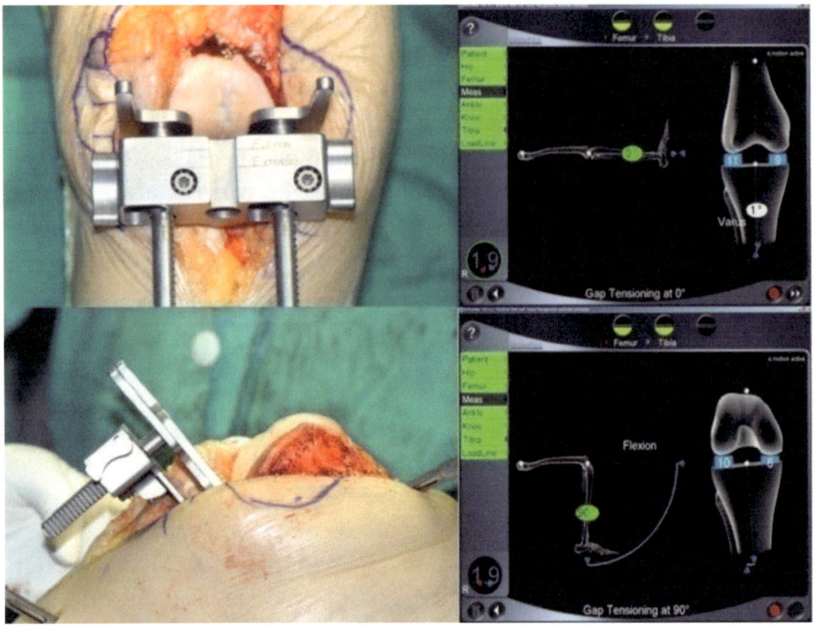

Fig. 6. After proximal tibial bone cutting while preserving the posterior cruciate ligament under navigation and before femoral bone cutting, flexion, and extension gaps were measured at full extension and at 90° of flexion using a tensioning device and a special torque wrench set at 50lb/inch (precutting flexion and extension gaps).

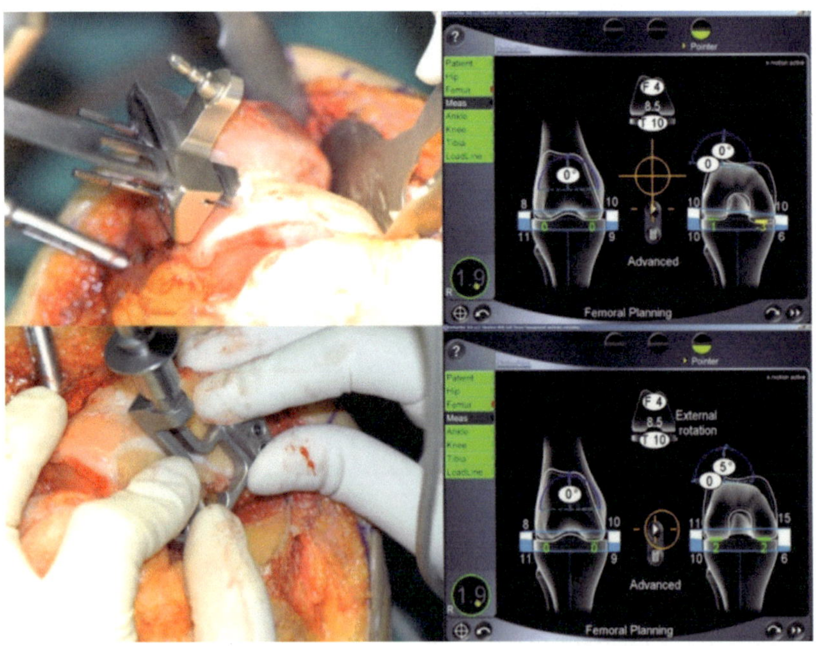

Fig. 7. Levels of distal and posterior femoral cuts and amounts of femoral component rotation were planned based on extension-flexion and medial-lateral gap differences.

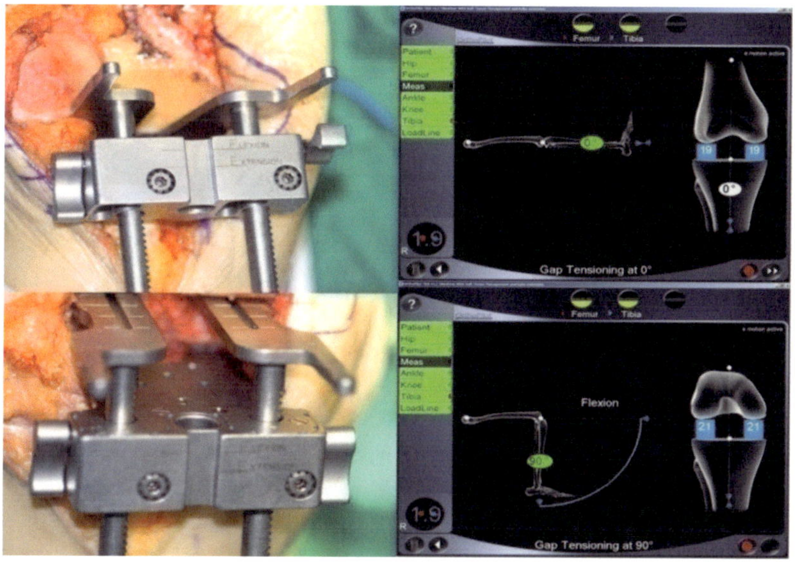

Fig. 8. Following final bone cuts and soft tissue release, flexion and extension gaps were reassessed (final flexion and extension gaps).

3.4 Clinical outcomes

Many reports have concluded that computer-assisted TKA produces consistent results, reduces malalignment and inappropriate prosthesis placement, and promotes rapid recovery and rehabilitation after surgery. Rosenberger et al.(Rosenberger et al., 2008) investigated 100 patients, and found that 50 patients who underwent navigation assisted TKA showed an average varus angle of 0.28°, whereas patients who underwent conventional TKA showed 1.88° in the coronal plane. The ideal prosthesis location was achieved in 16 cases (32%) in the conventional TKA group, and in 31 cases (62%) in the navigation assisted TKA group. These results show that navigation assisted surgery is a straightforward, stable, useful procedure for total knee arthroplasty.

Seon and Song et al.(Seon et al., 2009) investigated 43 cases in a 2-year follow up study, and found that Hospital for Special Surgery(HSS) and Western Ontario and McMaster University (WOMAC) scores were increased in both the navigation assisted and conventional groups, the scores were non-significantly different in both groups. Ranges of knee joint movement were also similar, but limb and prostheses alignments were better in the navigation assisted group.

However, others have reported that the conventional and navigational methods are no different with respect to pain, range of motion, ankylosis knee scores, and patient satisfaction. Spencer et al.(Spencer et al., 2007) reported that after a 2-year follow up of 71 patients with navigation assisted TKA group showed better alignment, but other factors such as functional assessments failed to reveal any significant difference.

4. Robotic-assisted TKA

4.1 Introduction to robot systems

Robotic surgery systems can be classified according to level of function, into three groups, that is, as passive types, active types, or semi-active types, and further devided into image based or image free systems. Passive types guide the surgeon through the fixation and cutting block resection stages - the actual cutting and drilling processes are executed by the surgeon. Navigation systems are passive types. Whereas active robotic types prepare and execute the operation process entirely or in part, and perform the bone cutting. Initially, these robots were custom-made in small numbers, but many others originated from larger industrial robots.

The ROBODOC® (Integrated Surgical Systems, Davis, CA), and the CASPAR® (URS Ortho Rastatt, Germany) are typical commercial TKA robotic systems. ROBODOC was the first of its kind, and is the only system used in South Korea. The system is composed of two main parts; Orthodoc, a supercomputer which plans and executes surgery, and ROBODOC, which has robot arms and performs the surgery (Fig. 9). Orthodoc uses pre-operative CT images to analyze anatomy, to choose a prosthesis of the right size, a prosthesis location, to plan cutting, drilling, and finally to register the data in ROBODOC for execution.

The development of the CASPAR® system was inspired by the commercial success of ROBODOC in Germany, and was first developed by OrtoMaquet (a subsidiary of Maquet). This system uses infrared cameras and reflective trackers to track limb positions. The system is designed to stop if excessive limb movement is detected during surgery. Care is required during operation to ensure that bone debris or fluid spatter on reflective tracker is removed; splash-guards may be needed. However, the ROBODOC system uses bone motion detectors fixed about 5mm deep in bone, which are not compromised by debris or fluid.

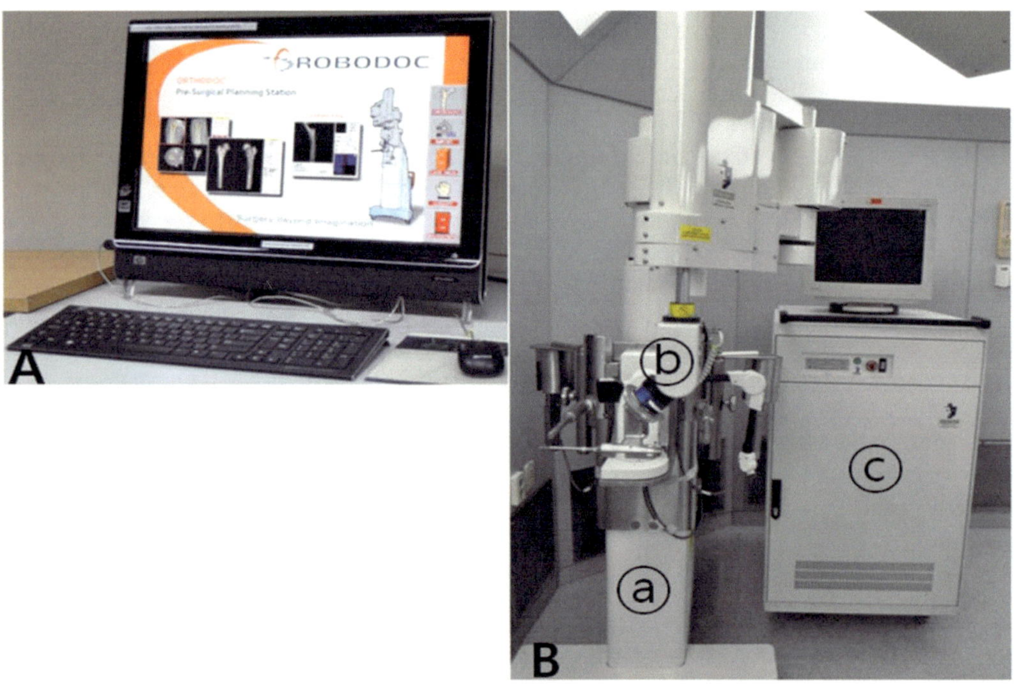

Fig. 9. ROBODOC ® system (Integrated Surgical Systems, Davis, CA) is composed of two primary components. (A) CT-based preoperative planning using ORTHODOC, and (B) Robot-assisted surgery using the ROBODOC surgical assistant (ⓐ = robot base, ⓑ = robot arm, ⓒ = the control computer)

Semi-active systems are a combination of the passive and active types, whereby a robot guides the cutting tools within specific ranges, and the operator controls robot arms within these ranges to process bone. The Acrobot® system (Acrobot Co. Ltd., London) and the MAKO Tactile Guidance System (TGS) (MAKO Surgical Corp., Fort Lauderdale, Fla)(Fig. 10) are semi-active types, and are often used for conducting unicompartmental knee arthroplasty.

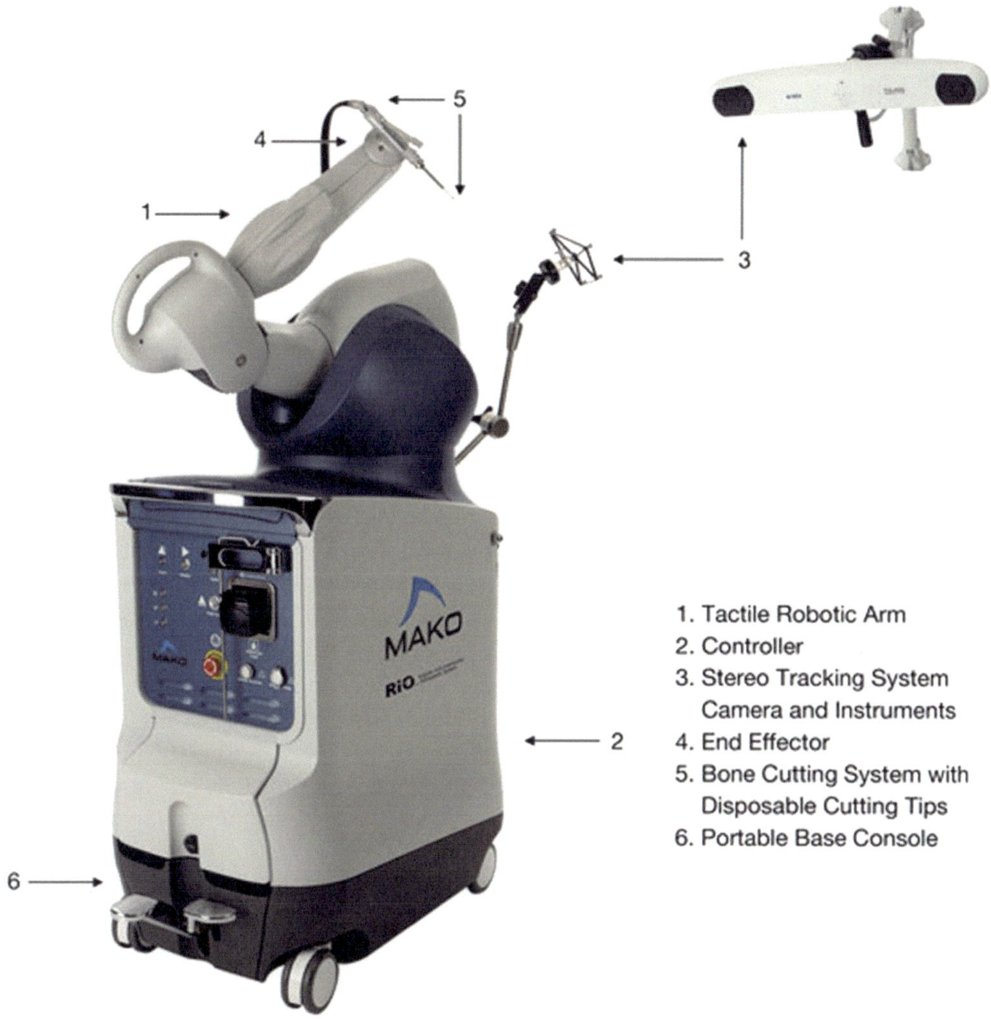

Fig. 10. MAKO Tactile Guidance System (TGS) (MAKO Surgical Corp., Fort Lauderdale, Fla)

The Acrobot system was developed at Imperial College (London) and was the first of its kind in the TKA field. According to this semi-active system, cutting tools are located within the dimensional range of bone to be cut. The tools are controlled by an Active Constraint Control™ system. At first Acrobot was used for TKA, but now it is more often used for unicompartmental knee arthroplasty. The robot software limits the movements of cutting tools within a pre-set range, and the operator resects bone to the planned extent in this range. The developers of the Acrobot system believe that it will be more attractive to surgeons than active systems like ROBODOC or CASPAR. The Acrobot® system consists of two robots; a large robot which functions as a gross positioning device, and a smaller robot which controls the active constraint function; technically, Acrobot refers to the smaller robot. The Acrobot has a spherical kinematic design that contains two rotational axes (yaw and pitch) and one prismatic axis (extension). The handle is equipped with a sensor that measures the force applied by the operator and controls the power output of the robot arm. The gross positioning device holds the limb in a manner that enables positioning of Acrobot near the cut volume. A six-axis gross positioning device is used for TKA, and a three-axis device for UKA. Anatomical data is registered using pre-op CT images; the operator marks 20-30 dots on the bone surface, and matching of the 3D-CT image and actual bone is then performed.

4.2 Surgical procedure (ROBODOC®)

Robotic TKA is composed of two steps; pre-op preparation (during which operation plans are determined based on CT images) and robot-assisted surgery.

CT images are acquired with the knee joint flexed at 15~20°. A calibration rod is attached to the limb, and CT scans are acquired at five different levels (the foot joint, mid tibia, the knee joint, mid femur, and the femoral head). When acquiring images of the distal femur and proximal tibia, slice thickness is reduced to 0.625 mm to improve accuracy.

Orthodoc reconstructs sagittal images and 3D images (surface models of the tibia and the femur) from acquired coronal CT images. The mechanical axis of the virtual 3D bone models is then set using the centers of hip, knee, and ankle joints. The virtual femur and tibia are then set parallel to the mechanical axis. Subsequently, suitable femoral and tibial prostheses, in terms of extent of resection, prosthesis size, and degree of external rotation, are then placed. The tibial prosthesis is placed on the line between the center of the posterior cruciate ligament's origin and the medial 1/3 of the tibial tuberosity. Finally, Orthodoc performs virtual surgery to confirm prosthesis alignment (Fig. 11). A supercomputer then determines exact sites and the extent of bone resection, the information saved on a disc, is delivered to ROBODOC. This preparatory step takes about 15~30 minutes.

The operation begins by fixing the robot to the subject knee, and this is followed by a verification process, during which correspondences are determined between anatomical bone surfaces and virtual bone. Bone resection and prosthesis insertion are then executed (Fig. 12).

Before surgery, a calibration process is initiated to achieve a precision of less than 0.2 mm. Robotic surgery is conducted, like conventional surgery, using a medial parapatellar approach. The approach is conducted by the surgeon. The patella is then everted to expose the knee joint, and the joint is fixed at 90~120°. The robot then inserts a Schanz pin in the proximal tibia and in the distal femur, and two straight beams are used to connect the limb. Traction devices (two curved S pins) are then attached to pull soft tissue and achieve maximum exposure. These devices are placed so as not to interfere with movement of the cutting arm. Next, the recovery markers, a screw and a pin, are fixed to the femur and tibia respectively. These markers enable the robot to sense unwanted limb movements (if movement exceeds 2 mm the robot will stop). This connecting step takes about 5-10 minutes (Fig. 13).

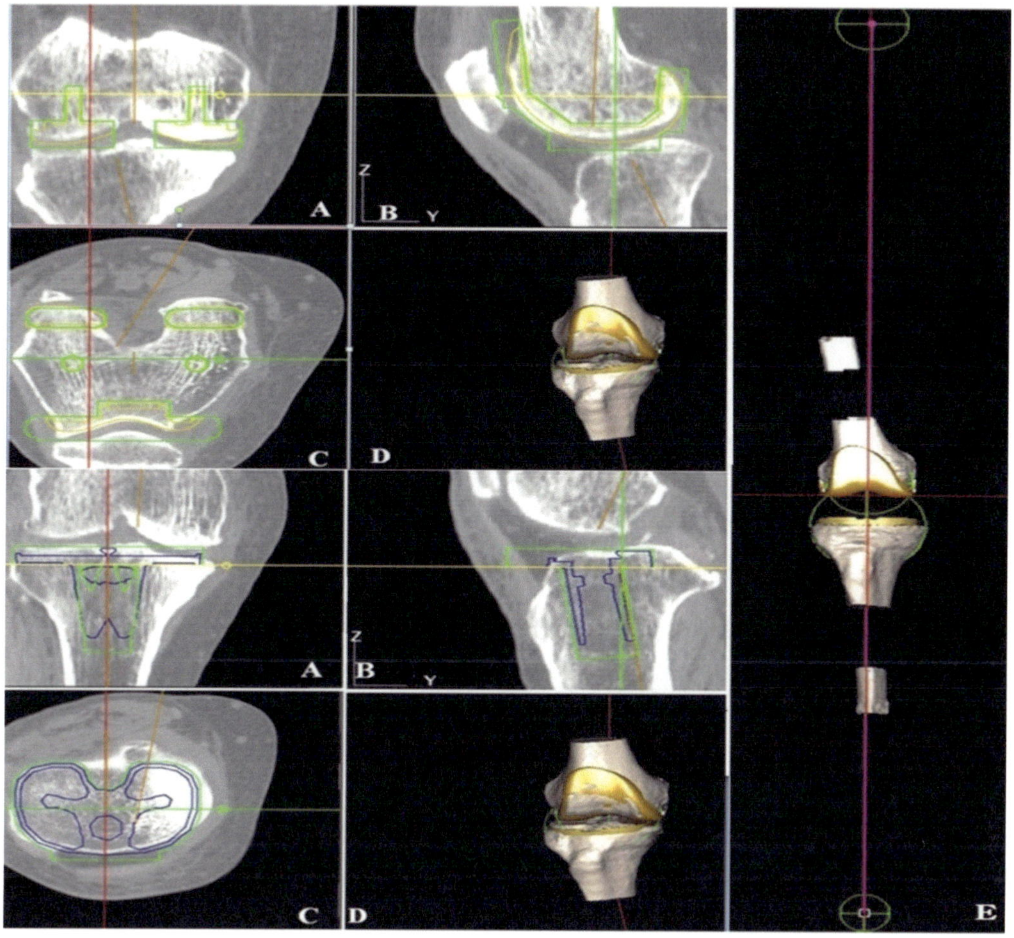

Fig. 11. Preoperative planning of the insertion of a femoral and tibial prosthesis using ORTHODOC. A= frontal plane; B= sagittal plane; C = transverse plane; and D= three-dimensional bone model of the femur and tibia; E= virtual surgery was conducted to verify femoral and tibial alignments and sizes with respect to the established femoral and tibial mechanical axes

Registration then performed. Actual knee joint bone surfaces are matched to the data saved in ROBODOC. This process is involves making the ball probe of the robot contact each of 97 contact points in 28 different locations as indicated by the computer program. After this process has been completed, which takes 5-10 minutes, the robot can recognize anatomical landmarks and bone spatial details.

After verifying data, physiological saline is applied continuously for cooling and irrigation, and the robot begins milling the femur and the tibia. The milling sequence proceeds in the following order; distal femur, anterior femur, posterior medial condyle, and posterior lateral condyle. At the tibia, milling begins at the tibial plateau, and after milling, pilot holes are drilled. The saw is replaced with a smaller one to make the peg holes and tibial flanges. The whole milling process takes about 20 minutes. The robot's job ends here.

The surgeon proceeds with trimming of the resection margin. Soft tissue is then relaxed and balanced. The knee is flexed and extended, from 0° to 90° to check for soft tissue stretching, and if soft tissue balance is adequate, the prostheses are inserted.

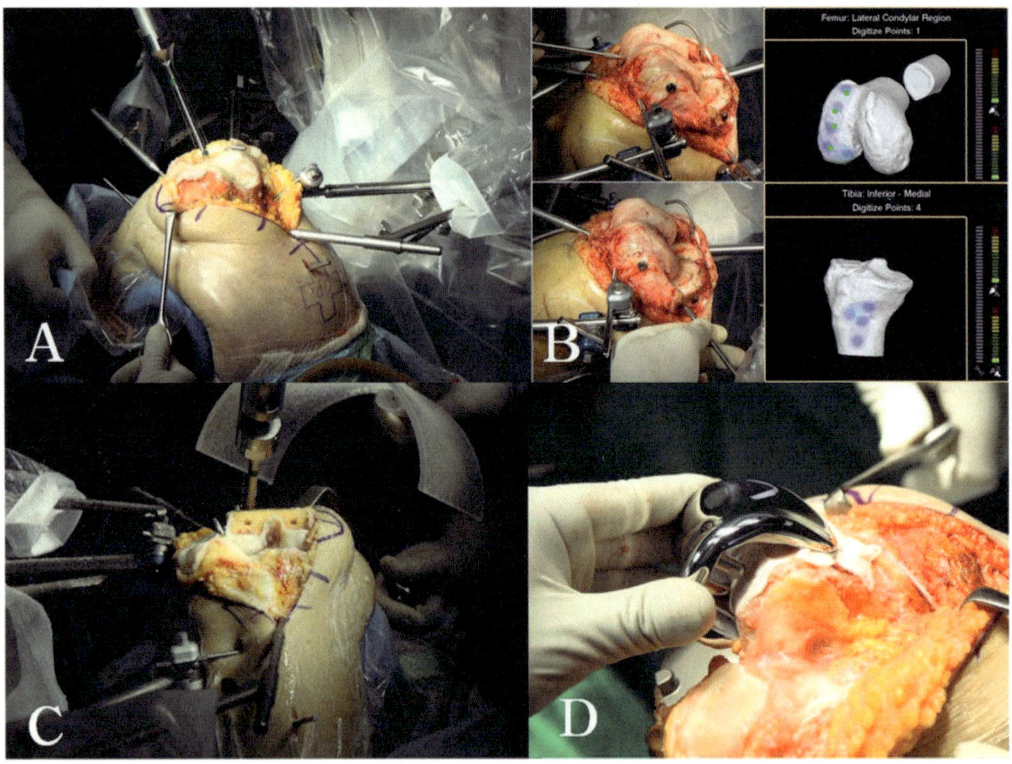

Fig. 12. Photographs showing the ROBODOC surgical procedure; Fixation between the patient's leg and surgical robot (A), Registration (B), Milling by the surgical robot (C), Implantation (D). During pinless registration (B), the digitizer arm is guided by the surgeon to certain points on the distal femur or proximal tibia. Digitized points are shown on the computer monitor. A correct hit is indicated when the point concerned turns green.

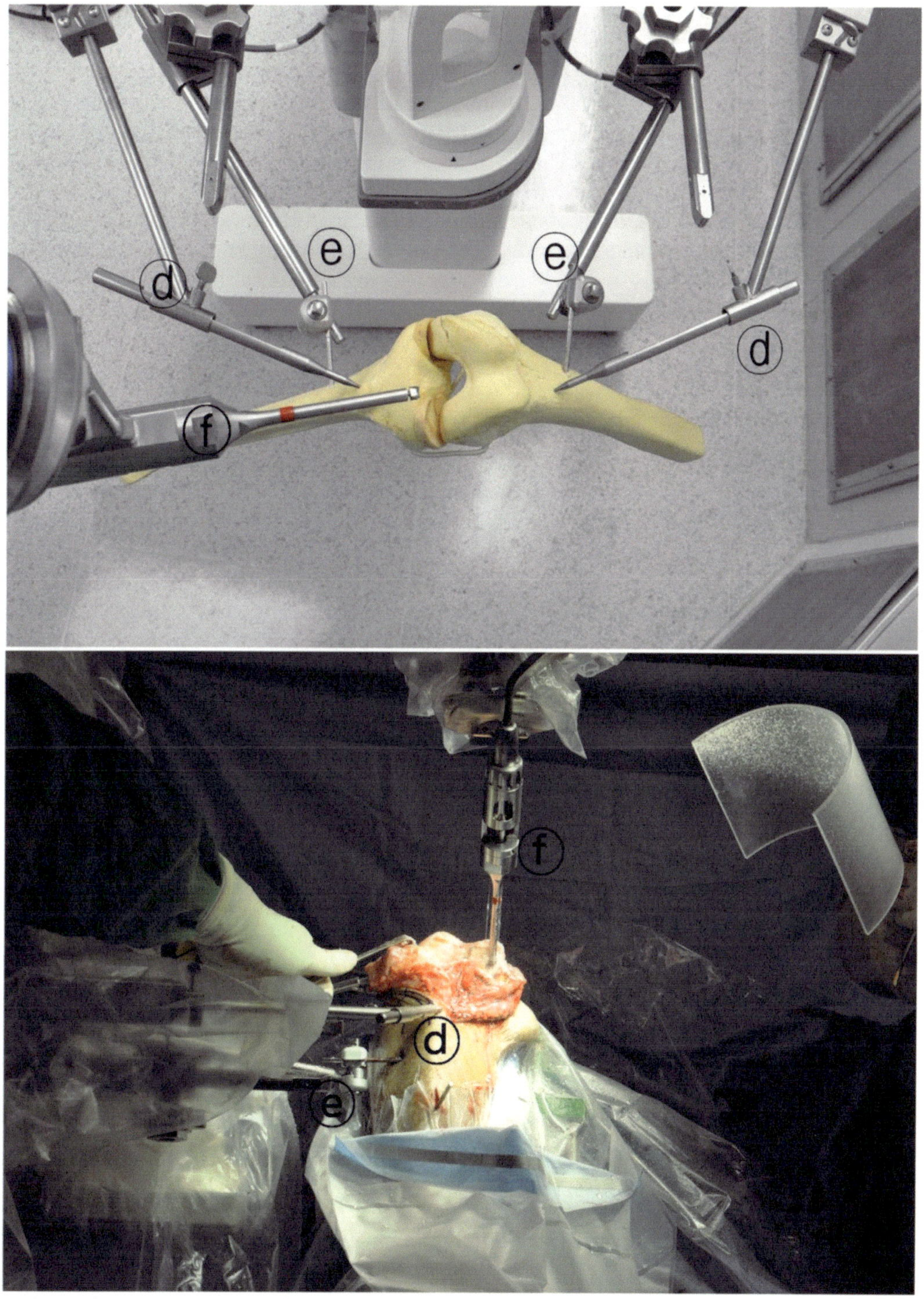

Fig. 13. The ROBODOC surgical robot. ⓐ, ⓑ, ⓒ (see Fig. 9), ⓓ = bone-motion detector, ⓔ = femoral and tibial fixators, ⓕ = the bone milling cutter.

4.3 Advantages and disadvantages of robotic-assisted TKA

4.3.1 Advantages

The robot surgery can be planned with greater precision than conventional surgery. Drills are guided with pin-point accuracy and bone milling is performed without any shaking or vibration. Ideal prostheses alignments and mechanical axes can be achieved and verified on CT or weight-bearing x-ray images. Furthermore, results consistent with the operation plan are consistently achieved with almost no outliers.

Siebert et al. (Siebert et al., 2002) also mentioned that inadvertent injuries of ligaments, vessels, or nerves can be avoided, because movement of the cutting arm is precisely planned and calculated, as are the resections. For example, during robotic surgery, the insertion site of the posterior cruciate ligament always remains intact. In addition, milled surfaces almost perfectly fit prostheses, and the amount of resected bone is minimized, which makes potential revision surgery less complicated.

4.3.2 Disadvantages

Coon(Coon, 2009) remarked that bone registration, burr exchanging, and a long milling time limit the efficiency of workflow during robot-assisted surgery. In addition, the author criticized the robot's design, especially the unnecessarily long arms, which make it difficult to appropriately deploy, sterilize, and drape. Bellmans et al. (Bellmans et al., 2007) discontinued robot-assisted surgery due to longer surgery time (over 30 min.), the need for highly experienced personnel, and higher costs, and Borner et al.(Borner et al., 2010) reported of the first 100 cases of ROBODOC assisted surgery, about 5% were converted to conventional surgery due to technical problems, such as, digitization error, calibration error, or bone motion.

Park and Lee(Park & Lee, 2007) found that the large pins required and the wide radius of robot arm movements made robot surgery unsuitable for minimally invasive surgery. They reported that of the first 32 patients that underwent robot surgery, 6 experienced complications, such as, superficial infections, rupture of the patellar ligament, dislocation of the patella, supracondylar fracture, or peroneal nerve injury.

Decking et al. (Decking et al., 2004) commented that before it could be viewed as an integrated method for total arthroplasty, robot surgery should be quicker, cheaper, smaller, and include an integrated soft tissue balancing process without losing its integrity.

Currently, we lack evidence that superior accuracy improves clinical outcomes, and thus, more investigations are required.

4.4 Clinical outcomes

Little information is available on the clinical outcomes of robot-assisted TKA. In a cadaver-based study undertaken to evaluate the accuracy of a robot system, alignment errors of the mechanical axis averaged 1° and ranged up to 2°, and average prosthetic displacement was 1mm with a maximum of 2mm. 3D CT pre-operative planning and the precision of the robot made ideal prosthesis placement possible. Decking et al.(Decking et al., 2004) acquired similar results using the CASPAR system. In this study, 13 patients underwent TKA and CT images acquired preop and 10 days postop were compared. Average mechanical axis discrepancy, as compared with preop images, was 0.2°. The accuracies of prostheses alignments in the coronal, sagittal, and axial planes were ±1.2°, whereas accuracies of linear alignments (anteroposterior, mediolateral, and craniocaudal) were ±1.1 mm. The authors concluded that robot-assisted TKA enables much more precise placement of prostheses. However, the authors added that the robotic procedure should include soft tissue balancing, and that robotic surgery should be quicker and less expensive to ensure its adoption.

Siebert et al. (Siebert et al., 2002) reported that in 70 cases of robot-assisted surgery, the average mechanical axis error was 0.8° and that the average operation time was 135 minutes. Furthermore, the conventional method had an average axis error of 2.6°, whereas robot surgery was more accurate. The authors mentioned that surgical precision (based on comparisons with pre-op CT images) was a strong point, but that the insertion and placement of markers, the longer operation time, and higher costs were weak points of the technique.

Borner et al.(Borner et al., 2004) reported 100 cases of ROBODOC assisted TKA. Mechanical axis errors were all within 3° and operations took only 90~100 minutes after sufficient experience. Precision beyond that achieved by the conventional technique has not been proven to be a requirement of TKAs, but it appears reasonable to believe that long term outcomes will surpass those of conventional surgery. Although most TKAs are viable for at least 15 years, robot-assisted surgery provides better axis alignment, and thus, minimizes prostheses wear and bone osteolysis, which should prolong the life spans of replaced knees.

Bellmans et al. (Bellmans et al., 2007) investigated 25 patients who underwent robotic TKA using the CASPER system. In this average 5-year follow up study, mechanical axis errors, alignments of prostheses in the coronal/sagittal planes, and rotation angles of femoral prosthesis were all < 1°.

Park and Lee(Park & Lee, 2007) compared 30 cases treated using the conventional method with 32 cases of ROBODOC assisted surgery and concluded that the robotic system offers - accurate procedural planning, precise resection of bone, and accurate alignments and locations of prostheses and axes. They also mentioned that big pins and the robot's wide arm radius are not suitable for minimally invasive surgery.

Song et al.(Song et al., 2009) found in a minimum 3-year follow up study of 50 ROBODOC-surgery patients that mechanical axes were corrected 0.49° varus on average, and that they were within 2° in 46 patients and within 3° in the remaining four. Average angles of femoral and tibial prostheses in the coronal plane were 89.5° and 90.1°, respectively, and average gradients in the sagittal plane were 1.06° and 85.56° respectively. The accuracies of coronal and sagittal plane were within 2°.

In a later study, Song et al.(Song et al., 2011) investigated 30 cases of bilateral degenerative arthritis of the knee in a randomized, prospective, comparative trial of robot-assisted and conventional surgery. One knee was operated on using ROBODOC, and the other was treated conventionally. Patients were followed up for at least 2 years. Clinical scores and ranges of movement were not significantly different in the two groups. Moreover, when patients were surveyed for pain, joint stability, joint weakness, snapping, swelling, and unexplained discomfort, 11 preferred the ROBODOC operated knee, 13 expressed no preference, and 6 preferred the conventionally operated side. However, in terms of mechanical axis alignments, whereas as the conventional method had 7 outliers, ROBODOC had none, and in terms of tibial prosthesis alignments, there were six outliers in the conventional group, and none in the ROBODOC group. The authors concluded that robot-assisted surgery produces better clinical and radiologic outcomes.

4.5 Future directions

Computer assisted orthopedic surgeries are being rapidly developed, and the future of navigation assisted surgery appears bright. In particular, if the physical sizes of these systems could be reduced they would be more useful for minimally invasive surgery. Furthermore, accuracies will undoubtedly be improved and errors will become infinitesimal.

The ROBODOC and CASPAR systems have achieved commercial success, and are now used in more than 100 European institutes. Furthermore, in South Korea, 10 institutions now routinely use the ROBODOC system. As was mentioned above, neither the ROBODOC nor the CASPAR system reduce operation costs, although robot supporters claim that by not using manual instrumentation the expenses of sterilization are saved, and that the superior clinical outcomes (lower revision operation rates, faster recovery, return to society, and others) offer across the board savings. However, there is insufficiency of the objective, and currently, it cannot be said that the superior accuracy provided by robot systems leads to better clinical outcomes.

5. Conclusion

In the orthopedic surgery field, navigation assisted surgery provides real-time alignment values, and allows the intra-operative evaluation and adjustment of prosthesis placement. Furthermore, computer-assisted surgery methods are expected to improve the qualities of surgical procedures. The majority of orthopedic surgeons believe that a computer system is needed during TKA to provide axis alignment, whereas others believe that computer-assisted surgery provides results that are effectively similar to those of conventional surgery. However, navigation assisted TKA provides precise information about femoral and tibial prostheses, enables optimal prosthesis sizes to be chosen for individual patients, and provides better range of knee movement after surgery. Furthermore, it improves the surgical experience for both the surgeon and patient.

In the operation room, robots have no limits regarding bone resection, which is why robot systems have been adopted in the orthopedic surgery field. In the TKA field, currently available robotic systems require more operative time and are more expensive than conventional surgery, but even at this stage of development they offer much more precise pre-operative planning.

6. Index

Knee joint, Osteoarthritis, Navigation, Kinematic registration, Surface registration, Infra-red, Optical system, Electromagnetic system, Light-emitting diodes, Ligament balancing, Tensioner, Real-time information, Robot, ROBODOC, ORTHODOC, Preoperative planning, Computer tomography, Passive system, Active system, Milling, Verification, Calibration, Bone motion, Mechanical alignment method, Anatomical alignment method

7. References

Bathis H, Perlick L, Tingart M, Luring C, Zurakowski D, Grifka J. Alignment in total knee arthroplasty. A comparison of computer-assisted surgery with the conventional technique. J Bone Joint Surg Br. 2004;86(5):682-687.

Bellemans J, Vandenneucker H, Vanlauwe J. Robot-assisted total knee arthroplasty. Clin Orthop Relat Res. 2007;464:111-116.

Borner M, Wiesel U, Ditzen W. Clinical experience with Robodoc and the Duracon Total Knee. In: Stiehl J, Konermann W, Haaker R(eds). Navigation and Robotics in Total joint and Spine Surgery. Berlin, Germany: Springer-Verlag. 2004:362-366.

Browne JA, Cook C, Hofmann AA, Bolognesi MP. Postoperative morbidity and mortality following total knee arthroplasty with computer navigation. Knee. 2010;17(2):152-156.

Chauhan SK, Scott RG, Breidahl W, Beaver RJ. Computer-assisted knee arthroplasty versus a conventional jig-based technique. A randomized, prospective trial. J Bone Joint Surg Br. 2004;86(3):372-377.

Choong PF, Dowsey MM, Stoney JD. Does accurate anatomical alignment result in better function and quality of life? Comparing conventional and computer-assisted total knee arthroplasty. J Arthroplasty. 2009;24(4):560-569.

Coon Thomas M. Integrating robotic technology into the operating room. Am J Orthop. 2009;38(2 Suppl):7-9.

Decking J, Theis C, Achenbach T, Roth E, Nafe B, Eckardt A. Robotic total knee arthroplasty: the accuracy of CT-based component placement. Acta Orthop Scand. 2004;75(5):573-579.

Ensini A, Catani F, Leardini A, Romagnoli M, Giannini S. Alignments and clinical results in conventional and navigated total knee arthroplasty. Clin Orthop Relat Res. 2007;457:156-162.

Fadda M, Marcacci M, Toksvig-Larsen S, Wang T, Meneghello R. Improving accuracy of bone resections using robotics tool holder and a high speed milling cutting tool. J Med Eng Technol. 1998;22(6):280-284.

Haaker RG, Stockheim M, Kamp M, Proff G, Breitenfelder J, Ottersbach A. Computer-assisted navigation increases precision of component placement in total knee arthroplasty. Clin Orthop Relat Res. 2005(433):152-159.

Kalairajah Y, Cossey AJ, Verrall GM, Ludbrook G, Spriggins AJ. Are systemic emboli reduced in computer-assisted knee surgery?: A prospective, randomised, clinical trial. J Bone Joint Surg Br. 2006;88(2):198-202.

Knutson K, Lindstrand A and Lidgren L. Survival of knee arthroplasties, a nation-wide multicenter investigation of 8,000 cases. J Bone Joint Surg. 1986; 68-B: 795-803.

Laskin RS. Alignment of total knee components. Orthopedics. 1984; 7:62.

Lehnen K, Giesinger K, Warschkow R, Porter M, Koch E, Kuster MS. Clinical outcome using a ligament referencing technique in CAS versus conventional technique. Knee Surg Sports Traumatol Arthrosc. 2010.

Matziolis G, Krocker D, Weiss U, Tohtz S, Perka C. A prospective, randomized study of computer-assisted and conventional total knee arthroplasty. Three-dimensional evaluation of implant alignment and rotation. J Bone Joint Surg Am. 2007;89(2):236-243.

Mullaji A, Kanna R, Marawar S, Kohli A, Sharma A. Comparison of limb and component alignment using computer-assisted navigation versus image intensifier-guided conventional total knee arthroplasty: a prospective, randomized, single-surgeon study of 467 knees. J Arthroplasty. 2007;22(7):953-959.

Park SE, Lee CT. Comparison of robotic-assisted and conventional manual implantation of a primary total knee arthroplasty. J Arthroplasty. 2007;22(7):1054-1059.

Plaskos C, Hodgson AJ, Inkpen K, McGraw RW. Bone cutting errors in total knee arthroplasty. J Arthroplasty. 2002;17(6):698-705.

Ranawat CS, Flynn WF, Saddler S, Hansraj KH, Maynhard MJ. Long-term results of total condylar knee arthroplasty. A 12-years survivorship study. Clin Orthop. 1993; 286: 94-102.

Ritter MA, Faris PM, Keating EM, Meding JB. Postoperative alignment of total knee replacement its effect on survival. Clin Orthop. 1994;299: 153-156.

Rosenberger RE, Hoser C, Quirbach S, Attal R, Hennerbichler A, Fink C. Improved accuracy of component alignment with the implementation of image-free navigation in total knee arthroplasty. Knee Surg Sports Traumatol Arthrosc. 2008;16(3):249-257.

Schnurr C, Csecsei G, Eysel P, Konig DP. The effect of computer navigation on blood loss and transfusion rate in TKA. Orthopedics. 2010;33(7):474

Scuderi GR, Insall JN, Windsor RE, Moran MC. Survivorship analysis of cemented knee replacement. J Bone Joint Surg. 1989;71-B:798-809

Seon JK, Park SJ, Lee KB, Li G, Kozanek M, Song EK. Functional comparison of total knee arthroplasty performed with and without a navigation system. Int Orthop. 2009;33(4):987-990.

Seon JK, Song EK. The Accuracy of Lower Extremity Alignment in a Total Knee Arthroplasty Using Computer-Assisted Navigation System. J of Korean Orthop Assoc 2004;39:566~571.

Siebert W, Mai S, Kober R, Heeckt PF. Technique and first clinical results of robot-assisted total knee replacement. Knee. 2002;9(3):173-180.

Sikorski JM. Computer-assisted revision total knee replacement. J Bone Joint Surg Br. 2004;86(4):510-514.

Song EK, Seon JK, Park SJ, Jung WB, Park HW, Lee GW. Simultaneous bilateral total knee arthroplasty with robotic and conventional techniques: a prospective, randomized study. 1. Knee Surg Sports Traumatol Arthrosc. 2011 Feb 11. [Epub ahead of print]

Song EK, Seon JK, Park SJ, Park JK, Park CH. Robotic Total Knee Arthroplasty - Minimal Follow-up of 3 Years - J Korean Knee Soc 2009;21:251~257.

Song EK, Seon JK, Yoon TR, Park SJ, Bae BH, Cho SG. Functional results of navigated minimally invasive and conventional total knee arthroplasty: a comparison in bilateral cases. Orthopedics. 2006;29(10 Suppl):S145-147.

Spencer JM, Chauhan SK, Sloan K, Taylor A, Beaver RJ. Computer navigation versus conventional total knee replacement: no difference in functional results at two years. J Bone Joint Surg Br. 2007;89(4):477-480.

Stulberg SD, Loan P, Sarin V. Computer-assisted navigation in total knee replacement: results of an initial experience in thirty-five patients. J Bone Joint Surg Am. 2002;84-A Suppl 2:90-98.

Teter KE, Bregman D, Colwell CW, Jr. Accuracy of intramedullary versus extramedullary tibial alignment cutting systems in total knee arthroplasty. Clin Orthop Relat Res. 1995(321):106-110.

Tria AJ, Jr. The evolving role of navigation in minimally invasive total knee arthroplasty. Am J Orthop (Belle Mead NJ). 2006;35(7 Suppl):18-22.

Van Ham G, Denis K, Vander Sloten J, Van Audekercke R, Van der Perre G, De Schutter J, Aertbelien E, Demey S, Bellemans J. Machining and accuracy studies for a tibial knee implant using a force-controlled robot. Comput Aided Surg. 1998;3(3):123-133.

29

Computer Assisted Total Knee Arthroplasty – The Learning Curve

Jean-Claude Bové
Multispecialties Private Hospital Clinique du Val de Sambre Maubeuge
France

1. Introduction

Over the last decades, orthopedic surgery has encountered a growing development that remains unfailing today.
Particularly in the field of total joint replacement, it is indeed a functional surgery aimed at a rather elderly population whose functional demand is increasing.
It is undeniable that a senior aged 60 in 2011 is very different from the senior suffering physical or psychological constraints caused by the ageing of his body about thirty years ago.
Nowadays, many seniors are willing to have an active lifestyle or even practice sport on a regular basis.
In the field of total joint replacement, that demand generates steady progress, which can come up to that expectation.
Among all orthopedic interventions that marked the twentieth century, total hip and knee arthroplasties are the most important.
Total hip replacement has even been labeled "intervention of the century."
Many forms specifically aiming to improve the quality of life have been incorporated into the various protocols for total prostheses monitoring (SF 16, HSS).
They accurately reflect the increasing demand of patients, which currently consists of simply forgetting the presence of the prosthetic joint.
This growing demand requires the constant search for improved joint replacement outcomes. That improvement is necessary to gradually reduce the rate of complications or imperfect results found in the literature.
Although few interventions have so much improved the quality of life for patients, much progress is still needed in order to increase the percentage of patients satisfied with their prosthesis.
The goal of arthroplasty is to obtain a joint which will be and remain mobile and painless as long as possible.
However, some studies [1-3] estimate that more than ten percent of the number of total knee prostheses do not fully come up to the patients' expectations, particularly in terms of residual pain.
The ideal thing would be to replace in due course the osteoarthritic joint (joint whose cartilage is worn) with the prosthesis and to obtain a prosthesis which would be functional all throughout the patient's life.

In other words, total joint replacement would be performed once and for all, and its sufficient longevity would prevent all prosthetic revision imposed by the failure or wear of the implant.
However, it is clear that the current average lifespan [4-5] of prostheses does not allow to avoid that revision among relatively young patients, that is to say patients who are younger than 50 years old.
Considering the gradual increase in the population's life expectancy and the more intensive use of the prosthesis among younger patients, one or two prosthetic changes are frequently required in such cases.
At the beginning of the twenty-first century, improving prosthetic longevity is still an absolute necessity.
This improvement in the lifespan of the implant must be combined with an improvement in the functional outcomes of arthroplasty, making some daily life activities easier to carry out thanks to the increase in prosthetic knee flexion, the opportunity to squat or kneel, to drive or practice some more demanding sport activities.
But how can that prosthetic function be improved as well as the prosthetic longevity of the implant?
First by working on the prosthetic design in order to increase its functional capabilities.
Much progress has been made in prosthetic design (design of the total hip prosthesis femoral stem, femoral offset, metaphyseal filling, anti-rotation wings,etc., radii of curvature of the total knee prosthesis femoral condyles, femoral offset, posterior slope of the tibial component, trochlear design, etc.).
Therefore we are currently moving towards an almost uniform design, gradually tending towards an almost unanimous prosthetic shape.
Progress will probably be made in that field in the coming years but the major part seems to have been done.
Similarly, many studies have been conducted to improve prosthetic anchorage (cemented prosthesis or not, press-fit effect, screwed prostheses, etc.) and many others will still have to be conducted in the future.
It is in the field of tribology, that is to say the science of the materials used in friction couples, that discussions are still lively, especially between the advocates of "hard-hard" and those of "hard-soft".
After decades of "hard-soft" corresponding to the first years of total joint replacement, roughly to the polyethylene-metal friction couple, the hard-hard friction couple appeared in the 1980s and 1990s (mainly alumina ceramic/alumina ceramic, metal/metal), those friction couples permitting to reduce the volume of wear debris, which are responsible for the so-called "aseptic" loosening.
Indeed the regular production of wear particles (cement, polyethylene, metal) will initiate a macrophage reaction of resorption, which when increasing, will compromise the prosthetic anchoring.
A certain number of complications of 'hard/hard' couples (breakage of ceramics, dissemination of metal ions in the body) has made the debate a little more lively but it is still not resolved. Some operators prefer so-called "hybrid" couples (alumina ceramic/polyethylene).
Improving the manufacturing techniques of various materials used is certainly an argument in the debate (maximum purity of ceramics limiting the risk of breakage, cross-linked polyethylene for superior mechanical resistance, etc.).

As it can be noted, contrary to the field of prosthetic design, significant progress is still desirable in the field of tribology.
The improvement in the technical realization of total joint replacement remains a key-issue.
This improvement in the insertion technique is a major factor to lengthen prosthetic longevity.
In the field of total knee arthroplasty, improving the accuracy of bone cuts is bound to have consequences on prosthetic stability (ligament balancing) and overall alignment of the lower limb on which prosthetic longevity depends [6-7].
Improving the arthroplasty's accuracy means improving the equipment used for the implantation of the prosthesis, which is called "ancillary equipment".
Over the last decade, new ancillaries have emerged, which allow to carry out knee arthroplasty minimizing the damage to soft tissues and exposure of bone ends, in a view to simplify the postoperative course. These techniques are known as "minimally invasive" [8-9].
The length of surgical incisions was significantly reduced, limiting the aggression of the surrounding soft tissues (skin, subcutaneous cellular tissue, muscles and tendons). Some operators limit their incision to a few centimeters (approximately half a conventional incision).
Clinical improvement was described in the immediate aftermath of these minimally invasive techniques. Studies are currently being carried out to confirm such progress.
Computer-assisted surgery is the second line of research to improve the ancillary equipment.
The computer appeared in operating rooms in the early 1990s under the leadership of neurosurgeons. The precursor surgical intervention was the computer-assisted transpedicular spine surgery, then, in the mid-1990s, it was followed by the computer-navigated total knee arthroplasty performed in France by the Grenoble university surgical team [10].
From the beginning, two systems were used, one using pre-operative imaging (CT), the other one using "bone-morphing" TM.
At the time, the computer created practical difficulties because of its volume and the numerous cables required by a complex connection.
An immediate preoperative tedious calibration of the ancillary equipment considerably lengthens operating time.
For simplicity, concerning total knee arthroplasty, computer-assisted surgery must be regarded as a tool aiming to bring improved accuracy in the realization of bone cuts, leading to a better ligament balancing of the prosthetic knee and a global alignment of the lower limb being more frequently close to the vertical (the ideal range of the angle between the femoral mechanical axis and the tibial mechanical axis extending from 3 degrees of varus to 3 degrees of valgus).
The so-called femoral mechanical axis is the line joining the center of the femoral head and the center of the knee; the tibial mechanical axis connects the middle of the tibial plateaus and the center of the ankle joint.
Thanks to that regularity in the alignment, the unexplained outliers of the overall mechanical axis of the lower limb are scarce.
With the help of a stereoscopic infrared camera, the rays being reflected by optically reflective balls, it is possible to obtain a virtual anatomical reconstruction of the operated knee. The software, using an extensive database, then guides the various bone cuts via a

graphical user interface (screen) and benchmarks for instant viewing of the various cutting blocks.
This is seen as an aid to surgery and not a robot automation of the surgical gesture. The surgeon remains the master of the surgical gesture, following on the screen the computer's visual indications to guide and set the different cutting blocks.
As mentioned above, this improvement in cutting accuracy induces a better ligament balancing and an alignment of the lower limb more consistently correct, which should increase prosthetic longevity.
However no study has so far clinically demonstrated any lengthening of the lifespan of a so-called "navigated" total knee prosthesis.
The follow-up is too short, which explains this gap. Indeed, computer navigation is still, in terms of its regular practice, in its infancy.
Therefore the success is less massive than expected with the improvements achieved during surgery. Among the reasons for this limited development, the cost of materials [11] is mentioned, given its limited distribution. Longer operative time with the addition of specific technical steps required by the computer, leading to an increased septic risk, and finally difficulty of learning the technique, even for a trained operator. Given his experience and the excellent results of the so-called conventional prosthetic surgery, the operator is not always convinced that new technique is really useful.
It seemed interesting to mention our personal experience of learning computer-assisted surgery in the field of total knee replacement.
Indeed, the obstacles seemed to be overcome without great difficulty. Using more user friendly and easier systems, we were even able to modify our practice as our experience grew.
A comparison of operating times enabled us to demonstrate the permanent aspect of learning by making our adaption to a totally new and unknown computer system easier and easier.

2. Materials and methods

In February 2003 we achieved our first computer-assisted total knee arthroplasty.
Two implantations were performed during the same operating session in the Val de Sambre clinic in Maubeuge.
At the time, concerning the primary knee arthroplasty, the author exclusively used the Natural Knee II TM sliding prosthesis (Zimmer, Warsaw, Indiana, USA).
The provision on a trial basis of the Navitrack Navigation System TM (Orthosoft, Zimmer) allowed those first two projects.
It is an imageless system requiring the calibration of computer tools (pointer, and cutting blocks) (Fig. 1) during the operation and not involving the bone morphing TM.
It was actually a simplified bone morphing including deposition of "computer chips" on the screen allowing to adjust cutting thickness (Fig. 2).
The graphical user interface not being interactive, the use of keyboards and pedals in the immediate vicinity or in direct contact with the operative field was a source of congestion and increased the risk of lack of asepsis.
After those two trials which were considered conclusive, the decision to purchase the equipment was made and, from September 2003, all primary knee arthroplasties were performed by the author using that system.

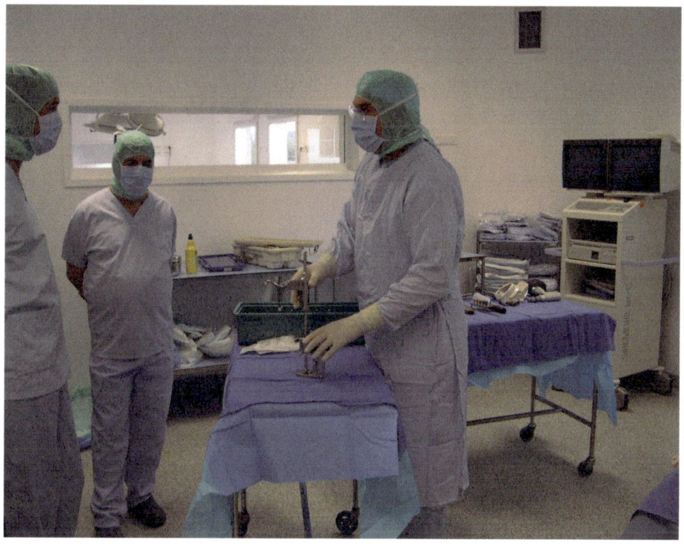

Fig. 1.

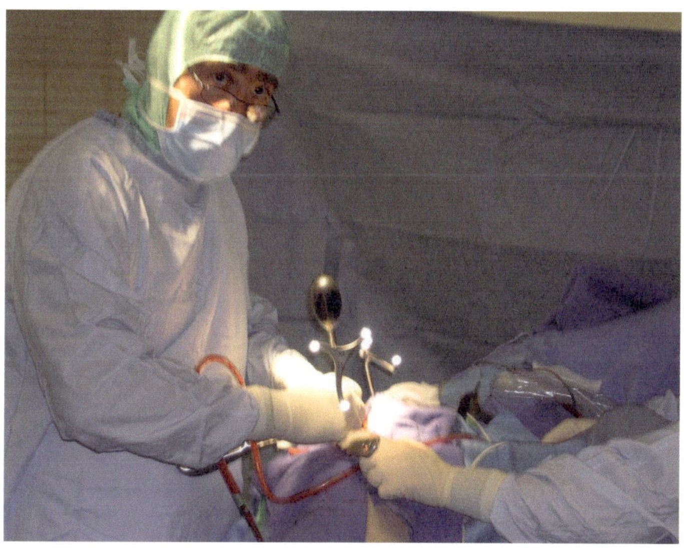

Fig. 2.

Computer-assisted surgery has been exclusively used whereas conventional surgery was only used for revision arthroplasty surgery.
Thus more than 200 total knee prostheses were implanted with a system that may now seem outdated, but which, at that time, gave entire satisfaction from September 2003 to July 2006.
The duration of the intervention and more specifically the time of tourniquet were studied [12] at the beginning and end of the user experience (Fig. 3) of this system.
In July 2006, we decided to use a more user-friendly system including a touch screen covered with a sterile drape allowing us to avoid cumbersome cables and pedals. It is also

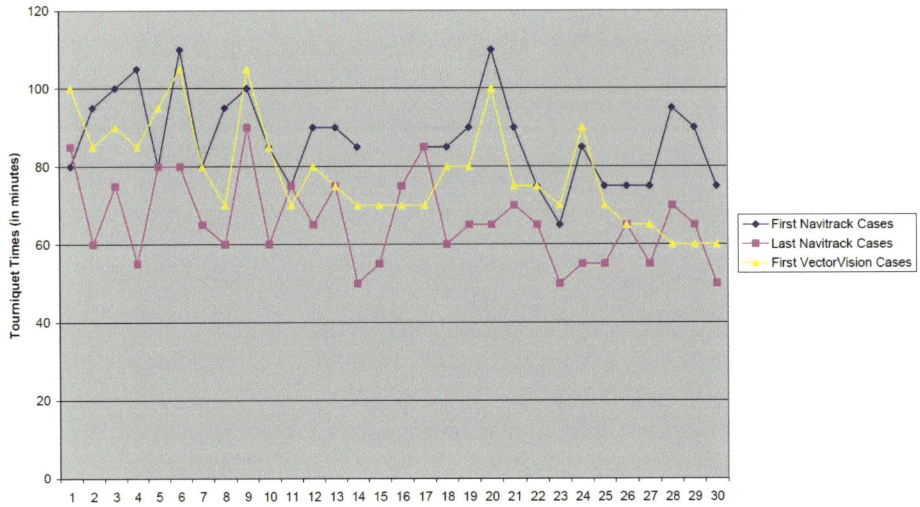

Fig. 3. Tourniquet Time

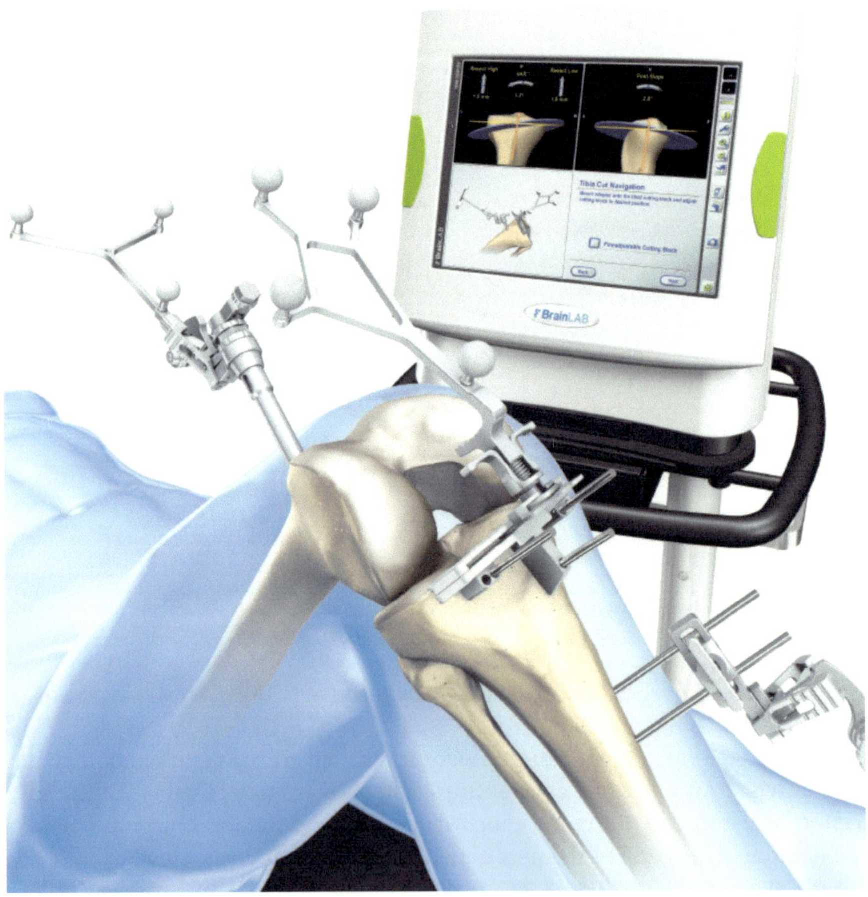

Fig. 4.

an imageless system based on a standardized bone morphing carried out using a pointer fitted with reflective balls and not requiring time-consuming instrumental calibration (VectorVision, Brainlab, Munich, Germany) (Fig. 4).
A "coloring" of the reference bone surfaces using a computer pointer (stylus provided with reflective balls) permits to transmit essential anatomical data to the computer. The data allows the operator to choose a knee anatomical model being as close as possible to the operated knee in a huge database.
More than 300 arthroplasties have been carried out so far using that system, which is still used in the service now.

3. Results

When using the computer system, an average lengthening of time tourniquet of 18 minutes has been noticed (range 0-45 minutes), which is likely to increase the septic risk. That average lengthening refers to the average tourniquet time of "conventional" total knee arthroplasties performed by the author during the previous five years.
The more detailed analysis of the curves indirectly shows the technical difficulties experienced by the operator since, for an average tourniquet time of 87 minutes during the very first use of navigation (first 30 implantations with the Navitrack system), we observe that in 4 out of the first 10 cases, 100 minutes are reached or exceeded.
This period of 100 minutes is critical because it jeopardizes the achievement of the entire knee arthroplasty under pneumatic tourniquet, because the latter cannot be maintained more than 120 minutes or it can cause complications. The tourniquet release before the setting of cement may compromise the prosthetic anchorage, although for some operators the procedure is performed without any tourniquet.
When examining the curves, we can notice a progressive decrease in the time of tourniquet as the operator's experience and mastery of the technique develops.
Last but not least, a comparison of tourniquet time in the series performed using the second system has identified a more rapid decrease in additional operative time induced by the use of the computer ancillary, which supports the working hypothesis of the study, namely the maintenance of the operator's knowledge.
That situation could be compared to driving : the successive adaptation to a different vehicle is done gradually with less difficulty as the driving technique improves.
Over the last eight years, no specific complication to navigation has been deplored, except, at the beginning of our practice, some cases of transitory inflammation or suppuration of the holes of the tibial antenna fixation pins.
These were probably caused by the excessive overheating of the drilling, which caused neighboring bone necrosis. The problem was solved by the use of tibial fixation rods with a 3.5 mm diameter.
We observed no supracondylar fracture on way to the fixing pin of the femoral rigid body and a single non-displaced tibial fracture, which rapidly consolidated.
Particular care is brought to the precise location of the fixing rods to reduce the risk of fracture [13].
Similarly, the average rate of postoperative prosthetic sepsis (less than one percent in the literature and personal experience) has not been modified by the lengthening of operating time.

The functional results and the possible and expected lengthening of computer-assisted arthroplasty longevity will be clinically studied as soon as the mean perspective of the series will be sufficient to be scientifically exploited.

4. Discussion

As seen, after studying of the duration of the learning curve, we can consider this learning difficulty as easily surmountable.
The reluctance of some practitioners, experienced in the practice of orthopedic joint replacement, to perform computer-assisted surgery is mainly due to the supposed difficulty of learning an innovative technology, with all the constraints that it brings, and not to the duration of the learning curve itself.
In addition, the computer ancillary equipment itself, tends to annoy or frighten those trained operators who only consider that equipment as an additional constraint.
Actually the major obstacle now seems to be the cost of equipment and particularly in France since the supervisory bodies consider that the benefit induced by the technique is not sufficient to support the extra cost induced by the purchase and use of computer equipment.
That benefit will only be found and admitted through the rigorous exploitation of satisfactory scientific studies. To be useful, such studies must always have sufficient perspective (10-year-follow-up minimum), but computer-assisted surgery started being used on a regular basis about 12 years ago. In the coming years, exploitable series should appear.
Similarly, the proliferation of studies on the comparative functional results of conventional arthroplasties versus navigated arthroplasties should rapidly lead to interesting conclusions.
It is mainly in the private sector that the financial aspect has the greatest impact. Indeed, in a context of economic crisis, the health system severely suffers from the decline of its funding due to a reduction in social contributions, if only because of rising unemployment.
The financial investors involved in the management of the private health care system in France are increasingly careful with potential investments such as the purchase of a new ancillary equipment.
The need for learning computer-assisted surgery, considered by some operators as tedious, with the costs incurred by the purchase of computer equipment (hardware and software), is currently a major obstacle to the further development of that promising technique.
However, that development will itself lead to a consequent decrease in acquisition costs through the diffusion of technology.
Similarly, the different national science societies for computer-assisted surgery will have to continue their efforts of representation, for educational purposes, including in university education.

5. Conclusion

In our view, and especially in the field of total hip and knee arthroplasties, computer-assisted surgery represents a promising technique, able to bring significant progress in terms of function and prosthetic longevity.
These improvements will meet the needs of elderly patients, who are more and more numerous, more and more demanding about maintaining a good quality of life and sometimes wishing to practice sport on a regular basis.

Similarly, younger and younger patients will take advantage of that technical progress.
To allow further development of computer navigated surgery, a reduction of costs is necessary and will only be obtained thanks to the diffusion of the technique and the improved support of those costs by supervisory bodies, once they have been convinced of the reality of the benefit provided by the computer.
To achieve this goal, the proliferation of scientific studies is essential. Those studies must be very serious, have a sufficient perspective, and be rigorously statistically exploited.
In those conditions, the expected improvement in terms of longevity and prosthetic function will be clearly demonstrated and allow the financial support of supervisory bodies.
As for the supposed inconvenience of learning time, our study has shown that it is minimal. On the one hand, a limited number of implantations is necessary to that learning (about 30 cases) and on the other hand, the growing experience allows the operator to adapt more easily to any new computer ancillary.
Finally, the educational value of the material is undeniable. Young operators should not be trained to the exclusive practice of computer-aided prosthetic surgery but their introduction to that technique should enable them to have a more rigorous, thoughtful and interactive approach of the different stages of arthroplasty surgery, which could improve their reasoning.

6. References

[1] Sun ZH, Liu J, Tian MQ, Zhang Y, Zhao HW, Zhu RS. Management of post operative pain after total knee arthroplasty. Zhonghua Wai Ke Za Zhi. 2011 Mar 1; 49 (3): 222-6.
[2] Jacofsky DJ, Della Valle CJ, Meneghini RM, Sporer SM, Cercek RM. Revision total knee arthroplasty: what the practicing orthopaedic surgeon needs to know. Instr Course Lect. 2011; 60: 269-81.
[3] Bonnin MP, Basiglini L, Archbold HA. What are the factors of residual pain after uncomplicated TKA? Knee Surg Sports Traumatol Arthrosc. 2011 May 20 [Epub ahead of print].
[4] Keeney JA, Eunice S, Pashos G, Wright RW, Clohisy JC. What is the evidence for total knee arthroplasty in young patients?: a systematic review of the literature. Clin Orthop Relat Res; 2011 Feb; 469 (2): 574-83.
[5] Ritter MA, Meneghini RM. Twenty-year survivorship of cementless anatomic graduated component total knee arthroplasty. J Arthroplasty. 2010 Jun; 25(4): 507-13.
[6] Rosenberger RE, Hoser C, Quirbach S, Attal R, Hennerbichler A, Fink C. Improved accuracy ofcomponent alignment with the implementation of image-free navigation in total knee arthroplasty. Knee Surg Sports Traumatol Arthrosc. 2008 Mar; 16(3): 249-57.
[7] El Masri F, Rammal H, Ghanem I, El Hage S, El Abiad R, Kharrat K, Dagher F. Computer-assistedsurgery in total knee replacement. Preliminary results: report of 60 cases. Rev Chir Orthop Reparatrice Appar Mot. 2008 May; 94(3): 261-67.
[8] Watanabe T, Muneta T, Ishizuki M. Is a minimally invasive approach superior to a conventional approach for total knee arthroplasty? Early outcome and 2 to 4 year follow-up. J Orthop Sci. 2009 Sep; 14(5): 589-95.
[9] Tria AJ Jr. Minimally invasive total knee arthroplasty: past, present and future. Am J Orthop (Belle Mead NJ). 2007 Sep; 36 (9 Suppl): 6-7.

[10] Saragaglia D. Computer-assisted total knee arthroplasty: 12 years experience in Grenoble. Bull Acad Natl Med. 2009 Jan; 193 (1): 91-104; discussion 104-5.
[11] Rivkin G, Liebergall M. Challenges of technology integration and computer-assisted surgery. J Bone Joint Surg AM. 2009 Feb; 91 Suppl 1: 13-6.
[12] Bové JC. Computer-assisted total knee arthroplasty. Comparison of two successive systems. Learning curve. Rev Chir Orthop Reparatrice Appar Mot. 2008 May; 94(3): 252-60.
[13] Beldame J, Boisrenoult P, Beaufils P. Pin track induced fractures around computer-assisted TKA. Orthop Traumatol Surg Res; 2010 May; 96(3): 249-55.